ABDOMINAL ULTRASOUND
A Basic Textbook

ABDOMINAL ULTRASOUND
A Basic Textbook

Morimichi Fukuda, M.D., Ph.D.
Professor Emeritus, Department of Ultrasound and Medical Electronics,
Sapporo Medical University Hospital, Sapporo, Japan

David O. Cosgrove, M.A., M.Sc., F.R.C.P., F.R.C.R.
Professor of Clinical Ultrasound, Department of Imaging,
Royal Postgraduate Medical School at Hammersmith Hospital, London, U.K.

IGAKU-SHOIN Tokyo·New York

Addresses of Authors

Morimichi Fukuda, M.D., Ph.D.
Professor Emeritus
Department of Ultrasound and Medical Electronics
Sapporo Medical University Hospital
S-1, W-16, Chuo-ku, Sapporo 060, Japan
E-mail: fukuda@sapmed.ac.jp

David O. Cosgrove, M.A., M.Sc., F.R.C.P., F.R.C.R.
Professor of Clinical Ultrasound
Department of Imaging
Royal Postgraduate Medical School at Hammersmith Hospital
Du Cane Road
London W12 0NN
United Kingdom
E-mail: d.cosgrove@rpms.ac.uk

Published and distributed by

IGAKU-SHOIN Ltd.
5-24-3 Hongo, Bunkyo-ku, Tokyo

IGAKU-SHOIN Medical Publishers, Inc.
One Madison Avenue, New York, N.Y. 10010

Library of Congress Cataloging-in-Publication Data

Fukuda, Morimichi.
Abdominal Ultrasound:a basic textbook / Morimichi Fukuda,
David O. Cosgrove.
p. cm.
Includes bibliographical references and index.
ISBN 4-260-14345-X.—ISBN 0-89640-345-9
1. Abdomen—Ultrasonic imaging. I. Cosgrove, David O. II. Title
[DNLM : 1. Abdomen—ultrasonography. 2. Ultrasonography—methods.
WI 900 F9612a 1997]
RC944. F836 1997
617. 5'507543—dc21
DNLM / DLC 96-52000
for Library of Congress CIP

ISBN 4-260-14345-X (Tokyo)
ISBN 0-89640-345-9 (New York)

Printed and bound in Japan

PREFACE

Real-time ultrasound, an automated ultrasonic scanning system, has today become almost a synonymous with ultrasound imaging, in spite of the extensive use of the contact compound scanning method in the past. Although in the very early days real-time ultrasound tended to be awkward in appearance, thanks to the rapid evolution of sophisticated equipment, it now produces images with improved resolution and gray scaling. In spite of sophisticated imaging modalities such as x-ray computed tomography and magnetic resonance imaging, ultrasound still holds a very superficial organs and even in the gastrointestinal tract within the reach of intraluminal scanning.

Ultrasound examination seems like a very simple technique because of the absence of any invasive effects on the side of a person being examined, compared to the other imaging modalities presently available. It is, however, not necessarily simple nor easy to interpret imaging data because of the necessity to have a thorough comprehension of anatomy as well as pathophysiology in order to understand the image that appears during the actual manipulation of the scanning head. It is also necessary to understand fully on possible occurrence of artifacts during ultrasound scanning for the elucidation of diagnostically useful informations. The economy of the method is indeed the reason to choose the ultrasound as the primary diagnostic tool in a variety of clinical conditions, however, it is also true that the equipment with better performance invariably gives better diagnostic informations in a number of clinical situations.

This book was written for the audience who indeed starts learning of abdominal ultrasound using real-time equipment. In order to allow the reader to persue the subjects in more detail, each chapter contains selected references.

It is indeed the wish of the authors that this rather introductory handbook will serve as a basic reference on abdominal ultrasound where the method still holds as one of the very best methods of medical imaging in solving the problems of differential diagnosis.

Finally, the authors are extremely grateful for the very delicate illustrations by Mrs. Hisako Kobayashi, and to the staffs of the publisher, Igaku-Shoin, who patiently followed the time consuming processes of editing the manuscripts and made this publication possible.

Morimichi Fukuda, M.D., Ph.D.
David O. Cosgrove, M.A., M.Sc., F.R.C.P., F.R.C.R.

CONTENTS

CHAPTER 1

THE HISTORICAL DEVELOPMENT OF REAL-TIME ULTRASOUND

ULTRASOUND TECHNIQUES

While the theoretical basis of the behavior of ultrasound had been thoroughly worked out by Lord Rayleigh (England, 1842-1919) in the late nineteenth century,[24] means of generating these high-frequency waves depended on two technical advances: suitable transducers had to be manufactured and the electronics both to drive them and to receive the signals had to be developed. The origin of modern transducers was the discovery of the piezoelectric properties of quartz in 1880 by Pierre Curie (France, 1859-1906).[4] It was a distinguished student and colleague of the Curie brothers, Paul Langevin (France, 1872-1946), who first produced ultrasound waves and set them to work as an underwater detector.[3] At first, he used a condenser as a transmitter and a microphone as a receiver, but he soon developed a piezoelectric quartz device for both functions. His work had been stimulated by the disastrous loss of the *Titanic* (1912) and was intended as an iceberg locator; it operated in the upper kilohertz range using continuous waves, which meant that no range information was available.

Improved electronics (a spinoff of RADAR methods) allowed pulsed ultrasound generators to be built. This led to SONAR (SOund Navigation And Ranging), which became important in the Second World War as a submarine echo locator. The concept of employing the same echo principle in solid materials as a flaw detector was proposed by Sergei Sokolov (USSR, 1897-1957).[21] Both of these applications were important for defense, so that research was classified, but information became available in 1946.[5,9] The "Reflectoscope" developed by Firestone (USA) was used for nondestructive testing (NDT) to detect flaws in metal castings. This use of ultrasound has become extremely important in industry.

Thus the basis for practical diagnostic imaging was laid in military and industrial development, first using continuous wave and later pulse-echo ultrasound waves.[26]

DIAGNOSTIC APPLICATIONS

The first diagnostic attempts with ultrasound, modeled on the experience with x-rays, were transmission shadowgrams. They were first used on the head and were developed by an Austrian physicist (F. Dussik) and his brother (K.T. Dussik), a psychiatrist.[8] They produced images on which they considered they had demonstrated brain tissue. In fact, it was later shown that these images consisted largely of artifacts caused by the barrier of the skull bones. This phenomenon is now readily understandable, but the problem caused considerable confusion at the time. Transmission techniques were abandoned after this attempt, though they still hold promise for soft tissue imaging in restricted anatomical areas.

Another military development was an Air Force trainer consisting of a tank with simulated terrain that was "flown over" by an ultrasound pulse-echo transducer. The images produced simulated in miniature the conditions a pilot would encounter using RADAR. After World War II, John Wild (UK/USA) obtained the first human echo images with this device.[10, 27] In 1950 he scanned bowel wall and measured its thickness, and in 1952, working with Jack Reid (USA), he obtained images of the breast in which he was able to demonstrate a tumor lying deep to the nipple.

Exploitation of the NDT flaw detector principle occurred at several sites simultaneously. Work at the Massachusetts Institute of Technology on the brain had demonstrated echoes from the midline of the brain. Leksell (Sweden) repeated these studies through a burr hole, obtaining a more detailed display of brain structure.[17] R. Turner (England) obtained clear midline brain echoes through the skull in 1952.[1] This work was taken up in neurosurgery, and midline echo location became an important clinical application. Both neurosurgical and cardiological applications have continued to provide the impetus for many of the developments in ultrasound, including real time.

Douglas Howry (USA, died 1969) developed a water bath system with a motor-driven transducer which produced compounded images showing the major tissue interfaces in the limbs and neck with impressive detail.[13] Ian Donald (Scotland, died 1987) and Tom Brown (Scotland) used an industrial flaw detector from the Glasgow dockyards for gynecological and, later, obstetrical problems.[6, 7] This device was developed into the first commercial B-scanner, manufactured by Nuclear Enterprises of Scotland. These early systems were cumbersome but remarkably effective clinically and set the scene for the progressive acceptance of ultrasound in diagnosis.

The images produced were of excellent quality, but only the major body interfaces (specular reflectors) were displayed. The presence of weaker echoes from the parenchyma of organs was reported in 1969 by Peter Wells (England).[26] Their display in tomograms was developed by George Kossoff (Australia) in the mid-1970s, using compression amplification techniques to form "gray-scale" ultrasound images with wide dynamic range.[15] Because these images were easier to understand and relate to x-rays, they were readily accepted by diagnosticians. Rapid, extensive expansion of their use followed in the late 1970s and early 1980s.

REAL-TIME SCANNERS

Display of movement in one line of sight was the basis of the earliest SONAR and clinical diagnostic systems. Wild's two-dimensional images could be repeated rapidly enough to show tissue movement. The earliest cardiac scans using NDT devices showed vascular movement (Figure 1-1), though it was not until some 20 years later that the great clinical potential of real time was appreciated.

The need to display the movement of the heart was self-evident but the first attempts to achieve this with two-dimensional tomography relied on electrocardiographic (ECG) gating to redisplay a series of static frames. The approach was clumsy and viewing in real time was not immediately available, so the interactiveness of M-mode work was forfeited. Åsberg first attemped to produce moving images directly, using a large mirror-operated system (Figure 1-2) which produced seven frames per second, hardly adequate for the heart.[2] The system was never developed further.

Work in Siemens' laboratories in Germany in 1961-1962 led to the development of the first practical real-time scanner for the abdomen.[20] Calculations based on the limiting factor, the speed of sound in tissue, indicated that it should be possible to produce an image some 12 cm in width, repeated 15 times/sec with a line density of 1 per mm. This would be sufficient if a weakly focused transducer was used. To move a transducer assembly across 12 cm 15 times/sec was obviously impractical, so designs that avoided translation movement were explored.

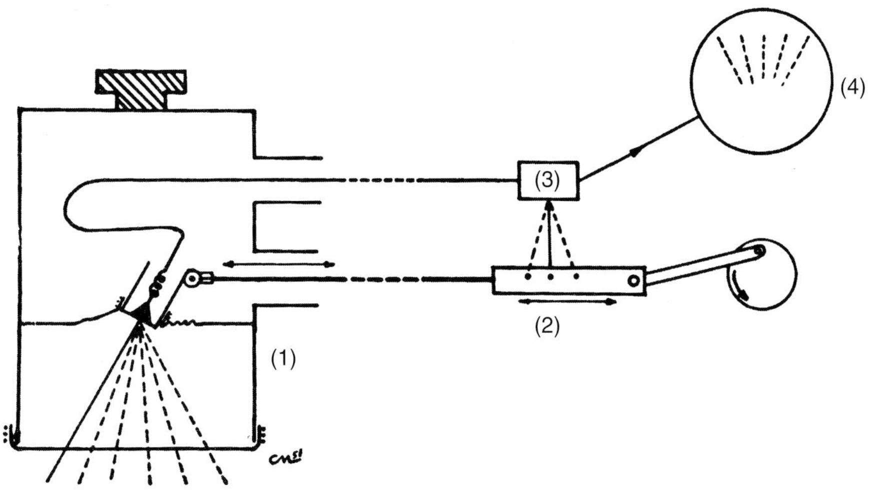

Figure 1-1. Water bath scanner with mechanical action by Wild and Reid.
This device, built by John Wild and Jack Reid in the early 1950s, gave sector scans that were capable of sufficiently rapid repetition to be considered as "real time." The transducer was housed in a water bath (1) and moved in an oscillatory fashion by a motor drive (2). The signals display on the cathode ray tube (4) was controlled by a sensor (3) on the motor drive. The design was never further developed. (Reprinted with permission from Wild JJ, Reid JM: Application of echo-ranging techniques to the determination of structure of biological tissues. Science 115 : 226-228, 1952. Copyright 1952 American Association for the Advancement of Science.)

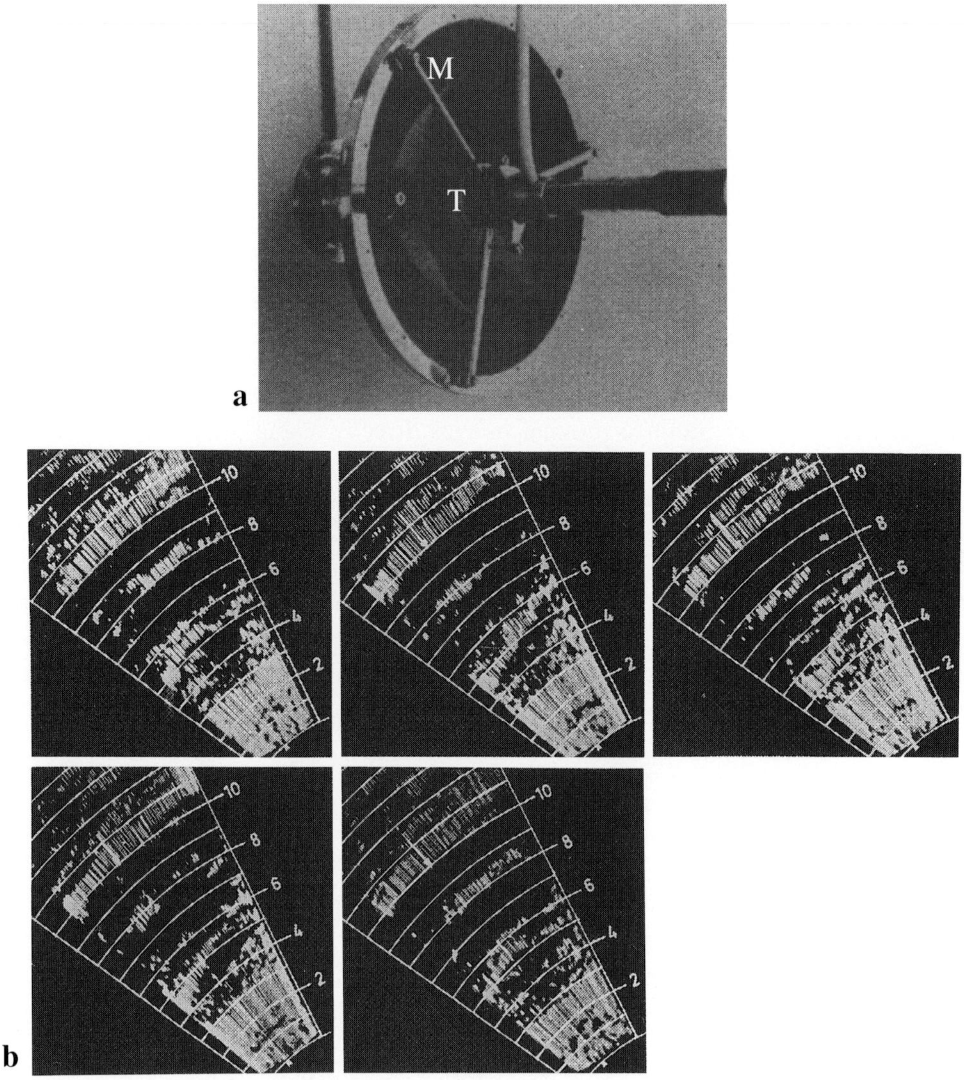

Figure 1-2. A real-time cardiac imager by Åsberg, 1963.
Using a large mirror (M) to produce a well-defined ultrasound beam from a small transducer (T), this whole device was oscillated in contact with the skin to produce narrow-angle sector scans. Åsberg published the design in 1963 for cardiac work. Serial frames from a moving sequence are shown in (b). (From Olofsson, Hertz, Åsberg, 1963.)

The final design employed a pair of rotating transducers which swept the beam across a parabolic acoustic mirror to produce a set of parallel ultrasound lines (Figure 1-3). The entire device was enclosed in a water bath with a soft plastic membrane to contact the patient's skin. The first prototype "Vidoson" scanner entered clinical trials in 1962. Its size and weight necessitated a supporting stand. The electronics was adapted from an NDT device. It operated at 2.5 MHz, with a frame rate of 16/sec and gave a rectangular gray-scale image of 12×16 cm.

There was initial resistance by potential users until its impact in obstetrics and gynecology was appreciated by Hoffman and Hollander in 1965, and later by Demling and Rettenmeier for abdominal use. The catch phrase "real time" was never applied to the Vidoson, and this seemingly trivial fact partly accounts for the lack of recognition of its innovativeness. Failure to appreciate the importance of the display of movement slowed the acceptance of the technique.

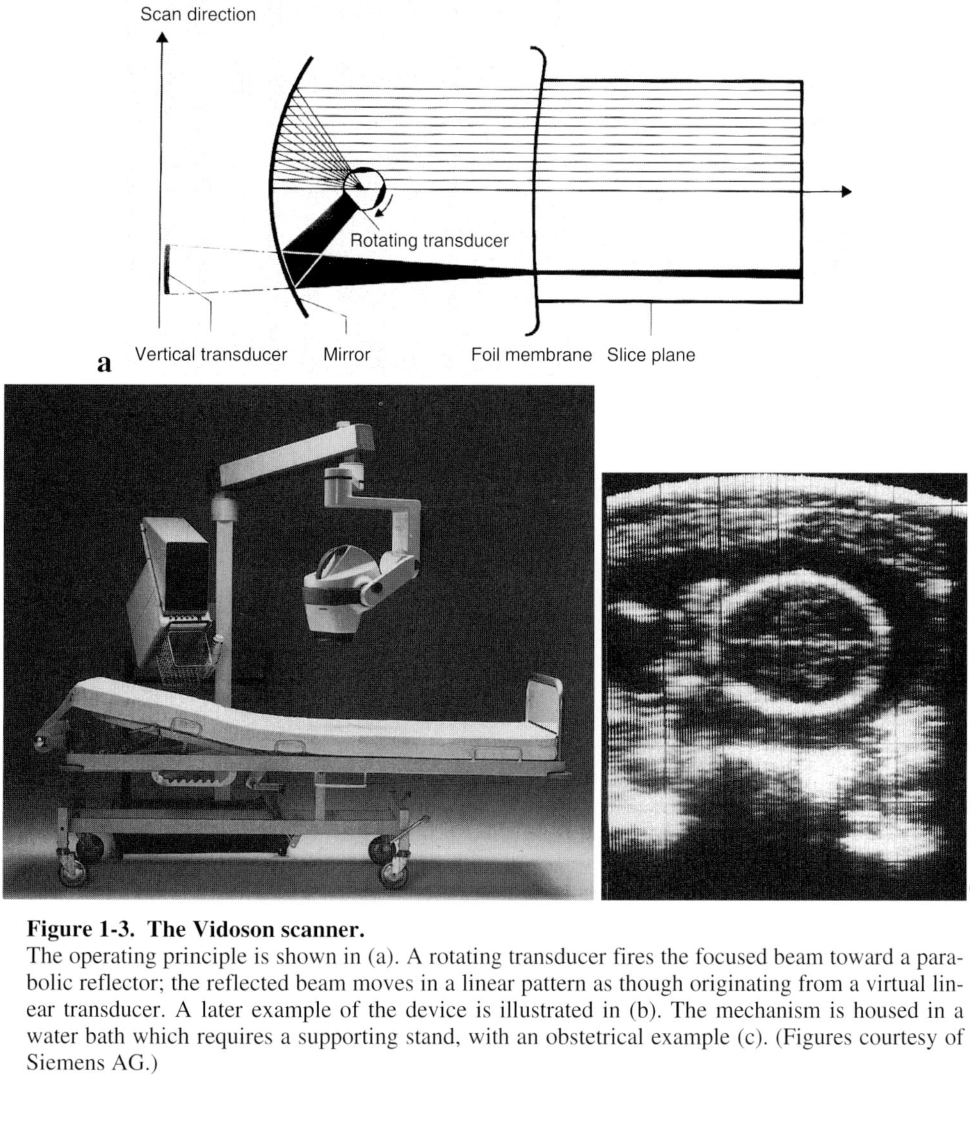

a b c

Figure 1-3. The Vidoson scanner.
The operating principle is shown in (a). A rotating transducer fires the focused beam toward a parabolic reflector; the reflected beam moves in a linear pattern as though originating from a virtual linear transducer. A later example of the device is illustrated in (b). The mechanism is housed in a water bath which requires a supporting stand, with an obstetrical example (c). (Figures courtesy of Siemens AG.)

Although this mechanical design was very effective and ultimately successful, with more than 3,000 installations, the water bath scan head was bulky and cumbersome. A much more compact version that could be hand-held was developed by Norman McDicken (Scotland) in 1974 [18] (Figure 1-4a). The intention was to retain the flexibility of the scanning procedure that is so important in M-mode work. It used a single conventional transducer element which was oscillated through an arc of 90° to give a sector scan. It was coupled to the patient's skin through a film of oil about 1 mm in thickness so that the problems of direct contact between the transducer and the skin were avoided. It operated at 3.5 MHz and could provide 15 frames per second.

At the same time, Griffith and Henry (USA) were developing an oscillating system based on an Echoline 20A cardiac device.[12] A simple gear arrangement moved the 2.25-MHz transducer assembly through 30° to give 30 frames/sec. There were 66 lines per frame, but because of the simple harmonic motion of the drive, they were not uniformly distributed across the image, being sparser centrally. A rotation sensor was used to control the position of the lines on the display. It was used in cardiac studies and gave images with good resolution, though without gray scaling.

Subsequently, McDicken developed an alternative design using four small crystals mounted on a rotating wheel in a miniature water bath [19] (Figure 1-4b). This had a smoother action with the rather large transducers that were available at the time. By mounting the wheel in a small oil bath, the transducer could be rotated rapidly, safely separated from the patient's skin by a rigid window. This device was capable of providing 30 frames/sec, and again gave a 90° field of view and operated at 3.5 MHz (Figure 1-4c). Commercial introduction came first from EMI (Nuclear Enterprises) and almost simultaneously from companies in the United States (Advanced Technology Laboratories) and Europe (Bruel and Kjaer, Kretz).

The development of all-electronic systems appears to have been a Dutch initiative. Jan Somer, working at the Institute of Medical Physics (TNO) in Utrecht in 1964, was disappointed by the poor two-dimensional images of the head obtained with static scanners compared with the useful information available from A-scans. He speculated that the apparent degradation might be due to irregularities of the velocity of ultrasound through different parts of the skull. If so, the problem could be minimized by forming a two-dimensional image from a point. This would produce a sector scan with display of movement. Adapting the beam-steering methods developed for SONAR, he designed and built a phased-array sector scanner by 1967 [11, 22, 23] (Figure 1-5).

Somer built an array with 21 elements, each 0.5 mm in width. It was 11 mm long by 10 mm across, operating at 1.3 MHz, and produced a 90° sector image of 128 lines (comprising four separate acoustic fields which were interlaced) at a rate of 30 frames/sec. Each element was driven by its own pulser, and the time delays were controlled by varicap diodes. Although the probe itself was small, the associated electronics were cumbersome by modern standards; however, the images of the head were superior to those available from static scanners.[14] The general advantages of the system were not appreciated by clinicians until it was used in the heart. Somer's device was briefly marketed by the Diagnostic Electronics Corporation in Massachusetts. The same basic principles were later developed by Thurstone (USA) and utilized in the Grumman and Varian systems.[25] Subsequently the phased-array scanner was refined. It forms the basis for modern sophisticated devices.

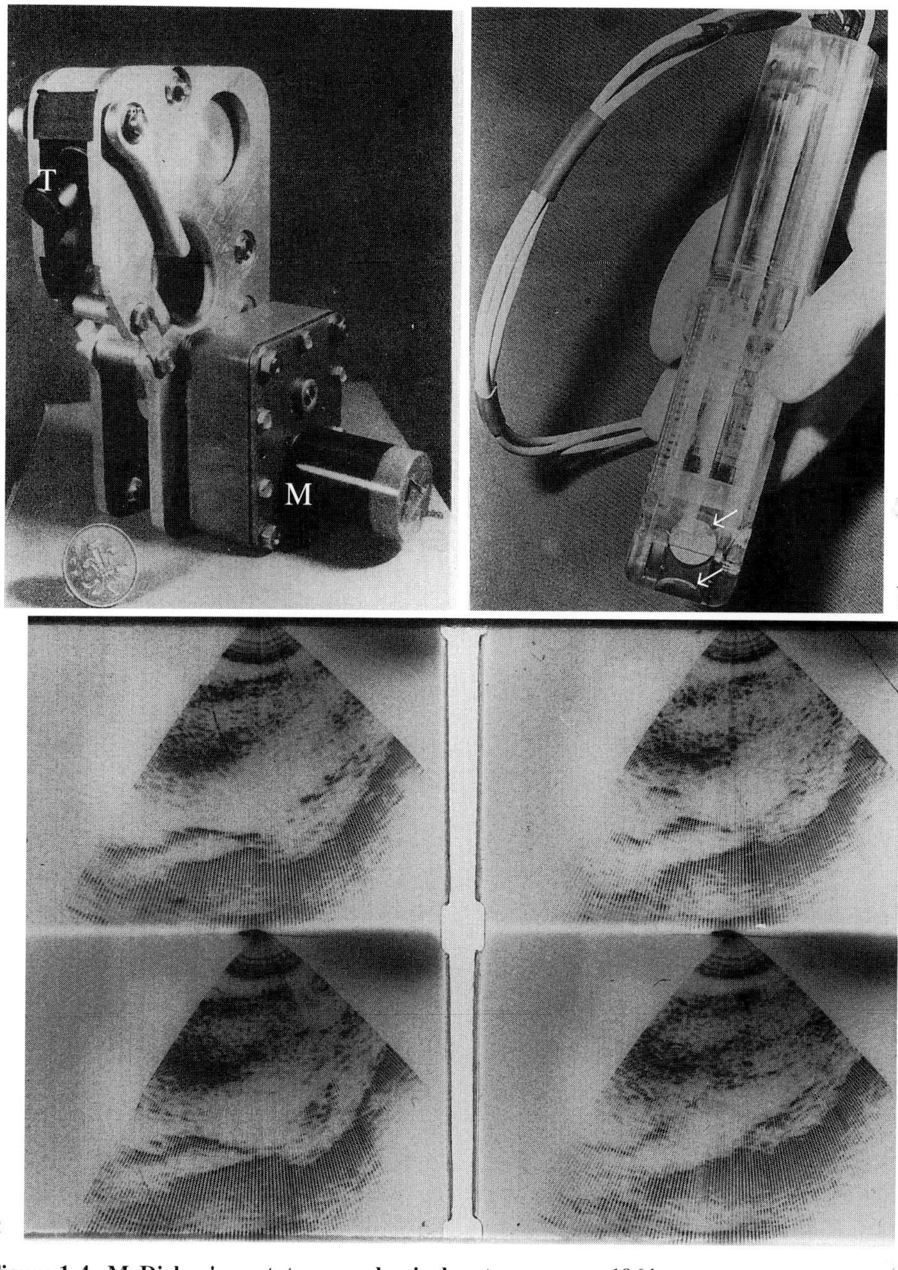

a b c

Figure 1-4. McDicken's prototype mechanical sector scanner, 1964.
The initial design (a) used a conventional transducer (T) mounted on an oscillating cam driven by a motor (M) (two-pence coin, 27 mm). Direct skin contact was inconvenient, so a water bath was added. To achieve a higher frame rate, a special rotating transducer assembly was built (b) containing four crystals (arrows). The probe was conveniently small. Four still frames from a cardiac sequence are shown in (c). (Figures courtesy of Dr. Norman McDicken.)

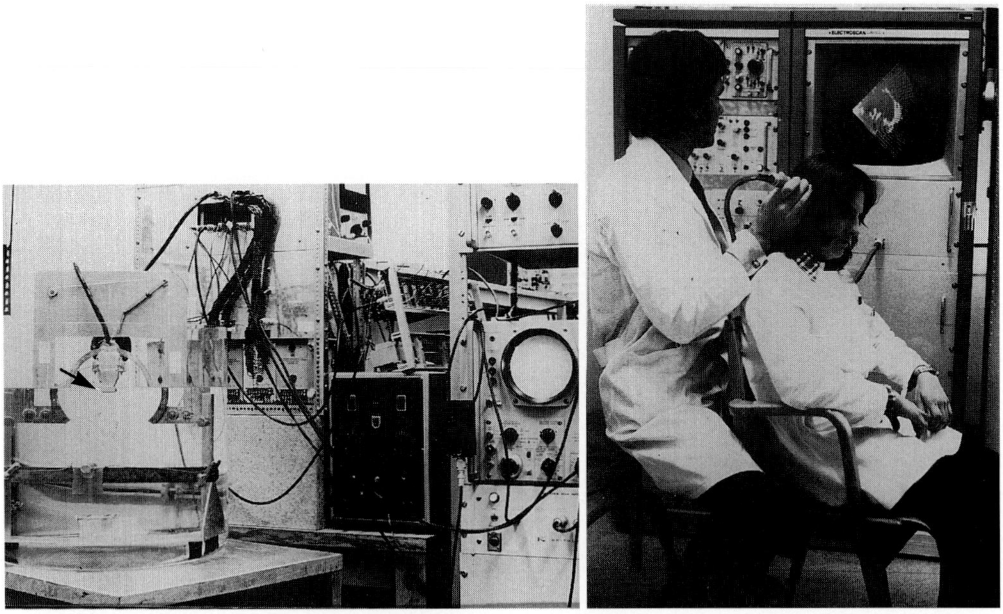

a b

Figure 1-5. Somer's prototype phased-array scanner, 1967.
The array transducer (arrow in a) is shown scanning a test object in a water bath. Notice the complexity of the cabling and electronic signal processing, which was refined in the prototype clinical version (b). (Figures courtesy of Dr. Jan Somer.)

Though in principle somewhat simpler, application of linear arrays to ultrasound began later. Nicholaas Bom, who had been working with underwater acoustics for NATO in Italy in the 1960s, moved to the Thorax Center in Rotterdam and set out to apply the SONAR work to cardiology. He designed and built the first linear-array scanner in 1969-70 (Figure 1-6a,b) (patented in 1971).[14] It consisted of 20 small elements which were fabricated separately and assembled into an array using epoxy (Araldite) cement. It operated at 2.25 MHz and produced 100 frames/sec. Each element was fired individually to form an acoustic beam so that the picture was somewhat crude, beam shape and direction being poorly controlled, and with few lines. Nonetheless, the device worked well enough to provide diagnoses that aroused intense interest among clinical cardiologists (Figure 1-6c). One on the first cases where it proved useful was in a patient critically ill with a pericardial effusion that was not diagnosed until the linear-array scanner was used. Such experiences provided the impetus for further developments to improve resolution and image quality. The eventual true clinical applications of these systems were a little lower in the body than the inventor's intention: Somer's phased array was conceived as a neurological scanner but is most useful in cardiology and in the abdomen, the latter being the most useful application of Bom's linear array, which was originally designed for the heart.

Bom's linear array was commercially produced by Organon Technika, which also made a remarkably compact, battery-driven version of the same device using a miniature TV screen; the entire scanner could be hand-held. Small, portable scanners of this general type are still being used in clinics and emergency units. More sophisticated versions were soon developed by American and Japanese manufacturers. One of the earliest of these was successfully marketed by Advanced Dynamic Research. Improved arrays with more closely

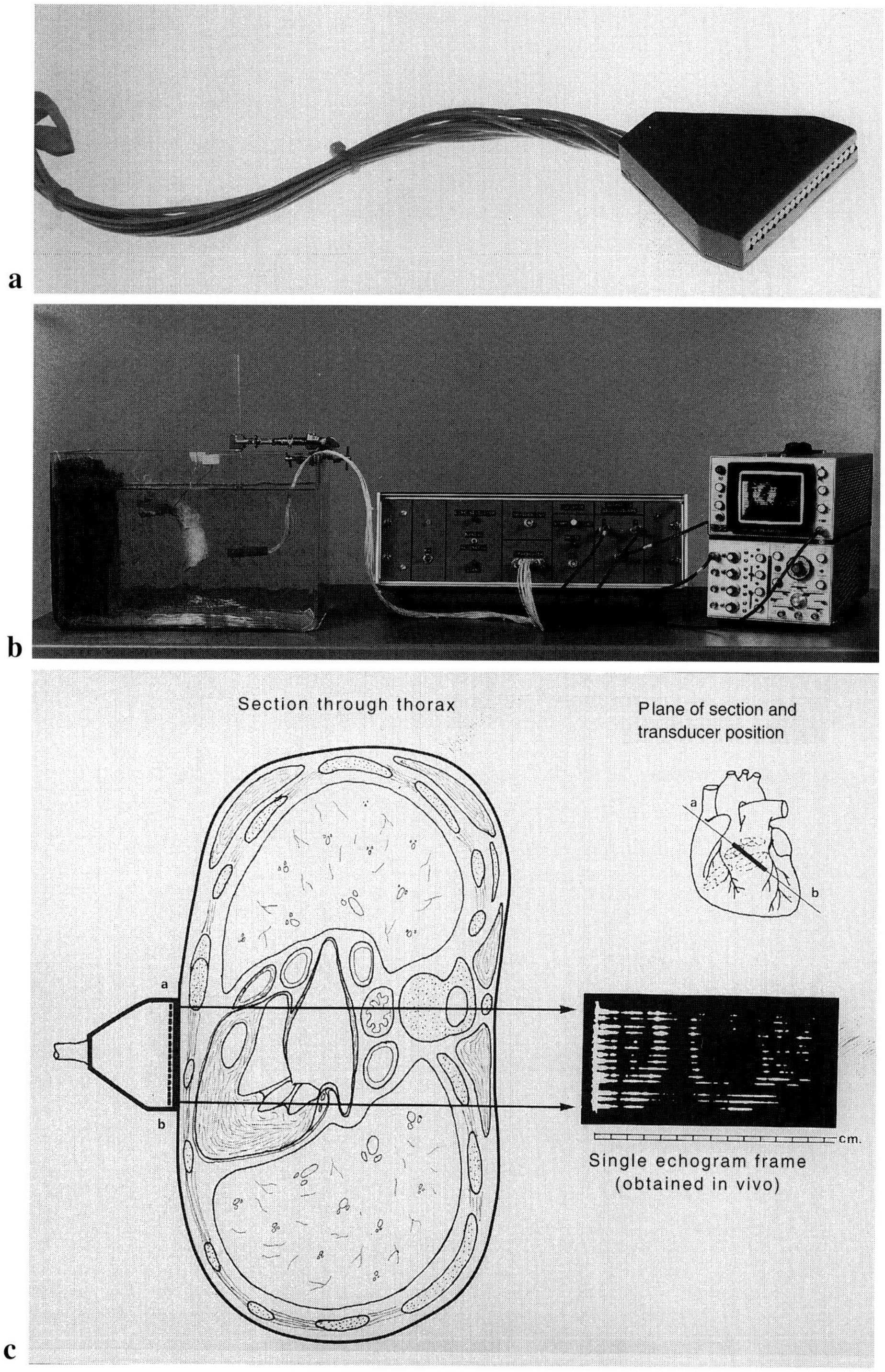

Figure 1-6. Bom's linear array, 1969.
The elements and cable arrangement can be seen in the close-up view of the first linear-array transducer (a). In (b) it is being used to scan an excised heart in a water tank. A frame from an *in vivo* moving cardiac sequence is shown in (c) together with a diagram of its orientation. (Figures courtesy of Dr. Nicholaas Bom.)

spaced elements, using electronic focusing, have been produced by several manufacturers and the images have improved greatly.

Bom also developed a miniature (3-mm) array mounted on a cardiac catheter for endocardiac scanning. This approach led to the development of small, specialized versions for intracavitary use as endoprobes and intraoperative scanning.

An important step was the introduction of digital systems, both for short-term image storage (digital scan converters) and as delay lines for dynamic focusing. Improved arrays with electronic focusing and improved images were produced by a number of commercial firms.

The history of the development of ultrasound has followed a pattern [28] of laboratory work by dedicated physicists, often encouraged by perspicacious clinicians, leading to commercial production of the successful designs by small manufacturing companies, often sponsored by the innovators themselves. Ultrasound has lent itself well to this form of low-investment development, since the unit cost of a scanner is low by comparison with that of other imaging technologies. It has produced a market with numerous small, specialized manufacturers with products that fill a niche, often even localized geographically. Ultrasound has come of age and is now an accepted part of the imager's repertoire. In addition, the rate of progress in image quality has slowed, so that there is much less difference between images from different products at a given price level than previously. Thus ultrasound has entered a somewhat different and more competitive phase in which the traditional manufacturers of diagnostic equipment are taking the lead and the choice between different scanners is made on the basis of cost and convenience rather than image quality. There is every likelihood that some of the traditional names in the ultrasound industry will have disappeared by the end of the decade. It is to be hoped that this will not deprive users and their patients of the benefits of the specialized, innovative systems that have been such a feature of this flexible and versatile imaging modality.

REFERENCES

1. Annon: Annual Report of the British Empire Cancer Campaign, 1952, p52.
2. Åsberg A: Ultrasonic cinematography of the living heart. Ultrasonics 5 : 113-117, 1967.
3. Chilowsky C, Langevin MP: Procedes et appareils pour la production de signaux sous-marins diriges et pour la localisation a distance d'obstacles sous-marins. French Patent No.502913, 1916.
4. Curie J, Curie P: Sur l'electricite polaire dans cristaux hemiedres a face inclinees. Comptes Rendues Seances Acad Sci 91 : 383-386, 1880.
5. Desch CH, Sproule DD, Dawson WJ: The detection of cracks in steel by means of supersonic waves. J Iron Steel Industry (Lond) 153 : 319-323, 1946.
6. Donald I, McVicar J, Brown TG: Investigation of abdominal masses by pulsed ultrasound. Lancet 1188-1195, 1958.
7. Donald I: Sonar: The story of an experiment. Ultrasound Med Biol 1 : 109-115,1974.
8. Dussik KT, Dussik F, Wyt L: Auf dem Wege zur Hyperphonographie des Gehirnes. Wein Med Wochenschr 97 : 14-17, 1947.
9. Firestone FA: The supersonic reflectoscope. J Acoust Soc Am 17 : 287-291, 1946.
10. French LA, Wild JJ, Neal D: Detection of cerebral tumours by ultrasonic pulses. Cancer 3 : 705-707, 1950.
11. Freund HJ, Somer JC, Kendel KH, et al: Electronic sector scanning in the diagnosis of cerebrovascular disease and space-occupying processes. Neurology 22 : 1147-1159, 1973.
12. Griffith JM, Henry WL: A sector scanner for real time two-dimensional echocardiography. Circulation 49 : 1147-1152, 1974.

13. Howry DH, Bliss HL: Ultrasonic visualisation of soft tissue structures of the body. J Lab Clin Med 40 : 579-592, 1952.
14. Kamphuisen HAC, Somer JC, Oosterbaan WA: Two-dimensional echo-encephalography with electronic sector scanning. J Neurol Neurosurg Psychiatry 35 : 912-918, 1972.
15. Kossoff G, Garrett WJ: Ultrasonic film echoscopy for placental localisation. Aust NZ J Obstet Gynaecol 12 : 117-119, 1972.
16. Krause WEE, Soldner RE: Ultrasonic imaging technique with high image rate for medical diagnosis. Digest of the Seventh International Congress of Biological and Medical Engineering. Stockholm, Almqvist & Wiksell, 1967, p315.
17. Leksell L: Echo-encephalography: Detection of intracranial complications following head injury. Acta Chir Scand 110 : 301-304, 1956.
18. McDicken WN, Bruff K, Paton J: An ultrasonic instrument for rapid B-scanning of the heart. Ultrasonics 12 : 269-272, 1974.
19. McDicken WN, Anderson T, McHugh R, et al: An ultrasonic real-time scanner. Ultrasound Med Biol 4 : 333-339, 1979.
20. Patzold J, Krause W, Kresse H, et al: Present state of an ultrasound cross-section procedure with a rapid image rate. IEEE Trans Biomed Eng 17 : 263-265, 1970.
21. Sokolov SY: The ultra-acoustic microscope. Zh Tech Fiz 19 : 271-273, 1949.
22. Somer JC: Instantaneous and continuous pictures obtained by a new two-dimensional scan technique with a stationary transducer, in Kazner E, Schiefer W, Zulch KJ (eds): Proceedings in Echo-encephalography, 1968, pp234-238.
23. Somer JC: Electronic sector scanner for ultrasonic diagnosis. Ultrasonics 6 : 153-159, 1968.
24. Strutt JW, Third Baron Rayleigh: The Theory of Sound, Vols 1 and 2. London, Macmillan, 1877-1878.
25. Thurstone FL, Von Ramm OT: Electronic beam steering for imaging. Rotterdam, Ultrasonics in Medicine, 1973, pp43-48.
26. Wells PNT: Developments in medical ultrasonics. World Med Electronics 4 : 272-276, 1966.
27. Wild JJ, Reid JM: Applications of echo-ranging techniques to the determination of structure of biological tissues. Science 115 : 226-228, 1952.
28. White DN: Historical survey, in White DN (ed): Ultrasound in Medical Diagnosis. Kingston, Ontario, Ultramedison, 1976, Chap. 1.

CHAPTER 2

INSTRUMENTATION AND INTERPRETATION

NATURE OF REAL-TIME SCANNING

An ultrasound image consists of the echo information along a series of contiguous scan lines displayed in their proper relationships. This is the static *B-scan*. For the moving picture version of this scan, a series of frames must be repeated and displayed rapidly enough to produce a flicker-free image. This is known as *real-time* scanning. The principle is the same as that of cine film. In many respects, the term *cine SONAR* is more aposite than *real-time*.

The image is usually displayed on a TV monitor so the display rate is determined by the video system used (NTSC = 60 frames/sec, PAL = 50 frames/sec). Both of these are adequate for a flicker-free display. Some experimental scanners used an *X-Y* display when the repetition rate was set by the manufacturer; higher rates are possible than with a TV system, though generally unnecessary. This type of screen avoids the TV raster pattern, but those with a good gray scale tend to be expensive. They are also incompatible with standard video recorders and so have fallen out of use.

The ultrasonic frame rate is constrained by the fact that time must be allowed for the most distant echoes from a pulse to return before the next pulse is transmitted. Thus the speed of sound in tissue and the depth of tissue to be imaged limit the pulse repetition frequency. For deep abdominal scanning, thc pulsc repetition frequency (PRF) must not exceed 3,000/sec, but it may be faster for superficial organs. These 3,000 lines can be distributed in space or time, depending on the overriding requirement for resolution. Thus, where spatial resolution is paramount, one might opt for 300 lines/image and accept the slow frame rate of 10/sec. Where rapid movements must be displayed, frame rates of 30 or 60/sec are required, but there can only be 100 or 50 lines/image. Thus temporal and spatial resolution are mutually exclusive. For the abdomen, the latter is usually more important and slow frame rates are accepted. The reverse is true for the heart.

The 300 lines of the image arrived at in this way for abdominal scanning can be tightly packed to form a smooth, line-free image with a small field of view, or they can be spread to form a larger field of view with a coarse line structure. The best compromise depends on the clinical problem, since a small image is more acceptable in some situations than others. For sector scanning a 90° field of view is the minimum practicable in the abdomen.

Thus it can be seen that the need to allow a pulse to fade before the next one is sent sets severe limits on real-time scanning. Interesting attempts to solve this problem have been proposed. One idea is to encode sequential pulses (e.g., by giving them different frequencies or pulse lengths) so that two pulses can overlap. Another is to send simultaneous pulses in different directions such that there is no overlap between them. One version of this method is to transmit an unfocused beam, but to focus down several different lines during the receive phase so that one pulse produces 2, 4, or more image lines. Solutions to this problem are likely to be featured in the next generation of ultrasound scanners.

Real-Time Scanning Methods

The basic technique employed in all real-time scanners is an automatic system to sweep the ultrasound beam repeatedly across the anatomy to be studied. Mechanical or electronic solutions have been developed, and the beam can be swept either in a line, to produce a rectangular image, or in an arc, giving a sector or triangular image (Table 2-1).

Table 2-1. Real-time scanning systems.

System	Beam Pattern	Image Shape	Comments
Mechanical	Linear	Rectangular	Not widely used
	Sector	Triangular	Trapezoid with water bath
Electronic	Linear	Rectangular	Linear array
	Convex	Trapezoidal	Curved linear array
	Sector	Triangular	Phased array

The *mechanical systems* employ standard transducers and thus exploit the body of knowledge on optimal design compromises. In principle, the images should be as good as those of a static scanner. Though the best examples do come close, the line density is usually lower (because of the real time compromise discussed above), and because the eye tends to assess image grain in proportion to total image size, thus somewhat reducing the real and perceived quality of frozen images. In addition, it is necessary to separate the moving transducer from the patient's skin by small fluid bath; any reverberations or distortions of the beam thus produced degrade the image. The problems due to the obligatory fluid bath can be minimized by keeping the path length small, by using a fluid that absorbs ultrasound rapidly, by acoustic matching of the contact surface to the fluid and skin, and by avoiding any parallel reflecting surfaces that may cause multiple reverberations. Two basic designs are possible. If the probe travels along a rail, a *linear scan* is produced, giving a rectangular image. This approach is apt to be clumsy, but one version designed for carotid artery scanning was marketed (Picker Microview). In the more successful approach, the transducer is pivoted about a point to produce a *sector scan* . One arrangement uses a single crystal set on a yoke that allows it to oscillate to and fro (the "wobbler"). Another uses several crystals mounted on the edge of a rotating wheel (the "spinner"); each crystal is switched into operation as it passes the contact window, so that sequential frames are produced by different crystals. The *oscillating system* has the advantage of having only one crystal and thus can be made very small. The electrical contacts required are straightforward via a flexible cable. However, the oscillating movement produces a windshield wiper effect on the image which can be tiring for the operator, and if the mechanical linkages become loose, the beam will image slightly different tissue planes in the two directions of sweep. This "mechanical hysteresis" produces an unsteady, fluttering image that is tiring to watch and that may mask tissue movement, making it impossible to detect small peristaltic or vascular movements.

Fast frame rates are easier to achieve with *rotating system*, which also produce steadier images because of the regular sweep direction (Figure 2-1). However, precise matching of the characteristics of the multiple transducers (especially the beam direction but also the beam and pulse shape) is critical; inconsistencies here give a throbbing or fluttering quality to the moving image. The electrical contacts of rotating systems pose a problem. Slip rings are simple but intermittently poor contacts are a besetting weakness, while the more sophisticated alternatives, contactless inductive coils, are bulkier and more costly.

In most mechanical systems the beam passes directly to the contact membrane, but ingenious systems using acoustic mirrors have been developed. These allow the beam path to be folded and effectively position the transducer farther from the skin so that the very near field (where the beam shape is poor) is not used for imaging. The field of view becomes trapezoidal in shape, allowing better display of the superficial anatomy. The first real-time system introduced, the Siemens Vidoson, employed a parabolic mirror to produce a near-rectangular field of view (see Chapter 1). It also allowed a large transducer to be utilized, with its advantages of good focusing that were more fully exploited in another obsolete model, the Xonics 200. It was the large size of the scan head that rendered these systems obsolete.

The *electronic systems* likewise can be divided into linear and sector approaches, both having proved successful. In the simplest linear scanners, a rectangular block of transducer material some 10 mm in width is sliced across into strips so that the probe consists of an array of matchstick-shaped elements arranged alongside each other (Figure 2-2). Each element is separately connected and, when pulsed, produces its own ultrasound beam and therefore a line on the final image. The earliest linear arrays operated this way and were remarkable in their day, but the image was crude because of the paucity of lines and because the small elements necessarily produced poorly focused beams. Advances in manufacturing technology led to probes with many more and smaller elements (current versions have as many as 250 elements in a 5-cm array), solving the problem of a coarse line grain.

Focusing has been improved by firing groups of elements together. Small elements produce spreading beams that tend toward the omnidirectional beam pattern from a point source. Large transducers produce a narrow beam, which can be simulated in an array by using, say, seven elements together. If the second line is formed by element 2 to 8, and the third by elements 3 to 9, and so on, only two lines corresponding to the ends of the array are lost. The resulting image retains its high line density, and the resolution is improved by the focusing. A further improvement in focusing can be produced if the firing of the element used for each pulse can be precisely controlled. This method, known as *electronic focusing*, depends on the interaction of two ultrasound beams when they overlap (Figure 2-3a). Cancellation occurs when a compression and a rarefaction wave coincide, and summation occurs when the compressions or rarefactions are in phase. If, in our example, seven elements are being used to form a beam, and the outer two are triggered very slightly earlier than elements 2 and 6, with elements 3 and 5, and finally the central element 4, being progressively more delayed, then the phase relationships of the individual beams are such that, with the correct delays, the resultant beam is focused. The effect is the same as that produced by focusing a conventional transducer by means of a concave face. Here, the periphery is closer to the tissue being imaged, so the ultrasound waves from there are "ahead" of those from more central parts. Electronic focusing using time delays can be thought of as electronically curving the transducer face. This system is most commonly used in linear arrays, but a disc transducer can be cut into a set of concentric rings to form an annular array and electronically focused in the same way (Figure 2-4).

A major advantage of electronic focusing is that the effective curvature, and therefore the focal zone, can be changed simply by altering the phase delays between the elements. Thus the position of the focal zone can be adjusted very easily, and many such scanners have a user control for this purpose. In the most sophisticated developments of this approach, each pulse is repeated at different focuses and only the portion of the echo within the focal zone is used for the image; thus the final image is a composite, with perhaps four bands at different depths, each from a different pulse, and each with optimal focusing (Figure 2-3b-d). The necessary penalty for this improvement in image quality is a drop in frame rate (1/4 if four zones are used).

In exactly the same way, focusing can be applied when the transducer is being used as a receiver. However, since the echoes from different depths are received sequentially, it is possible to sweep the focal zone progressively during receipt of the echoes from each pulse to optimize it continuously for all depths. This is known as *dynamic focusing*.

Linear arrays known as *curvilinear* or *convex arrays* can be constructed with a built-in curvature. These probes operate in the same manner as flat linear arrays, but they give a trapezoidal field of view with a good display of the superficial tissues and a wider exposure of the deeper tissues.

These methods for improving focusing of linear arrays operate only along the array, that is, in the *scanned plane*. In the other direction, called the *orthogonal plane*, these maneuvers have no effect. Happily, the lozenge shape of the array elements means that the beam is intrinsically better in the orthogonal plane. It can be improved in the conventional manner by concave shaping, but only for a fixed focal zone. The overall beam shape for such an array is asymmetrical around the beam axis, unlike the symmetrical beam of a conventional disc-shaped transducer.

An additional problem afflicting arrays is that the presence of discrete elements produces peaks of sensitivity off the main beam axis. These are known as *grating lobes*.

All ultrasound transducers have side lobes; with conventional disc transducers, these are distributed uniformly around the beam, with a sensitivity less than 10 or 20 dB below the main beam. In addition, array transducers have grating lobes which result from interactions between the wavelength and the element size (they can be reduced by making the elements smaller; eventually this approximates to a continuous transducer, that is, when the element size is negligible in relation to the wavelength). For a linear array (conventional linear, curvilinear, or beam-steered phased array), the grating lobes lie within the scanned plane and may be almost as intense as the main beam, so that they can pose a serious problem. Grating lobes can be suppressed by using different transducer elements for transmit and receive to avoid superimposing the transmit grating lobe pattern on the receive grating lobe pattern. The same problem applies to annular arrays, but here the grating lobe pattern is symmetrical about the beam and, in practice, is likely to be more serious because of the difficulties of making annular arrays with sufficiently small elements. Grating lobe artifacts are distinct from those caused by the beam width (azimuthal or orthogonal beam width), which also produce partial volume problems. Beam width artifacts can be limited by focusing (using large apertures or by curving the transducer). Both are serious problems for arrays, especially when the transducer must be kept thin in order to make it manageable (e.g., in endoscopic ultrasound). Side lobes produce artifacts on the image in which strong reflectors lying to one side are superimposed on the directly imaged tissue. This is a form of noise (known as *clutter*, since it is structured rather than random); minimizing the effects of side lobes is an important aspect of array design.

Electronic sector systems are also multielement arrays, the beam being swept through an arc by phase delays. The array is made up of a set of small elements; in conventional scanners there may be 20 to 30 elements, but newer high-resolution systems employ up to 128. Generally all are triggered for each pulse, but with small, progressive delays applied to successive elements along the array. The same phase cancellation and summation effects that are employed for focusing a linear array act to direct the resultant beam to one side (Figure 2-5). At the next pulse, the delays are slightly reduced to redirect the beam, and, for the straight-ahead position, no delays are used. Reversing the delay pattern causes steering in the other direction, so that the beam is swept through an arc of typically 90°. Electronic and dynamic focusing can also be added, as well as transducer shaping for orthogonal focus.

The electronic sector scanners, often loosely called *phased arrays,* have some advantages over mechanical versions. Since there are no moving parts, they are more robust and the probes can be made small and light (Figure 2-6). Because beam control is instantaneous, they can exploit important time-sharing functions such as true, simultaneous B-mode and Doppler imaging, a feature that is particularly important for color Doppler. However, their electronics are more complex and costly, and there are problems with image quality due to side lobes and system noise.

In the new generation of high-resolution scanners, advanced electronic systems have been developed to reduce these effects. It seems likely that mechanical systems will eventually be replaced by electronic probes for all but the simplest scanners.

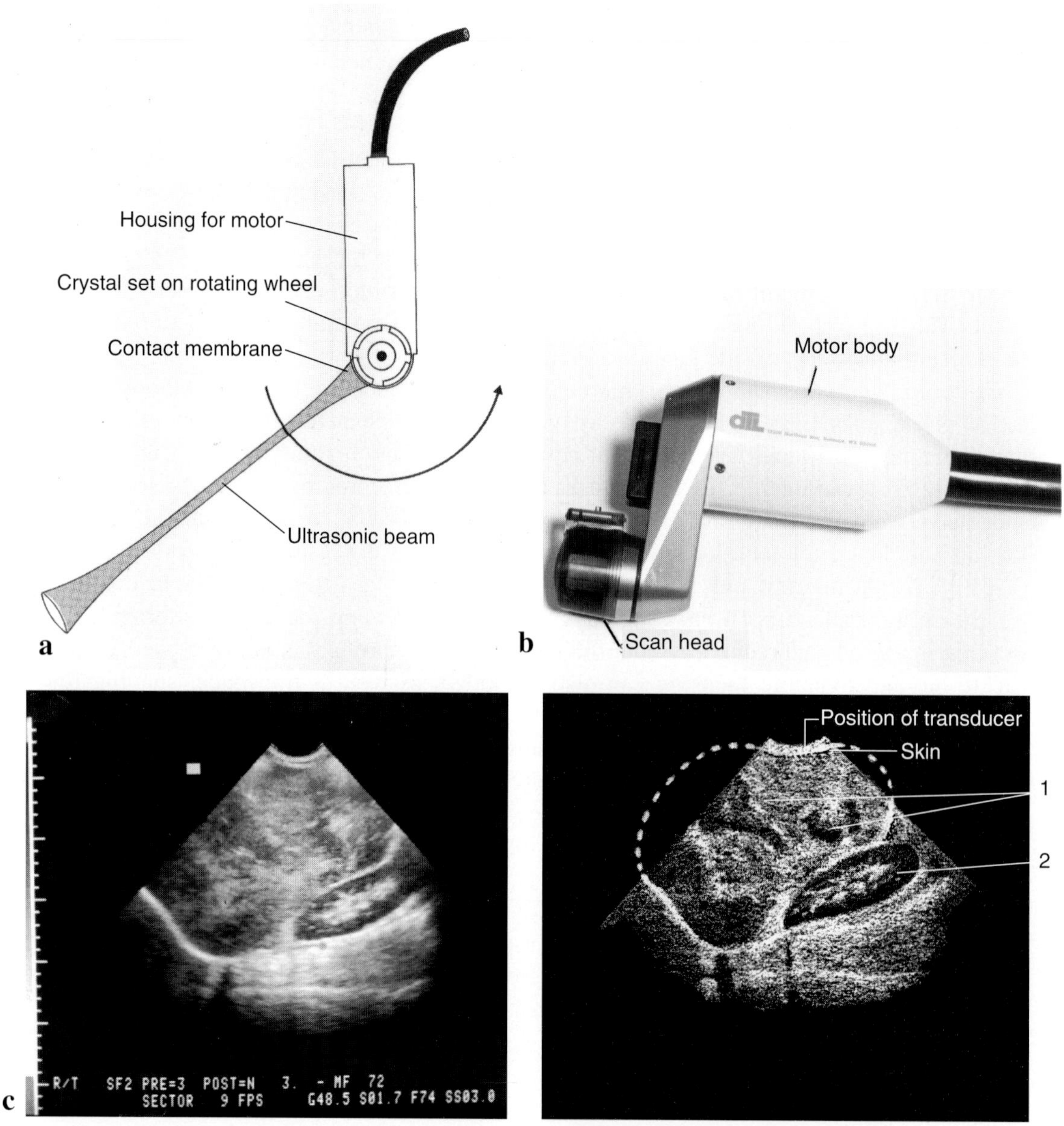

1. Metastases in liver 2. Right kidney

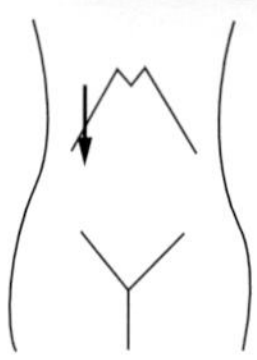

Figure 2-1. Real-time sector scanning.
In a typical rotating crystal transducer shown in diagrammatic form (a), the scan head contains several conventional crystals mounted on a wheel which spins in a fluid-filled housing. The motor and some electronic circuitry are contained within the hand-held body of the probe. An example is shown in (b) (A.T.L. probe; figure courtesy of Squibb Medical). The triangular geometry of the image produced by a sector probe is shown (c) in this sagittal view of the liver in a patient with multiple liver metastases. The 90° sector angle provides good visualization of the deeper tissues. (Image obtained on an I.G.E. Datason 3.5-MHz transducer.)

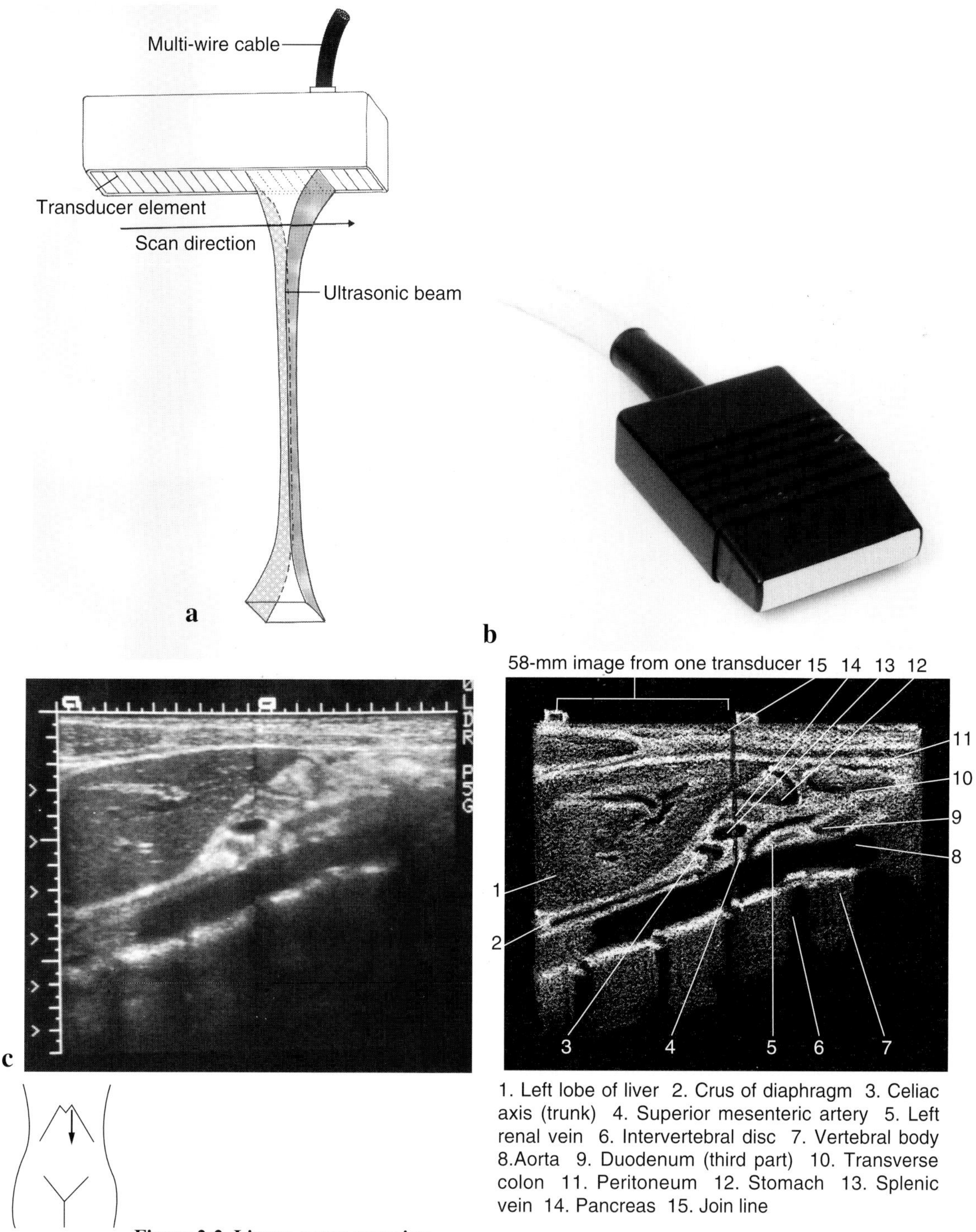

Figure 2-2. Linear-array scanning.
The array of elements is shown diagrammatically in (a). Parts of the amplifier chain are sited in the housing. A typical example is shown in (b). (5-MHz Acuson linear array; figure courtesy of Acuson.) Two contiguous images have been placed side by side to form the composite image in (c). The good display of superficial anatomy requires a contact window of 5.8 cm in this example. Shorter arrays are available, but the field of view is then smaller. (Images from Acuson 5-MHz 58-mm linear array transducer.)

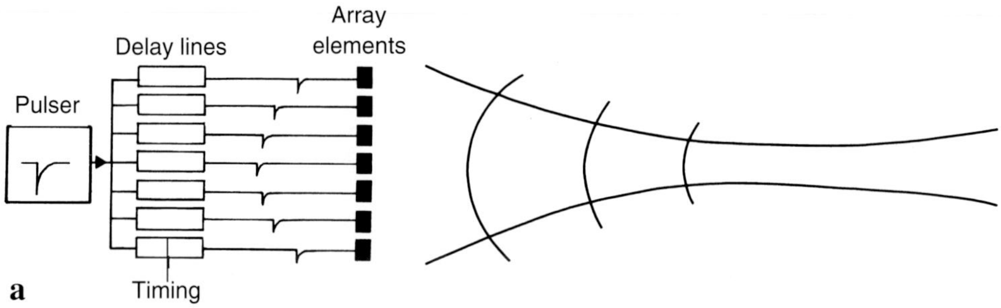

a

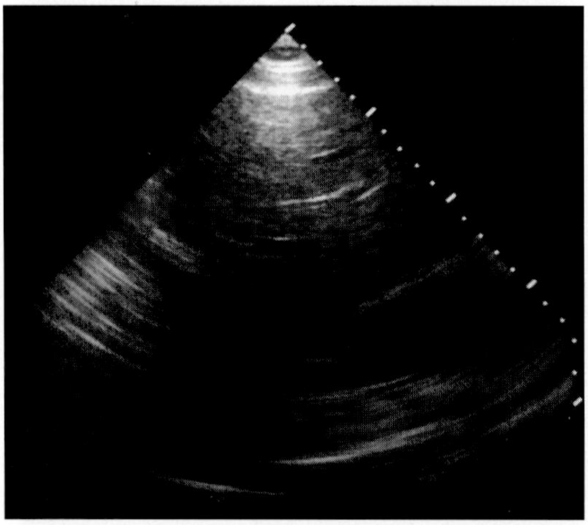

b

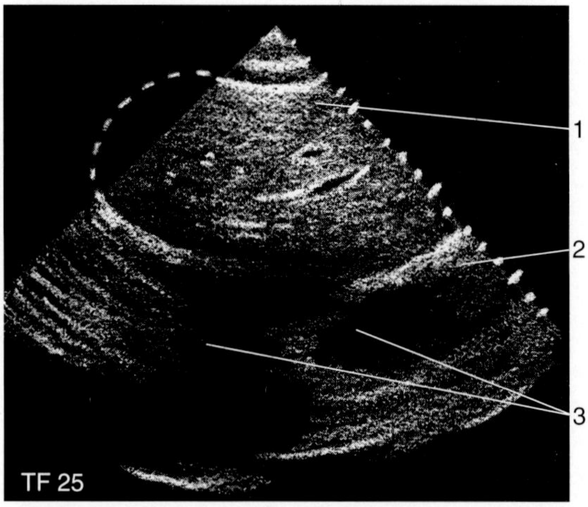

1. Liver 2. Kidney 3. Loss of detail

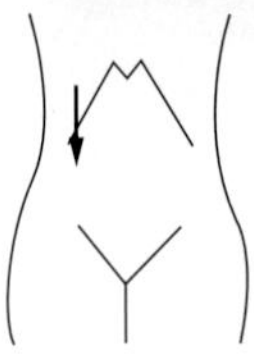

Figure 2-3. Electronic focusing.
Using a transducer with a multielement crystal, delays to the portion of the transmit pulse applied to the individual elements are used to control the beam shape. A section through a linear or an annular array is shown, with the outer elements triggered slightly earlier than the more central elements. The effect is the same as that produced by applying a lens to the transducer face, and the beam is focused. Electronic focusing of this sort, however, is more flexible, for the focal zone can be changed simply by altering the delays used. The same considerations apply while the transducer is being used as a receiver, except that in this mode the delays can be altered continuously to optimize the focus for the entire depth of tissue being imaged. (This bonus is impossible in the transmit mode because a pulse of ultrasound cannot be altered once it has left the transducer.)
The effects of transmit focus are apparent in these images of a right pleural effusion via the liver. In (b), with the focus set for the near zone (25 mm), the effusion is barely discernible; the improved resolution in the far field produced by selecting a deeper focal zone (120 mm in c) reveals the lesion clearly. With all zones selected (d), optimum clarity is achieved throughout the image. (Images from I.G.E. 3000 at 3.5 MHz.)

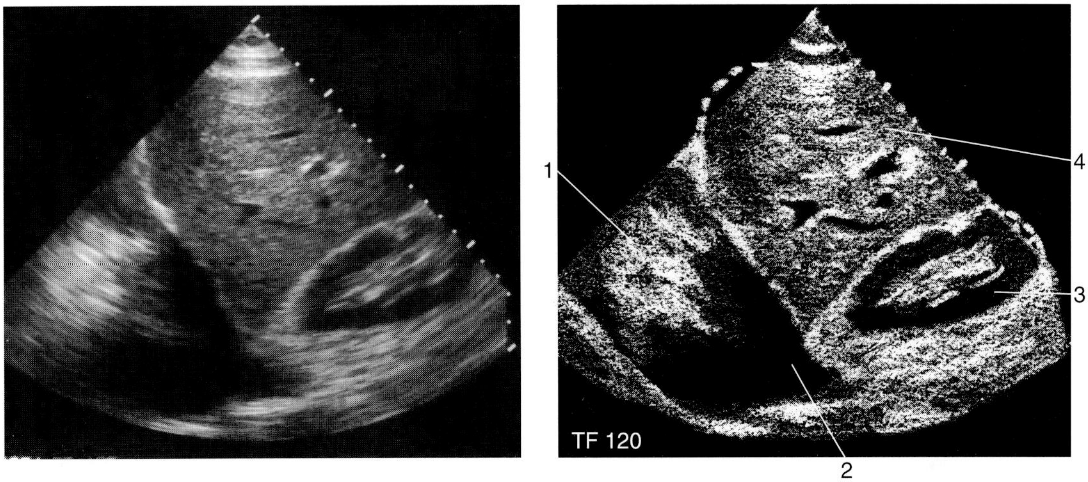

c

1. Lung 2. Effusion 3. Kidney 4. Liver

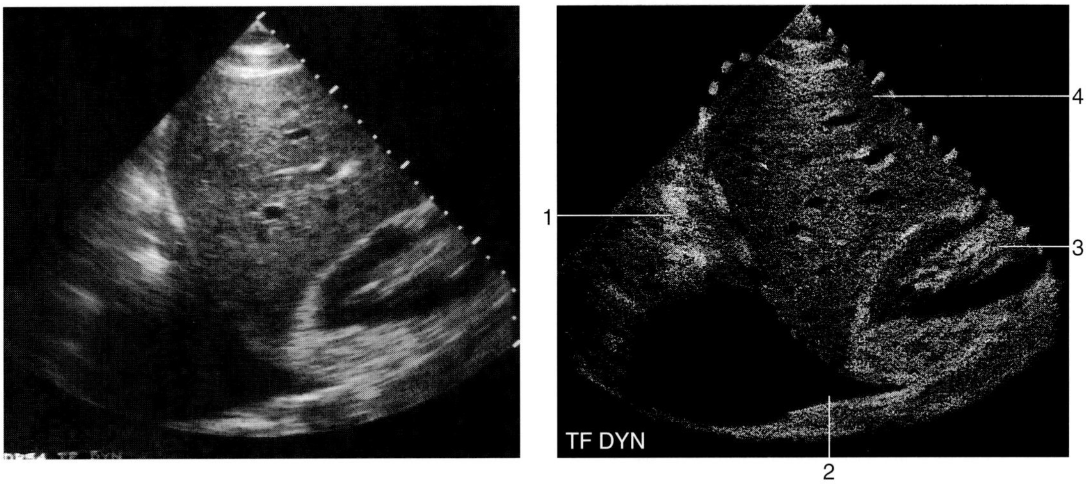

d

1. Lung 2. Effusion 3. Kidney 4. Liver

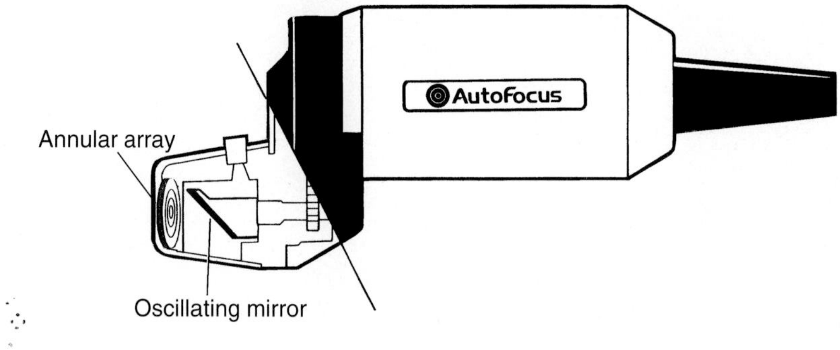

Figure 2-4. Annular array probe.
In this hand-held, real-time probe, the conventional crystal has been replaced by one that is cut into five rings. Each ring can be triggered separately, and the timing of their firing within a single ultrasound pulse shapes the beam in the same way as a lens, but with the added versatility that the focusing can be optimized for any depth. The same process in the receive period allows the focal zone to be swept throughout the depth range. This design uses a fixed crystal, the beam sweeping being performed by an oscillating mirror. (Autofocus probe; courtesy of Technicare Corporation.)

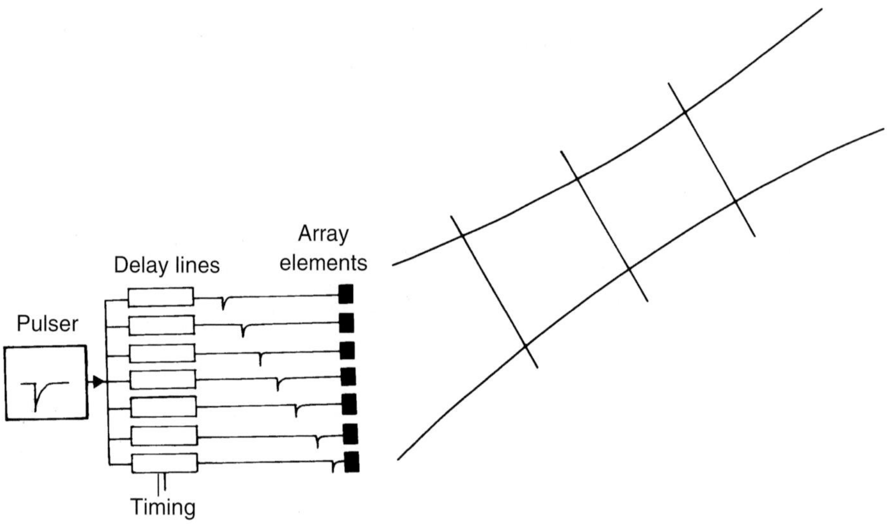

Figure 2-5. Electronic beam steering.
The elements of an array transducer are shown being triggered, with sequential delays from one end to the other. This has the effect of steering the beam to one side, the angle being controlled by the phase delays applied within a single pulse. By changing these delays progressively from pulse to pulse, the beam is swept through an arc to produce a sector scan (the so-called phased array). Electronic beam steering is usually combined with electronic focusing (see Figure 2-3).

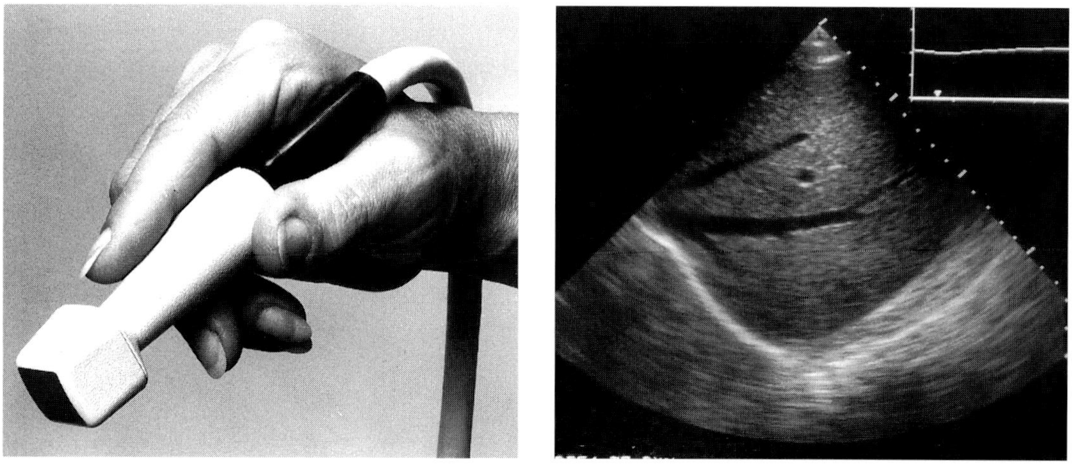

a b

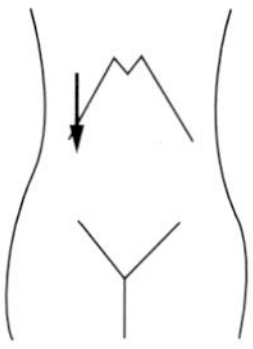

Figure 2-6. Phased-array transducer.
The small probe (a) achievable with electronic beam steering is a major clinical advantage in accessing all parts of the abdomen that are obscured by gas or bone. An intercostal view of the right lobe of the liver with parts of the right hepatic vein (b) demonstrates this facility. (I.G.E. 3000 probe.)

Linear and Sector Imaging

The two basic systems available have distinct mutual advantages and disadvantages which affect the selection of the optimal probe for clinical applications (Table 2-2). The image on linear scanners is of uniform quality (beam shape permitting) from skin to full depth, and the rectangular shape is more generally acceptable for viewing than the triangular one. The great advantage of sector scanning is the extent of deeper anatomy displayed, even with restricted access. However, the sector field means that superficial structures are poorly displayed, the field of view here being too small to cover a recognizable extent of anatomy. In addition, the spreading beam pattern produces a coarsening of the line structure with increasing depth. With a linear array, the whole length of the array (several centimeters) needs to be in contact with the skin to produce a complete image. Where access is easy, the linear systems are preferable. Obstetrics is the prime example, but small structures (including the breast), the kidneys, and the pancreas are also usually well displayed this way. For those regions where gas and bone limit acoustic access and one has to work through restricted "windows," sector scanners have a great advantage. Examples include the neonatal brain (via the anterior fontanel), the heart, the liver, the spleen and often also the kidneys, and the pelvis. The ideal scanner is equipped with both linear and sector probes.

Table 2-2. Sector vs. linear vs. convex transducers.

	Sector	Convex	Linear
Convenience of image shape	Poor	Good	Good
Access via restricted windows	Excellent	Variable	Variable
Display of superficial structures	Poor	Good	Good
Image quality	Moderate	Good	Excellent

Scanners giving a trapezoidal field of view form a halfway house in many clinical situations. A simple way to arrange this system is to use a sector scanner with a fluid stand-off. This can be built into the probe or consist of a detatchable water bath. Many sonographers simply use a part-full saline bag placed on the skin and work through it. Alternatively, if the crystals of a rotating mechanical scanner are mounted on a large wheel, each crystal sweeps out a trapezoidal image. Curvilinear or convex arrays combine some of the advantages of both types of electronic probes, being simpler than sector (phased array) systems but retaining their good display of anatomy that is difficult to access with a linear array (Figure 2-7). In all of these systems a larger window is required than for a true sector scanner, but the better field of view is an advantage.

a 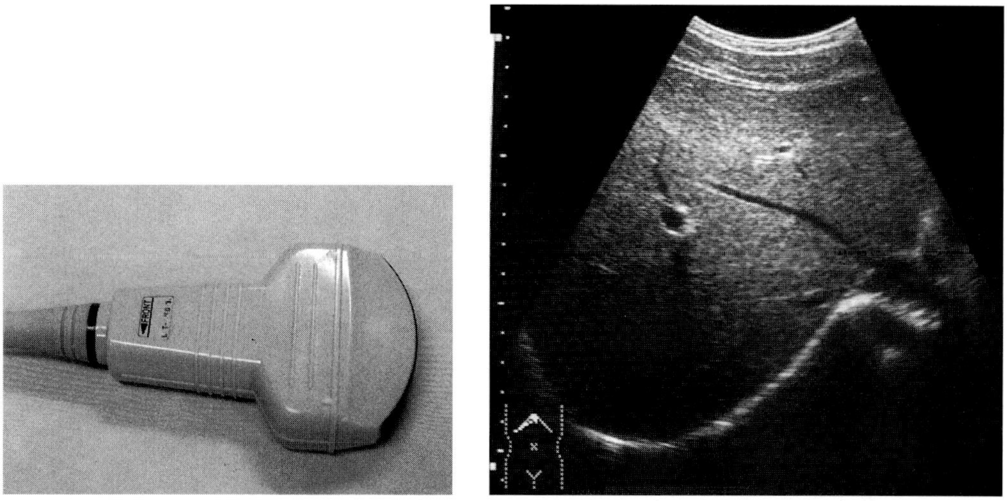 b

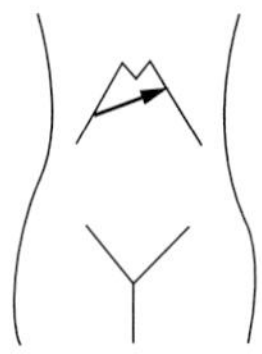

Figure 2-7. A convex array transducer and a sonogram of the liver obtained.
(a) Aloka SSD 650 convex array transducer containing 128 scanning chips. This transducer has the capabilities of dynamic frequency imaging and multizone dynamic focusing to bring about good resolution in both azithmal and axial directions.
(b) A liver sonogram recorded by the transducer shown in (a). Resolution and gray scale show marked improvement over the previously used electronic linear array scanner and also in the width of the scan field visualized.

Advantages of Real-Time Scanning

The advantages of real-time scanning compared with static scanning are so great that it has replaced static scanning all applications. Apart from its low cost (due mostly to elimination of the scanning gantry), its advantages may be considered under two headings, according to the way it is used. The obvious advantage of real-time scanning is its ability to display the movement of structures, the so-called study mode. Another category of advantages accrues from the freedom of movement of the probe, the so-called search mode (Table 2-3).

Table 2-3. Advantages of real-time scanning.

Search Mode
Ability to move the transducer freely, rapidly, and precisely over the examination field
Rapid coverage of extended anatomy
Unraveling of complex anatomy, exploiting hand-eye coordination
Precise positioning of tomograms for the best view
Ability to scan in unconventional projections
Sector scanning only: more complete display of inaccessible structures
Study Mode
Probe held still to evaluate tissue movement
Respiratory
Cardiovascular
Peristaltic
Postural
Interventional

In the *search mode,* the probe is moved over the skin to give an overview of the region of interest. An important hand-eye coordination link is formed, allowing the operator to "feel through" the probe. Its position is sensed by proprioception, and the visual information can be assembled to form an impression of the anatomy under study in its three-dimensional relationships. This allows complex structures to be unraveled in a way that is difficult and tedious with static tomography. Examples include the ability to trace tortuous tubular structures and to assess the interrelationships of complex fluid spaces such as abcesses and hydronephroses. The same facility allows the best view of an organ or lesion to be obtained. This may be required to display an anatomical or pathological feature or to make a measurement of a maximum diameter. The mobility of the probe also allows unconventional views to be used; some are possible but time-consuming with a static scanner (e.g., coronal projections), and others are impossible (e.g., transverse scans of the epigastrium with the patient upright, as used for the pancreas). Sector scanners further improve flexibility and versatility in imaging deeper structures because their triangular field allows 45° of extra viewing over the best views achievable with a static scanner. This is an important advantage where access is limited, such as when using intercostal and pelvic views.

In the *study mode,* the self-evident advantage of real-time scanning—the observation of movement—is exploited by holding the probe stationary. Various types of movement are of diagnostic significance. Cardiac-induced pulsation is ubiquitous and often obvious. Arteries too small to be visualized themselves can often be located by their rhythmic movement. Sometimes a small artery may be seen as a point which appears and disappears in time with the pulse: presumably the vessel moves into and out of the scan plane due to the lengthening that accompanies systole. Vein movement is often complex, especially near the right atrium, whose triphasic pressure changes are imposed, for example, on the inferior vena cava, just as they are on the jugular vein, as seen in the neck. Even larger veins may be empty in a dehydrated patient; here a Valsalva maneuver may help in their delineation, though it should be borne in mind that intra-abdominal pressure may be high during the straining phase of this maneuver, so that the expected dilatation may not occur until normal breathing is resumed.

Respiratory movement of the diaphragm is readily demonstrated; ultrasound is the simplest way of detecting phrenic palsy. Abdominal organs move in response to diaphragmatic contraction; this affects the more freely mobile intraperitoneal organs more than the retroperitoneum. For this reason, organs like the liver, spleen, and omentum tend to slide across the kidneys, adrenals, pancreas, and retroperitoneal lymph nodes. Careful observation of relative movements during respiration can help in the correct allocation of a difficult mass to its anatomical compartment or organ of origin. In a similar way, induced movement of a structure by probe compression or by palpation with the free hand can be invaluable in distinguishing relationships and in revealing otherwise inapparent boundaries.

The demonstration of peristalsis is proof that the structure in question is gut. This can be most helpful when adjacent gut loops might be confused with significant masses. Examples include the duodenum; the first and second parts are easily mistaken for a tumor at the head of the pancreas if they do not contain gas, while the fourth part can masquerade as a mass at the inferior border of the body of the pancreas. In the pelvis, gut loops can simulate malignant or inflammatory masses. This problem is exacerbated by previous surgery because gut adheres to incision sites. Patient observation for peristaltic movement will often solve the problem.

Postural changes will often cause calculi, gas, and fluids within body spaces to move in diagnostic ways. The sinking of gallstones to the dependent part of the gallbladder is a classic feature. A trace of ascites may be more readily demonstrated in Morison's pouch if the patient lies in the right decubitus position for a few minutes. The movement of fluid-fluid layers with posture can help distinguish them from artifacts and provide clues to the viscosity of the fluids. Gas can sometimes be moved out of the field of view by repositioning the patient. An important example is scanning the pancreas with the patient upright; one of the factors that makes this maneuver so useful is the movement of the gastric bubble to the fundus of the stomach. Gas in the biliary tree may obscure deeper parts of the liver. Rotating the patient may allow dependent parts of the liver to be imaged.

Interventional maneuvers include the obvious benefit in guided biopsies of being able to monitor the needle continuously. Simpler uses include palpation with the probe and combined probe and manual compression to elucidate relative movements of the tissues, referred to in the above discussion of respiratory movement. Simple contrast studies are useful, especially for the stomach and rectum. The stomach can pose a diagnostic problem, masquerading as a cystic or solid mass in the left upper quadrant. The dramatic appearance of the bubbles in water the patient drinks provides unequivocal identification of the stomach's position. It should be a working rule that no patient with an apparent lesion in the left upper quadrant leaves the scanning unit without having this simple test. Similarly, a water enema is useful to define the position of the rectum and even parts of the sigmoid colon. This may be helpful in evaluating a suspected pelvic mass.

The strong echoes due to gas bubbles also form the basis for ultrasound intravenous contrast agents. Almost any fluid, when injected, releases small gas bubbles which can be clearly visualized. Thus blood or saline injected into an arm vein or down a right atrial catheter fills the right atrium and ventricle with a shower of echoes. This is very useful in cardiology in evaluating such problems as complex malformations, tricuspid and pulmonary valve incompetence, and right-to-left shunts. Since the bubbles are filtered out by the pulmonary bed, this simple approach is not useful for the systemic circulation, but progress has been made in developing useful systemic contrast agents that exploit the intense reflections from gas bubbles to increase the reflectivity and Doppler signal strength from blood. Since bubbles of <10 micron diameter (small enough to cross the lung bed) dissolve rapidly under the influence of their surface tension, they require some form of stabilization if they are to give useful enhancement in the systemic circulation after intravenous injection of the methods that have been explored, coating the microbubbles, e.g., with albumin (Albunex™, MBI, San Diego) is the easier to understand. In the other approach (in Levovist™, Schering, Berlin) the surface tension of the bubbles is lowered by adding a surfactant, palmitic acid. In this preparation, the microbubbles' size is controlled by engineering crystalline galactose to form a matrix whose interstices, following solution in blood, leave microbubbles of the desired size range. Levovist produces useful and sometimes spectacular enhancement of Doppler signals even in small peripheral vessels; the increased reflectivity persists for several minutes.

Limitations of Real-Time Scanning

The major practical limitation of real-time scanning is the small field size. This may occasionally make it difficult to measure a large structure, but generally this is not a serious problem for the operator. However, when real-time images are to be interpreted later, or used to illustrate an anatomical or pathological point, the small field of view is a limitation. This is a particular problem for those unused to ultrasound images; physicians and surgeons, often find ultrasound images, especially real-time ones, unconvincing compared with x-rays, computed tomography (CT), or magnetic resonance images (MRI). An interesting compromise to produce a large field of view while preserving the flexibility of real time uses a sector probe attached to a gantry. It is used first to form a full-sized, static tomogram. Then the probe is moved back to the region of interest to give a sector real-time image, which is keyed into the static scan (Figure 2-8). The loss of probe mobility is a liability that detracts from any attempt to increase the field of view in real time.

Image quality in real-time scans tends to be slightly poorer than that of the best static scans. One factor is that because a real-time probe is relatively expensive, a scanner will usually be equipped with fewer of them than of the cheaper transducers for a static scanner. This means that in real-time scanning, one is less able to choose the optimal transducer for a particular problem. This limitation has been minimized by the development of wide band transducers whose frequency can be switched electronically. Another factor is the subjective effect that makes the same spot size seem larger in a small field of view than in a larger one. This makes real-time images appear coarser by comparison with static images. The limited number of lines in the image produce real coarsening, as does poor beam width. Beam control is often worse on real-time scans than on static scans, either because of the water bath used in mechanical systems or because of the effects of arrays (e.g., grating lobes). For arrays also, the beam is asymmetrical, so that focus in one plane is better than in the other. The noise floor tends to be higher for real-time systems because of the small size of the elements, difficulties with sliding contacts, and the proximity of the motor, causing interference. Many of these problems are being overcome, and there has been striking improvement in real-time image quality in recent years.

Real-time scanning is subject to all the artifacts of ultrasound in general, though most are in fact easier to recognize. Artifacts due to the display of movement are peculiar to real-time scans, though in practice, these seem to be of no significance in the abdomen. Theoretically, the frame rate must be twice as high as the fastest movement to be resolved. If the frame rate is too low, the speed or even the direction of movement will be misrepresented in exactly the same way that the frame rate of a cine-film causes chariot wheels to appear to stand still or to rotate in reverse. This phenomenon is known as *aliasing*. Since the movement of structures in the abdomen is slow, this is unlikely ever to be a problem, though it could be important in cardiology. One rather curious movement artifact does occur when the constituents of a rotating gray-scale target seem to move in the wrong direction in some parts of the image. This seems to be due to the interference of scattered echo information, with the progressive movement of the scattering matrix sending echoes back in unexpected directions. This paradoxical movement effect is worse for scanners with poorer resolution.

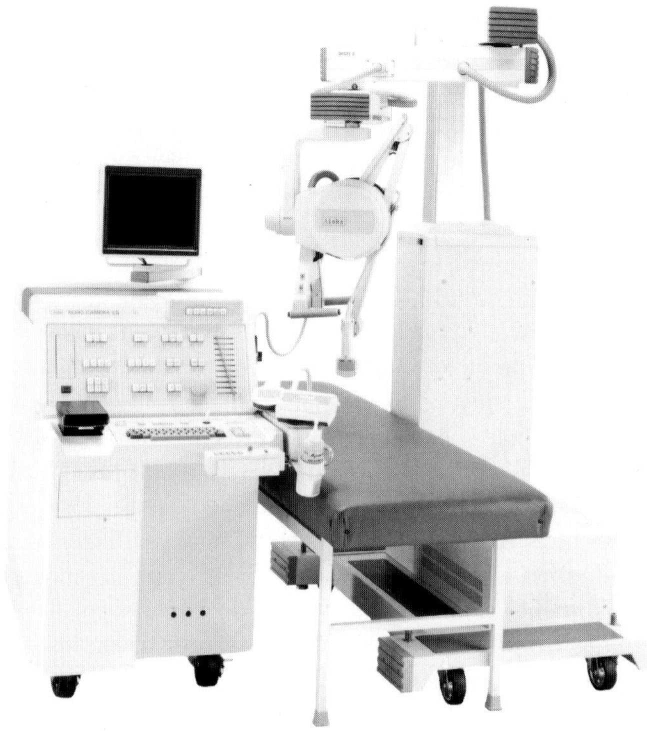

Figure 2-8a. A compound electronic contact compound scanner.
An electronic convex array probe is mounted on a scan arm to produce a complete compound tomogram semiautomatically (Aloka's Fansonic scanner).

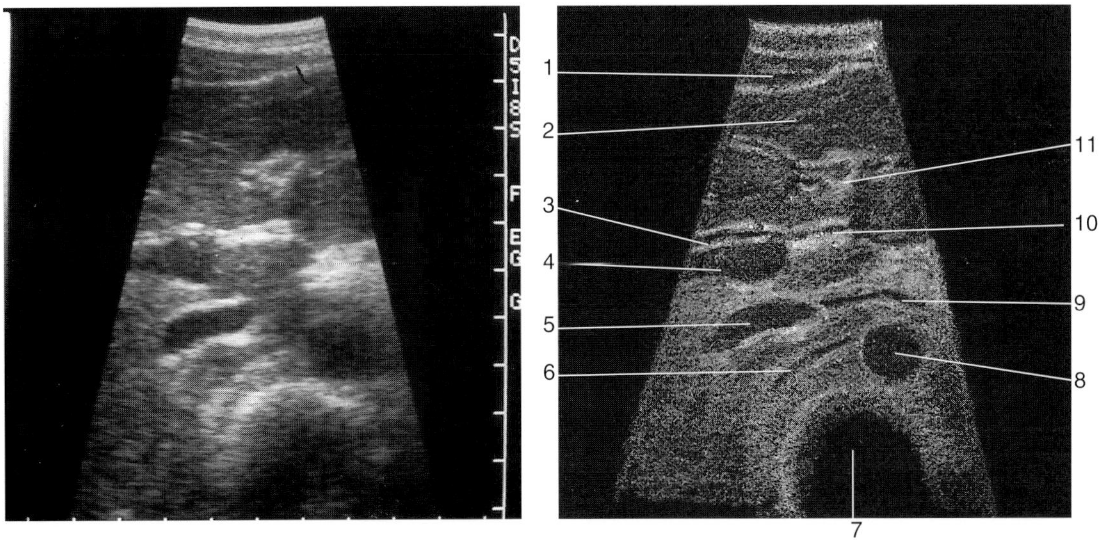

b

1. Right rectus sheath 2. Liver 3. Right hepatic duct 4. Portal vein 5. Inferior vena cava 6. Right renal artery 7. Vertebra 8. Aorta 9. Left renal vein 10. Left hepatic duct 11. Umbilical vein

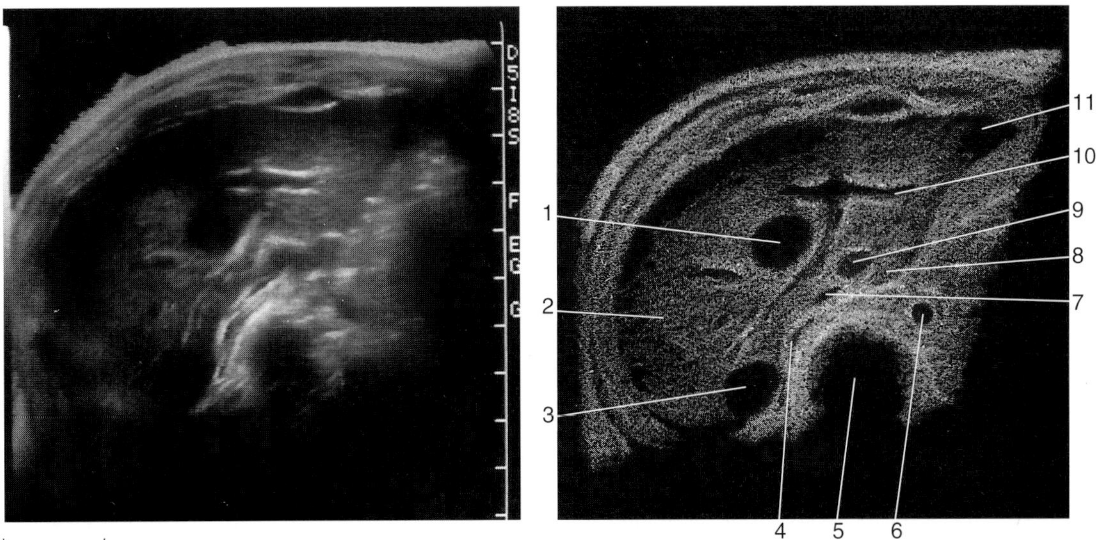

c

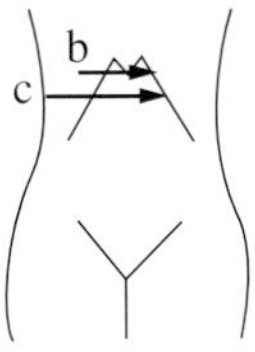

1. Gallbladder 2. Liver 3. Tip of right kidney 4. Renal vein 5. Vertebra 6. Aorta 7. Renal artery 8. Caudate lobe of liver 9. Inferior vena cava 10. Portal vein 11. Left lobe of liver

Figure 2-8b,c. Transverse tomograms of the upper abdomen obtained by the Fansonic instrument.

The upper figure shows a single-frame sonogram obtained at the mid epigastrium. The lower figure shows a compound sonogram obtained by the same instrument tracing the transverse plane of the upper abdomen. The resolution of the single image is better. Compounding produces slight smearing of the fine structures obtained by the single-frame scan.

DIAGNOSTIC PROBLEMS IN ULTRASOUND

Basic and Scanner Limitations

Intrinsic weaknesses in the ultrasound imaging system combine with operator errors (of technique and interpretation) to produce diagnostic errors. The intrinsic weaknesses include the limitations of the equipment and a number of artifacts. All of these problems need to be understood to be recognized, the vital step in avoiding pitfalls. Of the equipment limitations, the most important is the shape of the ultrasound pulse. The improvements in beam width that can be achieved by focusing leave the sonographer with a beam in which most of the energy passes along the central axis but which spreads, decreasing off-axis with a Gaussian distribution. The beam pattern is radially symmetrical for a simple transducer, but for arrays it has a complex shape, usually being wider in the orthogonal plane (across the imaged plane). Its overall width increases proximal and distal to the focal zone. Since a strong reflector will send back a detectable signal when further off-axis than a weaker one, the effective beam width for imaging is worse for strong than for weak reflectors. A precise value therefore cannot be given but, in general, using a 5-MHz probe, weak reflectors 1 mm or so apart can be resolved separately when they lie in the focal zone. Because it is registered off-axis, a strong point reflector appears as a streak across the beam instead of as a dot. This has two important effects on the image. Firstly, the lateral dimensions of a strongly reflecting object are exaggerated; secondly, two such strong reflectors, even when several millimeters apart, appear as a single object on the image. Thus, for brightly reflecting objects, neither size nor number can be assessed reliably. Gallstones are an example of this problem (Figure 2-9); the size of an individual gallstone cannot be measured accurately using ultrasound, and a group of stones may be seen as a continuous echogenic layer.

The partial volume effect is the expression of the same beam width limitation but in the orthogonal plane. It produces spurious images of structures lying beside the imaged plane and is most obvious where the curved wall of a fluid-filled structure is being scanned. The wall may appear as an indistinct layer across the fluid; this effect can simulate debris in the gallbladder.

Because of grating lobes (forms of discrete beam spreading), array transducers are sensitive to strong reflectors that lie a long way off-axis but within the scanned plane. This is a special problem for electronic sector (phased-array) scanners, in which spurious information on the scan may be produced by nearby reflectors which may even lie outside the field of view.

The pulse length also affects resolution but is less of a practical limitation since it is easily held to an order of magnitude better than the beam width.

Another general problem with real-time scanning is the relatively high noise level. Some noise is acoustic due to the small transducer elements used, and some is electronic due to the use of crystals without matching layers. Noise produces a snowstorm effect on the screen, which reduces perceived contrast and fills in echo-free regions. It usually worsens with depth because of extra time gain compensation (TGC) amplification. The localized spurious echoes due to side lobes are also a type of noise. Using real-time scanning both can be distinguished from genuine structures by the way they persist with time and despite changes in the angle of imaging.

Artifacts are a major difficulty in ultrasound. They may arise when the beam does not travel straight and directly to and from the echo-producing interface at constant velocity, the assumptions on which the image-forming process is based (Table 2-4). Beam refraction causes structures to be displayed alongside their true positions. It is mainly a problem in the pelvis, where it is due to the much lower velocity of the sound in fatty tissue than in watery soft tissue (1,340 and 1,640 mps, respectively). The arrangement of the abdominal muscles, especially the rectus muscle, and the associated fat tends to produce refractions giving double or laterally expanded images of pelvic structures. An apparently double uterus or prostate, as well as "bilobed" lesions, may be encountered. In obstetrics this can upset fetal biometry and can even give the false appearance of twin gestational sacs.

Table 2-4. Artifacts in ultrasound.

These arise from four erroneous assumptions relied on in the image-forming process:

1. Ultrasound beams are narrow and well defined.
2. Ultrasound beams travel in a straight line.
3. Ultrasound beams travel in a direct path to and from the reflecting interface.
4. Ultrasound beams travel at constant velocity.

The low velocity of sound in fat leads to structures lying deep to a fat layer being displayed as falsely remote from the probe. Generally, the effect is minimal, but for large fatty masses it can distort the image, so that, for example, significant mispositioning can occur distal to angiomyolipomas.

Refraction also accounts for the fine shadows falling behind the edges of strongly curved structures (Figure 2-10). As the beam traverses a cystic structure, for example, part of the ultrasound is refracted at the edges so that the beam is defocussed. Thus less ultrasound reaches the tissues deep to the cyst margins, and an echo-poor band is produced. Solid structures within well-defined, curved margins may have similar edge shadows; tumors and the fetal skull are examples.

Generally, in ultrasound imaging, the beam is reflected only once before being received by the transducer. This is because of the rapid attenuation in ultrasound by tissues and the fact that most surfaces reflect only a small proportion of the beam. However, multiple reflections can occur when strongly reflecting objects are encountered. A common situation occurs at the diaphragm when the right lobe of the liver is imaged. Ultrasound striking the air-pleural interface is reflected back into the liver, with little loss of intensity. There it behaves exactly as a beam originating above the diaphragm, and the liver reflectors return echoes back toward the diaphragm. They then retrace their path, being reflected off the diaphragm back to the transducer. They are displayed as though the pulses had traveled in a straight line, that is, as being due to intrathoracic structures! (Figure 2-11) In this way, both normal liver and focal lesions can be falsely projected in the right lower zone, the air surface of the lung acting as a mirror. A pleural effusion, by moving the lung away, destroys the mirror, as expected, and genuine intrathoracic anatomy is then seen. A similar but more confusing situation occurs in the pelvis when gas in the bowel forms a layer behind the bladder. The bladder space is then double-imaged as an echo-poor mass deep in the pelvis (Figure 2-12). This appearance is easily mistaken for a genuine mass.

The transducer-skin interface itself is a strong reflector; only part of the returning echoes actually enter the transducer, some being returned to the tissues. (Matching layers on transducers are designed to reduce this problem.) If a strong reflector in the tissue lies parallel to the transducer, the ultrasound can be reflected repeatedly between the two surfaces, producing a series of mirror copies of the tissue interface; they fade with time according to the attenuation of the interface tissue. This produces a series of equally spaced bands on the image, which become fainter with depth (Figure 2-13). (Because fainter objects seem narrower on ultrasound, the bands also become progressively narrower with depth.) The effect is the same as that in a hall of mirrors, where one stands between a pair of parallel mirrors and sees a series of reflections fading into the distance. Multiple reverberations of this type are seen with gas-containing structures, and are routinely observed if the lung is imaged intercostally and when gas-containing bowel is scanned.

An important related phenomenon affects the display of flat surfaces when they lie approximately along the beam direction. In this arrangement, even a well-defined surface may not give a reflection and so may not be detected on the image (Figure 2-14). Viewing from another angle will reveal the surface. Awareness of absent information requires a high level of sensitivity on the part of the operator.

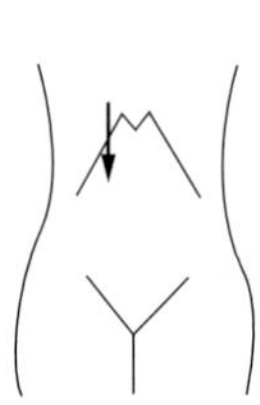

Figure 2-9. The beam width effect.
The finite width of the ultrasound beam leads to relatively poor lateral resolution. Echogenic targets are most seriously affected. Thus a collection of gallstones appears as a smear (a) but is better resolved into its components by the finer beam of progressively higher-frequency transducers (b and c). Similarly, the acoustic shadowing that is obvious with the higher frequencies is marginal at 3 MHz. The 4- and 5-MHz probes also give a more detailed picture of the anatomy displayed (compare the detail of the cystic duct region in the three images) but fail to penetrate to the deeper structures. Probes whose frequency can be switched are a practical solution to this problem. ►

a

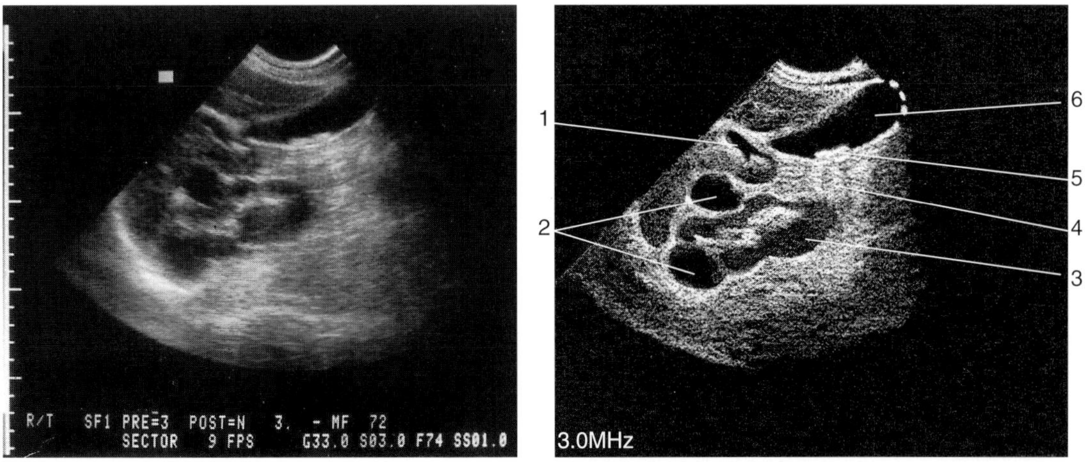

1. Portal vein 2. Renal cysts 3. Kidney 4. Shadow 5. Echogenic material 6. Gallbladder

b

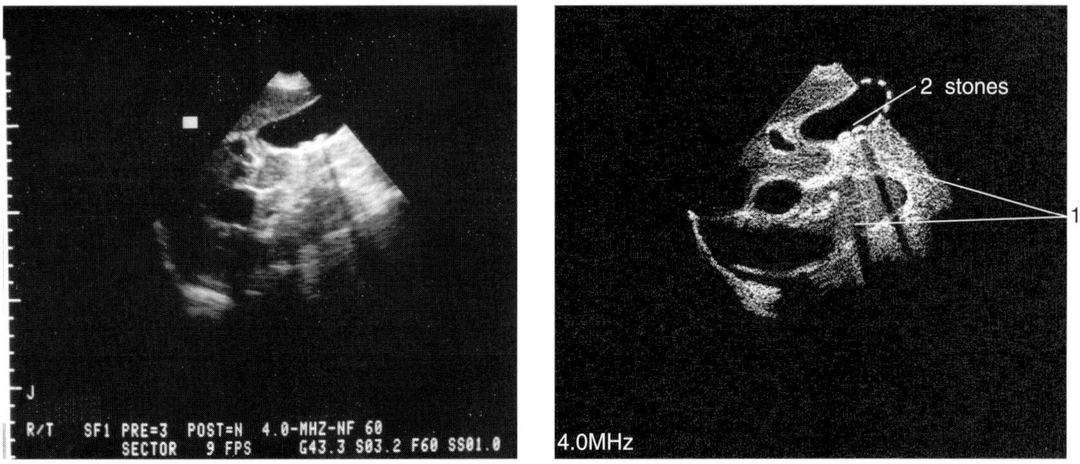

1. Shadow

c

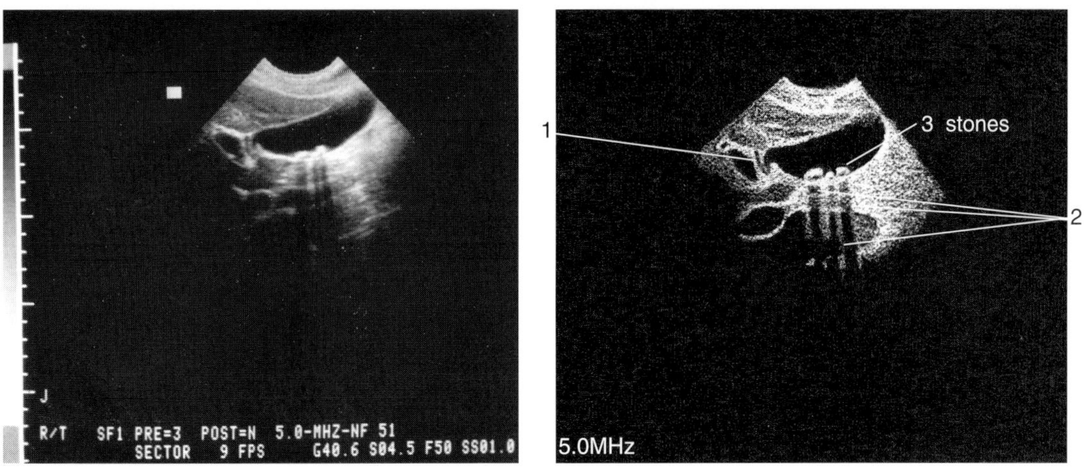

1. Spiral valve 2. Shadows

Figure 2-9. (See legend on opposite page)

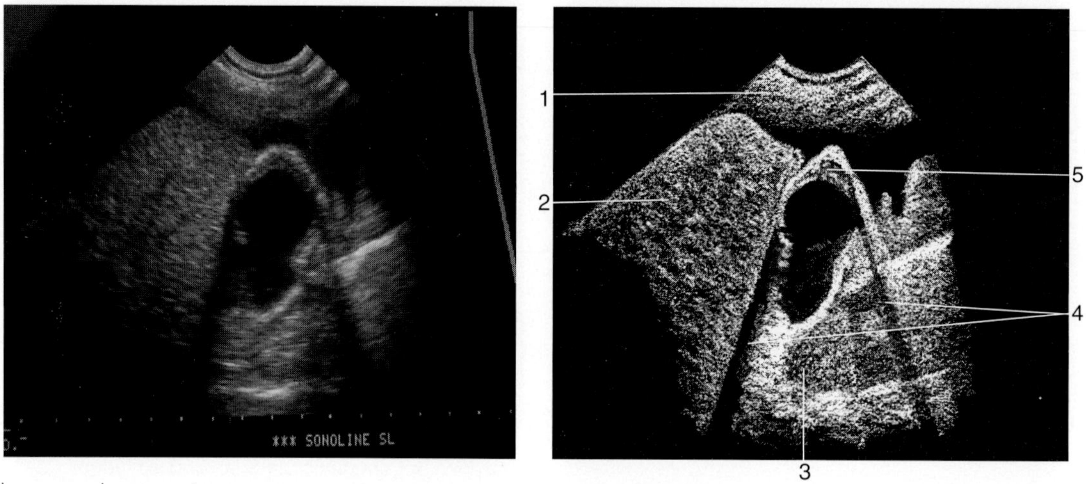

1. Ascites 2. Liver 3. Kidney 4. Refractive shadows 5. Gallbladder

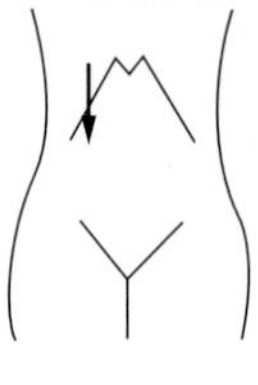

Figure 2-10. Refractive shadows.
The structures deep to the edges of the gallbladder are shadowed due to refractive effects from the strongly curved surfaces. They are typical of fluid-filled structures but also occur deep to curved edges of solid structures. In this patient with malignant ascites, the gallbladder wall appears thickened; this common feature does not necessarily indicate cholecystitis (see Chapter 4).

a

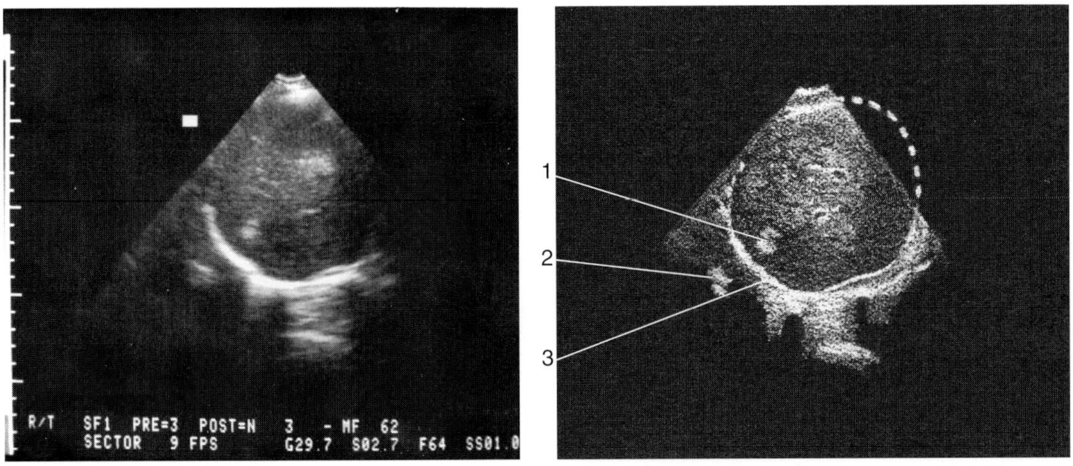

1. Mirror image of hemangioma 2. Diaphragm
3. Hemangioma

b

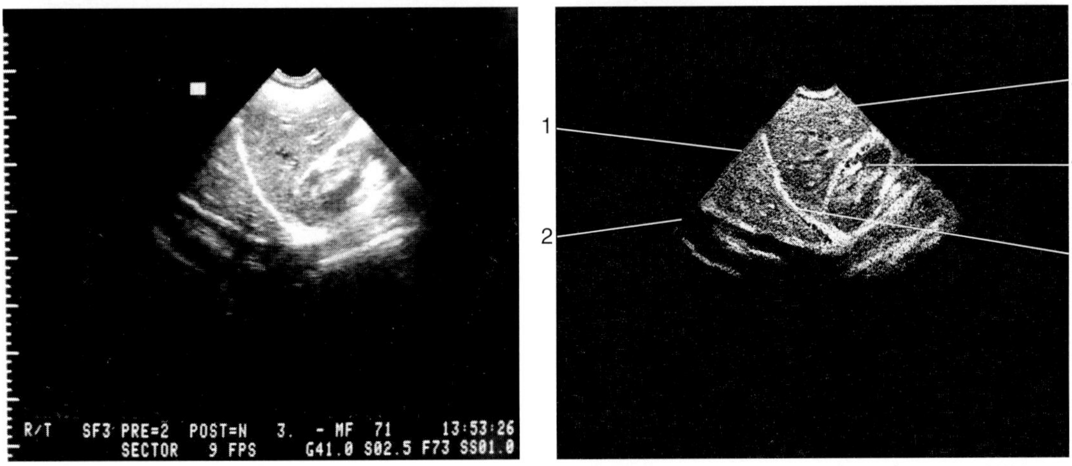

1. Mirror image of liver 2. Mirror image of kidney
3. Diaphragm 4. Kidney 5. Liver

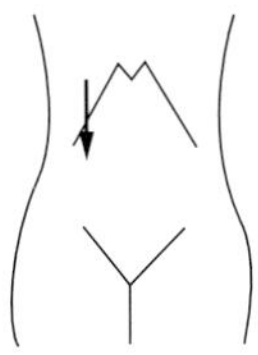

Figure 2-11. Mirror images.
Strong reflectors return so much of the incident ultrasound beam that they can act as acoustic mirrors. The diaphragm is a typical example; the air surface of the lung acts as the reflector. Subdiaphragmatic tissues are double-imaged, the mirror image appearing in the lower zone of the lung. A hemangioma and a normal lung and kidney are shown in these two examples.

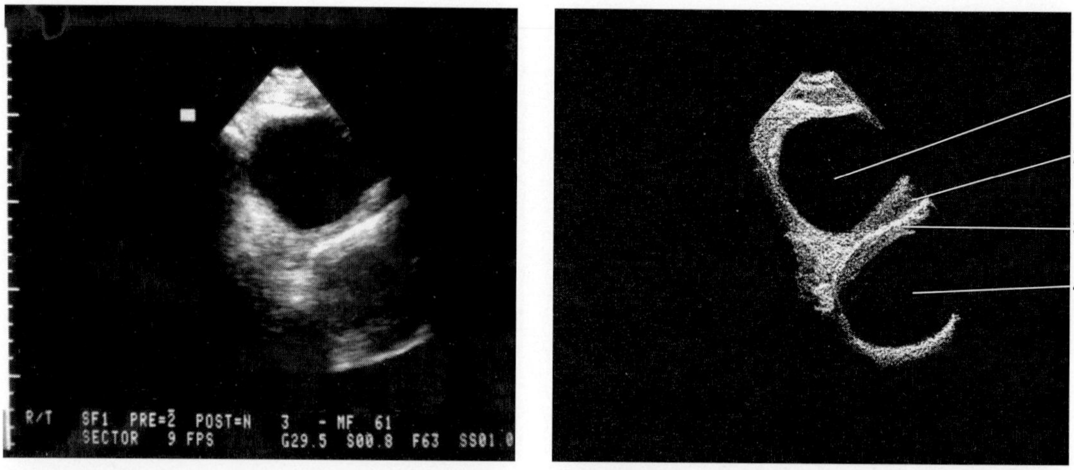

a

1. Pseudomass 2. Rectum 3. Vagina 4. Bladder

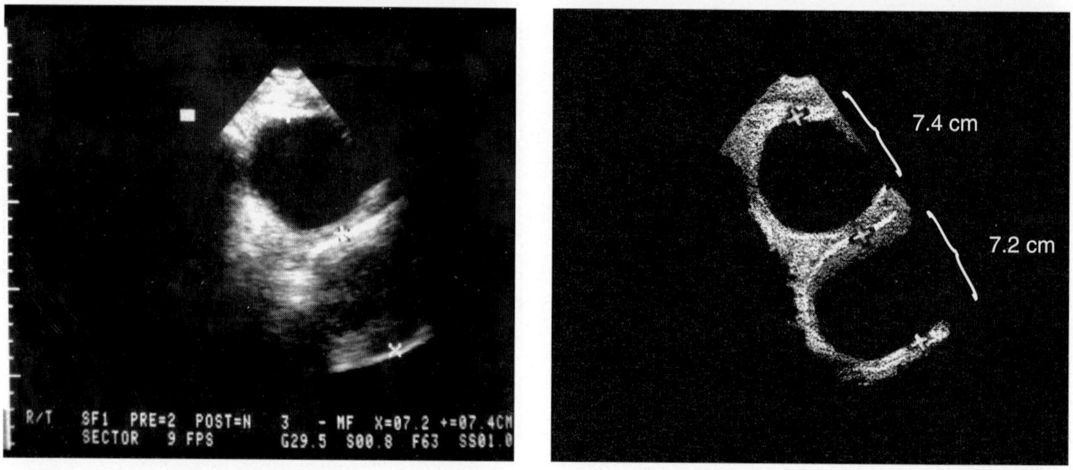

b

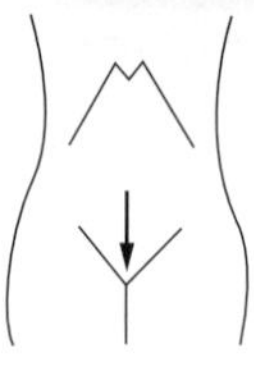

Figure 2-12. False mass.
Gas in bowel can act as an acoustic mirror. Here the rectum returns a mirror image of the bladder, which might be mistaken for an echo-poor mass. Knowledge of the normal anatomy helps avoid the potential error (there is no room for a mass of this size behind the rectum), and the fact that the "mass" and the bladder are equidistant from the rectum is an important clue.

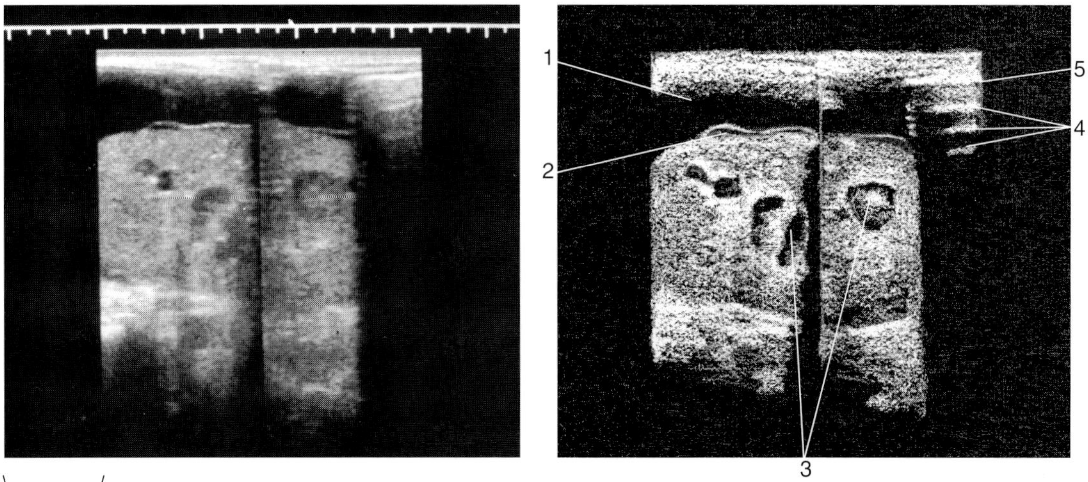

1. Ascites 2. Adhesions 3. Liver metastases
4. Reverberations 5. Gas in colon

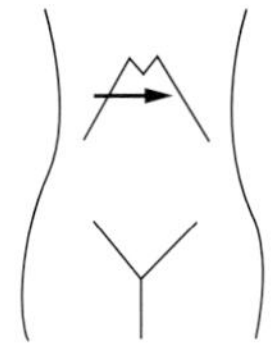

Figure 2-13. Parallel mirror artifacts.
The ultrasound echoes from a strong gas interface are reflected back into the tissue; repetition of this process from the two parallel, mirror-like surfaces gives rise to a repeated series of banded reverberation echoes.

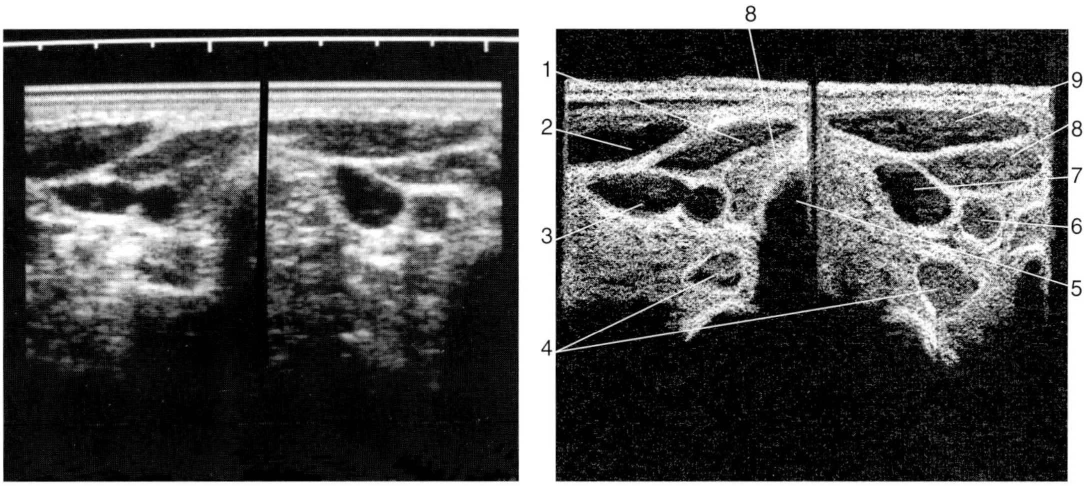

1. Lobe of thyroid 2. Sternomastoid muscle 3. Vessel 4. Longus colli muscle 5. Trachea 6. Right carotid artery 7. Internal jugular vein 8. Right lobe of thyroid 9. Sternomastoid muscle

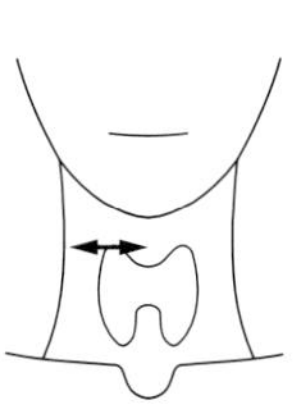

Figure 2-14. Missed septum.
Even well-defined structures may be missed on ultrasound if they lie along the beam direction. The interface between the right carotid artery and the internal jugular vein is not displayed in the left sonogram because the ultrasound beam passes along the surface. Altering the beam direction reveals the missing interface (right). Failure to recognize this artifact can lead to serious misinterpretation.

Scanning Technique

Scanning technique with real-time systems is easier than with static systems, but correct use of electronic settings and the choice and use of the probes remain important. The prime objective in setting the scanner controls is to display the region of interest as mid-gray. The transmit power and receive gain are used for this. For most purposes the two can be treated as equivalent, though a high power could increase any theoretical risk of damage to the patient (not a particular concern in abdominal scanning), and a high receive gain makes the scanner sensitive to electronic noise. The midpart of the display gray scale is chosen because it gives maximum sensitivity to differences in reflectivity and therefore reveals texture best. If the region of interest is set too bright or dark, texture and, at the extremes, resolution, are lost.

A second objective is to obtain as even a picture as possible. The TGC is used for this purpose and should be adjusted to balance the deep and superficial parts of the image for the effects of attenuation. The best setting is easily achieved with real time because it is so interactive, but the effect of too steep a TGC setting may be confusing (Figure 2-15). The TGC amplifier (like all amplifiers) has a maximum gain, beyond which no further amplification is available. Deep to the corresponding point in the image, correction for attenuation is no longer being applied and the image becomes progressively darker. If this appearance is thought to be due to too little TGC, an understandable error, and the slope is further increased, the saturation point is brought closer to the skin. The deeper tissues then become further darkened, and a bright band is produced in the midzone of the image. Too low a TGC, of course, makes the image darken progressively from the skin. Adjustment of the TGC is made more flexible if a segmented control rather than a single control is provided. Effective automatic TGC systems are being introduced and should provide a welcome simplification of real-time scanning.

The only other control affecting the image that is required routinely is postprocessing, which alters the allocation of echo levels to the gray scale. Slight adjustments can be useful to change the contrast for an improved display of pathology. Extreme changes make interpretation more difficult. Similarly, edge enhancement applied discreetly can improve the subjective quality of the image but in excess is confusing.

Some real-time scanners allow the user to change the frame rate. A high rate gives a better display of tissue movement; a low rate gives more ultrasound lines and therefore improves spatial resolution. These considerations dictate the optimal setting. In a similar way, controls for dynamic focusing may allow multiple zones to be chosen for the best lateral resolution, but at the expense of frame rate.

Considerations of scanning technique include choice of the highest frequency that allows penetration to the full depth to be imaged, selection of the optimal focal zone, and the use of a stand-off for superficial structures. The choice of linear, curved or sector transducer is determined chiefly by the ease of accessibility, the linear or curved displays being preferred in general but the sector display being more useful in the abdomen because of better accessibility via limited windows.

The speed with which a real-time scan can be performed is a potential trap. The operator must be careful to allow time for the structures being scanned to be studied thoroughly.

It is possible to glimpse the entire upper abdomen with a single sweep of the transducer, but a proper study will take 10 to 20 min.

Some important points on technique have been mentioned in considering the applications of real-time scanning in general. These include ways to exploit respiratory, vascular, and peristaltic movements to their best diagnostic advantage, as well as the use of contrast in ultrasound. A further "golden rule" in ultrasound is to insist on visualizing a lesion in at least two planes before accepting it as genuine. This helps avoid some pitfalls due to artifacts, as well as providing a three-dimensional anatomical view of the pathology.

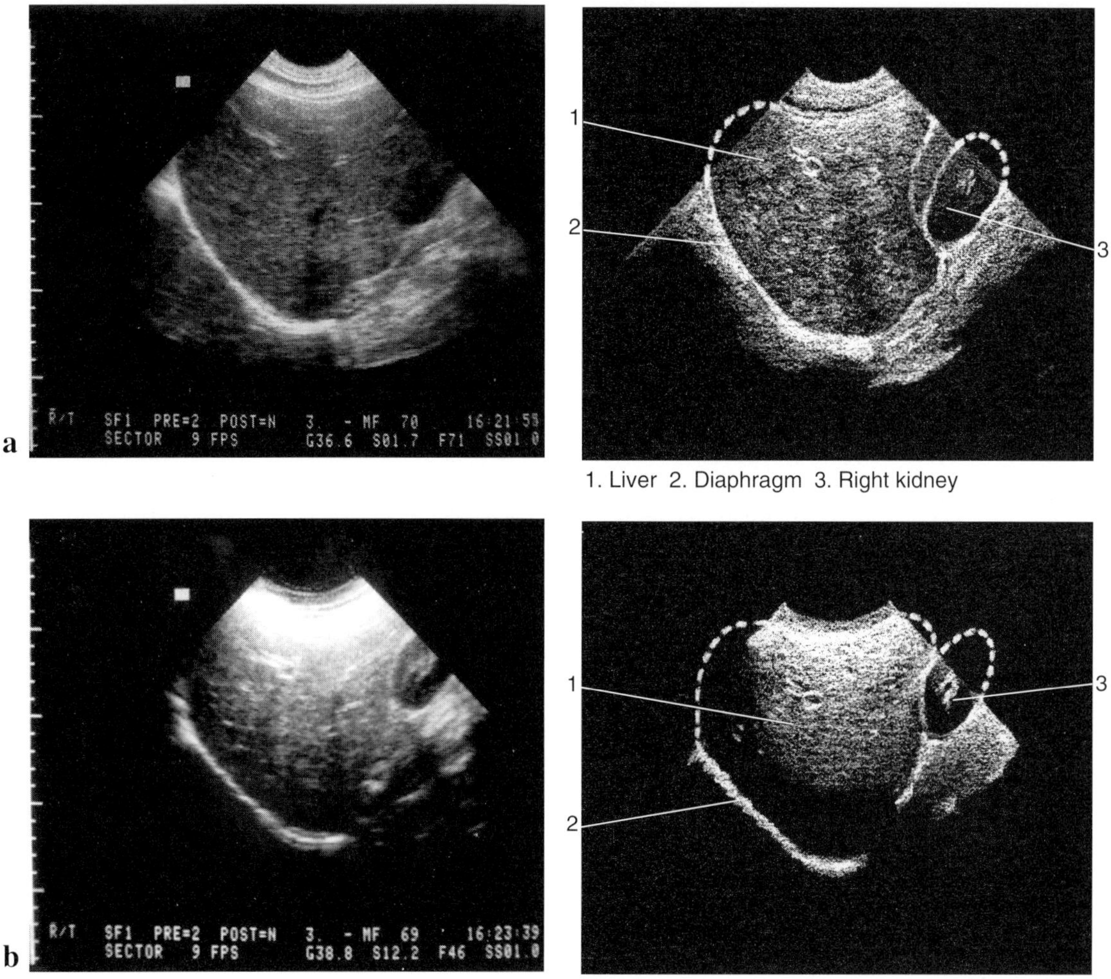

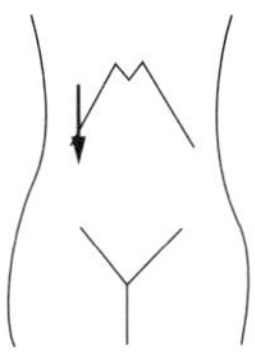

Figure 2-15. TGC setting errors.
A correctly set TGC gives an image that is balanced from front to back (a). Too low a setting leaves tissue attenuation uncompensated, so that the image darkens with depth (b). Too high a TGC, with an attempt to compensate for the overall excess gain this produces, gives a bright band in the mid-zone (c).

c

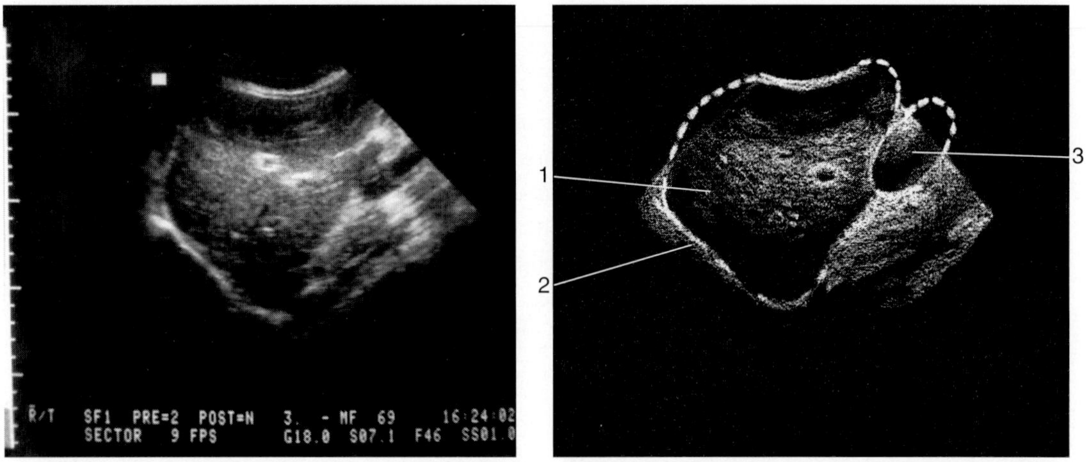

1. Liver 2. Diaphragm 3. Right kidney

Figure 2-15.

Interpretative Principles

Mistaken anatomy is probably the major cause of interpretative errors. For the most part, avoidance of this problem depends on having excellent knowledge of normal anatomy together with its variations, as well as the effects produced by masses (displacement and distortions). The excellent illustrated general sectional anatomy texts that are available are helpful for this purpose and enable most difficulties to be resolved. Three-dimensional models of key structures are also available. However, resort to actual dissection in the autopsy room can be a powerful educational experience and is strongly recommended.

Some particularly troublesome normal structures in the abdomen should be mentioned. The gut is a persistent interpretive problem for ultrasound (and indeed for CT also), especially when it does not contain gas. Recognition depends on knowing where to expect to find the gut and on the demonstration of peristalsis, which may require painstaking observation or even a rescan some hours later. The stomach can masquerade as a left upper quadrant mass, whether cystic or solid, echo-poor or echogenic, depending on the nature of its contents. The bubbles swallowed with a glass of water provide positive proof of its nature. This simple test should be used whenever there is the least doubt about a left upper quadrant mass.

A genuine mass lying posterior to the stomach may be obscured following a drink, leading to the conclusion that it is part of the stomach, so care must be taken that the bubbles fill the entire "mass." The esophagus is usually easy to identify by its position, but again, observation of gas transit following swallowing provides proof. The duodenum likewise can be more easily identified if filled with fluid; chilling the drinking water and lying the patient in the right decubitus position hasten transit. The first and second parts of the duodenum are easily confused with a mass in the head of the pancreas. The fourth part can simulate a mass in the pancreatic body inferiorly. Gut loops in the midabdomen can simulate masses. Careful observation is required to differentiate between them, especially in detecting thickening of the parietal peritoneum, where the superficial structures must be displayed well (using a high-frequency transducer or a water bath standoff). The main problem with the midabdominal gut is the masking effect, which obscures deeper-lying retroperitoneal structures. By tipping the patient decubitus and scanning in the coronal plane, this problem can be minimized, if not entirely eliminated. Gut in the pelvis can also be mistaken for mass lesions; again, patient observation will usually clarify its true nature. Failing this, a water enema will often be definitive.

Structures whose appearance is changed by enhancement or shadowing are sometimes a trap. The effect of ascites can often be dramatic, not only in opening up peritoneal planes that are normally not delineated but also in causing deep structures to appear with high-level echoes. Thus the kidney or pancreas, imaged via the nonattenuating ascitic fluid, can seem pathologically echogenic. Usually another projection can be found that allows a comparison with, say, the liver, without any intervening fluid. Ascites also makes some membranes seem thickened. The walls of the gallbladder and urinary bladder are examples (cf. Chapter 4).

Shadowing from fibrous or calcific structures can sometimes be confusing. The effect of the interlobar fissure making the caudate lobe of the liver echo-poor can simulate an abnormality. The left portal vein often runs transversely in the lateral segment of the left lobe of the liver and may shadow the posterior portion, so that it seems to be a totally separate structure. On intercostal views, rib shadowing can be confusing.

Shadowing and enhancement provide important diagnostic clues. A clean shadow due to calcification is sometimes more obvious than the lesion itself. Absorption and reflection together contribute to the intensity of the shadow. To produce shadowing, the lesion must interrupt the ultrasound beam. Therefore small foci will not shadow, so that, for example, ultrasound is insensitive to the punctate calcification typical of chronic pancreatitis. Gas also produces shadowing, but here due purely to reflection. For this reason, reverberations tend to fill in the shadow with structured (noisy) echoes, so that the shadowing is less clear than with calcium. Though this so-called dirty shadowing is typical of gas, it is not always seen.

Increased through transmission is the hallmark of fluid spaces and is due to the characteristically low attenuation of fluid. Generally, it is easily demonstrated, though when an intensely echogenic structure lies deep to the cyst, the increased through transmission is applied to echoes that already saturate the display, so it is undetectable. Cysts adjacent to the diaphragm (Figure 2-16) and those lying up against the renal sinus are examples. Cysts are typically echo-free, but fluid may return weak or strong echoes when it contains debris or particulate material. Hemorrhagic or purulent fluid spaces are examples. The presence of echoes does not mean that they are not fluid-filled. It is the distal echo enhancement which provides the clue.

When a mass is large or distorts nearby structures, its organ of origin may be unrecognizable. Large tumors may have this effect; giant cysts of the liver, spleen, or kidney are other common causes. Attention to the movements due to respiration or induced by bimanual palpation is helpful in allocating a mass to its correct anatomical compartment and defining its attachments to adjacent structures. Careful study of the associated blood vessels can provide clues to the organ of origin. A space-occupying lesion in the upper abdomen that lifts the splenic vein anteriorly, for example, is unlikely to have arisen in the pancreas, but it might represent enlargement of retroperitoneal lymph nodes or of the left adrenal gland.

Interpretation of echo levels is somewhat complex, but some general principles can be stated. High-level echoes result from marked changes in acoustic impedance corresponding approximately to changes in tissue rigidity. Among soft tissues, the most marked changes are due to fat and connective tissue. Adipose tissue and fatty infiltration give intense echoes. The collagen fibers around blood vessels are important determinants of the pattern and intensity of parenchymal echoes, though an exact correlation is by no means obvious. Fibrosis tends to produce high-level echoes. Separation of interfaces by edema tends to lower echo levels; this is why inflamed and malignant tissues are generally echo-poor, except where hemmorrhage or necrosis provides echo-producing interfaces. Much fundamental investigation is still required before a full understanding of the ultrasound appearances can be claimed.

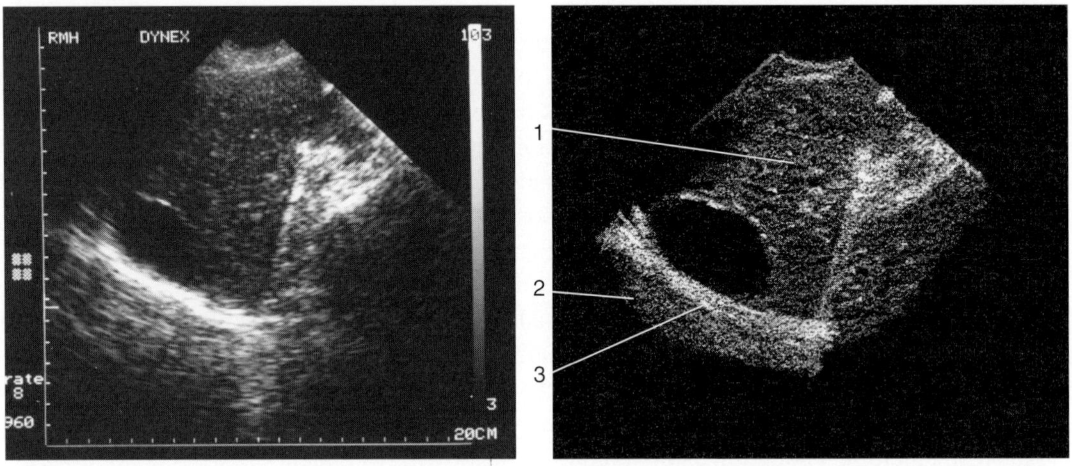

1. Liver 2. Cyst 3. Diaphragm

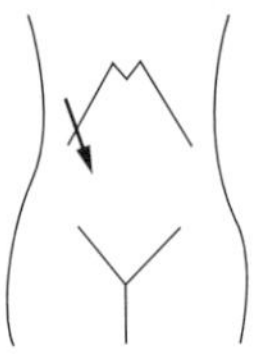

Figure 2-16. Concealed enhancement.
When the enhancement distal to a cyst falls across an intensely echogenic structure, it cannot be detected because the display screen cannot reveal the further increases in intensity. A cyst lying close to the diaphragm is a typical example.

FURTHER READING

Introduction:
Meire HB, Farrant P: Basic Clinical Ultrasound. London, British Institute of Radiology, 1982.

Physics:
Kremkau FW: Diagnostic Ultrasound: Physical Principles and Exercises. New York, Grune & Stratton, 1980.
Lu JY, Zou H, Greenleaf JF: Biomedical ultrasound beam forming. Ultrasound Med Biol 20 : 403-428, 1994.
McDicken WN: Diagnostic Ultrasonics: Principles and Use of Instruments, ed 2. New York, Wiley, 1981.
Wells PN, Harris RA, Halliwell M: The envelope that tissue imposes on achievable ultrasonic imaging. J Ultrasound Med 11 : 433-439, 1992.

Safety:
ter Haar G: Safety of medical ultrasound, in Kurjak A (ed), Progress in Medical Ultrasound, Vols 2 & 3. Amsterdam, Excerpta Medica, 1981/1982.
Nyborg WL: Scientifically based safety criteria for ultrasonography. J Ultrasound Med 11 : 425-432, 1992.

Anatomy and Pathology:
ESP Anatomical Models: Liver, Pancreas, Pelvis. Redhill, Surrey, UK, Educational and Scientific Plastics Ltd.
Hollinshead WH: Anatomy for Surgeons. Vol. 2, Thorax, Abdomen and Pelvis, ed 3. Philadelphia, JB Lippincott, 1982.
Lyons EA: A Color Atlas of Sectional Anatomy. St Louis, CV Mosby, 1978.
Morely P, Donald G, Sanders R: Ultrasound Sectional Anatomy. Edinburgh, Churchill Livingstone, 1983.
Sandritter W, Thomas C, Kirsten WH: Color Atlas and Textbook of Macropathology. Chicago, Yearbook, 1979.
Wagner MW, Lawson TL: Segmental Anatomy. New York, Macmillan, 1982.

Scanning Techniques:
Taylor KJ, Jacobson P, Talmont CA, et al: Manual of Ultrasonography. New York, Churchill Livingstone, 1982.

Clinical Interpretation:
Cosgrove DO, McCready VR: Ultrasound Imaging: Liver, Spleen, Pancreas. Chichester, UK, Wiley, 1982.
Cosgrove DO, Meire HB, Dewbury KCD (eds): Clinical Ultrasound: A Comprehensive Text (4 Vols). London, Churchill Livingstone, 1993.
Goldberg BB, Pettersson H (eds): Nicer Yearbook 1996: Ultrasonography. Oslo, Nicer Institute, 1996.
JAMA : Medical diagnostic ultrasound instrumentation and clinical interpretation. Report of the ultrasonography task force. Council on Scientific Affairs. JAMA 265 : 1155-1159, 1991.
Sanders RJ (ed): Ultrasound Quarterly, Vols 1 & 2. New York, Raven Press, 1983/1984. (Each issue explores a current topic in depth.)
Sarti DA, Sample WF: Diagnostic Ultrasound. Boston, GK Hall, 1980.
Weil FW: Ultrasonography of Digestive Diseases. St. Louis, CV Mosby, 1978.

CHAPTER 3

THE LIVER

NORMAL ANATOMY

The liver comprises a large right lobe and a smaller triangular left lobe (Figure 3-1). A line from the gallbladder fossa to the inferior vena cava separates them; the middle hepatic vein runs in this plane.[38, 55, 62, 79]

The anterior and superior surfaces are smooth and rounded to fit under the right hemidiaphragm, but the visceral surface (lying posteroinferiorly) is complex, since it contains the porta hepatis and impressions from contiguous organs such as the stomach and duodenum, the right kidney, and the hepatic flexure of the colon. Because the liver is soft, these indentations can be well marked and determine the liver's shape, which is therefore very variable, making assessment of liver size difficult.

Each lobe is separated into two segments. The boundary between the medial and lateral segments of the left lobe is the ligamentum teres, which is the remnant of the umbilical vein that returns placental blood from the fetus. It occludes in the neonatal period to leave a fibro-fatty strand that extends from the free edge of the liver to the left portal vein. Occasionally a minute vessel persists within it in the adult, and it may open or recanalize in portal hypertension (see the section "Diffuse Diseases"). The lateral segment is very variable in size, in some objects being rudimentary and in other extending inferiorly as a thinned plate as far as the umbilical level. The medial segment, lying between the ligamentum teres and the gallbladder fossa, is known as the *quadrate lobe* from its rectangular shape. Because of the lie of the liver with the right lobe situated relatively posteriorly, the quadrate lobe usually lies anterior to the medial part of the right lobe. A fissure commonly separates them.

The right lobe has anterior and posterior segments separated by the right hepatic vein, which usually runs in the coronal plane. There is no obvious indicator of this plane on the liver surface. A common and striking variant is inferior extension of the right lobe over the right kidney, known as *Reidel's lobe.*

The caudate lobe is a projection from the superior part of the visceral surface of the right lobe; it passes toward the left. It lies anterior to the inferior vena cava and is in contact with the posterior surface of the left lobe, the peritoneal layers that intervene forming the interlobar fissure. These consist of the lesser omentum (hepatogastric ligament) and the peritoneum covering the liver itself. Thus the caudate lobe lies in the lesser sac.

The porta is arranged approximately transversely and contains three sets of vessels. The largest is the portal vein, which divides into right and left branches at the porta just before entering the liver substance. The portal vein lumen usually measures some 10 mm in diameter, with an upper limit of normal of 15 mm.[64] Anterior to the portal vein line the hepatic artery medially and the biliary system laterally. These also have left and right branches and tributaries, respectively. The three sets of vessels, forming the portal triads, remain together through successive branchings. Because of the shape of the abdominal cavity (see Chapter 2), the left lobe lies more anteriorly than the right, so that the left portal vein curves anteriorly as it passes to the left. By contrast, the right portal vein passes directly laterally. The first main branches of the portal triads supply the liver segments; since the hepatic veins run along the lobar and segmental margins, these two sets of vessels interdigitate.

The veins draining the liver pass directly into the inferior vena cava just below the diaphragm. There are three major hepatic veins, the left and right draining those parts of the liver while the middle drains the midportion. The left and middle veins usually join to form a short common trunk before emptying into the inferior vena cava. Smaller, inferior hepatic veins drain the caudate and medial right lobes.

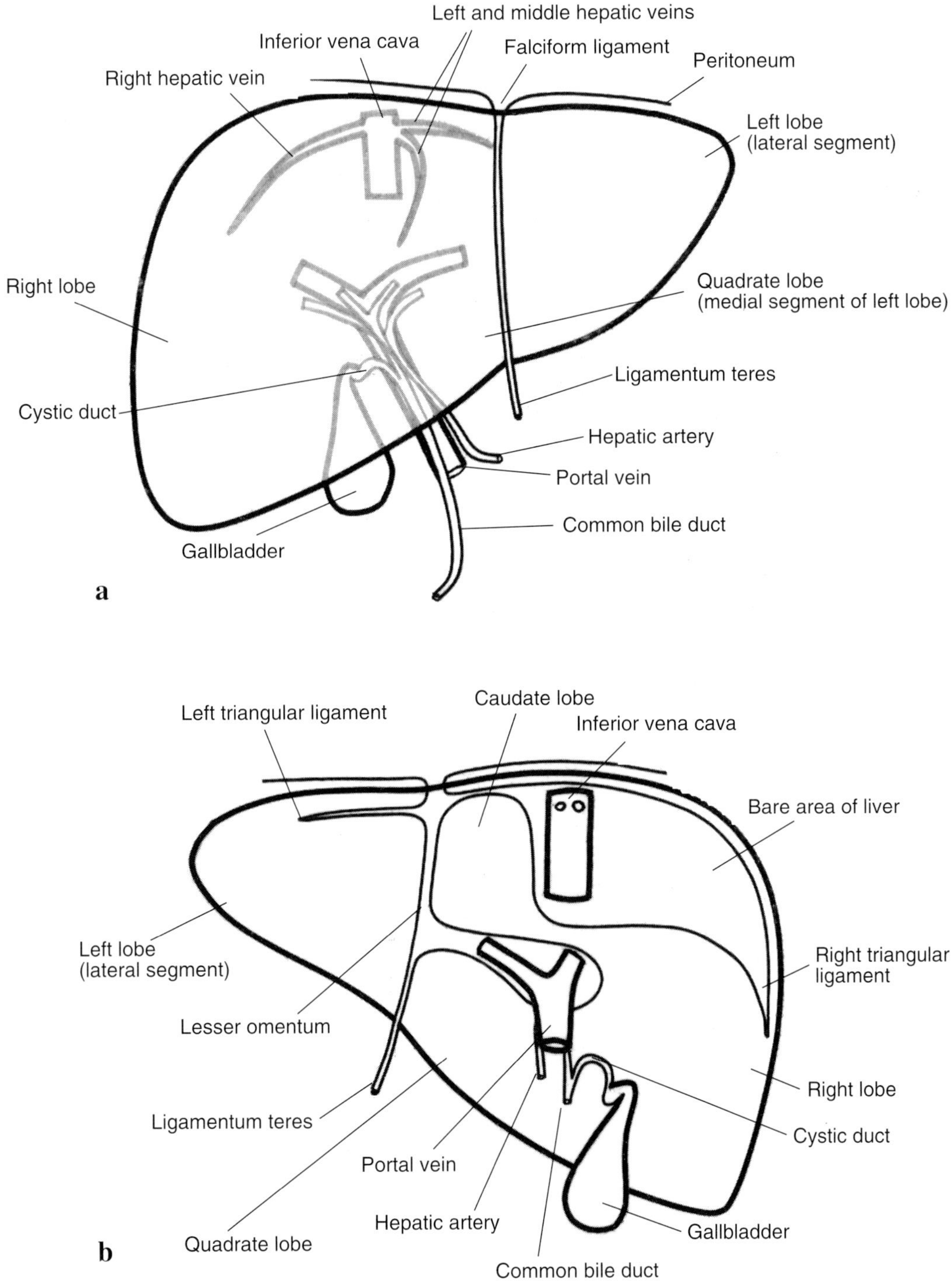

Figure 3-1. Liver anatomy.
Diaphragmatic views of the anterior (a) and visceral (b) surfaces of the liver show the portal vessels and the draining hepatic veins with the lobar divisions they define. The peritoneal reflections are indicated.

ULTRASOUND APPEARANCES

Sagittal ultrasound sections near the midline show the left lobe as a triangular structure, with the diaphragm and heart superiorly (Figure 3-2). The caudate lobe may be visualized posteriorly overlying the inferior vena cava or, when it is prominent, the aorta as well (Figures 3-4 and 3-5).[53, 54, 81] A little to the right, the left portal vein is encountered as a C-shaped, tubular structure curving anteriorly into the left lobe of the liver. The portal vein and its branches usually have a reflective cuff of surrounding tissue due to the associated arterial and biliary vessels together with fat and fibrous tissue. Farther to the right, the right portal vein is cut across and so is seen as a ring (Figure 3-3). At this point, the right hepatic artery is often visualized running parallel to the right portal vein and, lying anterior to both, part of the biliary system.[71] Often this portion of the bile duct is cut lengthwise, and its caliber is seen to increase inferiorly, suggesting that the upper part is in fact the right hepatic duct, with the point of enlargement corresponding to the junction of the two hepatic ducts. Thus the wider, inferior part is the common hepatic duct (see Chapter 4, page 113).

Sections farther to the right show the major part of the right lobe bounded superiorly by the strongly reflective diaphragm, with the right kidney posteriorly. The gallbladder may appear in this region. Often a fine reflective line can be identified linking the right portal vein with the neck of the gallbladder. This represents the fissure separating the quadrate lobe anteriorly from the right lobe. Inferiorly, the gas-containing bowel gives strong echoes with shadowing.

Transverse sections show the right lobe of the liver in close contact with the diaphragm (Figure 3-4) and the wedge-like left lobe extending anteriorly to the aorta, the stomach, and the pancreas. The caudate lobe can be seen as a tongue of liver projecting to the left from the upper part of the right lobe, superior to the porta (Figure 3-5).

The liver parenchyma is seen as a uniform, sponge-like texture of low-level gray. Passing through it are the blood vessels, which are seen as branching tubular structures that can be traced toward the porta (portal veins) or the inferior vena cava (hepatic veins) (Figure 3-6). Indentification of these two groups is facilitated by the fact that portal vein branches are usually surrounded by reflective tissue, whereas hepatic vein tributaries are not and appear as simple tubular defects. There are exceptions to this observation, for hepatic veins can have strong wall echoes where the beam strikes them at right angles.

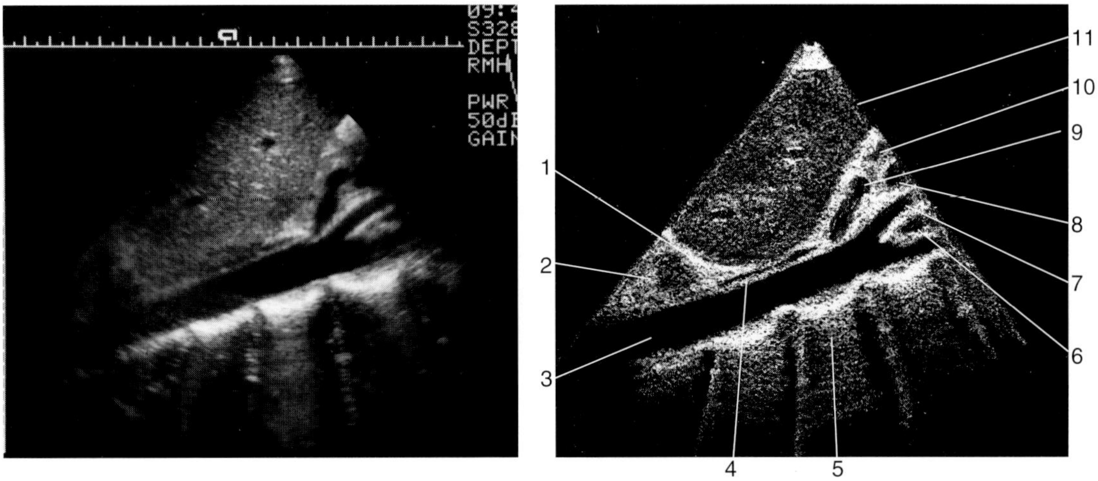

a

1. Esophagus 2. Heart 3. Aorta 4. Crus of diaphragm 5. Spine 6. Left renal vein 7. Superior mesenteric vein 8. Splenic vein 9. Celiac axis (trunk) 10. Stomach 11. Left lobe of liver

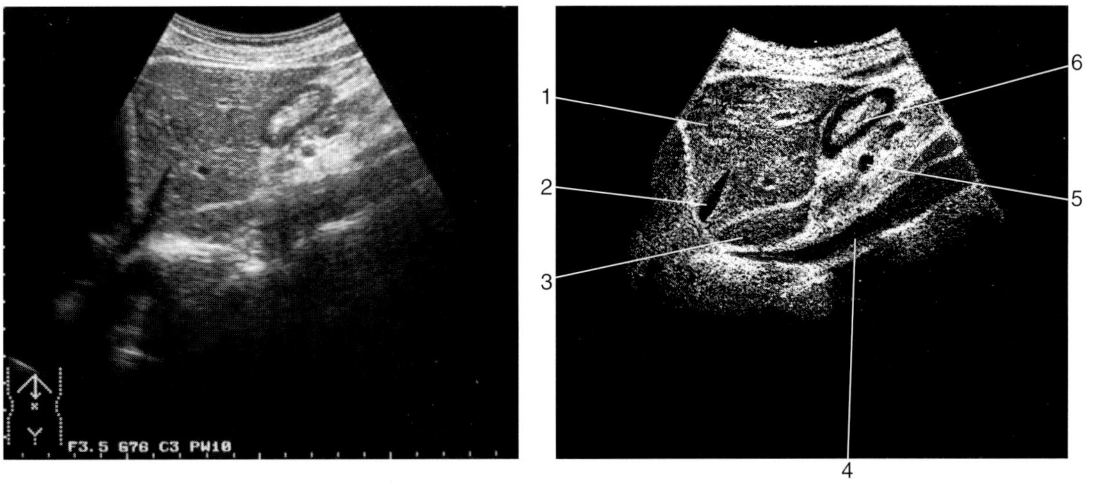

b

1. Left lobe of liver 2. Left hepatic vein 3. Caudate lobe of liver 4. Aorta 5. Splenic vein 6. Stomach

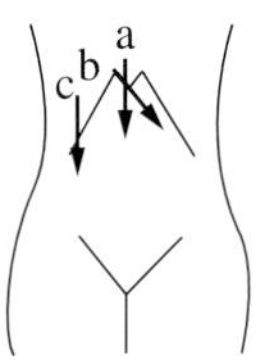

Figure 3-2. Sagittal sections of the left lobe of the liver.
The left lobe overlies the aorta and inferior vena cava and extends as far to the right as the aorta. Note its close relationship to the diaphragm superiorly and the stomach posteriorly. The fibro-fatty tissue around the portal vein may cause shadowing (c). The left portal vein characteristically has an anterior sweep, as in this example.

c

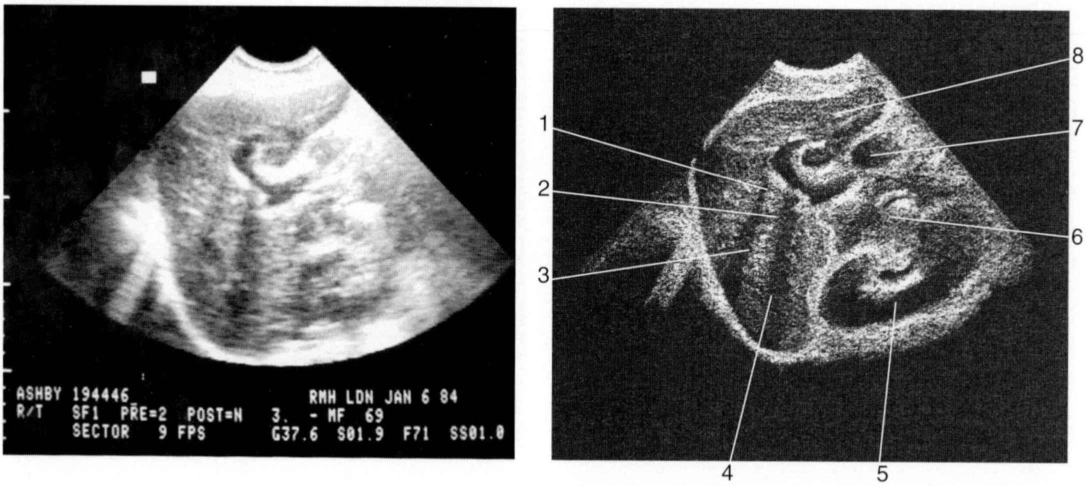

1. Left portal vein 2. Right portal vein 3. Enhancement 4. Shadowing 5. Right kidney 6. Colon 7. Antrum of stomach 8. Left lobe (quadrate lobe) of liver

Figure 3-2.

a

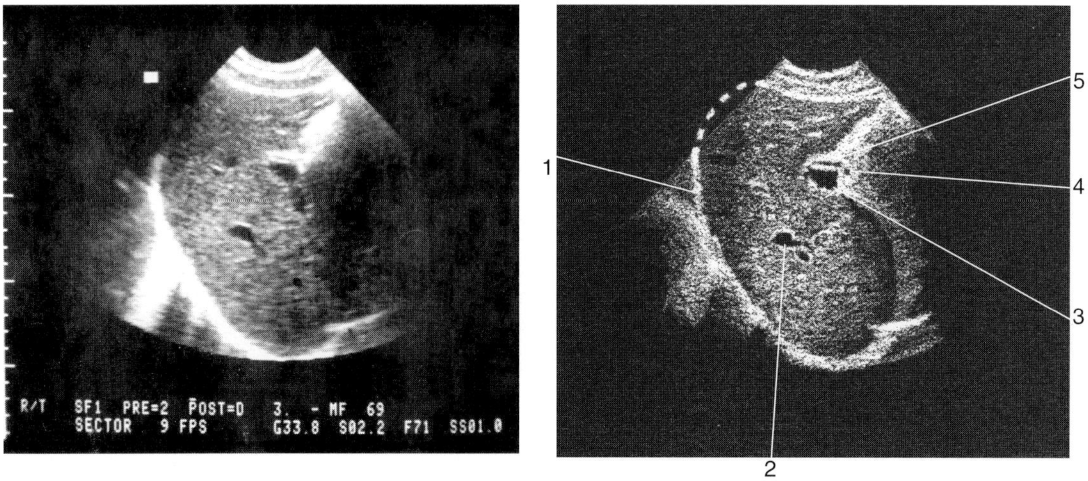

1. Diaphragm 2. Right hepatic vein 3. Right portal vein 4. Right hepatic artery 5. Common duct

b

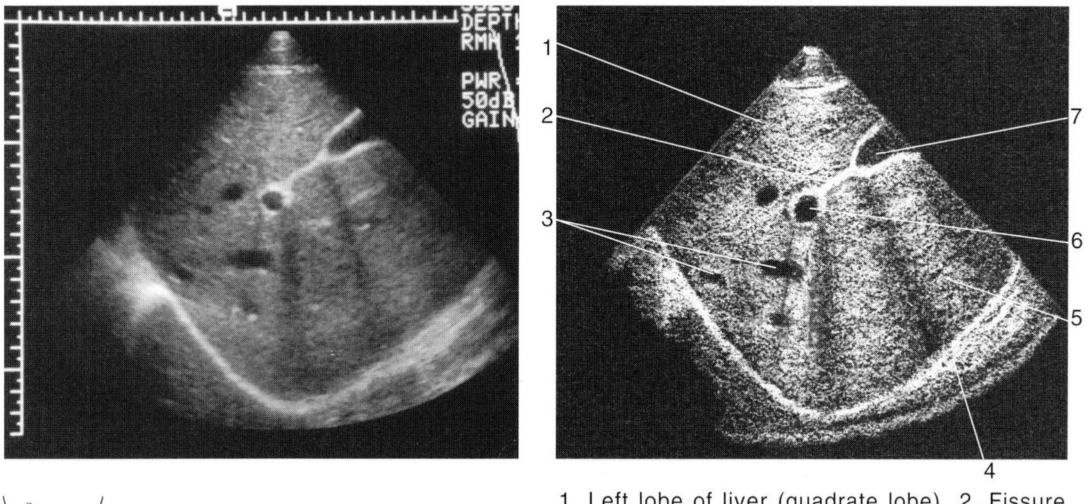

1. Left lobe of liver (quadrate lobe) 2. Fissure between left and right lobes 3. Hepatic vein radicals 4. Sacrospinalis muscle 5. Right lobe of liver 6. Portal vein 7. Gallbladder

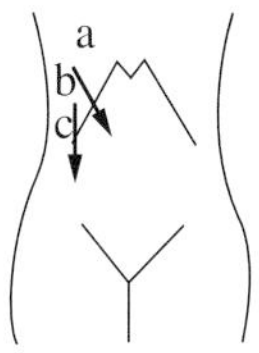

Figure 3-3. Sagittal sections of the right lobe of the liver.
Extending across from the porta, the right lobe is bounded superiorly by the diaphragm and is related inferiorly to the right kidney, the gallbladder, and the hepatic flexure of the colon. The bile duct is seen as a fine vessel lying anterior to the right portal vein (a). The echogenic band passing from the portal vein to the gallbladder neck (b) is the fissure separating the quadrate lobe anteriorly from the right lobe.

c

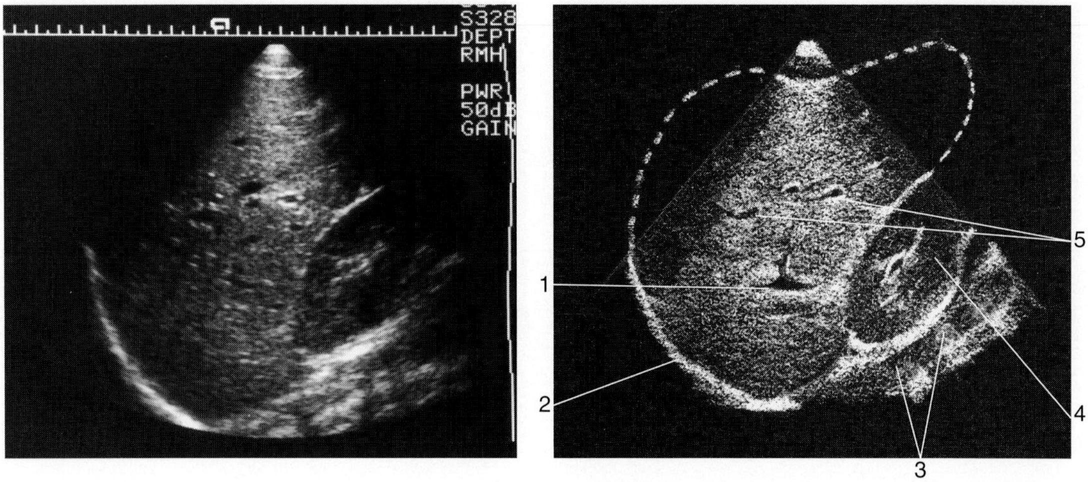

1. Hepatic vein 2. Diaphragm 3. Ribs 4. Right kidney 5. Right portal vein

Figure 3-3.

a

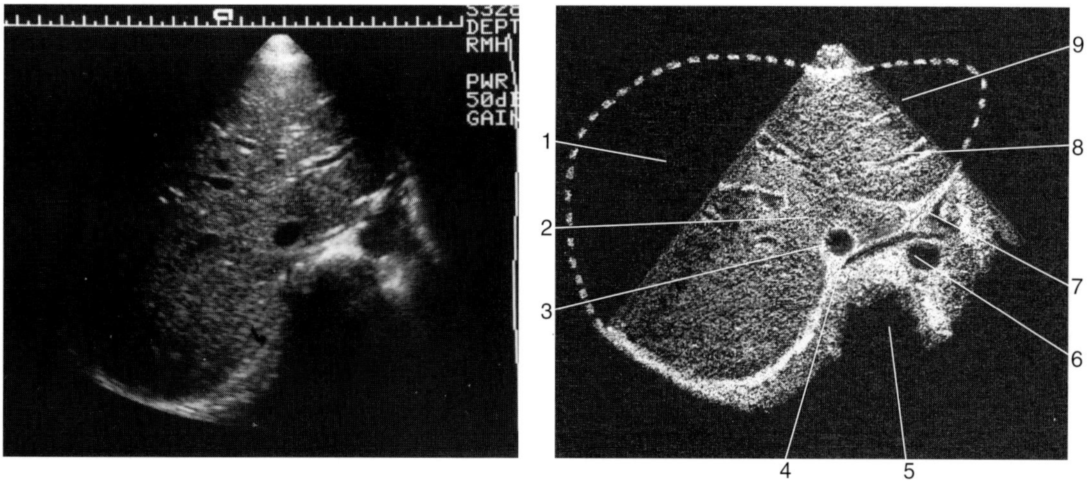

1. Right lobe of liver 2. Caudate lobe of liver 3. Inferior vena cava 4. Crus of diaphragm 5. Spine 6. Aorta 7. Esophagus 8. Left portal vein 9. Left lobe of liver

b

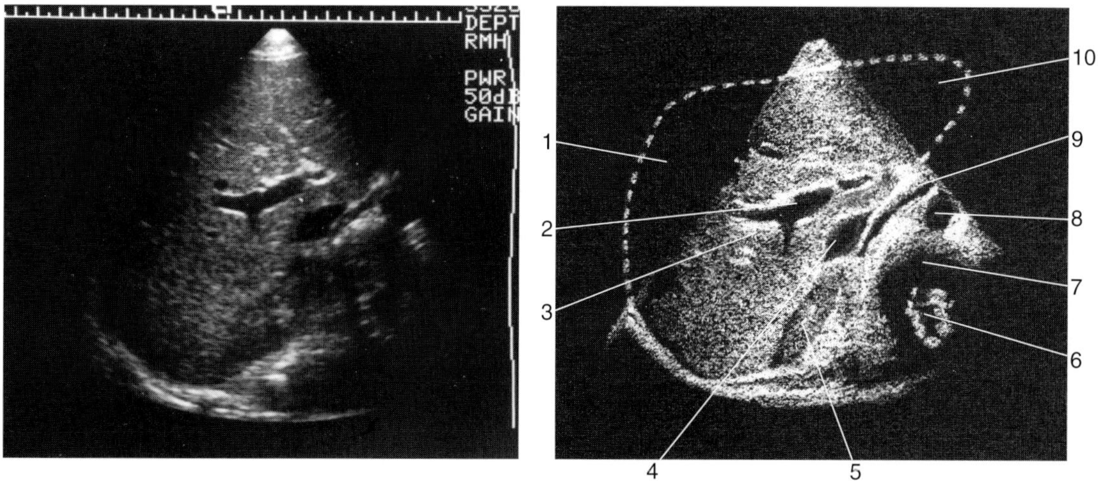

1. Right lobe of liver 2. Right portal vein 3. Division of right portal vein 4. Inferior vena cava 5. Upper pole of right kidney 6. Spinal canal 7. Intervertebral disc 8.Aorta 9. Crus of diaphragm 10. Left lobe of liver

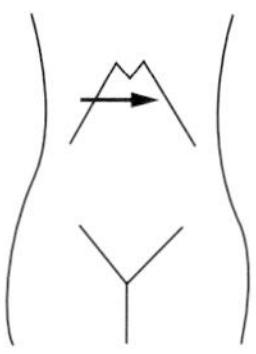

Figure 3-4. Transverse section of the liver.
The relatively posterior lie of the right lobe is seen in these views, with the right branch of the portal vein passing transversely. Note the crus overlying the lower thoracic aorta (a).

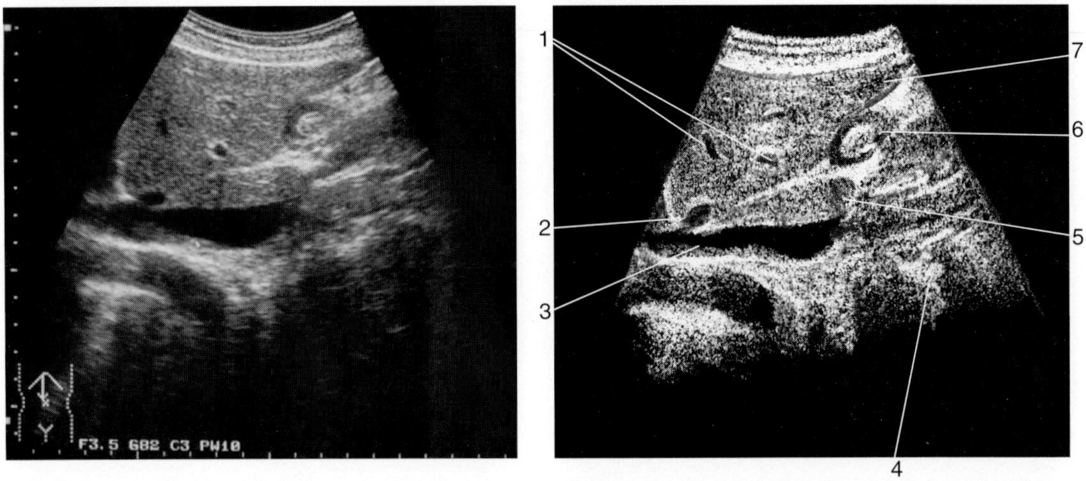

a

1. Branches of left portal vein 2. Left hepatic vein 3. Inferior vena cava 4. Spine 5. Caudate lobe of liver 6. Stomach 7. Left lobe of liver

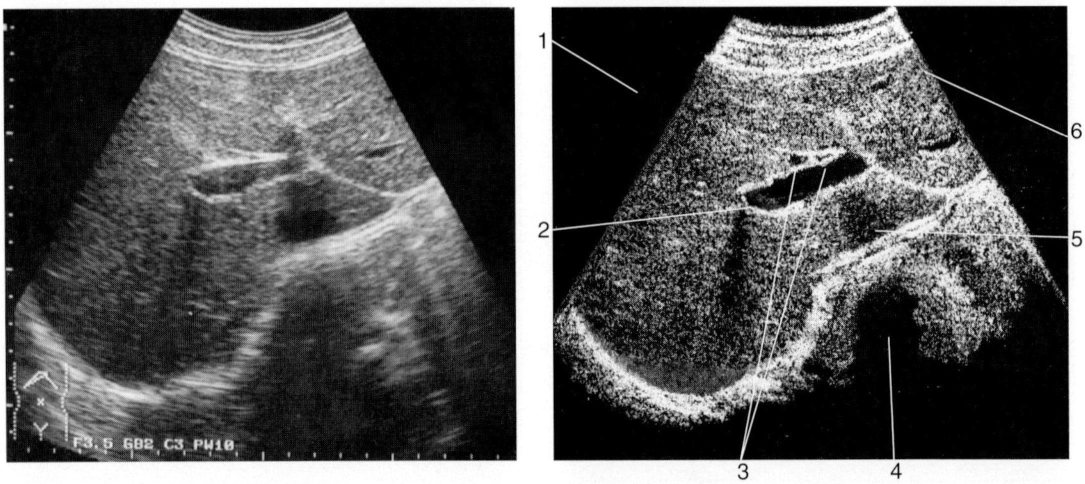

b

1. Right lobe of liver 2. Right portal vein 3. Common bile duct and hepatic artery 4. Spine 5. Caudate lobe of liver 6. Left lobe of liver

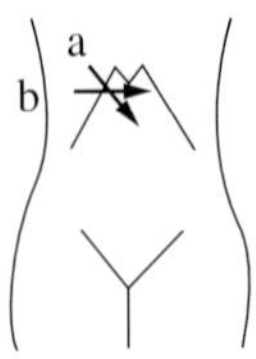

Figure 3-5. The caudate lobe.
In longitudinal section (a), the caudate lobe appears as an almond shape lying posterior to the left lobe. The inferior vena cava—and, if it is large, the aorta—also lie posterior to it. It is continuous laterally with the superior part of the right lobe (b) and is separated from the left lobe by the fissure that contains the lesser omentum.

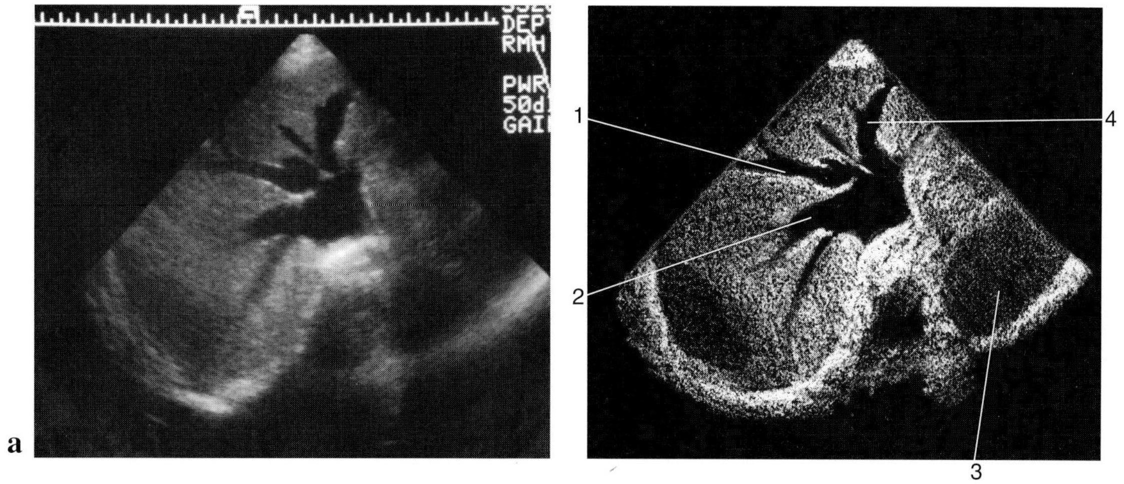

1. Middle hepatic vein 2. Right hepatic vein 3. Heart 4. Left hepatic vein

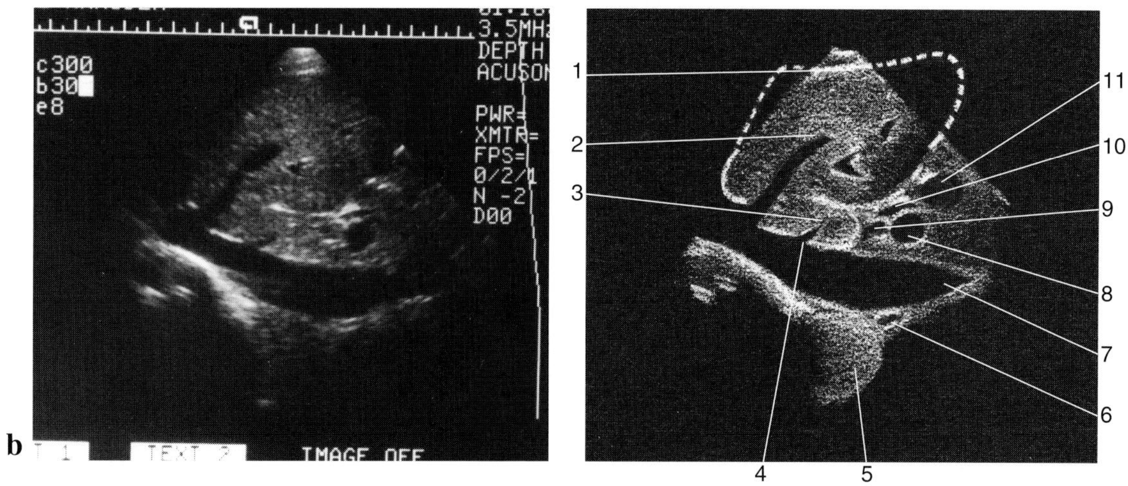

1. Left lobe of liver 2. Left hepatic vein 3. Caudate lobe of liver 4. Caudate lobe vein 5. Part of right lobe of liver 6. Right renal vein 7. Inferior vena cava 8. Head of pancreas 9. Splenic vein 10. Gastro-duodenal artery 11. Gastric antrum

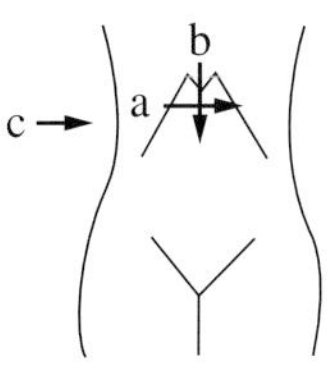

Figure 3-6. The hepatic veins.
The three main hepatic veins are best seen in cross section (a), interdigitating with the portal vein branches. The left and middle hepatic veins usually join to form a short common trunk before emptying into the upper part of the inferior vena cava (see Figure 3-2b). In the sagittal section through the inferior vena cava (b), the left or middle hepatic vein is often imaged. The right hepatic vein (c) usually runs in the coronal plane; it divides the anterior and posterior segments of the right lobe. The smaller, inferior hepatic veins, which drain the caudate lobe and the medial portion of the right lobe, are usually not imaged. Where high-resolution images can be obtained (b), they may be discerned.

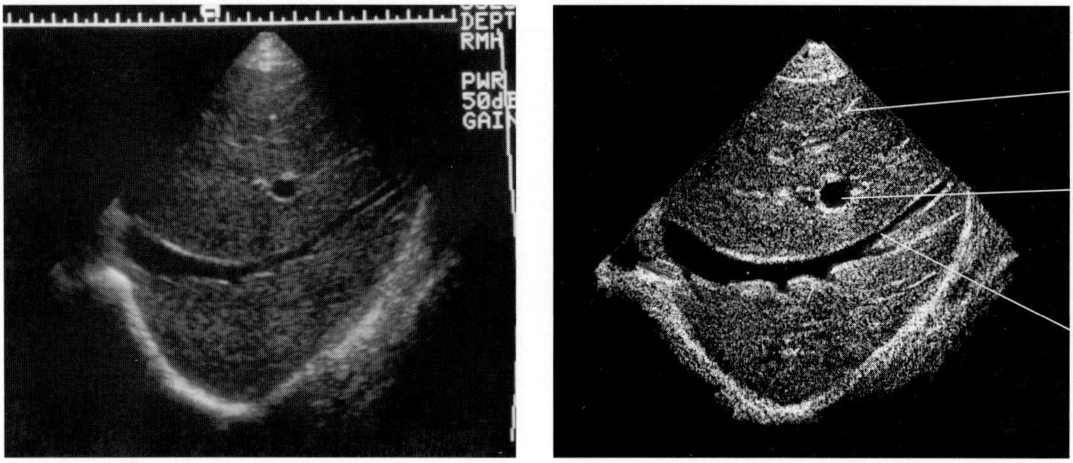

c

1. Liver 2. Portal vein 3. Right hepatic vein

Figure 3-6.

INTERPRETATIVE DIFFICULTIES

Some parts of the liver may cause difficulties in interpretation (Table 3-1). The neck of the gallbladder, the ligamentum teres, and the interlobar fissure (between the left and caudate lobes) may attenuate the sound beam sufficiently to cause shadowing of the deeper-lying portions of the liver.[59] Sometimes the main portal veins cause shadowing which must not be misinterpreted as representing a lesion. The tip of a Reidel's lobe often has a lower level of echoes than the remainder of the liver. The reasons for this are not understood. The deepest parts of the liver seem to have low-level echoes if the liver is highly attenuating (e.g., in fatty infiltration) or if the scanning technique is wrong (TGC misset or transducer of too high a frequency used).

Table 3-1. Pseudolesions in the liver.

- Echogenic
  - Ligamentum teres
  - Diaphragmatic leaflets
- Echo-poor
  - Shadowing
    - Caudate lobe
    - Posterior left lobe
    - Right lobe behind portal vein
  - Tip of Reidel's lobe
  - Deepest right lobe

The ligamentum teres is easily confused with an echogenic focal lesion in cross section (Figure 3-7). Since it often has an oblique path, it may be cut across in both transverse and longitudinal sections, which can be rather confusing. Oblique alignment of the transducer along its length will clarify the anatomy. Although the superior surface of the liver is usually quite smooth, if diaphragmatic leaflets hypertrophy, they indent the soft liver to produce cough furrows (Figure 3-8). Seen from inferiorly, they produce echogenic bands or foci in the liver and can be mistaken for focal lesions.

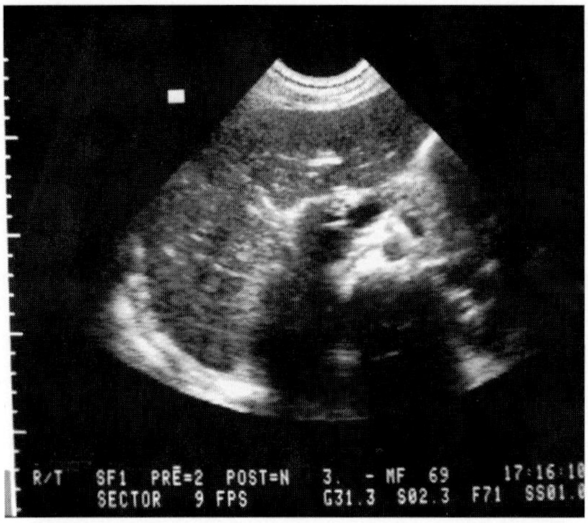

a

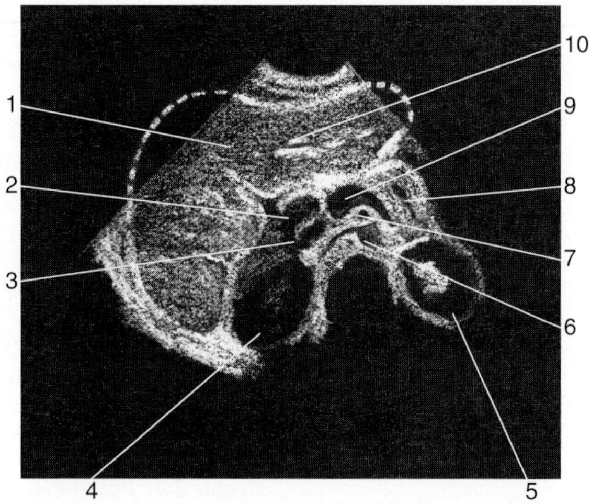

1. Quadrate lobe of liver 2. Duodenum 3. Inferior vena cava 4. Right kidney 5. Left kidney 6. Aorta and right renal vein 7. Superior mesenteric artery 8. Pancreas 9. Portal vein (origin) 10. Ligamentum teres

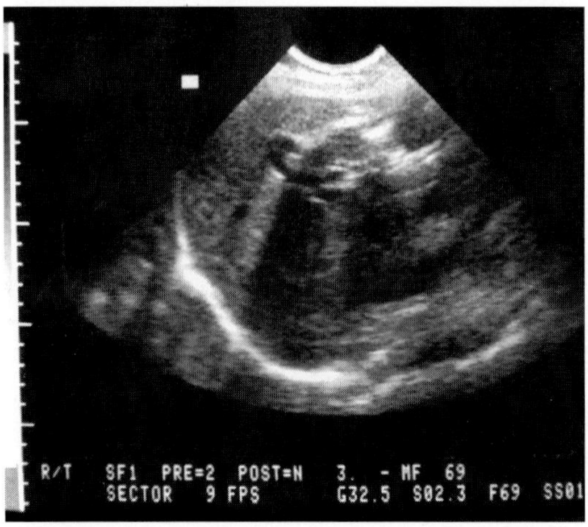

b

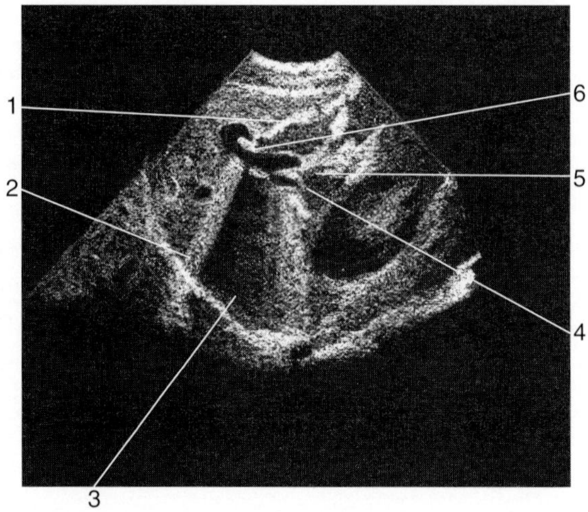

1. Ligamentum teres 2. Enhancement 3. Shadowing 4. Right portal vein 5. Porta hepatis 6. Left portal vein

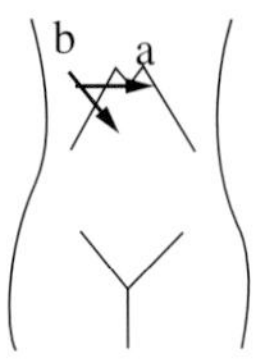

Figure 3-7. The ligamentum teres.
The ligamentum teres (round ligament) is often striking in transverse section as an echogenic focus within the left lobe (a). It may give rise to some shadowing. Since it crosses from midline to right as it passes to the left portal vein, an oblique tomogram (b) is required to image its full length.

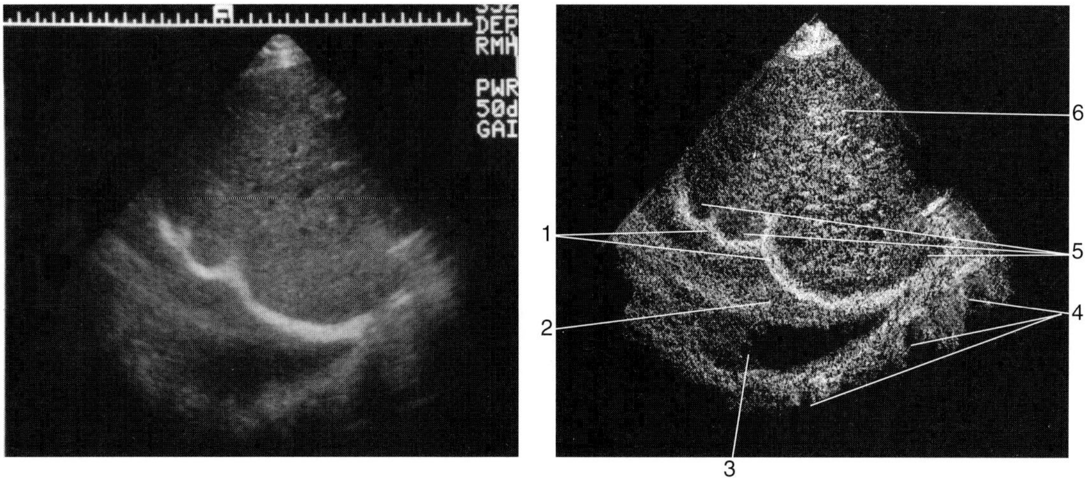

1. Diaphragmatic leaflets 2. Consolidated lung 3. Pleural effusion 4. Ribs 5. Liver humps 6. Right lobe of liver

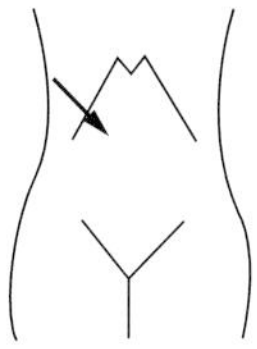

Figure 3-8. Diaphragmatic humps.
Hypertrophic diaphragmatic leaflets may indent the otherwise smooth upper surface of the right lobe of the liver. Seen from below, the intervening liver forms humps which must not be mistaken for mass lesions.

LIVER SIZE

Although its total volume is closely related to body weight, the liver is very variable in shape.[22, 31, 64] Thus any linear measurement or tomographic slice may give a misleading impression of its size. Assessment of hepatomegaly by ultrasound is therefore difficult, though it is often easy to be sure that the liver is not enlarged. In addition, an obvious cause of the clinically apparent hepatomegaly can be suggested; a Reidel's lobe or a prominent right kidney are typical examples.

Liver volume can be assessed accurately by taking serial sections and cumulating the areas, but this is a time-consuming procedure. The liver span, measured at the midclavicular line, forms a practical but not a very sensitive measure of liver size; the same measurement is useful for assessing changes.[31]

SCANNING TECHNIQUES

Because most of the liver is protected by the rib cage, access for ultrasound is limited. Therefore, sector or convex transducers are more useful than linear probes. The best views of the left lobe are obtained subcostally in longitudinal and transverse sections, with the patient holding inspiration if necessary. The same subcostal approach may be used on the right, though it is often simpler to exploit the windows provided by the intercostal spaces, which give good access without the need for patient cooperation. They are especially useful where the liver is high-riding or when the patient cannot hold a deep inspiration. The left decubitus posture causes the liver to drop below the costal margin and can greatly improve visualization. This is particularly helpful for the study of the porta and the common bile duct.

Where a linear array is used, views of the right lobe can be obtained with the probe held parallel to the costal margin and then angled up under it. This maneuver produces tomograms in planes lying between transverse and longitudinal and is sometimes referred to as the *recursive view*. The anatomical relationships may seem unfamiliar, but much of the liver can be covered in this way.

As with all ultrasound scanning, the highest-frequency transducer that can be used gives the best spatial resolution and gray-scale display. The effects of focal zone are important, especially where this is fixed, as in mechanical sector scanners. Use of a water bag to stand the transducer away from the skin can be helpful for superficial structures where the poor-quality near field may obscure lesions. The variable focus of electronically focused arrays on either sector or linear probes improves resolution and flexibility (see Chapter 2).

No preparation is required for liver scanning, though fasting is necessary for gallbladder studies (see Chapter 4).

FOCAL LIVER DISEASES

Simple liver cysts are common incidental findings.[7, 60, 75] Most are developmental, the cysts representing failed biliary ducts. Some represent persistent traumatic hematomas or remnants of abscesses, though often there is no history of the original event. Regardless of their origin, they appear as rounded, smooth-walled, echo-free spaces with marked distal enhancement (Figures 3-9 and 3-10). They are commonly loculated, and several may be found in the same patient. Necrotic tumor deposits and abscess cavities may also have fluid properties, but their walls are usually irregular (Figure 3-11). In difficult cases, careful study is necessary to elucidate such subtle but important differentiating features.

Like solitary cysts, polycystic liver disease is asymptomatic, though the renal cysts that usually coexist lead to progressive renal failure. The liver cysts have the same features as solitary cysts, except that they are often so packed together as to become polyhedral rather than rounded (Figure 3-12). They often have internal echoes due to hemorrhage. In Caroli's disease, a similar appearance is due to ectasia of the bile ducts [43, 59] (Figure 3-13). If their communication with the biliary tree can be demonstrated, the diagnosis can be made. The summed distal enhancement of these multiple cysts makes the normal parenchyma appear patchy, so that interpretation of coexisting significant lesions can be impossible. A similar problem applies in gross biliary tree distention.

Hydatid disease (due to *Echinococcus granulosus*) can produce a cystic lesion that is quite indistinguishable from a simple cyst (Figure 3-14a).[7, 19, 27, 34, 39, 42] However, when daughter hydatids bud from the wall of the cyst, irregularities of the wall are found. The earliest stages of this process produce small elevations of the germinal layer of the cyst; they appear as internal blebs along the cyst wall. These irregularities must be carefully searched for in any liver cyst, especially when the patient comes from a sheep-farming region. When mature, these irregularities form complete daughter cysts that on ultrasound look like cysts within cysts (Figure 3-14b). Eventually they may fill the mother cysts completely, showing a pathognomonic "cartwheel" pattern in which the spokes represent the walls of the compressed daughter cysts. Scolices may separate from the germinal matrix and lie in the cyst fluid. This forms "hydatid sand," which may layer in the dependent parts of the cyst.[74] Fine needle aspiration of hydatid cysts is considered safe, though it would seem prudent to confirm the diagnosis with a complement fixation test before intervening. Following treatment with an antihelminthic agent (e.g., albendazole), hydatids tend to become more echogenic as they shrink.

A more aggressive disease is produced by *E. multilocularis*, which is spread by dogs and foxes and is prevalent in eastern Europe and the former Soviet republics, Japan, and Australia. Since the daughter cysts bud outward, the disease spreads throughout the liver, giving irregular patchy changes (Figure 3-15).

The use of ultrasound in liver abscesses has changed the management of this dangerous condition.[16, 49, 60, 73] The right lobe is more commonly affected than the left. The majority of abscesses are due to infection ascending the biliary tree following cholecystitis or spreading up the portal vein from pelvic and appendiceal sepsis. The initial changes, seen in early cases before pus accumulates, are of an ill-defined solid mass lesion with reduced echoes[82] (Figure 3-16). The alteration in liver texture is often minimal and easily missed unless great care is taken with the scanning. Mature lesions are seen as a cortex of altered liver parenchymal echoes (darker than normal) a few millimeters thick surrounding a more or less echo-free central region, representing the pus. The shaggy-walled "capsule" represents inflamed but viable liver tissue. The affected region of the liver is often tender under the probe. The origin of the infection may also be detected on ultrasound. For example, a fluid collection in the right iliac fossa would indicate an appendix abscess, and one around the gallbladder a pericholicystitic abscess. Amebic and pyogenic liver abscesses have the same appearances.[3, 68] Gas may form within an abscess, giving rise to high-level echoes which may move with a change of posture (Figure 3-17a). On resolution, an abscess may disappear entirely or leave a cystic space which may persist indefinitely[69] (Figure 3-17b). Ultrasound is useful not only in detecting abscesses but also in guiding needle aspiration of their contents for bacteriological culture (anaerobic as well as aerobic).[48] Therapeutic drainage with a catheter can also be performed under ultrasound control when the lesion is accessible, but the large drain required is often more easily placed with fluoroscopy under general anesthesia.

Liver trauma may also be detected on ultrasound.[23, 33, 85, 90, 91] When there is a parenchymal hematoma, the appearance varies with the state of organization of the blood. Initially, it is seen as an echo-poor region (Figure 3-18); clotting and then fibrotic organization produce internal echoes. There may be distal enhancement. Eventual scarring leads to an echogenic linear band. Sometimes the blood products are reabsorbed to be replaced by serous fluid producing a posttraumatic cyst. When the liver capsule is ruptured, hemorrhage occurs into the peritoneal spaces surrounding the liver, where it may be indistinguishable from ascites. A high degree of suspicion of hemoperitoneum should be entertained when "ascites" is discovered following abdominal trauma.

Pneumobilia may occur spontaneously but is more often encountered in patients who have had surgery to the biliary tree, especially bypass procedures to relieve obstruction. The intense echoes due to the gas tend to lie in lines (string-of-beads pattern) and produce acoustic shadowing if the bubbles are large enough [13, 30] (Figure 3-19). This shadowing may obscure the deeper-lying parts of the liver, but the problem can usually be overcome by exploiting the effect of gravity. Rotating the patient decubitus will cause the gas to rise to the uppermost part of the liver so that more dependent parts can be imaged. The other decubitus position can then be used for the remaining liver.

Intrahepatic cholelithiasis has a similar appearance but does not show the same gravitational movement (Figure 3-20a). Calcification within the liver parenchyma has a more clumped appearance; it may be encountered in certain tumor types and in old inflammatory or traumatic lesions [40, 51] (Figure 3-20b). A plain x-ray may be required to establish the distinction from gas.

Hemangiomas are the most common benign liver tumor. When extensive, they may present with high-output heart failure in the neonate, but otherwise they are asymptomatic. Two histological types occur, the capillary type consisting of numerous malformed small vessels and the cavernous type consisting of lakes of blood. On ultrasound, the capillary type returns strong echoes while the cavernous type is relatively echo-free unless the vessels have thrombosed [8, 10, 24, 65, 83](Figures 3-21 and 3-22). Wide spread cavernous hemangiomas produces an irregular echo texture that is similar to the numerous other conditions causing the so-called "moth-eaten liver" (Table 3-2). Dynamic CT and angiography are the definitive investigations, but ultrasound can be a useful way to follow progress in the newborn.[61]

Echogenic hemangiomas cause confusion with echogenic metastases. Their rounded shape and uniform high reflectivity are often characteristic. They do not produce acoustic shadowing and they remain unchanged over months of follow-up. Angiography is the definitive test when the diagnosis remains a problem. Fine needle aspiration is surprisingly safe, though the cytologist may have difficulty in interpretation unless specifically alerted to the possibility of this diagnosis. Dynamic CT shows a characteristic pattern, with slow filling from the periphery, but these changes can be discerned only when the lesion is large.[21, 41] Doppler is usually unhelpful because the rate of blood flow is very low.[86]

Table 3-2. Moth-eaten liver.

Focal fatty change
Multiple hemangioma
Widespread focal necrosis
Alcoholic or viral hepatitis
Ascending cholangitis
Extensive malignant replacement
Hepatoma
Metastatic

Modified from Cosgrove DO, McCready VRM: Ultrasonic Imaging; Liver, Spleen, Pancreas. Chichester, UK, John Wiley, 1982, p190.

Benign tumors of the liver have become increasingly important, since at least one type, the true adenoma, is induced by long-term exposure to estrogens (usually in the form of contraceptives).[56, 93] On ultrasound these lesions are seen as masses of altered echo level, either of lower or, more usually, of higher level than the liver itself (Figure 3-23). The echo texture is rather heterogeneous because of hemorrhage into the lesions. The other tumor type, focal nodular hyperplasia, is a somewhat puzzling lesion, thought to represent an incomplete repair response to ischemia rather than a true tumor (Figure 3-24). It does not have the same association with estrogens as the adenoma, and may occur in children and males.[5, 12, 15, 72] It has a similar appearance on ultrasound but does not carry the same risk of hemorrhage. Because focal nodular hyperplasias usually contain Kupffer cells, they may take up sulfur colloid and thus show up on an isotope scan. The combination of a clear-cut CT or ultrasound lesion that is not represented by a cold area on an isotope scan is diagnostic of focal nodular hyperplasia, though not all cases fulfill these criteria. Both may show high flow on color Doppler.[86]

Hepatocellular carcinoma (hepatoma) most commonly produces a focal mass which is initially echo-poor but becomes more echogenic with increasing size (Figures 3-25 to 3-28). These carcinomas characteristically show a mosaic pattern, which is often accompanied by posterior echo enhancement and/or lateral shadowing. Ultrasound is particularly important in evaluating patients at risk of developing hepatomas (e.g., chronic hepatitis B or non-A, non-B, posttransfusional hepatitis and cirrhosis). In some cases, the tumor infiltrates widely through the liver substance, giving rise to an irregular pattern. Invasion of veins, both hepatic and portal, is commonly seen. The incidence of intra- and extrahepatic dissemination is high in this type of hepatocellular carcinoma.

Metastatic tumors are more common than primary hepatocellular carcinoma [6, 58, 87] (Figure 3-29). The most common appearance is that of multiple focal lesions of altered reflectivity [14] (Figures 3-30 to 3-32). The margins are poorly defined, and there is neither shadowing nor enhancement. The echoes are generally less intense than those of the surrounding liver, but many are more strongly reflective (echogenic). This type is usually due to deposits from urogenital or gastrointestinal tract primary tumors. When the tumor is extensive, the liver takes on a generalized patchy appearance often referred to as the *moth-eaten liver* (Table 3-2, Figure 3-33). In these extensively involved cases, it may be difficult to decide which part is tumor and even detection of the abnormality may be difficult. Additional imaging techniques, such as isotope or CT scans, may be more revealing.[58, 67]

Other patterns also occur in metastases, the *bull's-eye* or *target* lesion being the most dramatic (Figures 3-34 and 3-35). Here an echogenic central region is surrounded by a rim of echo-poor tissue. Fluid-filled deposits arise following central necrosis and metastases from mucin-secreting tumors (such as carcinoma of the ovary and pancreas) which retain the secretory function (Figure 3-36). They simulate simple cysts. Necrotic lesions have a shaggy wall and contain debris, the appearance being similar to that of an abscess. Calcification is most common in mucin-secreting tumors, such as those of the colon and pancreas, and produces extremely high reflectivity accompanied by shadowing [9] (Figure 3-37).

Reliable detection of liver malignancy is one of the more demanding applications of ultrasound. Attention to the mass effects of the expanding lesion is helpful. The gross changes of hepatomegaly and rounding of the liver's free margin are nonspecific and not always present, but their detection raises the suspicion of some type of liver pathology. More subtle effects are the presence of surface nodules overlying superficial deposits, distortion of blood vessels by masses, and obstruction to the biliary tree of lobar or lobular distribution (not necessarily accompanied by jaundice).[57]

Using all of these criteria and careful scanning technique with a good quality scanner, some 85 per cent of cases with liver metastases can be detected, with an almost negligible false-positive rate.[67] CT will often help in the eveluation of cases that are difficult to assess on ultrasound, though in general, ultrasound is just as accurate.[78] Equivocal areas can easily be biopsied under ultrasound control.

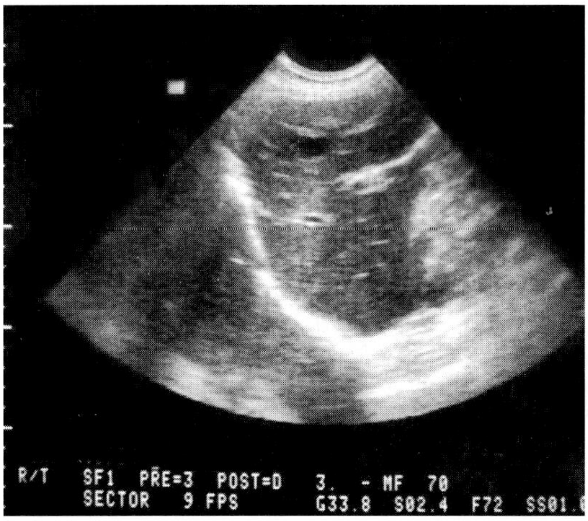

a

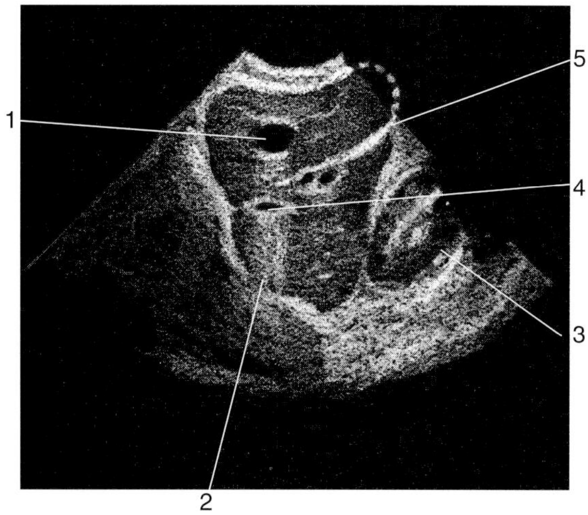

1. Cyst 2. Enhancement 3. Right kidney 4. Portal vein branches 5. Fissure

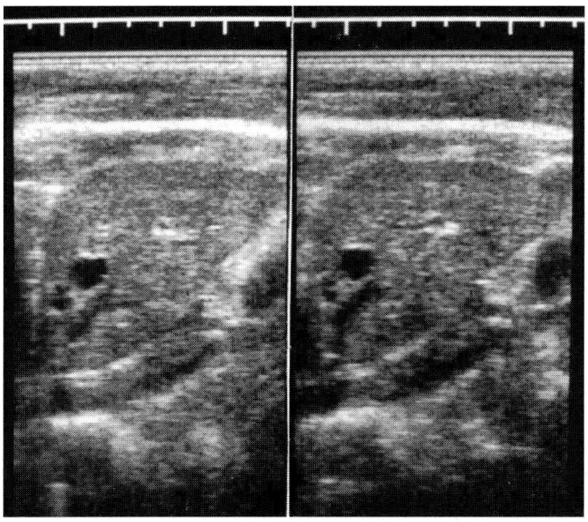

b

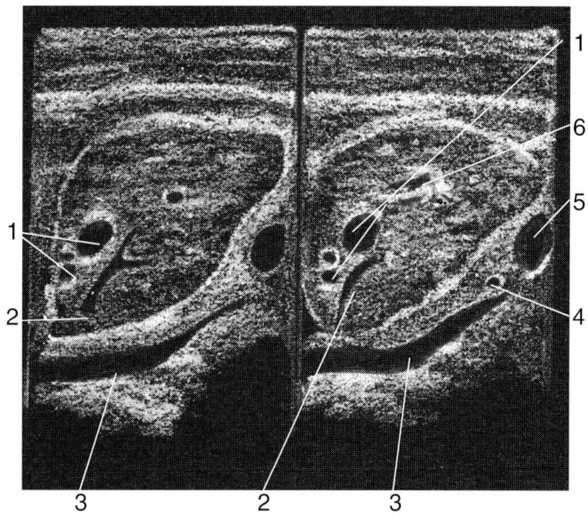

1. Cysts 2. Left hepatic vein 3. Inferior vena cava 4. Hepatic artery 5. Portal vein 6. Left portal vein

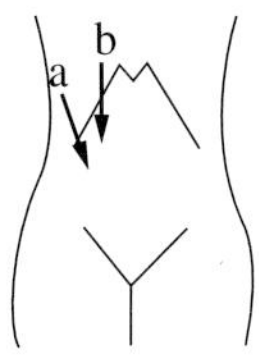

Figure 3-9. Simple cyst.
These rounded, smooth-walled lesions are typical of simple cysts (a). Enhancement is a characteristic feature indicating their fluid contents. However, with small cysts (b), it may be inapparent.

a

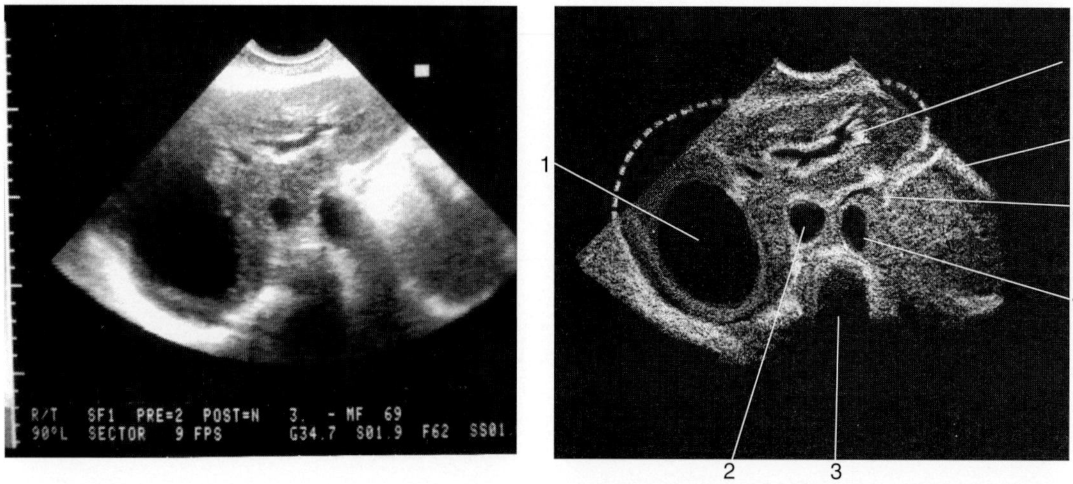

1. Cyst 2. Inferior vena cava 3. Spine 4. Aorta
5. Crus of diaphragm 6. Stomach 7. Left portal vein

b

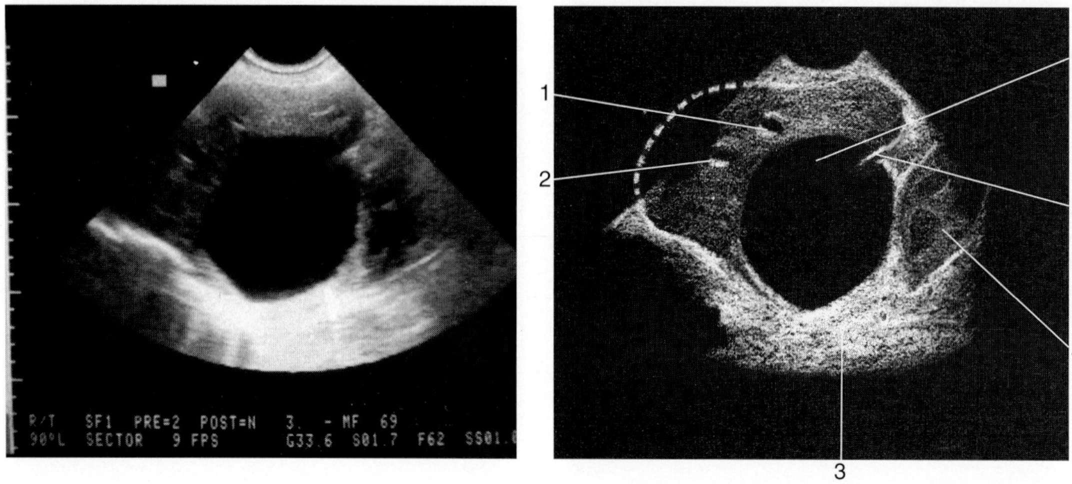

1. Portal vein 2. Hepatic vein 3. Enhancement
4. Right kidney 5. Hepatic flexure of colon 6. Cyst

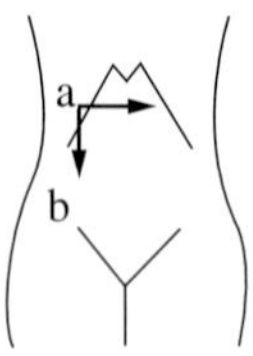

Figure 3-10. Giant simple cyst.
This large liver cyst has so distorted the local anatomy as to make confident determination of its origin difficult.

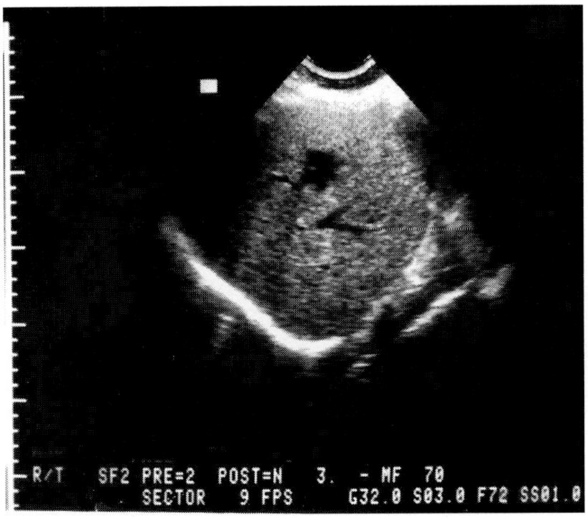

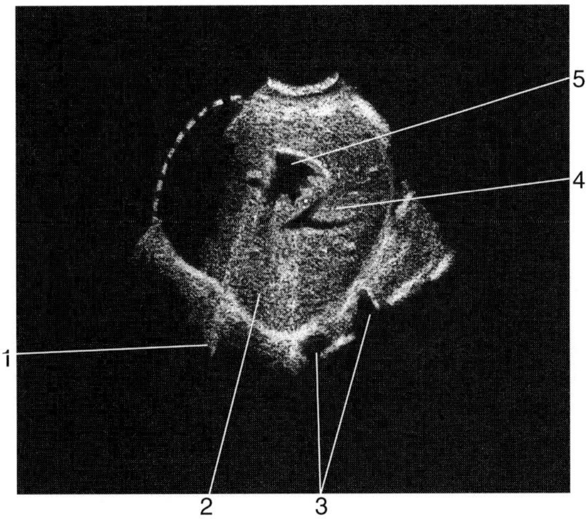

1. Edge shadows 2. Enhancement 3. Ribs 4. Hepatic vein 5. Cystic lesion

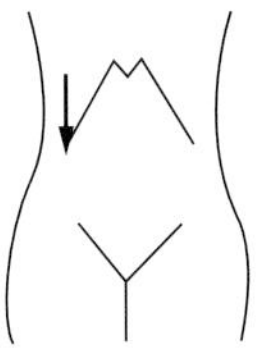

Figure 3-11. Nonsimple liver cyst.
The distal enhancement indicates that this is a fluid-filled lesion, but the irregular walls create doubt about its nature. Though a collapsed simple cyst could have this appearance, a necrotic tumor mass must be excluded, perhaps by a guided aspiration (see Figure 3-36b).

a

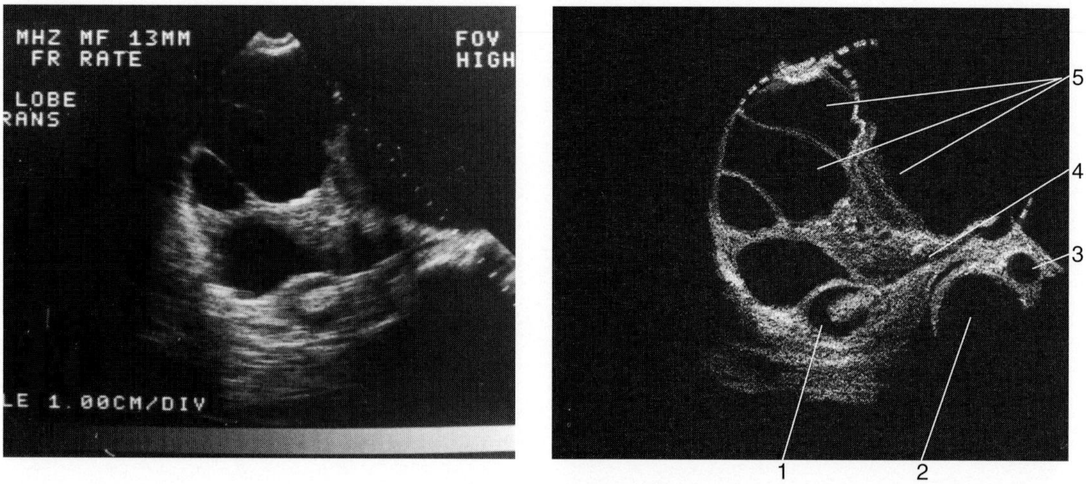

1. Right kidney 2. Spine 3. Aorta 4. Inferior vena cava 5. Cysts

b

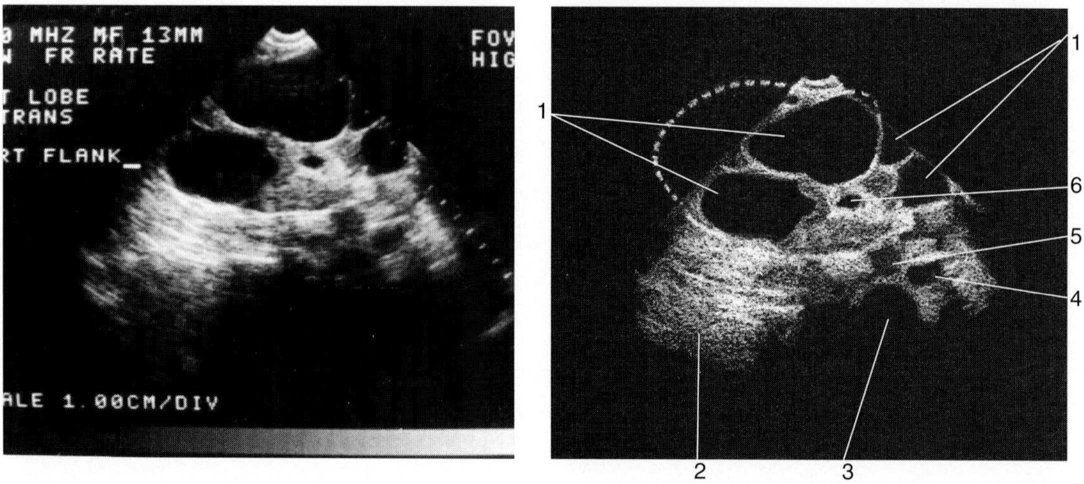

1. Cysts 2. Enhancement 3. Spine 4. Aorta 5. Inferior vena cava 6. Portal vein

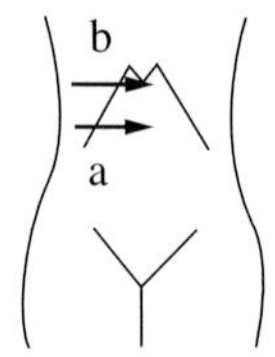

Figure 3-12. Polycystic disease.
A collection of liver cysts of varying sizes is a typical feature. The contiguity of the cysts compresses them into oval or polygonal shapes. Hemorrhage into a cyst gives low-level internal echoes. A coexisting lesion such as a tumor deposit would be very difficult to detect. (Figure courtesy of Dr. R. Obaro)

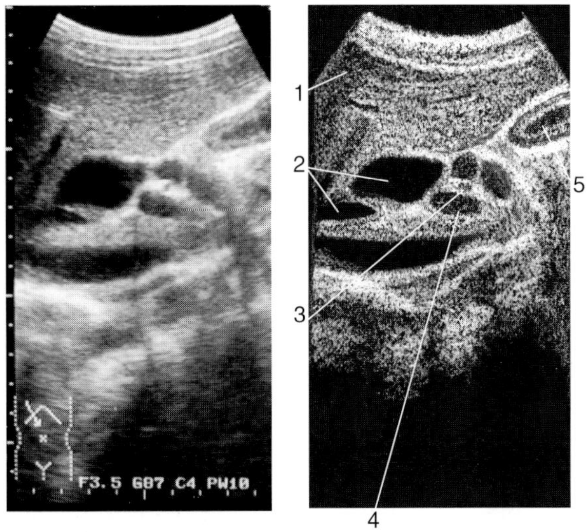

a

1. Left lobe of liver 2. Ectatic bile ducts 3. Hepatic artery 4. Portal vein 5. Stomach

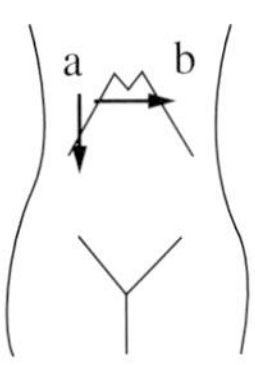

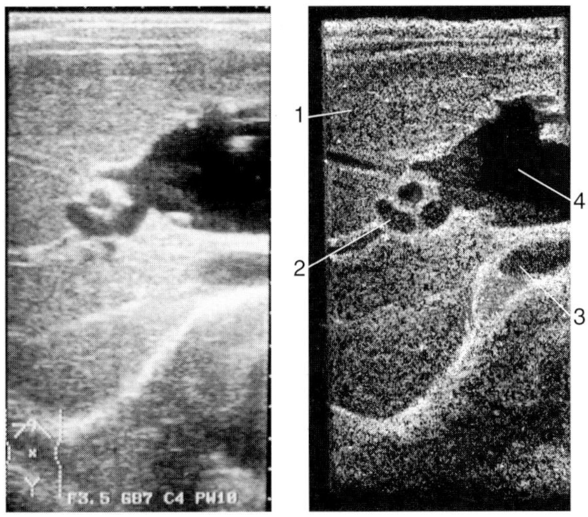

b

1. Right lobe of liver 2. Portal vein 3. Inferior vena cava 4. Ectatic bile duct

Figure 3-13. Caroli's disease.
The typical cystic dilatation of the intrahepatic biliary tree is shown in these sections in a patient with Caroli's disease. No stones were detected.

a

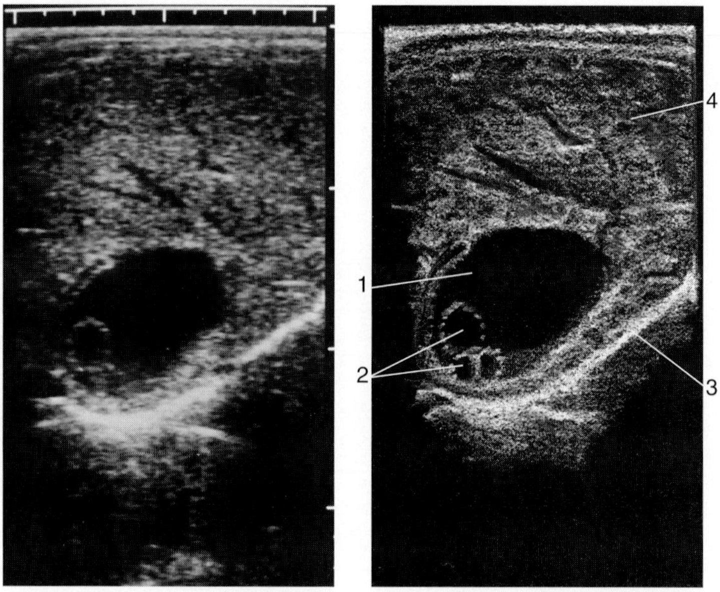

1. Echinococcal cyst 2. Daughter cysts 3. Diaphragm 4. Liver

b

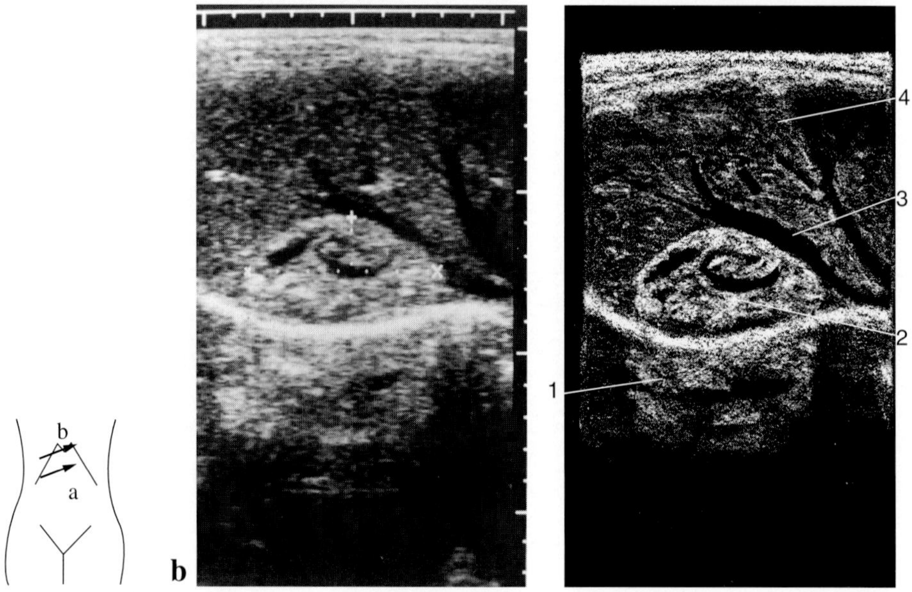

1. Mirror image 2. Echinococcal lesion 3. Right hepatic vein 4. Liver

Figure 3-14. Hydatid cysts.
The typical echo pattern of a hydatid cyst (*E. granulosus*) in the liver is shown in (a). A well-defined cyst containing small daughter cysts lies in the right lobe of the liver. Echinococcal infestation of the liver may also develop as a "solid" lesion. The subcostal scan in (b) shows an ovoid, echogenic lesion in the posterior portion of the right lobe of the liver; it has caused slight elevation of the adjacent hepatic vein. Despite its apparently solid nature, there is marked distal echo enhancement, suggesting that it is in fact fluid and that the echoes arise from numerous interfaces within it. (Figures courtesy of Dr. B. Frider, Buenos Aires)

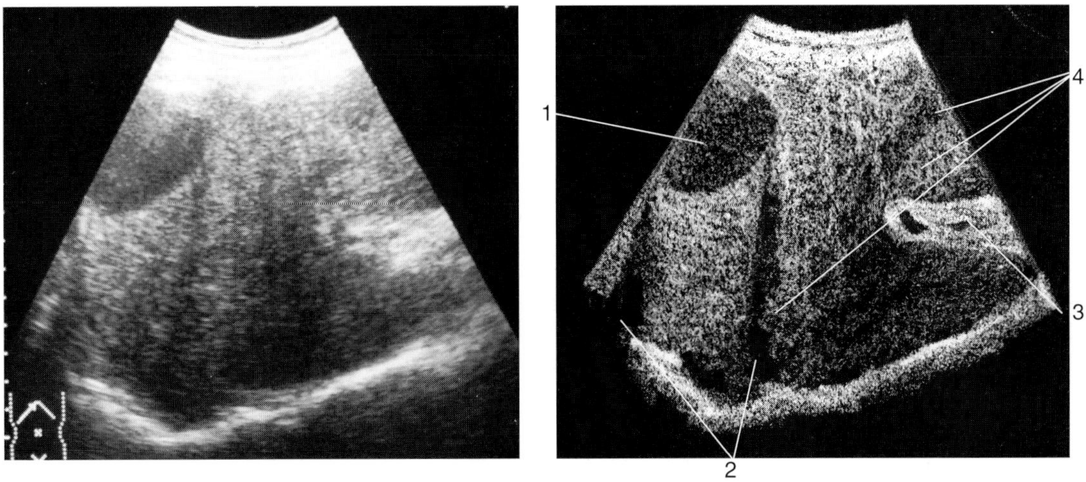

1. Hydatid mass 2. Edge shadows 3. Portahepatis
4. Irregular echoes

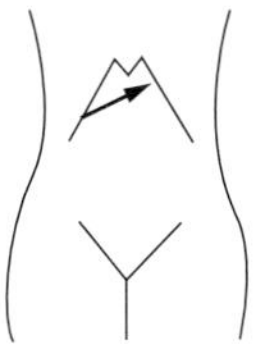

Figure 3-15. Echinococcosis of the liver, multilocular type.
E. multilocularis has a slow but relentlessly progressive course. This patient, a 62-years-old male, suffered from long-sustained, general malaise and weakness; a medium-sized cystic lesion in the right lobe of the liver was found on ultrasound. The entire right lobe of the liver showed irregular echogenic areas, with a mottled appearance but without cystic spaces. High attenuation was also noted. The left lobe showed compensatory enlargement.

a

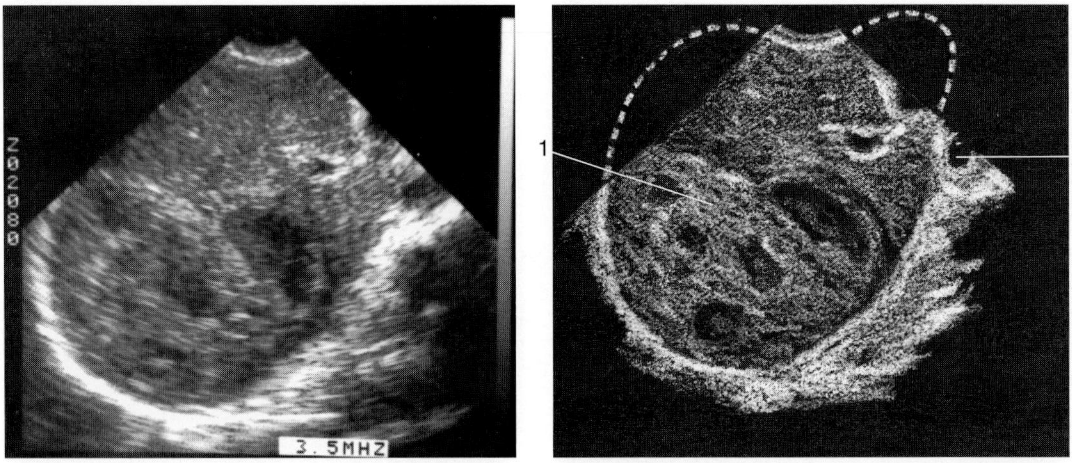

1. Abscess 2. Aorta

b

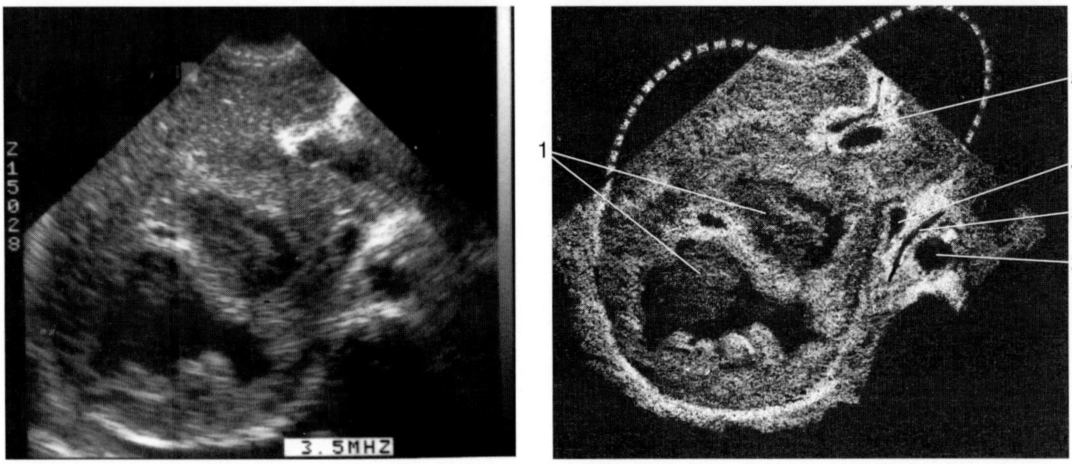

1. Abscess 2. Aorta 3. Crus of diaphragm
4. Inferior vena cava 5. Left portal vein

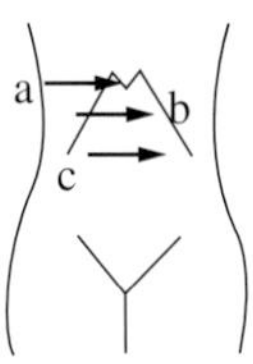

Figure 3-16. Liver abscess.
In the early stages of the development of an abscess, a solid inflammatory mass may be present (a, b). Distinction from other mass lesions depends on the clinical background or on aspiration biopsy. Later, as liquid purulent material forms (c), the appearance becomes more characteristic. (Figures courtesy of Dr. A.E. Joseph)

c

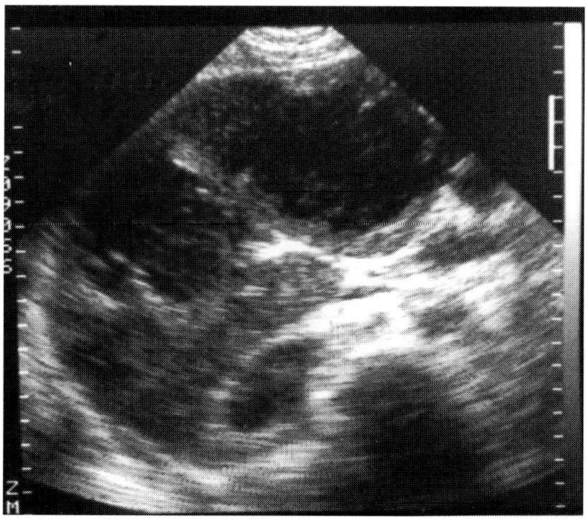

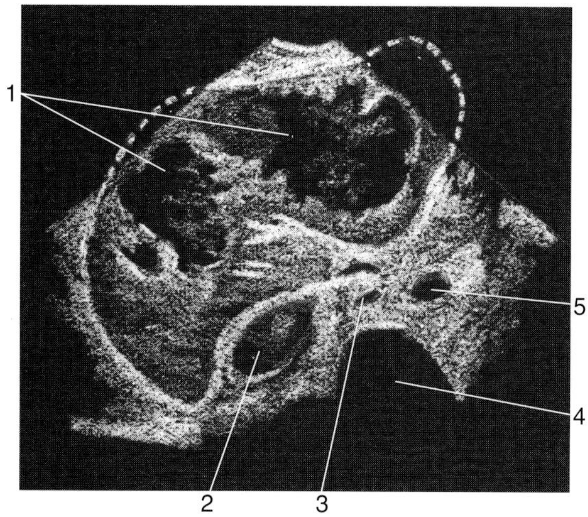

1. Abscess 2. Right kidney 3. Inferior vena cava
4. Vertebra 5. Aorta

a

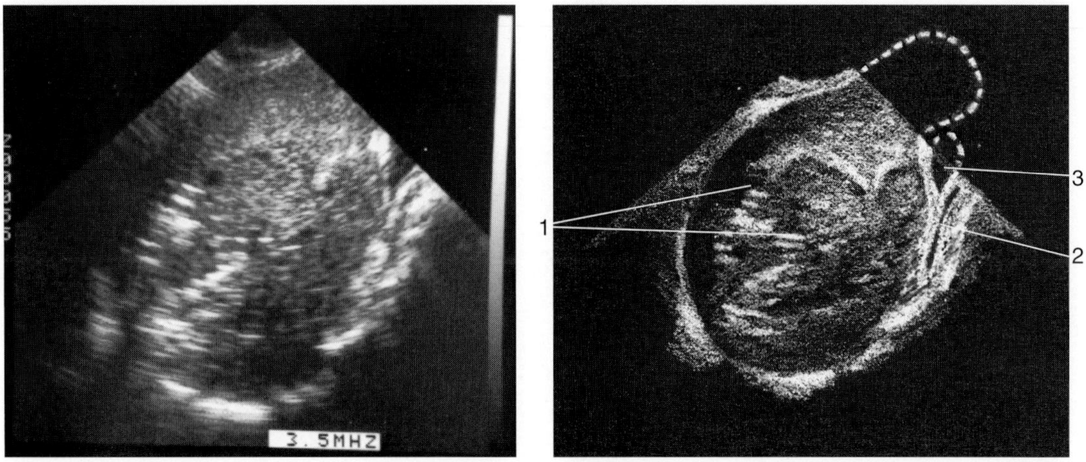

1. Gas bubbles 2. Crus of diaphragm 3. Inferior vena cava

b

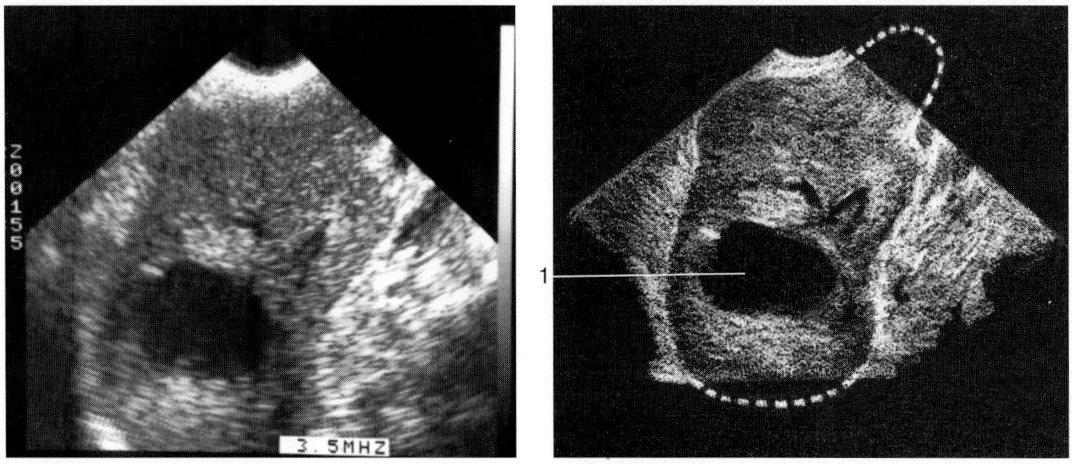

1. Abscess cavity

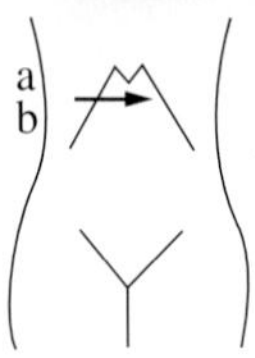

Figure 3-17. Liver abscess.
Gas may form within an abscess, giving rise to high-level echoes (a). With resolution, an abscess may absorb and disappear entirely, may form an echogenic scar, or may persist as a cystic space (b). (Figures courtesy of Dr. A.E. Joseph)

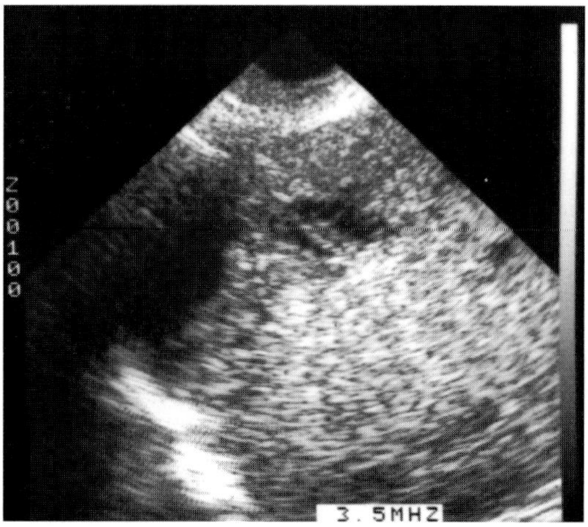

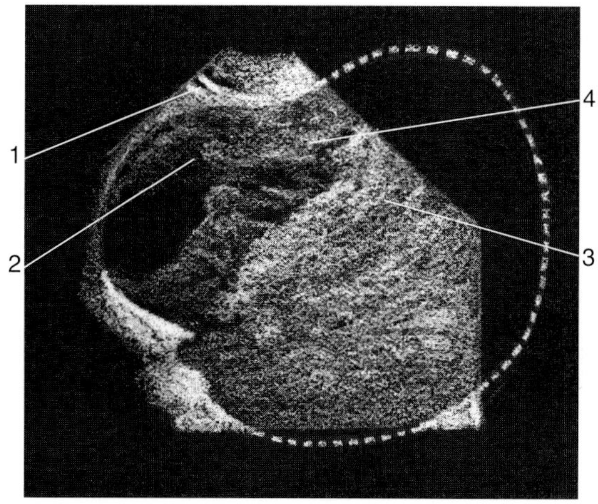

1. Lung surface 2. Hematoma 3. Intact liver
4. Damaged liver

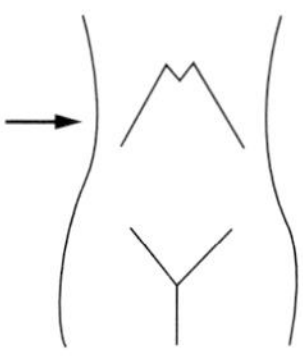

Figure 3-18. Trauma to the liver.
The edematous liver parenchyma returns low-level echoes, while hematoma may be anechoic in the early stages, as in this example. Later, with organization, echoes appear, and eventually scarring supervenes. (Figures courtesy of Dr. A.E. Joseph)

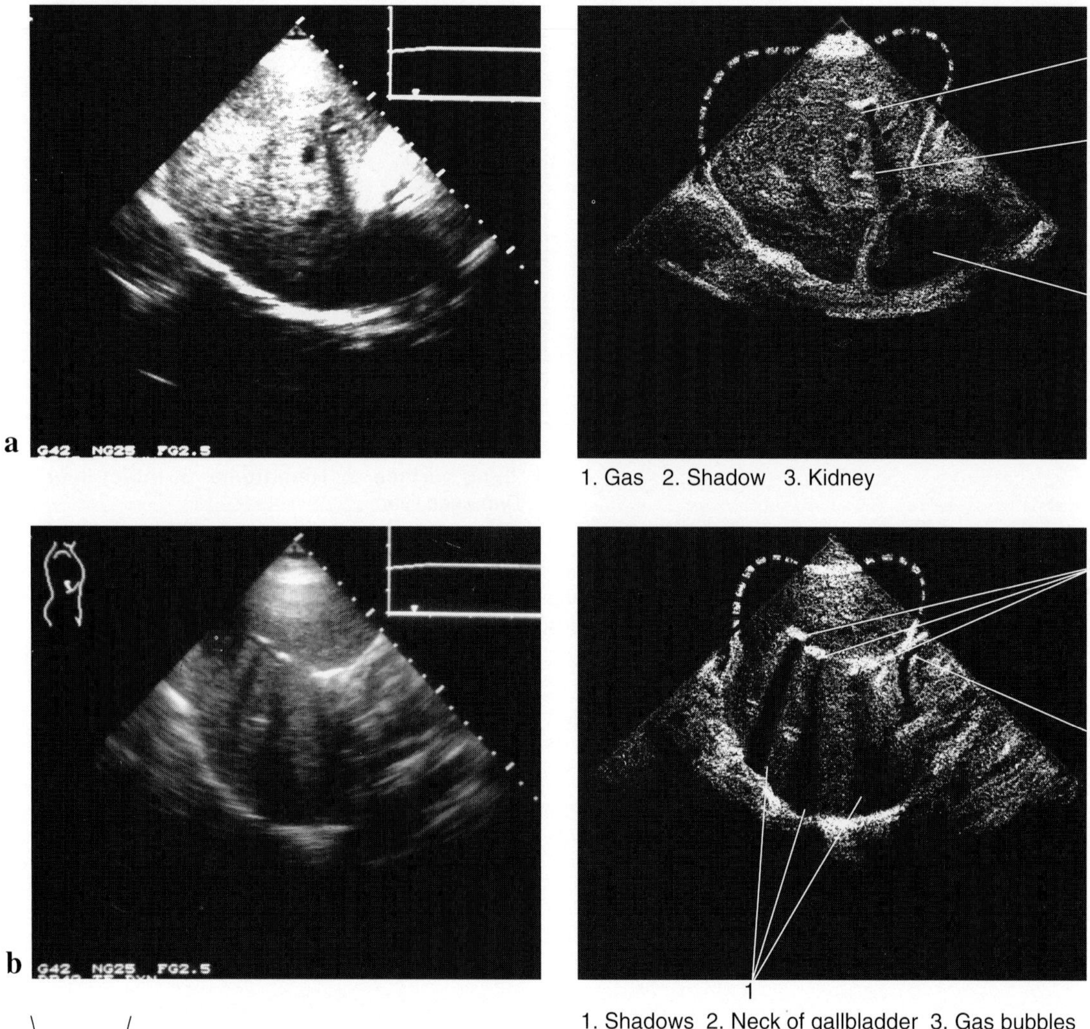

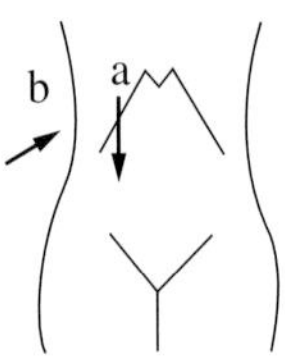

Figure 3-19. Pneumobilia.
Gas in the biliary tree gives the same strong echoes with distal shadowing seen elsewhere. These echoes tend to occur along the portal tracts and may be distinguished from intrahepatic biliary calculi by the way they rise when the patient is turned decubitus.

a

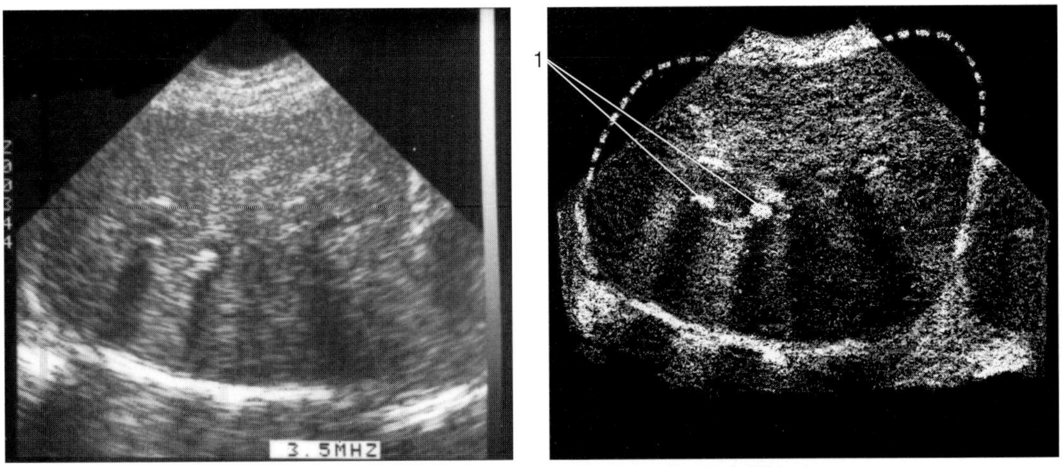

1. Intrahepatic cholelithiasis

b

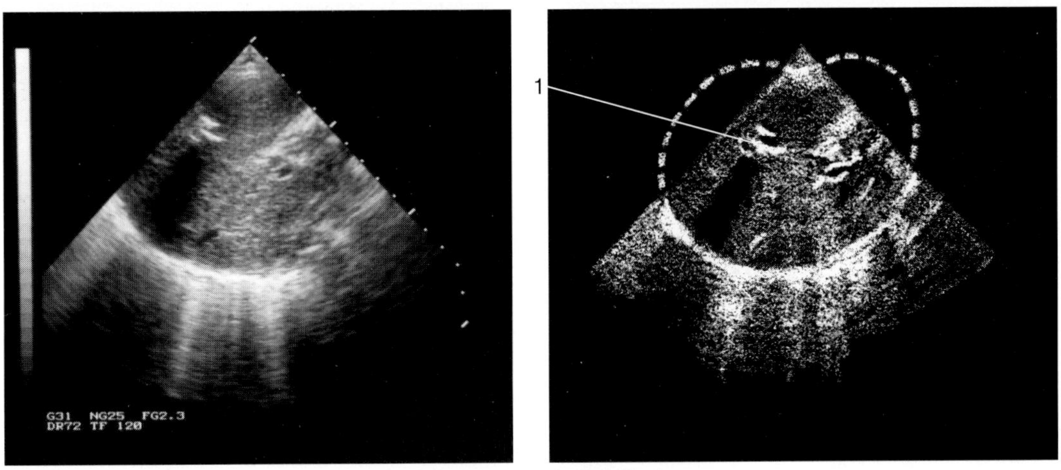

1. Calcific focus

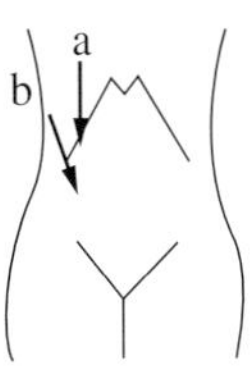

Figure 3-20. Intrahepatic calcification.
Intrahepatic cholelithiasis gives echogenic foci which cause shadowing if they are sufficiently large to interrupt the ultrasound beam, exactly like stones in the gallbladder. Because of their position within the bile ducts, they tend to lie in strings (a). (Figure courtesy of Dr. A.E. Joseph)
Parenchymal calcification forms irregular, clumped, echogenic masses, as in this example following old sepsis (b).

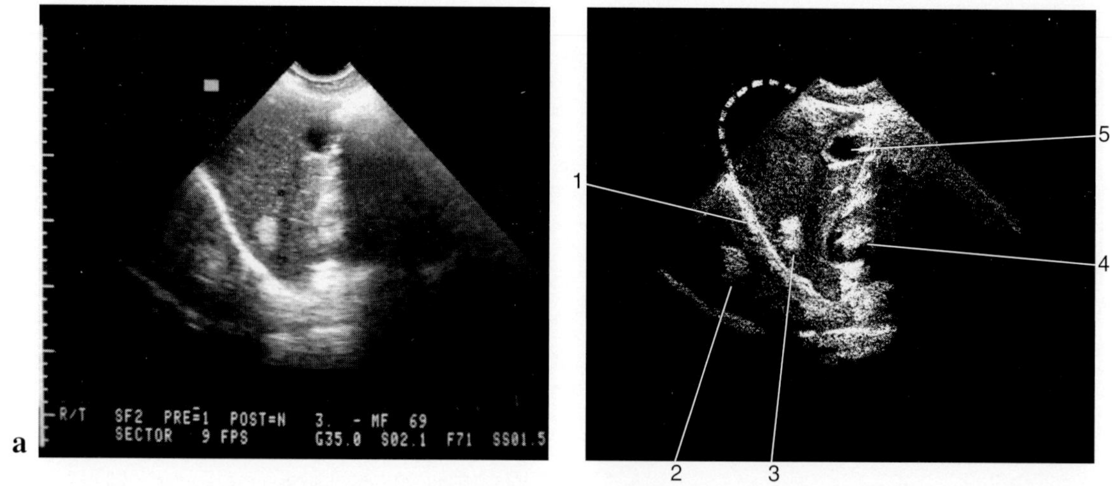

1. Diaphragm 2. Mirror image 3. Hemangioma 4. Kidney 5. Gallbladder

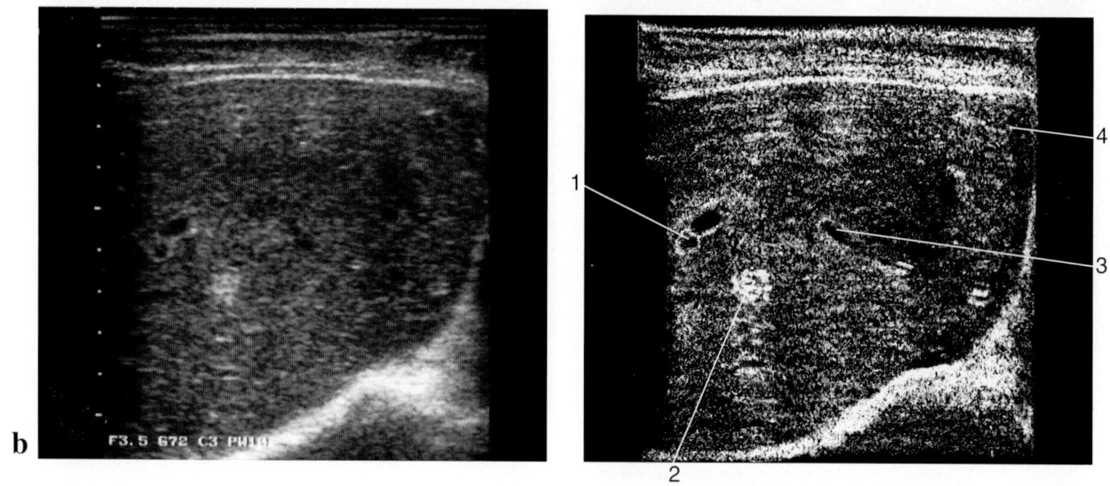

1. Portal vein branches 2. Hemangioma 3. Hepatic vein 4. Right lobe of liver

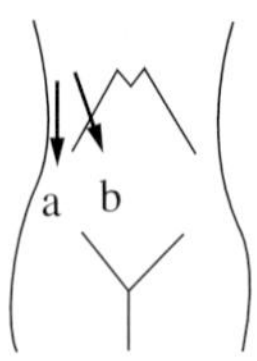

Figure 3-21. Hemangioma.
The adult type of these common lesions has strong echoes. The intensity of the echoes is a suggestive feature, and they are often found in a subcapsular position. Note in (a) the mirror image of the lesion projected into the right lower zone of the chest.

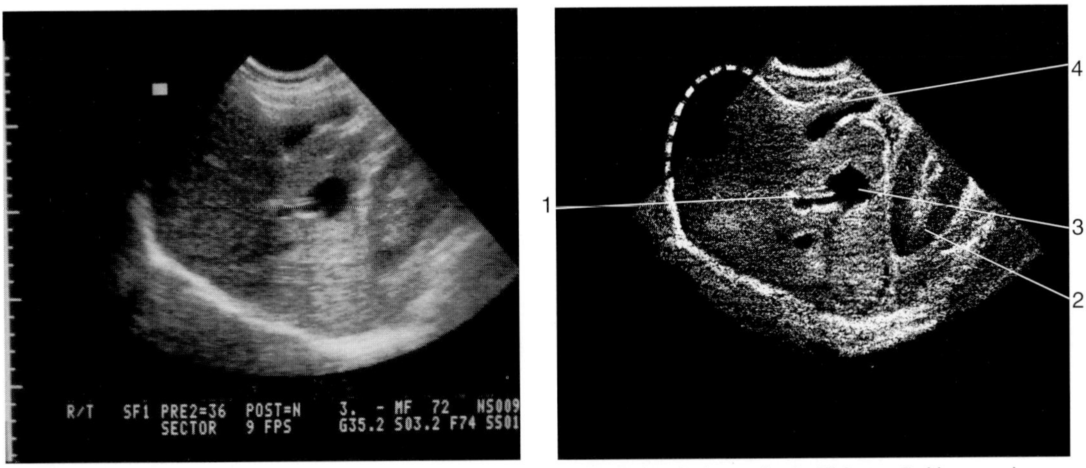

1. Portal vein branch 2. Kidney 3. Hemangioma
4. Edge of gallbladder

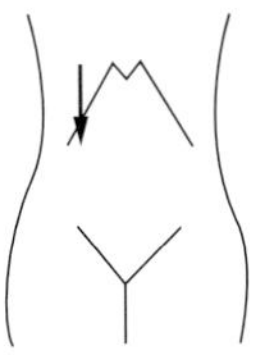

Figure 3-22. Hemangioma.
The cavernous hemangioma has low-level echoes and shows some distal enhancement. A feeding (or draining) vessel is seen.

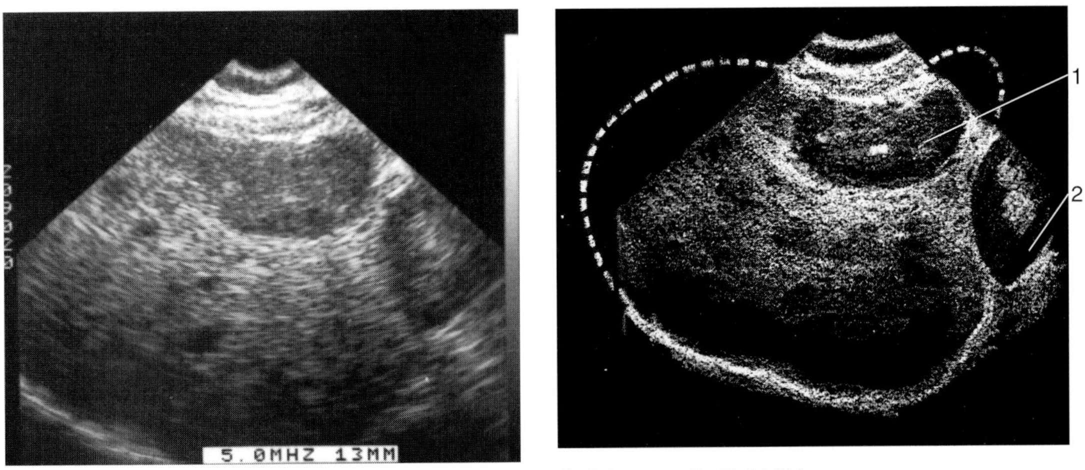

1. Adenoma 2. Right kidney

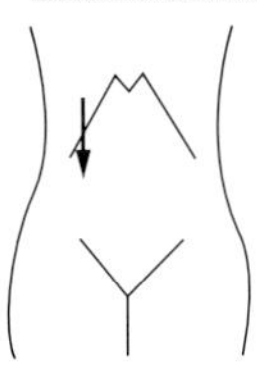

Figure 3-23. Estrogen adenoma.
This well-defined, somewhat heterogeneous mass was due to an estrogen adenoma. (Figure courtesy of Dr. A.E. Joseph)

a 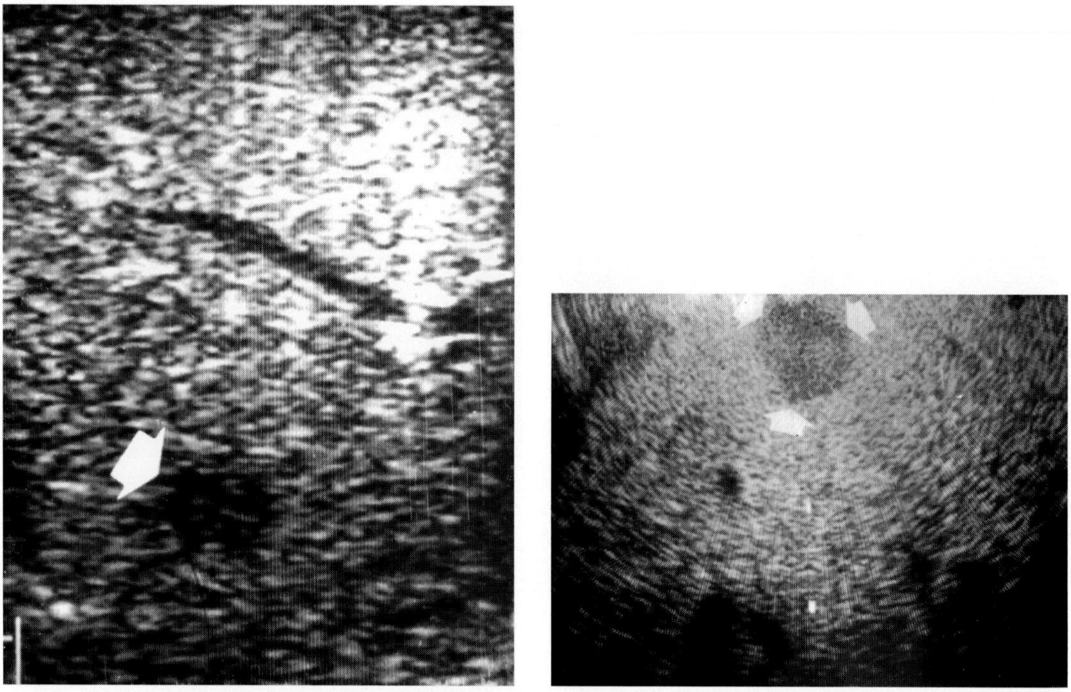 b

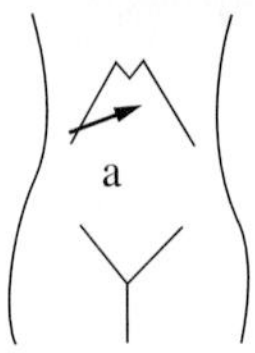

Figure 3-24. Focal nodular hyperplasia.
Multiple small, echo-poor lesions in the liver mimic hepatocellular carcinoma in this case of focal nodular hyperplasia (a). Although the appearance of the nodules is similar to that of primary hepatocellular carcinoma, the slight irregularity in contour and the strand-like structure in the mass (arrow) barely suggest the diagnosis. Laparoscopic ultrasound (b) with a 10-MHz transducer clearly demonstrates the characteristic ground-glass pattern of focal nodular hyperplasia (arrows).

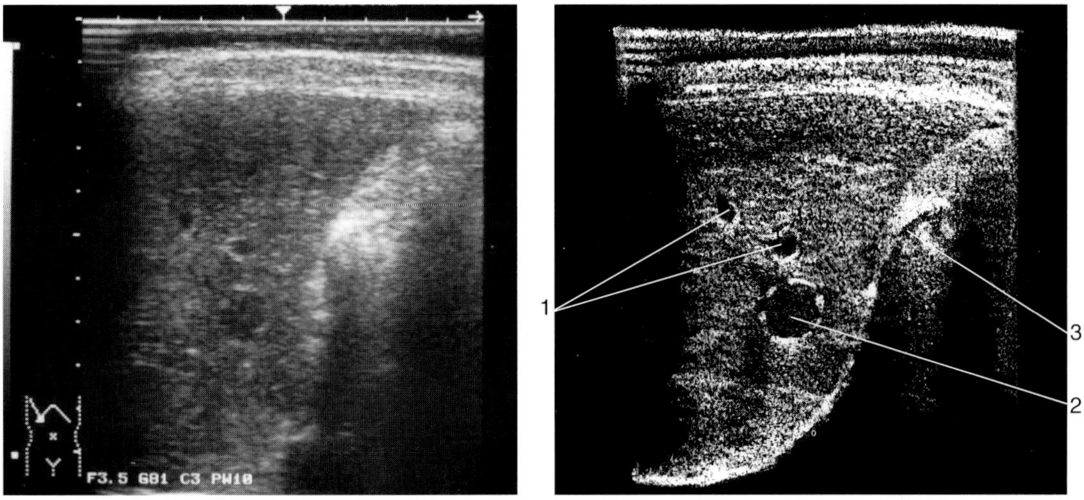

1. Portal vein branches 2. Hepatoma 3. Stomach/ colon

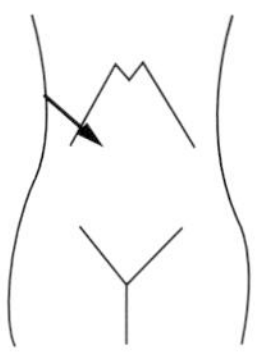

Figure 3-25. Hepatocellular carcinoma.
In the early stage of hepatocellular carcinoma, a slightly irregular, echo-poor nodule may be the sole sonographic sign, as in this patient. Usually the nature of the mass cannot be determined by ultrasound alone; more invasive modalities such as angiography, dynamic CT, or laparoscopy are usually needed for confirmation.

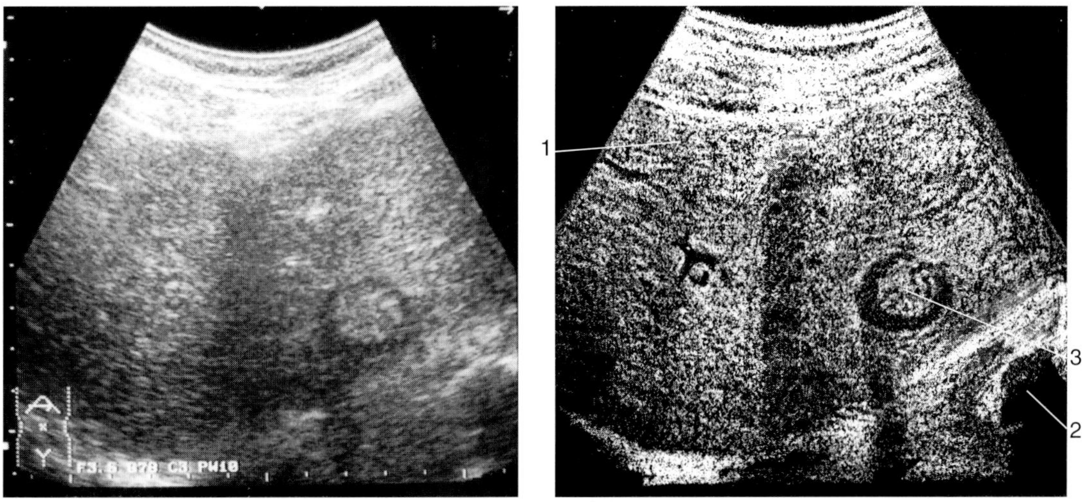

1. Right lobe of liver 2. Spine 3 .Hepatoma

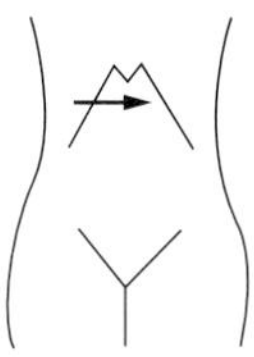

Figure 3-26. Hepatocellular carcinoma.
Hepatocellular carcinoma in its very early stage usually lacks the typical sonographic features of a poorly reflective mass with a mosaic pattern, posterior echo enhancement, or lateral shadowing originating from the less echogenic capsule. This patient suffered from posttransfusion chronic hepatitis. A small, well-demarcated, poorly echogenic mass with a halo developed in the subdiaphragmatic portion of the left lobe of the liver. The diagnosis of hepatocellular carcinoma was confirmed at surgery.

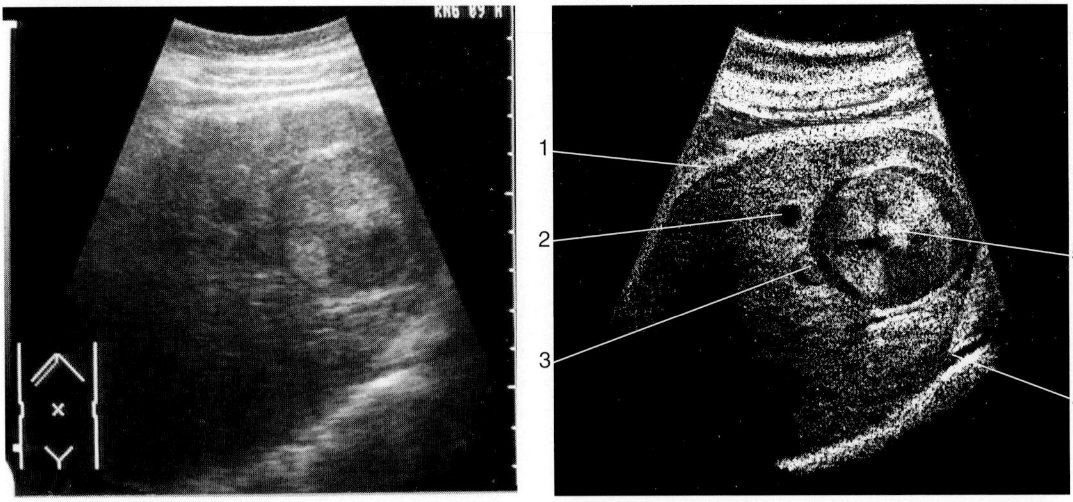

1. Liver 2. Hepatic vein 3. Thrombus in portal vein branch 4. Gut 5. Hepatoma

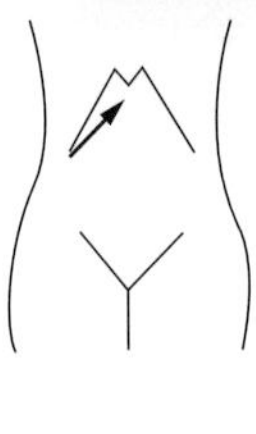

Figure 3-27. Hepatocellular carcinoma.
At a later stage of hepatoma development, the characteristic mosaic pattern is seen. Here the tumor texture consists of multiple separate regions representing nodules of differing reflectivity. In this example the tumor is spherical, with a thin, echo-poor rim. Intravascular tumor thrombi were also identified.

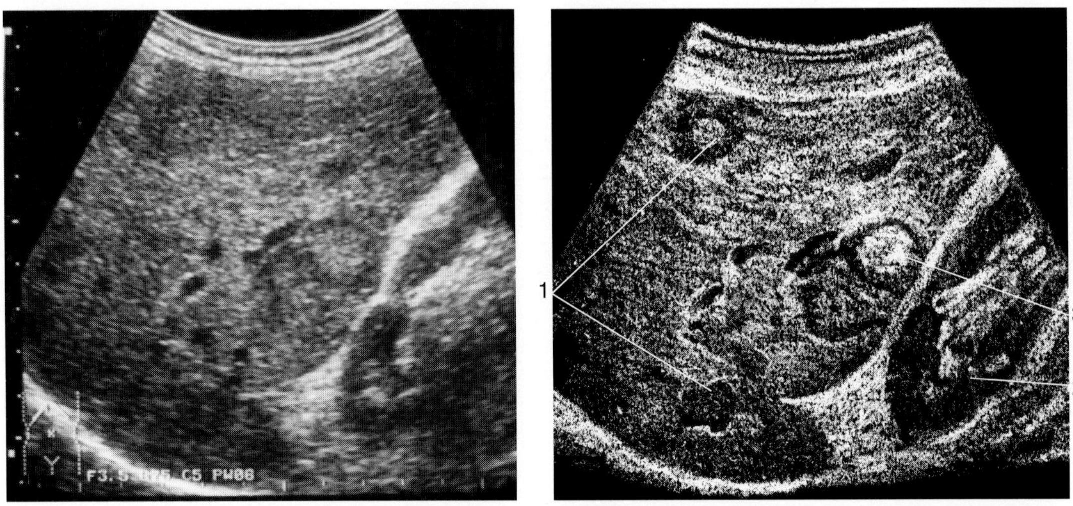

1. Mass 2. Right kidney 3. Hepatocellular carcinoma

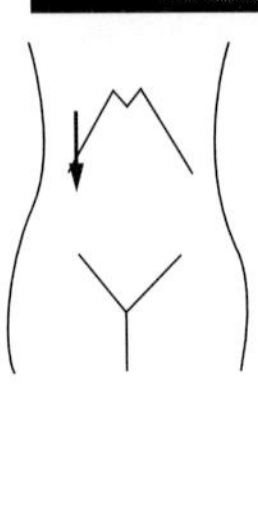

Figure 3-28. Hepatocellular carcinoma with distant metastases.
This patient was referred for ultrasound from the chest clinic when a biopsy of a pulmonary mass was found to contain metastatic hepatoma. A mass was demonstrated in the right lobe of the liver, with several smaller masses elsewhere. The main lesion is rather ill-defined, the poorly demarcated appearance being typical of a rapidly growing hepatocellualr carcinoma.

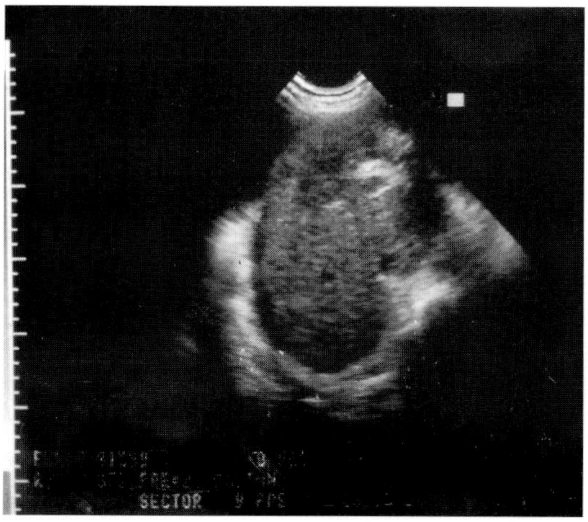

a

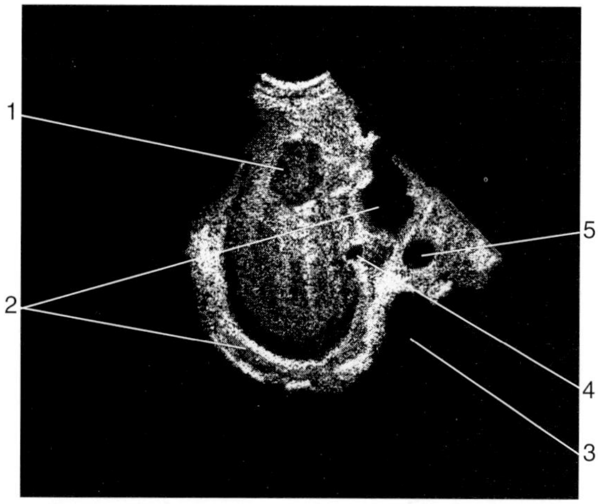

1. Lesion 2. Ascites 3. Spine 4. Inferior vena cava 5. Aorta

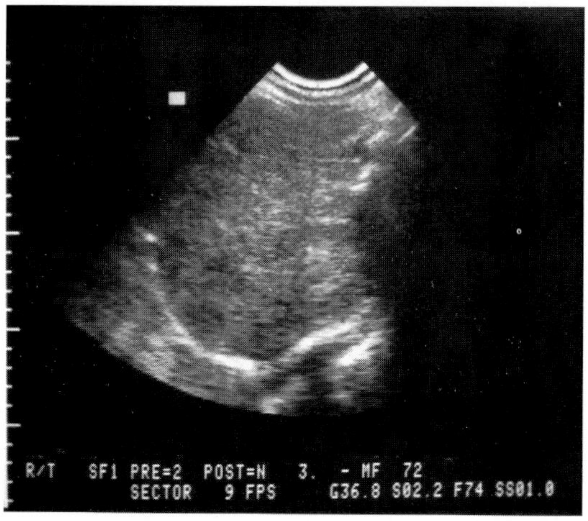

b

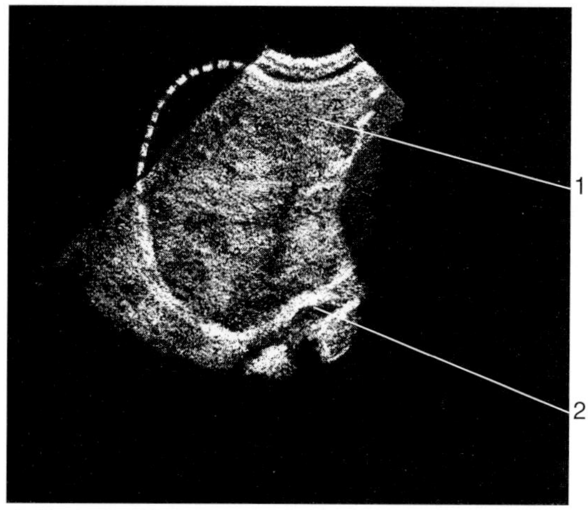

1. Liver 2. Rib

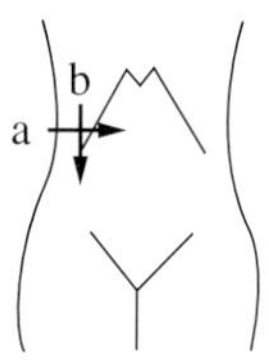

Figure 3-29. Hepatoma.
The echo-poor focal lesion in (a) is readily detected but is indistinguishable from a secondary deposit. Suspicion may be raised by demonstration of features of cirrhosis, such as the ascites seen in this case.
Diffuse hepatoma (b) is much more difficult to detect. All that is seen is an irregularity of the liver texture, which has a pattern very similar to that of cirrhosis.

a

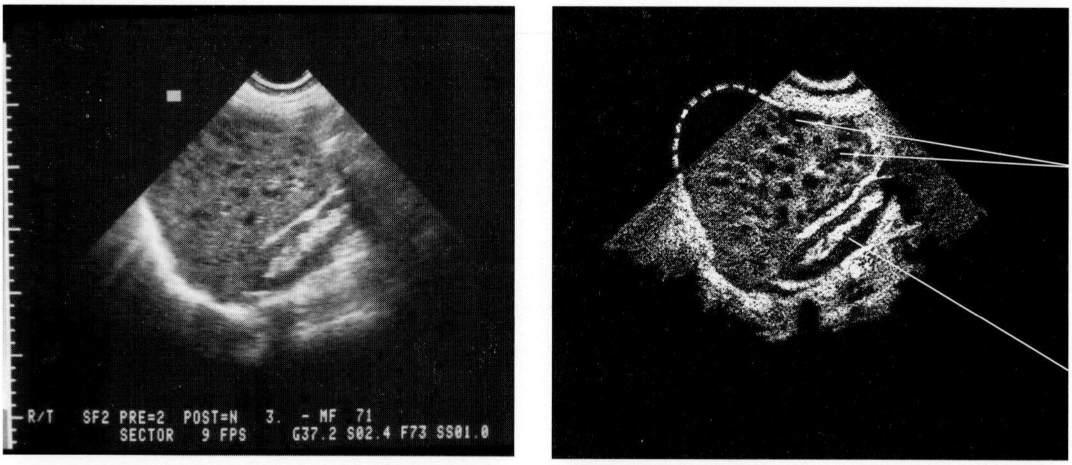

1. Deposits 2. Kidney

b

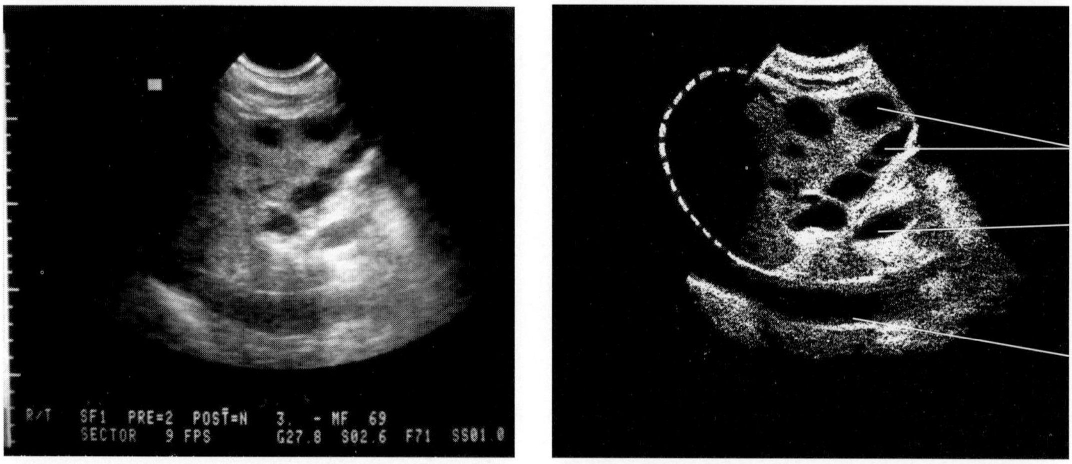

1. Deposits 2. Splenic vein 3. Inferior vena cava

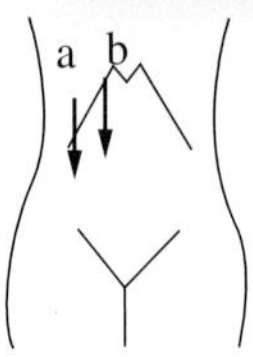

Figure 3-30. Metastases—echo-poor.
The most common variety of liver metastasis is the echo-poor type, in which rounded masses of reduced reflectivity are found. Note the hepatomegaly and blunting of the normally sharp free edge of the liver. In (b) the anterior surface is nodular.

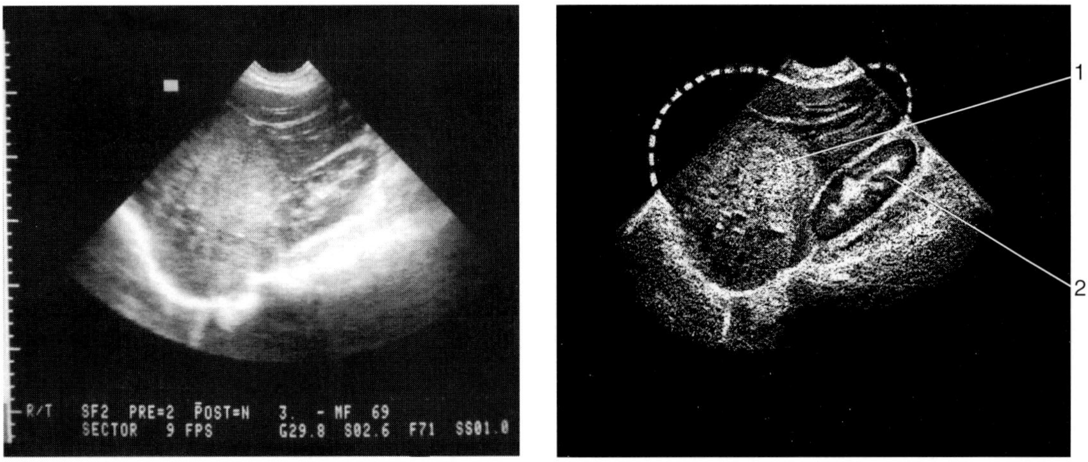

1. Deposit 2. Kidney

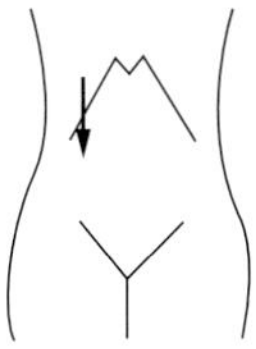

Figure 3-31. Metastasis—echogenic.
This large colonic metastasis shows the typical intense echoes.

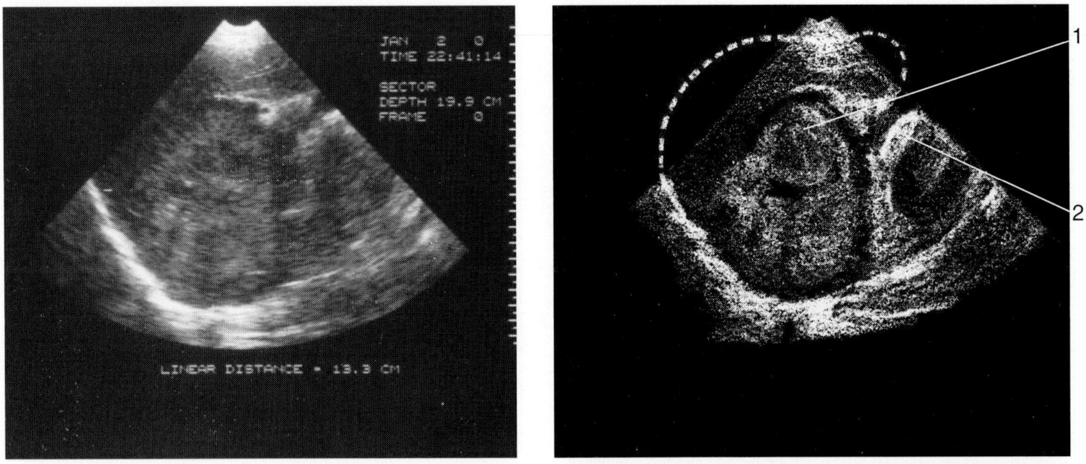

a

1. Large deposit 2. Hepatic flexure of colon

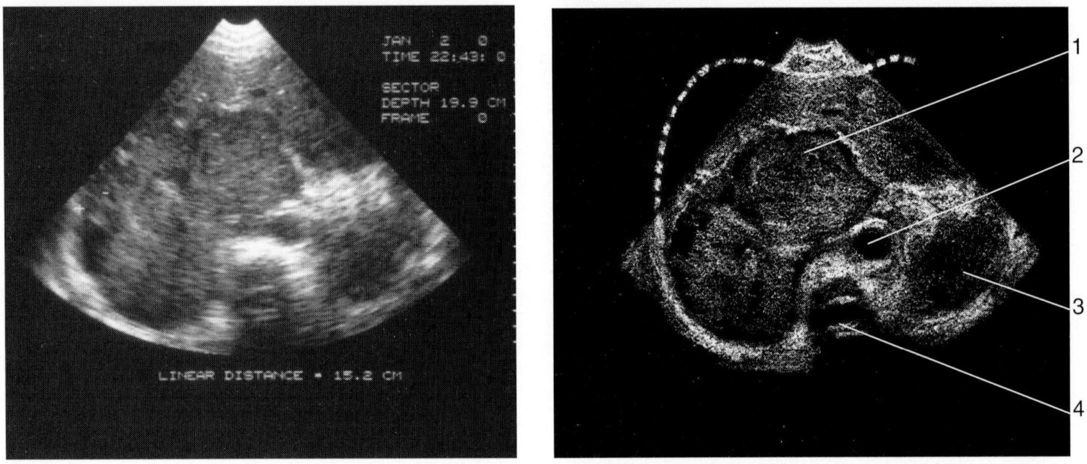

b

1. Large deposit 2. Aorta 3. Stomach 4. Spinal canal

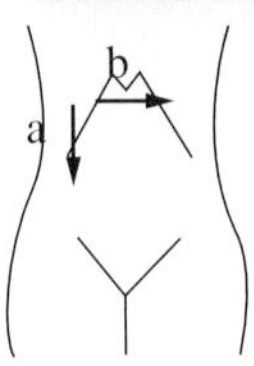

Figure 3-32. Metastasis—large, echo-poor.
Though extensive, this lesion is only slightly different in reflectivity from the surrounding liver. Such low-contrast lesions are easily missed altogether.

a

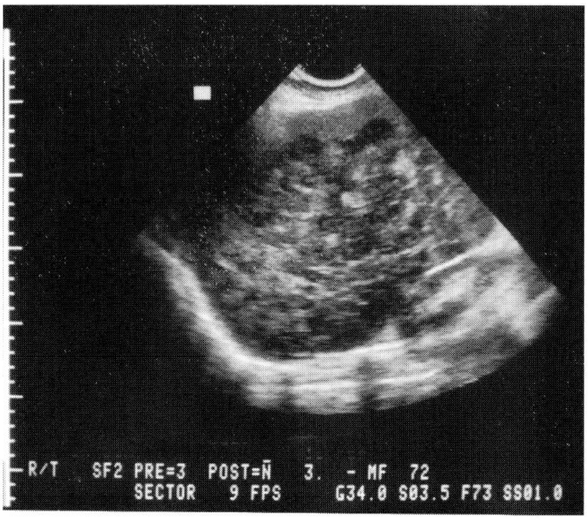

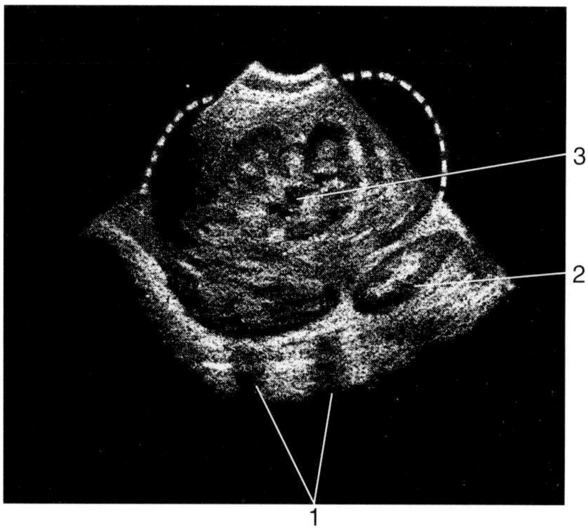

1. Ribs 2. Right kidney 3. Diffuse deposits

b

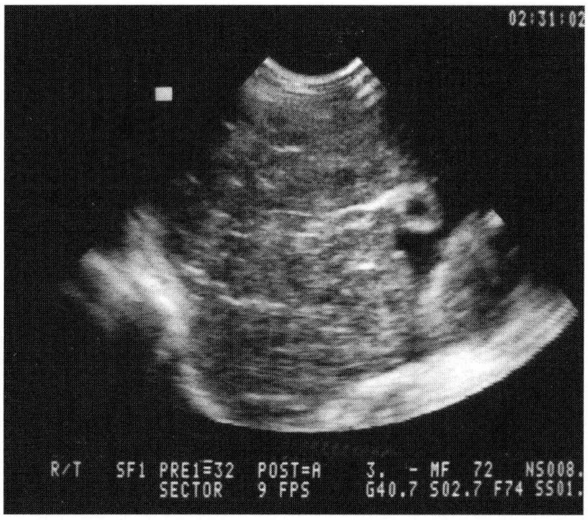

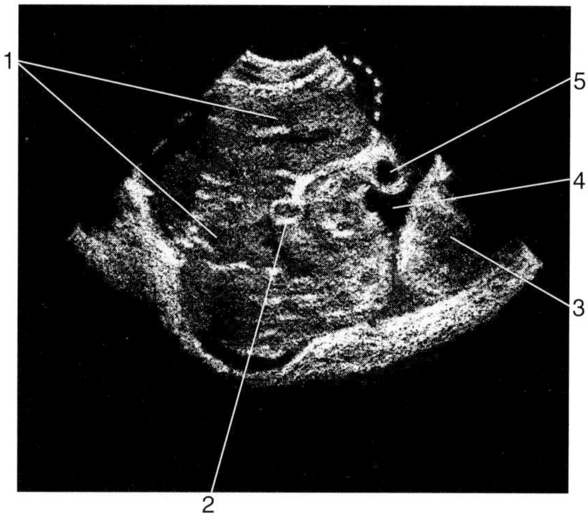

1. Diffuse deposits 2. Right portal vein 3. Ascending colon 4. Ascites 5. Gallbladder

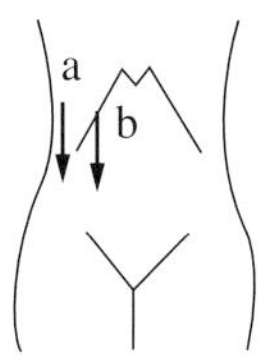

Figure 3-33. Metastases—diffuse.
Confluent, small lesions give an irregular, "moth-eaten" pattern to the liver. The abnormality is easily overlooked. Follow-up assessment is difficult in these cases because there is no discrete lesion that can be measured on serial scans.

a

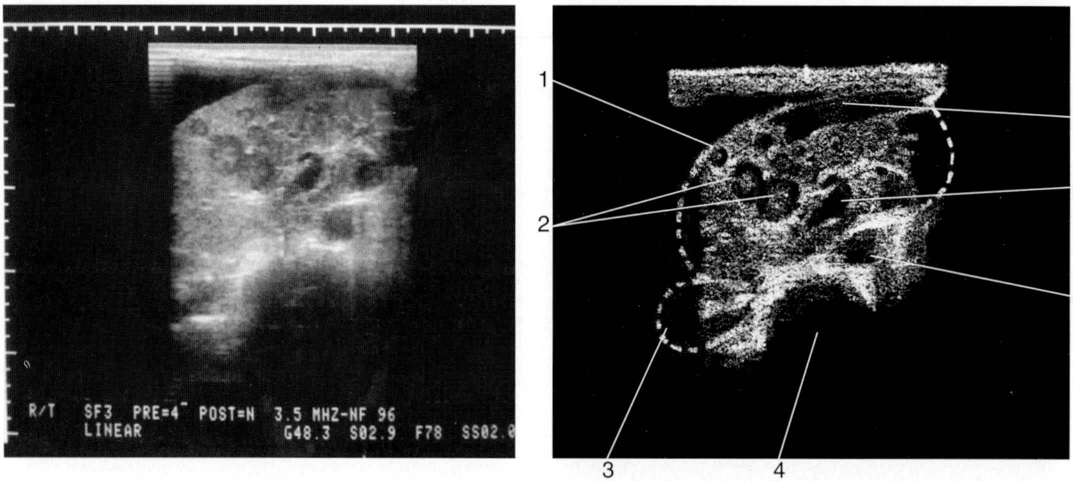

1. Ascites 2. Target lesions 3. Kidney 4. Spine
5. Aorta 6. Portal vein 7. Echo-poor lesion

b

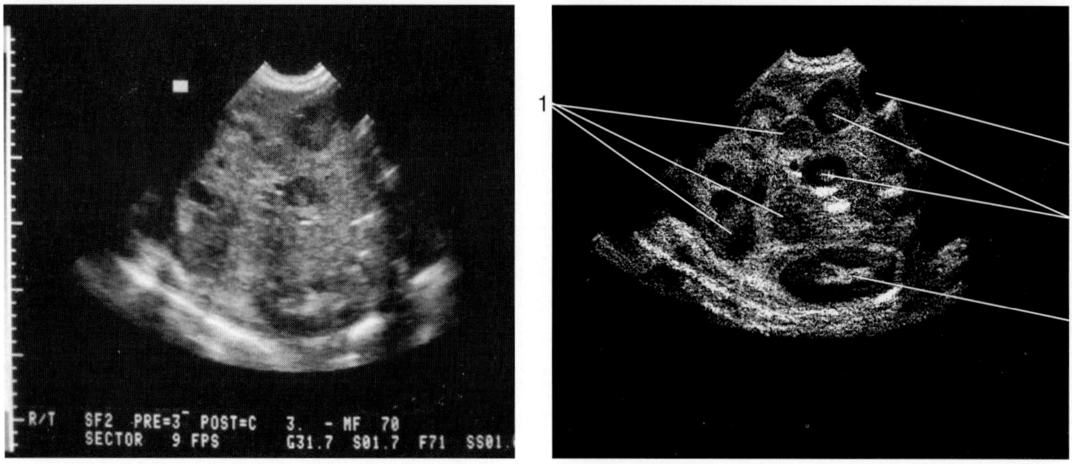

1. Echo-poor lesions 2. Kidney 3. Target lesions
4. Gallbladder

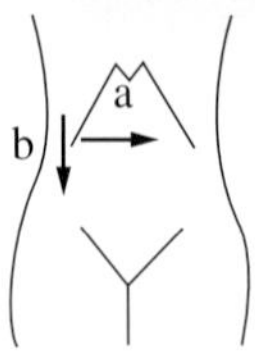

Figure 3-34. Metastases—target type.
Metastases with a concentric ring pattern form an eye-catching variety of liver deposit. Any type of tumor can assume this pattern.

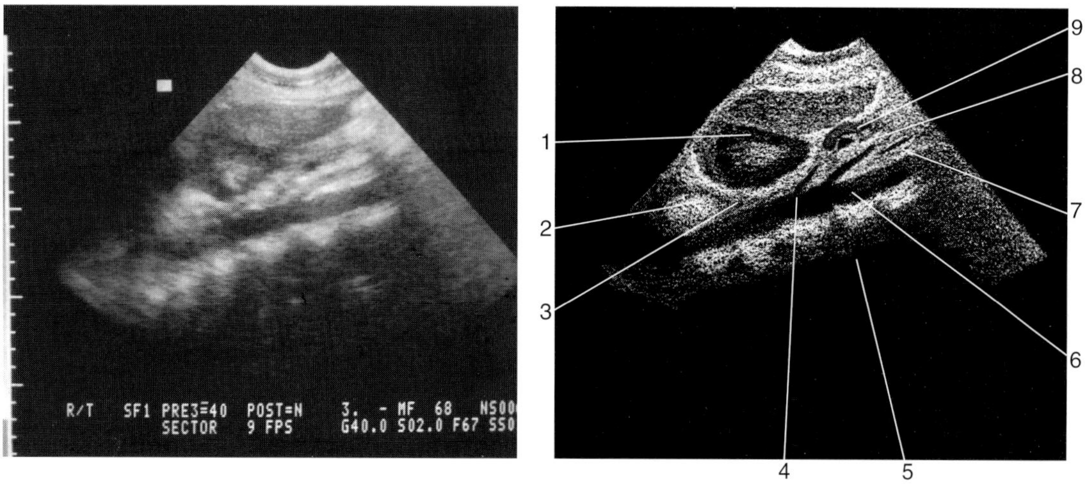

a

1. Target lesion 2. Esophagus 3. Crus of diaphragm 4. Celiac axis (trunk) 5. Spine 6. Aorta 7. Left renal vein 8. Superior mesenteric artery 9. Pancreas and splenic vein

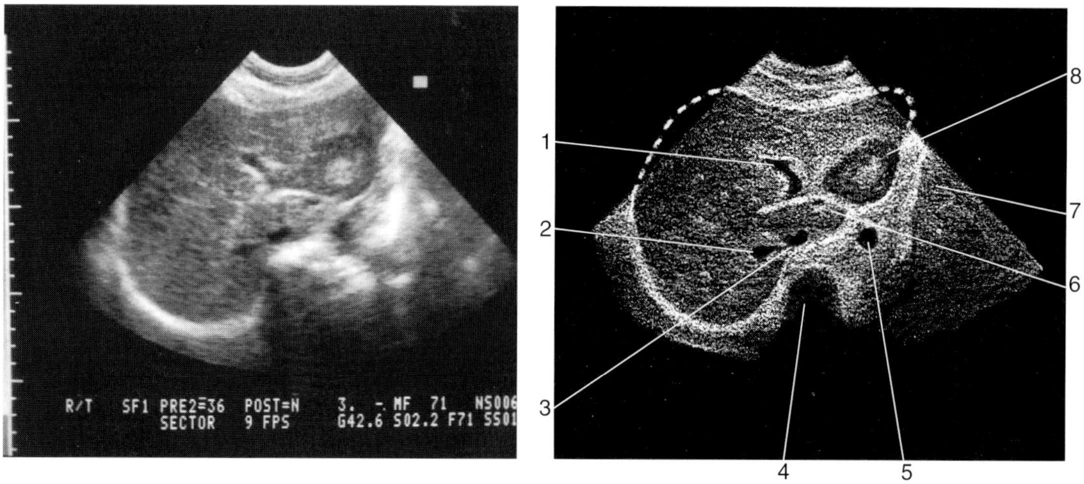

b

1. Portal vein 2. Right hepatic vein 3. Inferior vena cava 4. Spine 5. Aorta 6. Caudate lobe of liver 7. Stomach 8. Target lesion

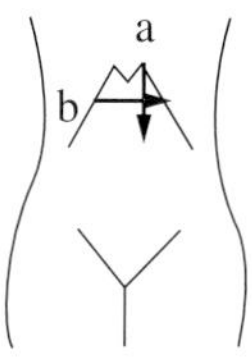

Figure 3-35. Metastasis—target type.
This large target or bull's-eye lesion in the left lobe shows the mass effect producing a nodule on the visceral surface of the liver.

a

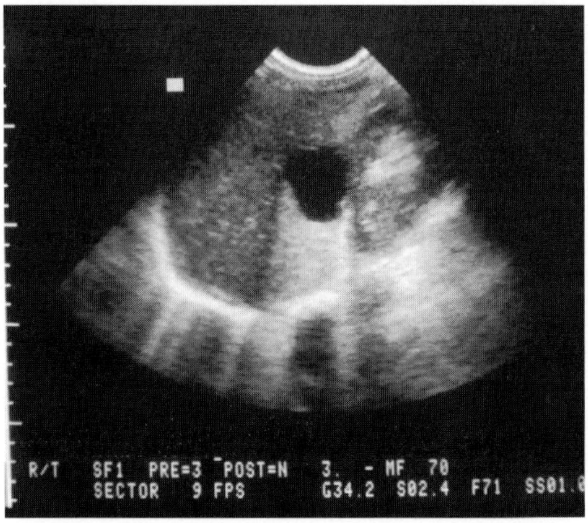

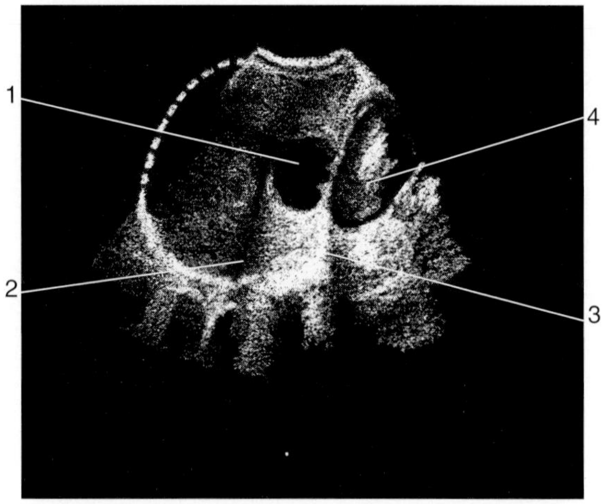

1. Cystic lesion 2. Refraction shadow 3. Enhancement 4. Kidney

b

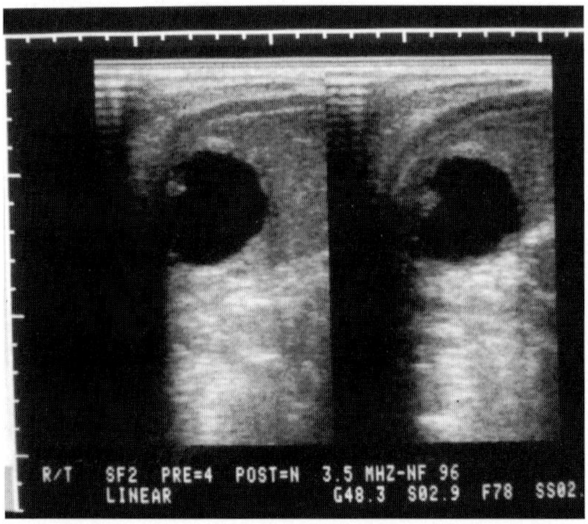

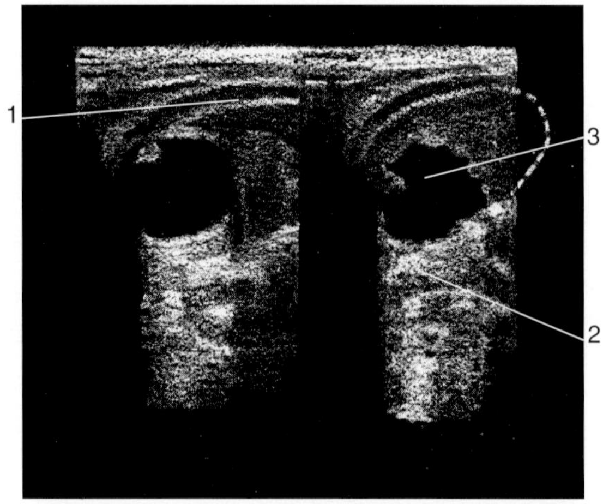

1. Left lobe of liver 2. Enhancement 3. Cystic lesion

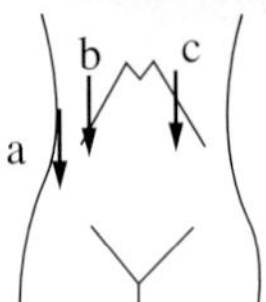

Figure 3-36. Metastases—cystic.
Cystic deposits may result from mucin-secreting tumors (a, b) or from necrosis within a deposit (c; see Figure 3-11). The former, usually arising from mucin-secreting primaries such as those of the pancreas, colon, or ovary, may have smooth walls, but usually there is some telltale irregularity. A thick, irregular wall is typical of the necrotic type (c), but all of these lesions may pose a diagnostic problem.

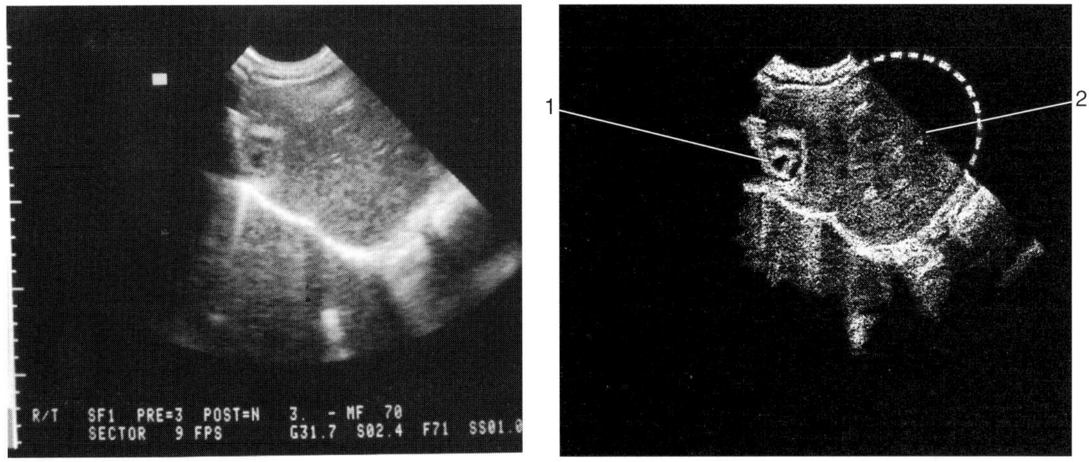

c

1. Central 'cyst' in complex lesion 2. Right lobe of liver

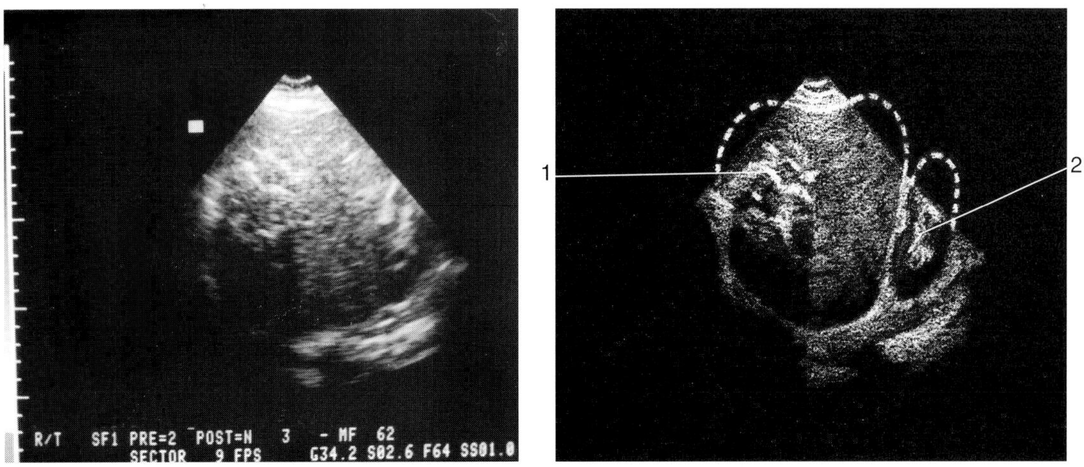

1. Calcific metastasis 2. Right kideny

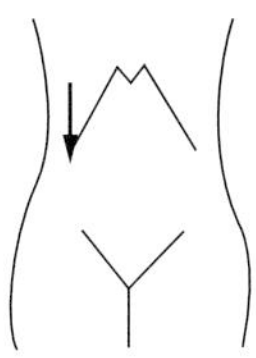

Figure 3-37. Metastasis—calcified.
Calcification gives strong echoes with distal shadowing, provided that the calcific foci are sufficiently large. This was a remnant from a healed teratomatous deposit. The calcification was more obvious on a CT scan.

DIFFUSE DISEASES

Two distinct patterns of diffuse disease with uniform alteration of liver reflectivity can be indentified: the so-called bright and dark livers in reference to the echo levels produced.

In the *bright liver* the overall echo levels are increased [17, 32, 44] (Figure 3-38). This change may be so marked as to be obvious on scanning, but references to internal landmarks improve diagnostic sensitivity. The kidney forms a useful internal standard. Usually the cortical echoes are somewhat lower than the liver echoes, but when liver reflectivity is increased, the difference increases, so that gain levels set to display the liver as a mid-gray make the renal cortex seem echo-free. Thus a dark-looking kidney is a clue to a bright liver. The other useful reference point is the normal periportal echoes. When the liver echoes are intense, they come to match these periportal echoes, which are then masked. The liver acquires a uniform "ground-glass" texture because of the loss of vascular markings.

The bright liver pattern is seen in a wide range of chronic diffuse condition[66] (Table 3-3). Fatty change is the most common; there may also be increased attenuation.[20] The increased echoes probably arise from the large number of interfaces produced by groups of fat-laden cells in a watery environment. Usually fatty change is uniform, but focal fatty change also occurs, presumably representing a stage in the development of general fatty change. A geographic pattern of high and low reflectivity is produced by adjacent lobules of normal and infiltrated liver.[80, 92] A single affected lobe gives a highly reflective patch of polygonal shape, the quadrate being the most common site. At the opposite extreme, a remaining spared lobule seems to be an echo-poor region against the reflective background (Figure 3-39). Attention to detail, including the geometric shape of the abnormality, provides the important clues. A biopsy of the echo-poor region will, of course, yield normal liver.

Table 3-3. Causes of bright liver.

Fatty change
Cirrhosis, fbrosis
Chronic hepatitis
Lipid and glycogen storage diseases
Hemochromatosis, hemosiderosis
Granulomata

Cirrhosis gives high echoes due to the presence of fibrous tissue in combination with any accompanying fatty change. There is often distinct enlargement of the caudate lobe, which is easily assessed in either sagittal or transverse section (Figure 3-40); the caudate lobe is usually less than half the width of the right lobe measured from the lateral margin of the porta.[35] In cirrhosis it may be of equal size; an upper limit of about two-thirds is suggested, and this can also be assessed in the anteroposterior dimension. Nodularity of the liver surface may be apparent.[18] It is more obvious when there is ascites, since the fluid reveals the liver surface more clearly [71] (Figure 3-41). The liver may be enlarged in the early stage, but later it shrinks.[94] In many cases of cirrhosis, the liver seems quite normal on ultrasound, so that only about 50 per cent of cases of cirrhosis can be detected by subjective criteria. Tissue characterization may improve sensitivity and may provide quantitative measures that could be useful in follow-up.[25, 26, 63]

Since regenerating nodules are rarely visualized (Figure 3-42), differential diagnosis is possible only if associated features of portal hypertension are present. Ascites and splenomegaly are the most obvious. Varices at the esophagus, the spleen, or the head of the pancreas can be demonstrated as tortous vascular spaces [37, 45, 46, 84] (Figure 3-43). More sensitivity is demonstrated with color Doppler. The umbilical vein may recanalize and form an obvious vessel within the ligamentum teres [29, 77] (Figure 3-44). The portal vein may dilate (the lumen is normally less than 15 mm), but this is not a frequent feature. Reduction of the portal blood velocity to below 13 cm/sec is an indicator of high pressure, and hepatofugal flow occurs in extreme cases. These measurements are facilitated if color Doppler is available.

Occlusion of the portal vein gives rise to prehepatic portal hypertension with varices but without the liver decompensation that dominates the clinical pattern in cirrhosis. Malignant, infective, and traumatic damage to the portal vein are the usual causes, carcinoma of the pancreas being most common in adults (Figure 3-45). Since fresh thrombus is usually echo-free, Doppler is required to establish the diagnosis. Mature thrombus and invading tumor are echogenic—demonstration of arterial Doppler signals within the latter establishes the free diagnosis. Reestablishment of effective portal flow may occur via a sheath of collaterals in the hepatic pedicle, producing the mistitled "cavernous transformation" of the portal vein.[47] This is well demonstrated on color Doppler.

Chronic hepatitis is another important cause of the bright liver pattern, the strong echoes here being due to fibrosis.[49] If the necrosis and scarring are nonuniform, the ultrasound picture is heterogeneous.

Schistosomiasis also produces a bright liver, but in addition, the periportal fibrosis may be evident (Figure 3-46). Two patterns occur; in *Schistosoma mansonii*, the larger, proximal veins are chiefly affected, producing thick, reflective walls to the portal veins close to the porta hepatis.[1, 2] The smaller ova of *S. japonicum* lodge deeper in the liver, so that more peripheral vessels are affected, and there may be calcification.[4]

The *dark liver* has the opposite features with low-level echoes such that the liver matches the renal cortex.[50] The dark liver throws the periportal echoes into relief, showing an apparent increase in the vascular marking and a streaky pattern (Figure 3-47). The conditions causing the dark liver (Table 3-4) are those associated with an increase in the water content of the liver; presumably the effect is due simply to increased separation between the echo-producing structures. It is commonly seen in congestive heart failure, where it may persist for surprisingly long periods after antifailure treatment. In the leukemias, infiltrating lymphocytes produce hepatomegaly with low-level echoes. The infiltrating cells may be neoplastic or reactive, so a specific diagnosis of liver involvement cannot be made without biopsy. In hepatitis, additional features are commonly noted, including thickening of the gallbladder walls, presumably due to direct extension of the inflammation, and hilar lymphadenopathy.[89]

Alcohol is the most common toxin causing hepatitis in most countries; often there is a background of cirrhosis or of fatty change due to malnutrition. The combination may produce an irregular, blotchy pattern, with geographic zones of interspersed high- and low-level echoes. Several other conditions produce this type of patchiness in the liver, especially diffuse or confluent malignant disease (see Table 3-2).

Table 3-4. Causes of dark liver.

Inflammatory
Acute hepatitis
Viral
Toxic
Congestive
Congestive heart failure
Infiltrative
Lymphoma
Leukemia

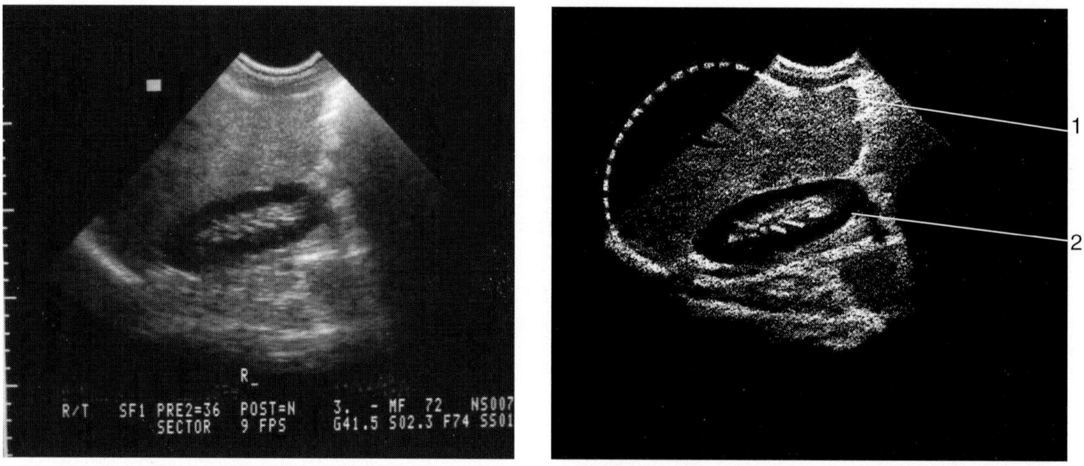

1. Liver 2. Right kidney

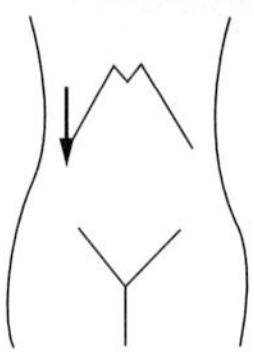

Figure 3-38. Bright liver.
The high level of echoes from the liver parenchyma exaggerates the contrast with the kidney so that this organ appears black. It also masks the periportal echoes giving the liver a smooth, ground-glass texture, with paucity of vascular markings. This was a patient with fatty change.

a

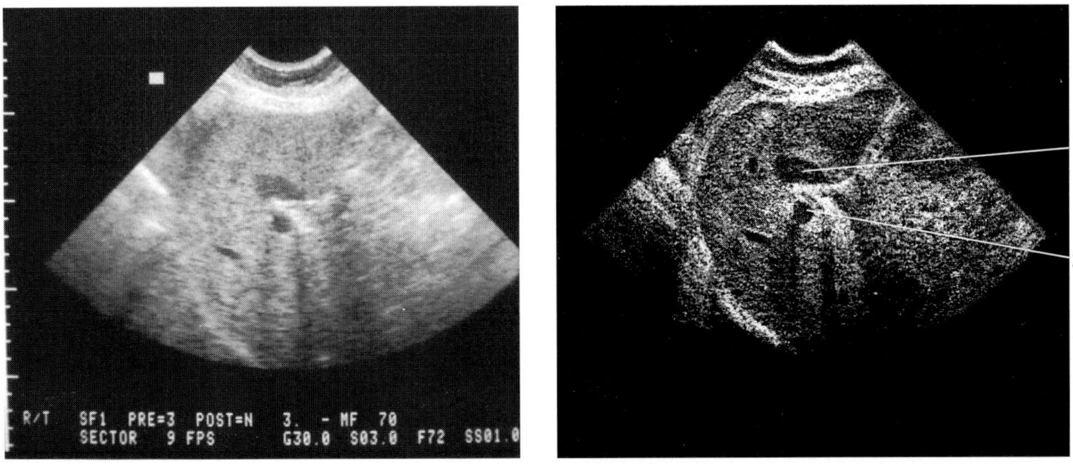

1. Echo-poor "lesion" 2. Porta hepatis

b

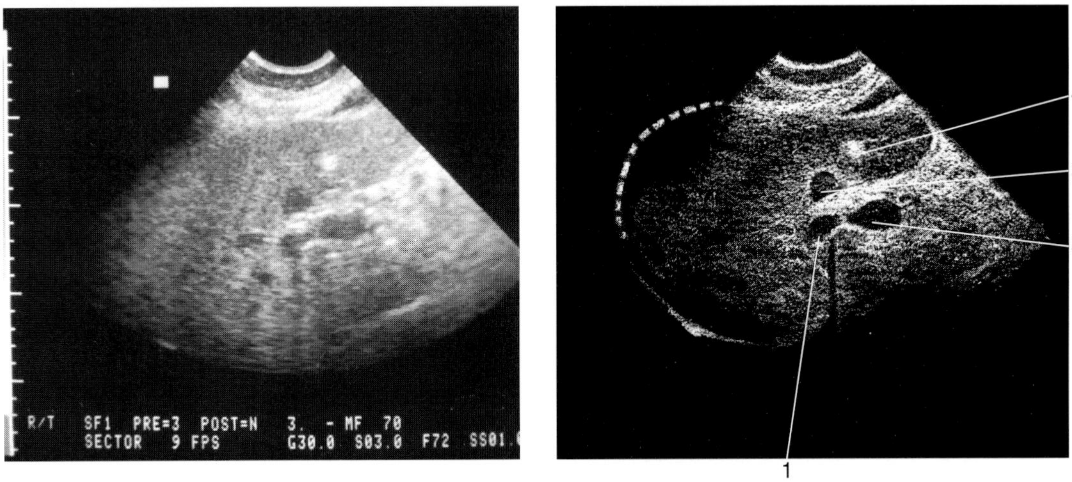

1. Inferior vena cava 2. Aorta 3. Echo-poor "lesion" 4. Ligamentum teres

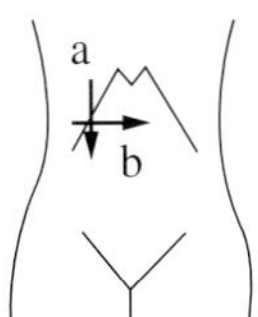

Figure 3-39. Focal fatty sparing.
Fatty change tends to develop in a segmental fashion, giving rectilinear regions of increased reflectivity. Here all of the liver is affected except for part of the quadrate lobe, which masquerades an echo-poor lesion. If this "lesion" is biopsied, normal liver will be obtained. The nearby liver shows fatty change.

a

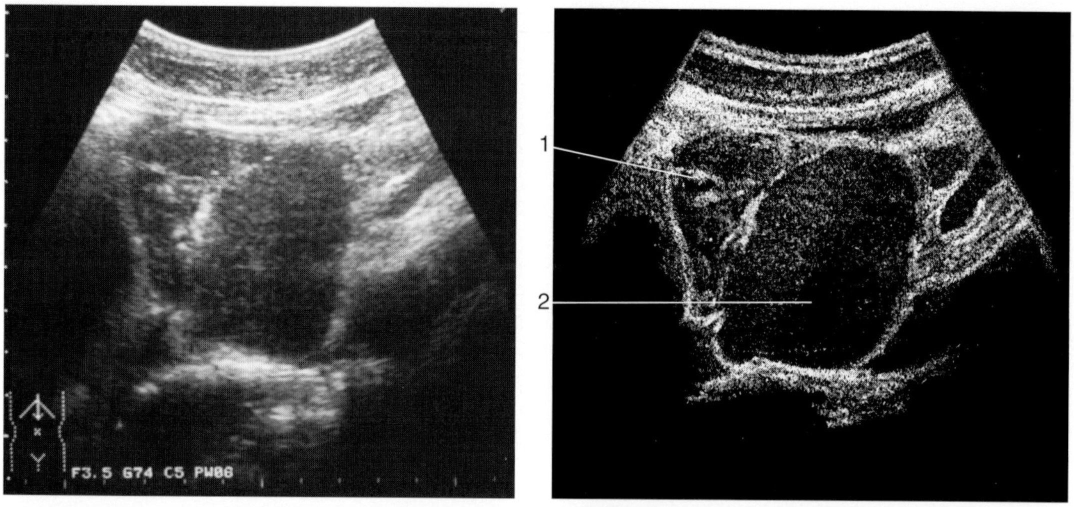

1. Left lobe of liver 2. Caudate lobe of liver

b

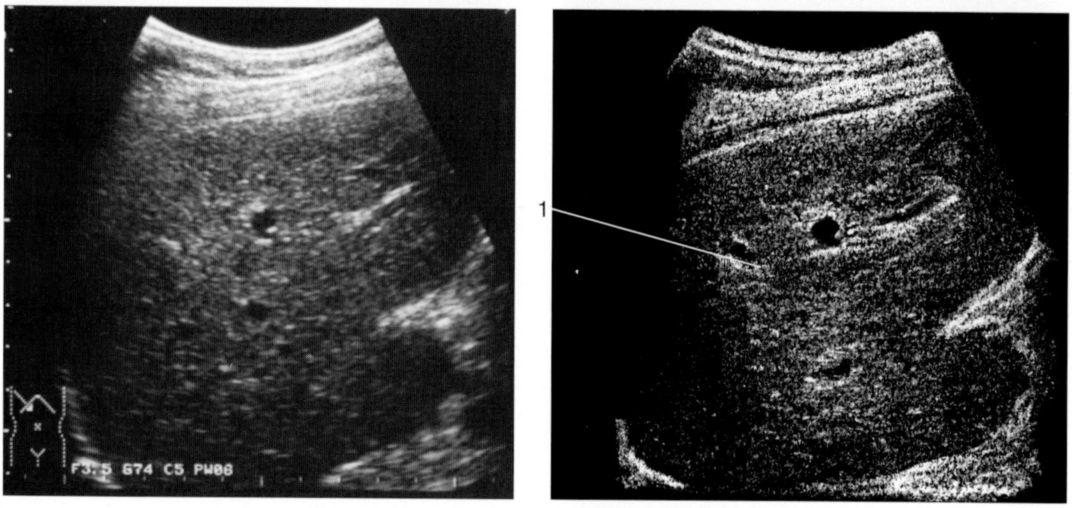

1. Right lobe of liver

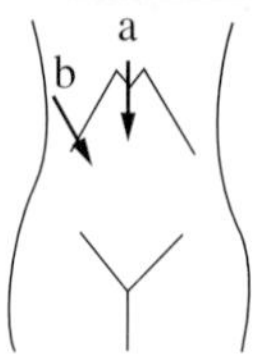

Figure 3-40. Hypertrophy of the caudate lobe in cirrhosis.
Hypertrophy of the caudate lobe of the liver occurs in most patients with cirrhosis, whether caused by alcohol abuse or consisting of the postnecrotic type following hepatitis (B or non-A, non-B). Presumably the special vascular pattern of the caudate underlies the hypertrophy. This patient was a 61-year-old female with a long history of chronic hepatitis. The atrophic left lobe of the liver is almost replaced by the large caudate.

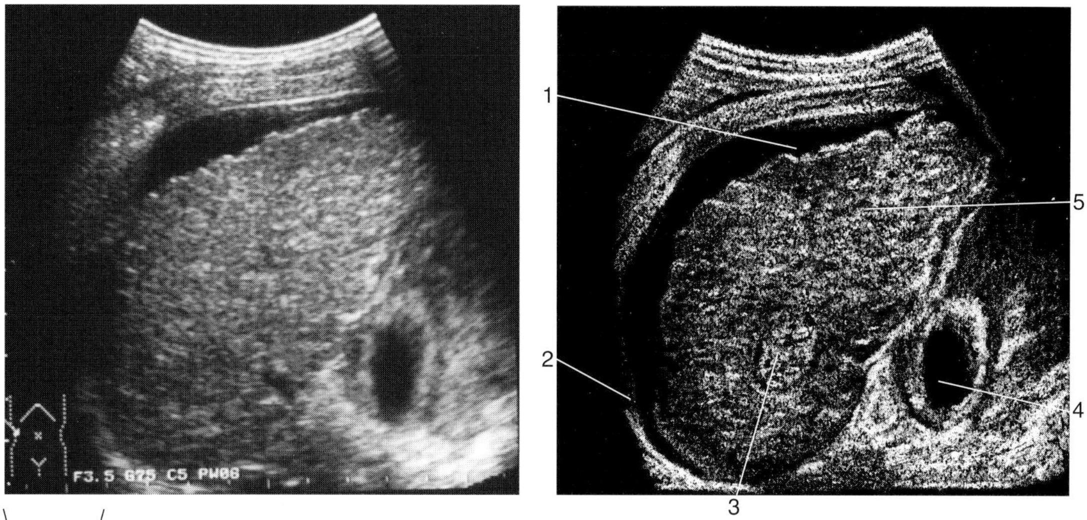

1. Ascites 2. Diaphragm 3. Hyperplastic nodule
4. Gallbladder 5. Left lobe of liver

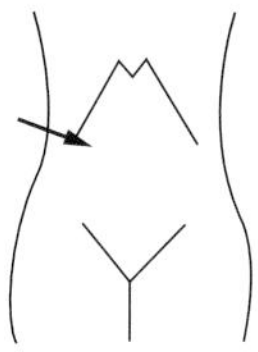

Figure 3-41. Cirrhotic nodules.
The surface irregularity characteristic of cirrhotic change is well shown in this case because of the surrounding ascites, which also demonstrates that the liver has undergone decompensation.

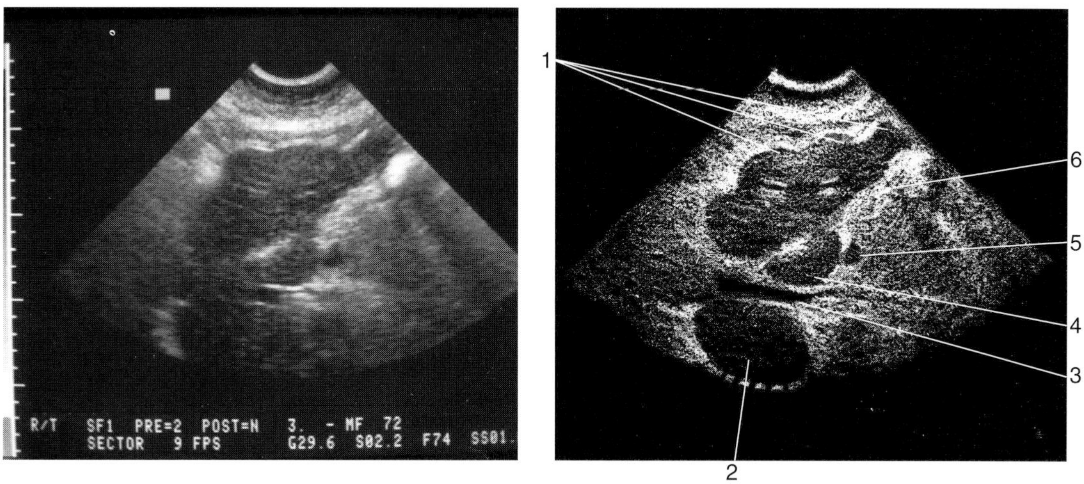

1. Nodular liver surface 2. Medial part of right lobe of liver 3. Inferior vena cava 4. Caudate lobe of liver 5. Splenic vein 6. Stomach

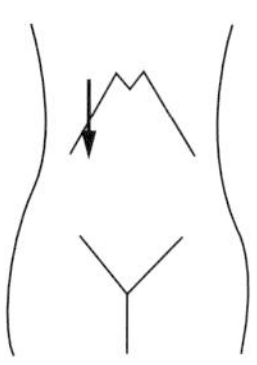

Figure 3-42. Cirrhosis.
In this case of macronodular cirrhosis, the regenerating nodules are sufficiently prominent to be visualized on the anterior surface of the liver. Unless gross, nodularity can only be defined when the liver is surrounded by ascites.

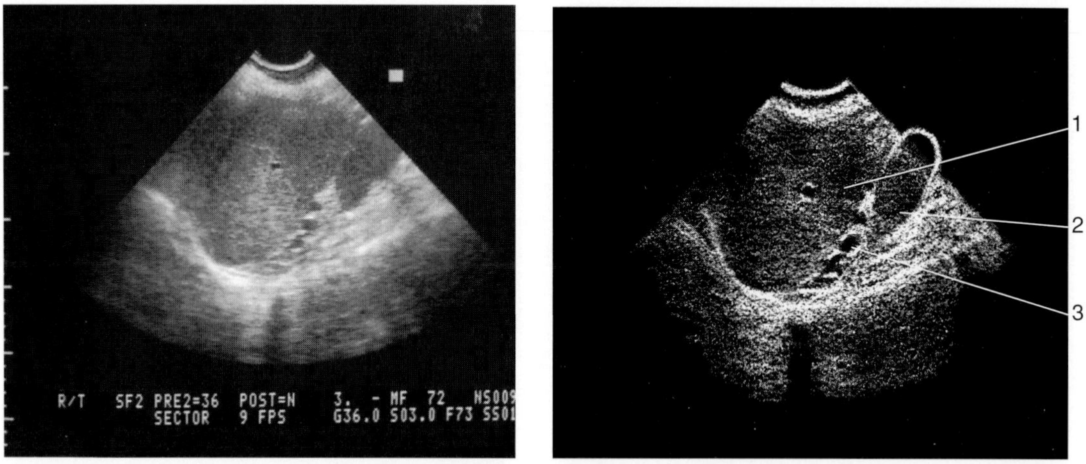

a

1. Spleen 2. Left kidney 3. Varices

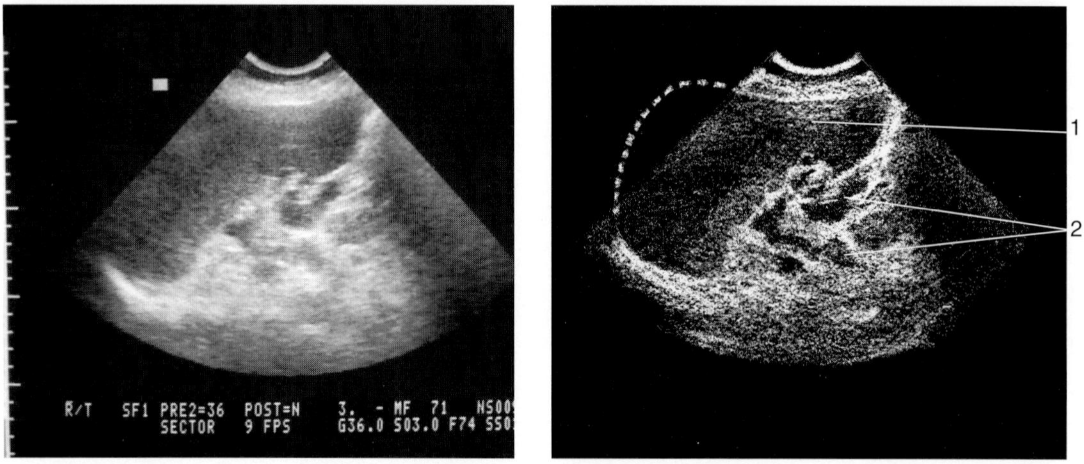

b

1. Spleen 2. Varices

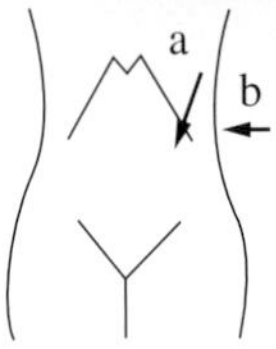

Figure 3-43. Varices around the spleen.
The dilated vessels near the splenic hilum represent variceal lienorenal and gastrosplenic anastomoses.

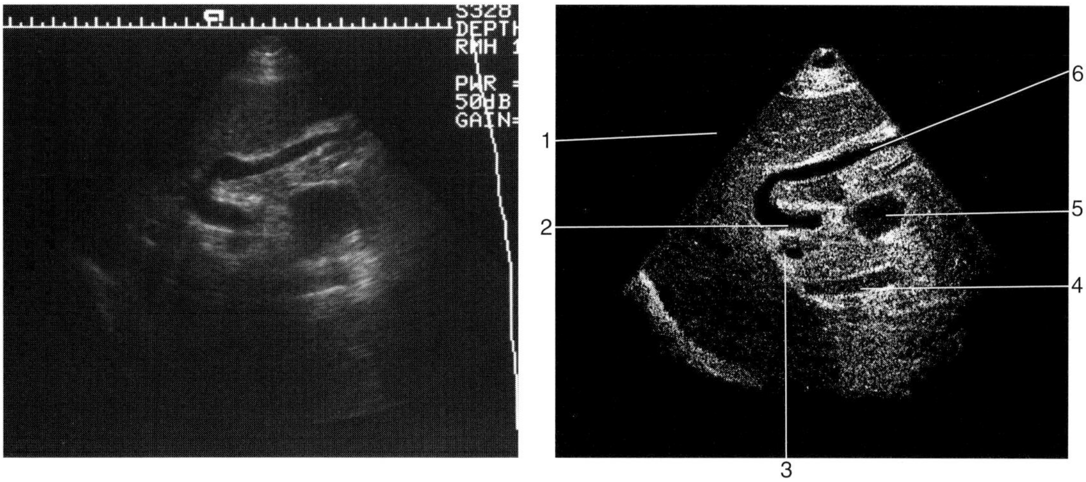

a

1. Left lobe of liver 2. Left portal vein 3. Hepatic artery 4. Inferior vena cava 5. Portal vein trunk 6. Recanalized umbilical vein

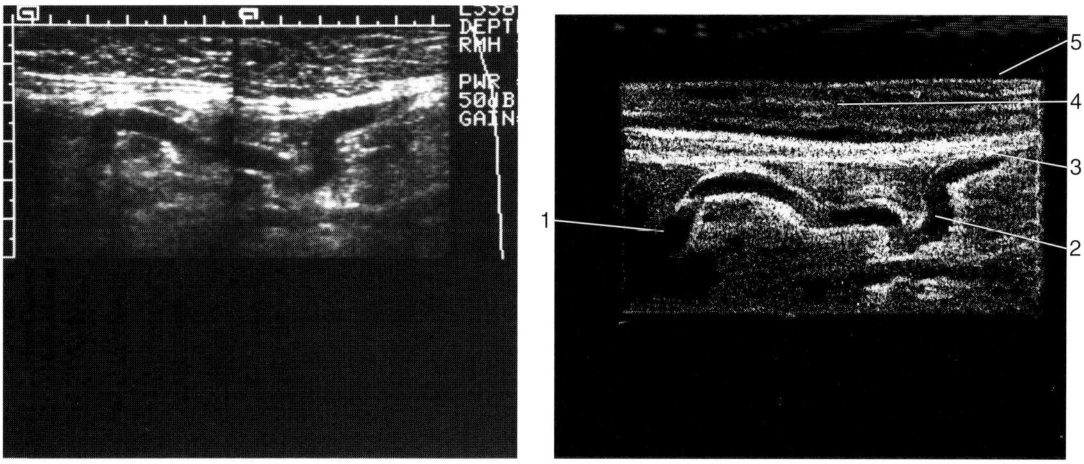

b

1. Left lobe of liver 2. Umbilicus 3. Peritoneum 4. Subcutaneous fat 5. Recanalized umbilical vein

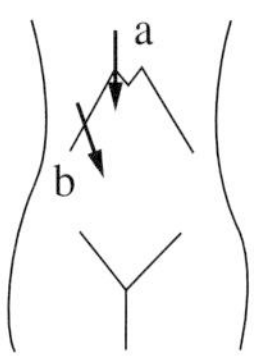

Figure 3-44. Recanalized "umbilical vein."
In this patient with portal hypertension due to cirrhosis, a prominent umbilical (or paraumbilical) vein could be traced, leaving the liver (a) and extending down to the umbilicus (b).

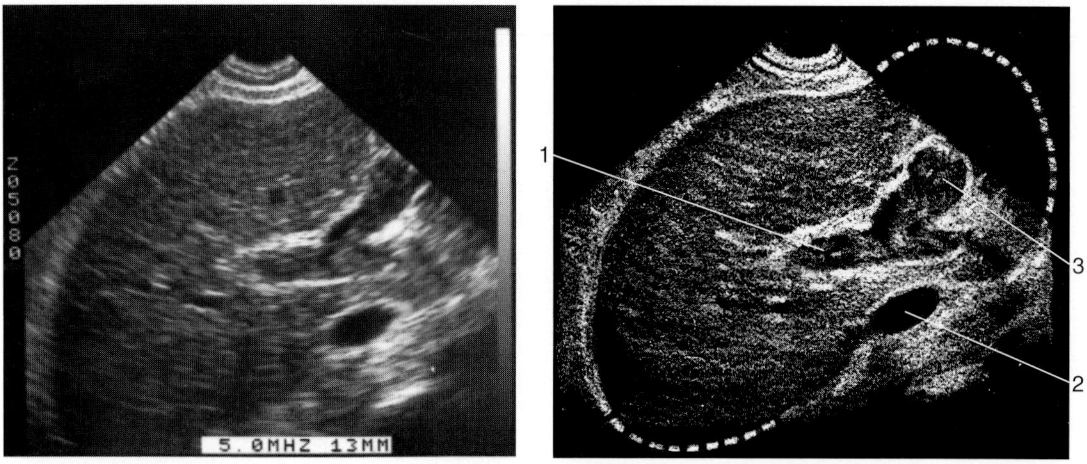

a

1. Thrombus in right portal vein 2. Inferior vena cava 3. Thrombus in left portal vein

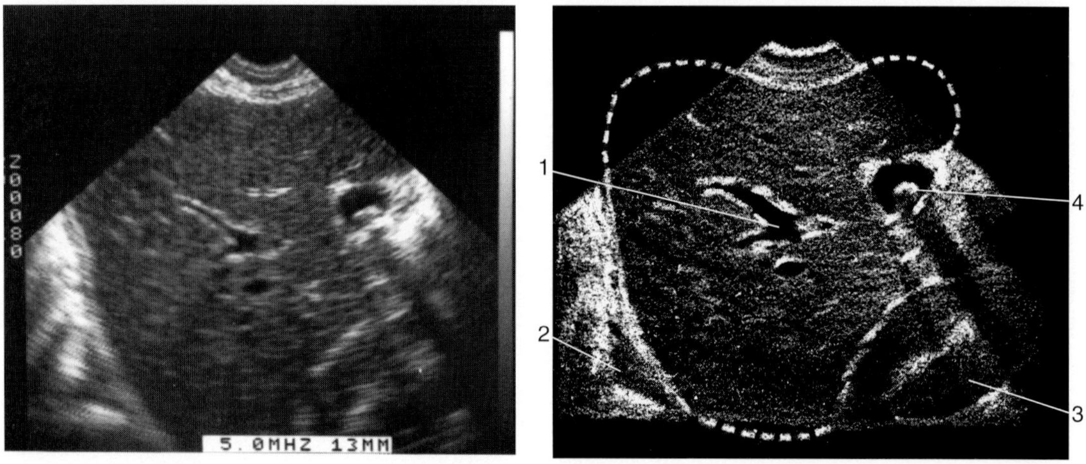

b

1. Thrombus in right portal vein 2. Pleural effusion 3. Right kidney 4. Gallbladder

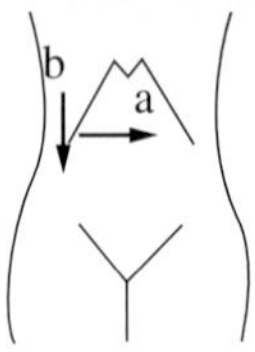

Figure 3-45. Thrombosed portal vein.
Intravascular thrombus appears as immobile, echogenic tissue within the vessel lumen. It is commonly seen with tumor invasion but also occurs with inflammatory processes.

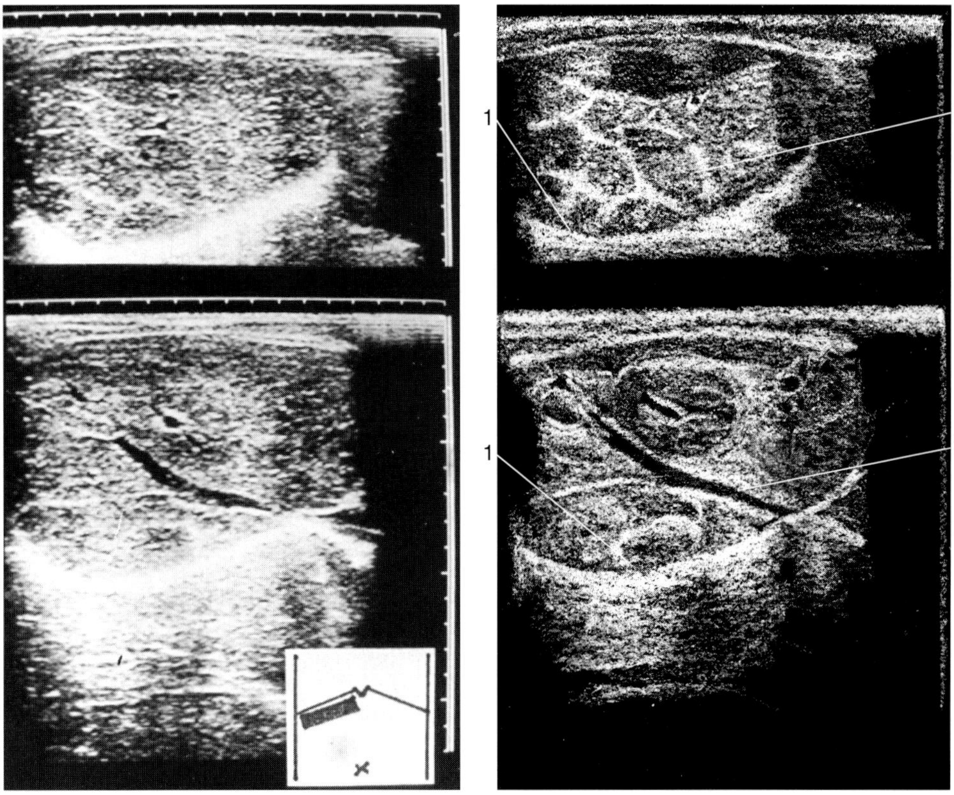

1. Diaphragm 2. Medial hepatic vein
3. Honeycomb-like marking caused by fibrosis

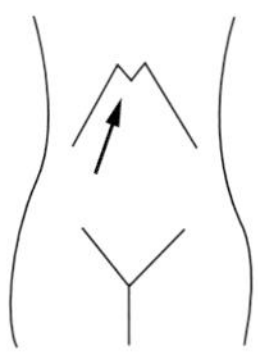

Figure 3-46. Hepatic schistosomiasis japonica.
Two tomograms from the same patient suffering from *Schistosoma japonicum* show its peculiar honeycomb appearance, with fibrotic network and cirrhotic changes in the liver parenchyma. The entire liver is affected so that the pattern is seldom mistaken for other types of cirrhosis. The disease is endemic in southwestern Japan and southern China. (Figures courtesy of Dr. Y. Majima, Kurume Medical School)

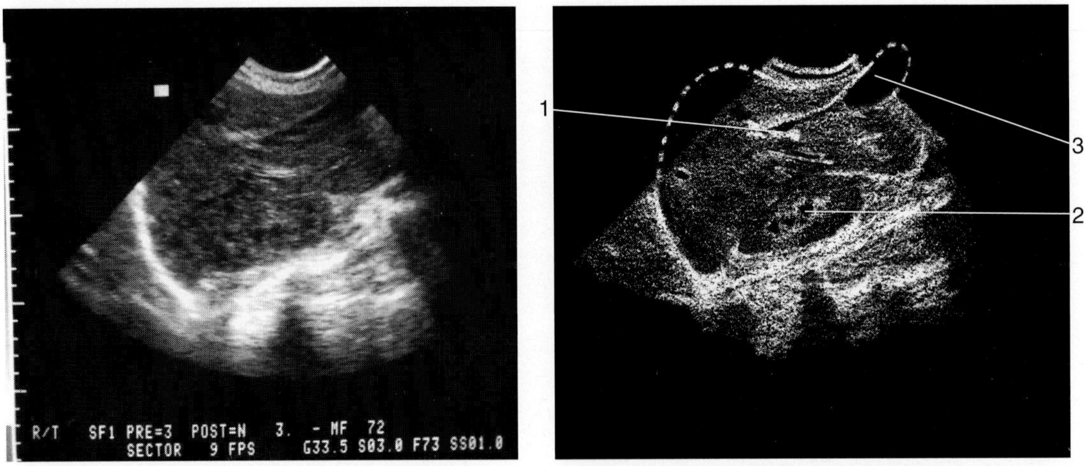

1. Portal triad 2. Kidney 3. Gallbladder

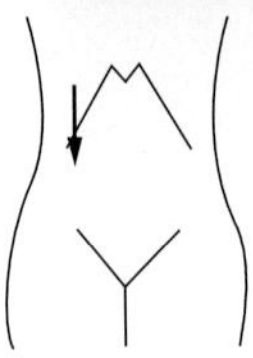

Figure 3-47. The dark liver.
The reduced echoes from the liver parenchyma may be equal to those from the kidney, so that the two seem to merge. The periportal echoes are highlighted, giving the impression of an increase in the number of vascular markings.

ABNORMALITIES AROUND THE LIVER

Ascites has a very characteristic appearance as fluid outlining the peritoneal spaces and forming pointed extremities as it passes between contiguous organs.[28] This is the "crescent moon sign," which is especially well seen in the hepatorenal angle. Since this is one of the most dependent parts of the peritoneum, fluid collects here readily (Figure 3-48). The retrovesical region in the pelvis is another dependent space where early ascites should be looked for. As the amount of ascites increases, the spaces fill and round off, so that intraperitoneal organs float in the "ascitic sea." The liver assumes a globular shape, losing much of its normal outline (which is chiefly maintained by pressure from adjacent organs). The gut wall thickens. Sometimes this is an effect of the cause of the ascites (e.g., hypoproteinemia, congestion in portal hypertension, direct involvement in peritoneal tumor), but there is probably an artifactual component as well.

Some normally invisible structures are revealed in ascites. The falciform ligament is inaptly named, since it consists only of a thin, double peritoneal layer. In ascites it can often be demonstrated as a strip passing from the anterior abdominal wall to the ligamentum teres in the left lobe of the liver. The lesser sac of the omentum may fill with ascitic fluid and then is imaged as a space separating the pancreas from the overlying stomach (Figure 3-49). The caudate lobe, lying in the lesser sac, is often outlined by fluid. It may be possible to demonstrate the lesser omentum itself as a sheet in the coronal plane with fluid to either side. Ultrasound is very sensitive to ascites, quantities as small as 100 ml being detectable. Such minute amounts are more easily seen if the patient is rotated to the right decubitus position to encourage pooling of the fluid in Morrison's pouch.

The cause of the ascites cannot usually be determined on ultrasound, though a clue may sometimes be obtained. Features of portal hypertension or congestive heart failure may be suggestive. Echoes within the fluid suggest the presence of cells, either malignant or inflammatory, and both of these processes may cause adhesion of bowel loops with attachment to the posterior abdominal wall. Normal bowel loops tend to float anteriorly; the observation that they are attached posteriorly suggests an inflammatory or a malignant cause. The latter conclusion is supported by the demonstration of tumor plaques on the peritoneal surfaces, most readily detected on the anterior parietal layer, though this requires care because even large masses can be obscured by the confused near field. Loculated ascites is common in both malignant and inflammatory peritonitis and produces rounded, walled-off fluid spaces that simulate cysts (Figure 3-50). The distinction from a cyst on the surface of an organ from cystic tumor deposits (e.g., in carcinoma of the ovary) requires aspiration biopsy. Hemoperitoneum can have exactly the same appearance as ascites; any clinical suspicion requires a diagnostic tap for confirmation.

Abscesses frequently collect around the liver because the distribution of the omental attachments tends to direct peritoneal fluid up to the right hemidiaphragm.[60] Common sites are the two subphrenic spaces (anterior and posterior) and the subhepatic space which is continuous with Morison's pouch in the hepatorenal angle. Phrenic palsy is usual, and a small reactive pleural effusion is commonly seen. Subphrenic abscesses have the same pattern as abscesses elsewhere, typically consisting of a thick-walled fluid space with a shaggy, poorly defined margin. The fluid contains a variable amount of echogenic debris. As with liver abscesses, ultrasound-guided sampling for confirmation and bacterial culture is readily performed. Definitive drainage is also possible and may be the best form of management in the weakened postoperative patient, but placement of the large drain required under local anesthesia is not always easy, and a general anesthetic may be preferred.[36]

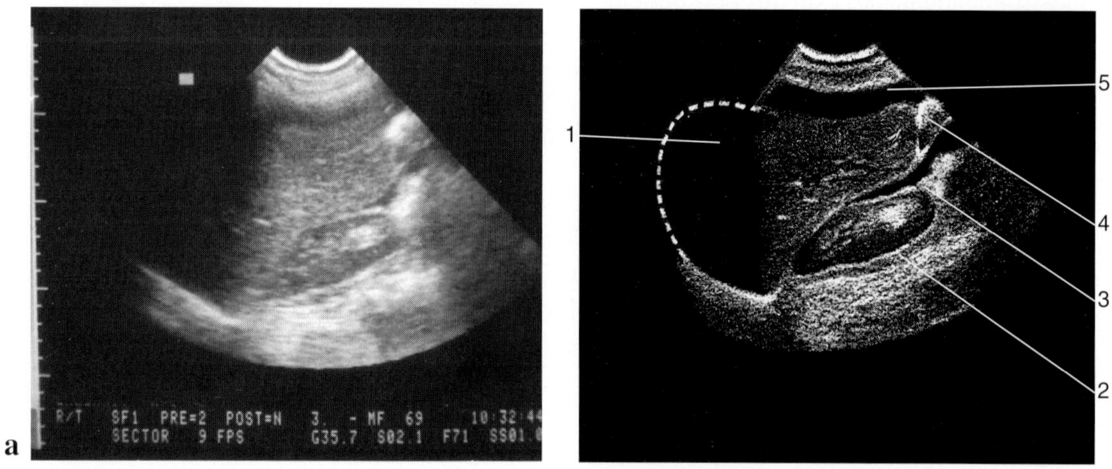

1. Liver 2. Kidney 3. Ascites in Morison's pouch
4. Hepatic flexure of colon 5. Ascites

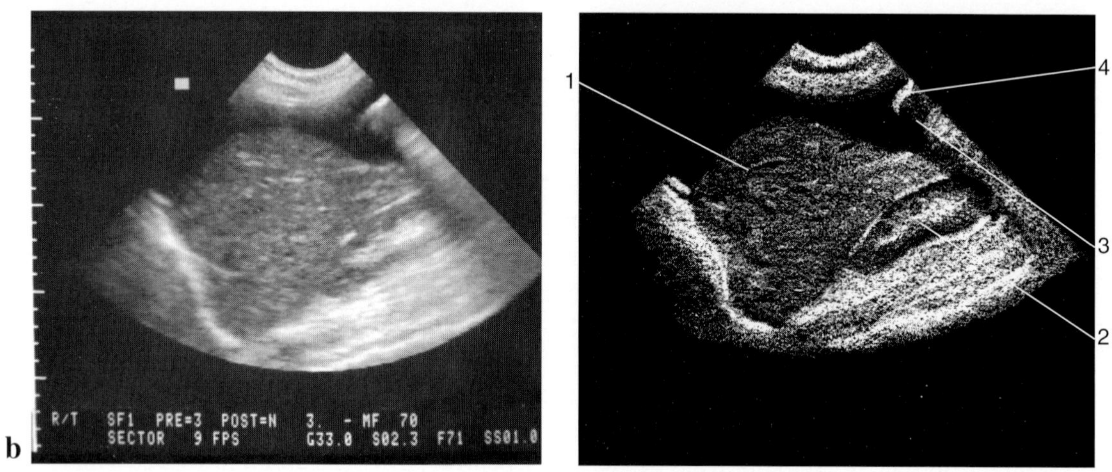

1. Liver 2. Kidney 3. Gut 4. Ascites

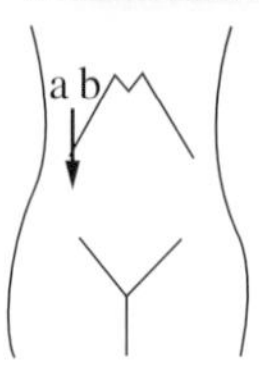

Figure 3-48. Ascites.
Early ascites pools in the hepatorenal angle (a) separating the right lobe of the liver and the right kidney with a fine, echo-free line. With increasing amounts of ascites (b), the liver tends to round off.

a

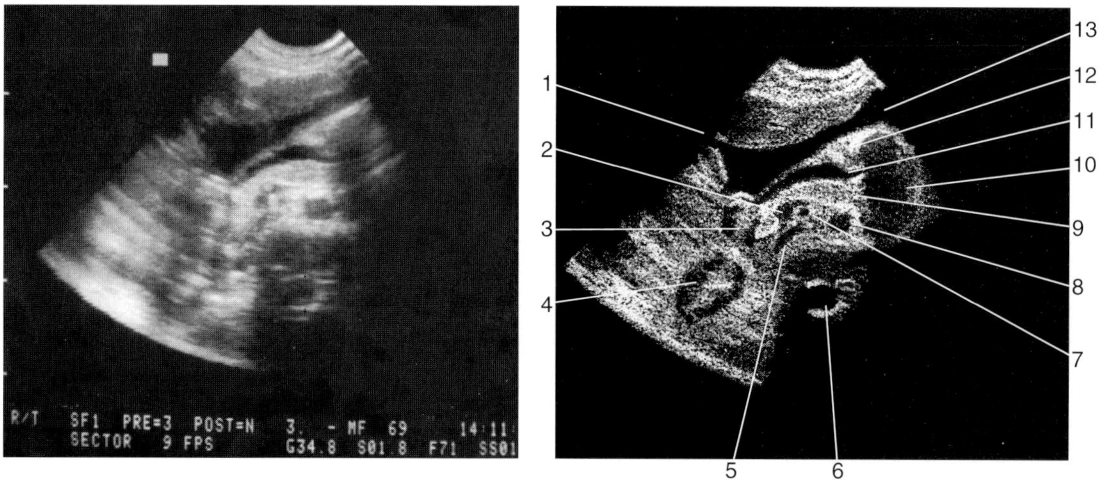

1. Liver 2. Superior mesenteric vein 3. Duodenum 4. Right kidney 5. Inferior vena cava 6. Spinal canal 7. Superior mesenteric artery 8. Aorta 9. Pancreas 10. Stomach 11. Ascites in lesser sac 12. Lesser omentum 13. Ascites in greater sac

b

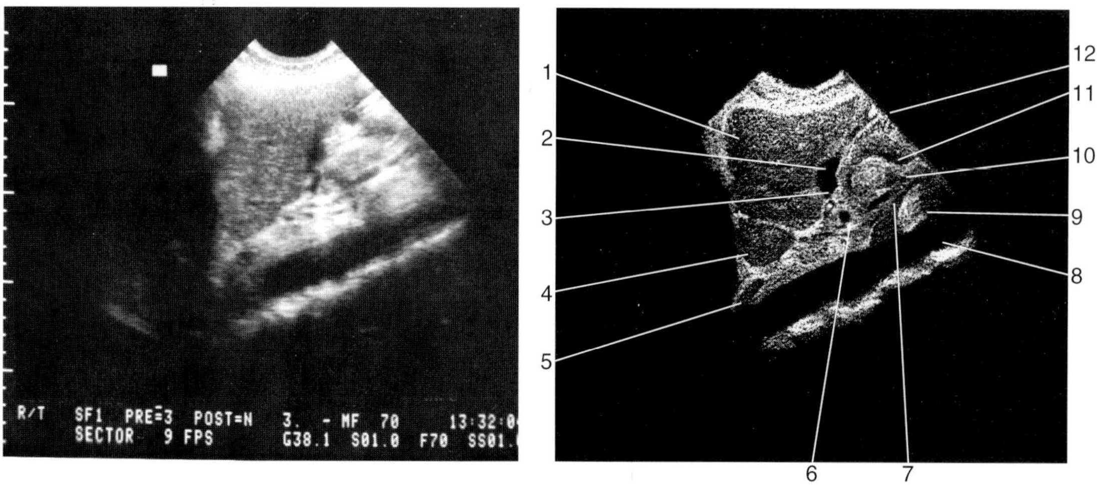

1. Left lobe of liver 2. Ascites in greater sac 3. Lesser omentum 4. Caudate lobe of liver 5. Esophagus 6. Splenic artery 7. Splenic vein 8. Aorta 9. Superior mesenteric artery 10. Pancreas 11. Ascites in lesser sac 12. Stomach

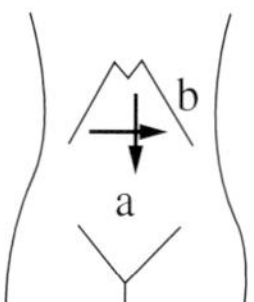

Figure 3-49. Ascites in the lesser sac.
The lesser omentum is outlined, extending from the lesser curve of the stomach to the fissure between the left and caudate lobes. Between it and the pancreas, fluid has accumulated in the lesser sac.

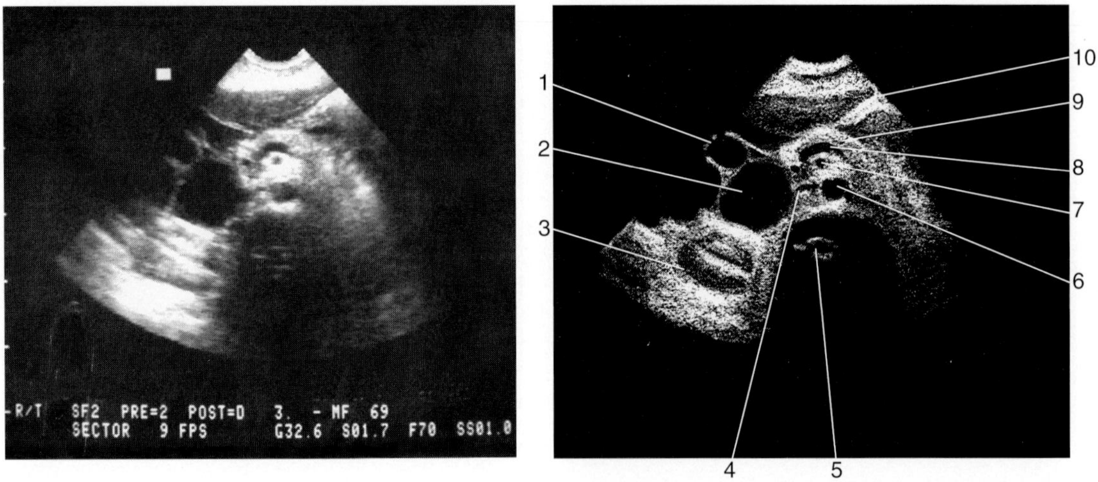

1. Gallbladder 2. Loculated ascites 3. Right kidney
4. Inferior vena cava 5. Spinal canal 6. Aorta
7. Superior mesenteric vein 8. Splenic vein
9. Pancreas 10. Stomach

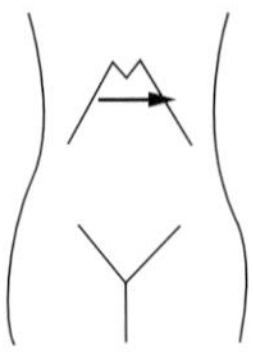

Figure 3-50. Loculated ascites.
Malignant and inflammatory ascites may become walled off to produce loculated fluid pockets. This example lies close to the head of the pancreas and anterior to the right kidney. It could easily be mistaken for a pancreatic pseudocyst. Note the common bile duct and the gastroduodenal artery cut in cross section at the head of the pancreas.

REFERENCES

1. Abdel-Latif Z, Abdel-Mahab MF, El-Kady NM: Evaluation of portal hypertension in cases of hepatosplenic schistosomiasis using ultrasound (abstract). Radiology 144 : 216, 1982.
2. Adel-Wahab MF, Esmat G, Narooz SI, et al: Sonographic studies of schoolchildren in a village endemic for Schistosoma mansoni. Trans R Soc Trop Med Hyg 84 : 69-73, 1990.
3. Ahmed L, El Rooby A, Kassem MI, et al: Ultrasonography in the diagnosis and management of 52 patients with amebic liver abscess in Cairo. Rev Infect Dis 12 : 330-337, 1990.
4. Albertyn LE, Ganguly BS, Cooper JE, et al: Turtleback liver on CT and ultrasound: Schistosoma japonica revisited. Australas Radiol 34 : 78-81, 1990.
5. Atkinson GO, Kodroff MB, Sones PJ, et al : Focal nodular hyperplasia of the liver in children: A report of three new cases. Radiology 137 : 171-177, 1980.
6. Atomi Y, Inoue S, Kawano N, et al: Hepatocellular carcinoma: Diagnosis by real-time ultrasonography, in Kossoff G, Fukuda M (eds), Ultrasonic Differential Diagnosis of Tumors. New York, Igaku-Shoin, 1984, pp108-122.
7. Beggs I: The radiological appearance of hydatid disease of the liver. Clin Radiol 34 : 555-563, 1983.
8. Bree RL, Schwabb RE, Neiman HL: Solitary echogenic spot in the liver: Is it diagnostic of a hemangioma? Am J Roentgenol 140 : 41-44, 1983.
9. Bruneton JN, Ladree D, Caramella E, et al: Ultrasonographic study of calcified hepatic metastases: A report of 13 cases. Gastrointest Radiol 7 : 61-63, 1982.
10. Bruneton JN, Douillard J, Fenart D, et al: Ultrasonography of hepatic cavernous haemangioma. Br J Radiol 56 : 783-791, 1983.
11. Bruneton JN, Eresue J, Caramella E, et al: Congenital cysts of the liver in echography. J Radiol 64 : 471-476, 1983.
12. Casarella W, Knowles D, Wolff M, et al: Focal nodular hyperplasia and liver cell adenoma. Am J Radiol 131 : 393-402, 1978.
13. Chu J, Husband JE, Cosgrove DO, et al: The B-scan appearance of gas in the biliary tree. Br J Radiol 51 : 728-730, 1978.
14. Cosgrove DO, McCready VRM: Ultrasonic Imaging: Liver, Spleen and Pancreas. Chichester, UK, Wiley, 1982.
15. Curtin NJ: Case of the spring season: Focal nodular hyperplasia. Semin Ultrasound 1 : 5-9, 1980.
16. Dewbury KC, Joseph AEA, Sadler GHM, et al: Ultrasound in the diagnosis of early liver abscess. Br J Radiol 53 : 1160-1167, 1980.
17. Dewbury KC, Clark BE: The accuracy of ultrasound in the detection of cirrhosis of the liver. Br J Radiol 52 : 945-950, 1980.
18. Di Lelio A, Cestari C, Lomazzi A, et al: Cirrhosis: Diagnosis with sonographic study of the liver surface. Radiology 172 : 389-392, 1989.
19. Esfahani F, Rooholamini SA, Vessal K: Ultrasonography of hepatic hydatid cysts: New diagnostic signs. J Ultrasound Med 7 : 443-450, 1988.
20. Foster KJ, Dewbury KC, Griffith AH, et al: Accuracy of ultrasound in the detection of fatty infiltration of the liver. Br J Radiol 53 : 440-448, 1980.
21. Freeny PC, Vimont TR, Barnett DC: Cavernous hemangioma of the liver: Ultrasonography, arteriography, and computed tomography. Radiology 132 : 143-150, 1979.
22. Fritschy P, Robotti G, Schneekloth G, et al: Measurement of liver volume by ultrasound and computed tomography. J Clin Ultrasound 11 : 299-303, 1983.
23. Froelich J, Simeone J, McKusick K, et al: Radionuclide imaging and ultrasound in liver/spleen trauma. Radiology 145 : 457-461, 1982.
24. Gandolfi L, Solmi L, Bolondi L, et al: The value of ultrasonography in the diagnosis of hepatic haemangiomas. Eur J Radiol 3 : 222-226, 1983.
25. Goyal AK, Pokharna DS, Sharma SK: Ultrasonic diagnosis of cirrhosis: Reference to quantitative measurements of hepatic dimensions. Gastrointest Radiol 15 : 32-34, 1990.
26. Hartman PC, Oosterveld BJ, Thijssen JM, et al: Detection and differentiation of diffuse liver disease by quantitative echography. A retrospective assessment. Invest Radiol 28 : 1-6, 1993.
27. Gharbi HA, Hassine W, Brauner MW: Ultrasound examination of the hydatid liver. Radiology 139 : 459-468, 1981.
28. Gefter WB, Arger PH, Edell SI: Sonographic patterns of ascites. Semin Ultrasound 2 : 226-241, 1981.
29. Glazer GM, Laing FC, Braun TW, et al: Sonographic demonstration of portal hypertension: Patent umbilical vein. Radiology 136 : 161-169, 1980.

30. Gosink BB: Intrahepatic gas: Differential diagnosis. Am J Roentgenol 137 : 763-779, 1981.
31. Gosink BB, Leymaster CE: Ultrasonic determination of hepatomegaly (abstract). Radiology 140 : 606, 1981.
32. Gosink BB, Lemon SK, Scheible W, et al: Accuracy of ultrasonography in diagnosis of hepatocellular disease. Am J Roentgenol 133 : 19-27, 1979.
33. Grabenwoger F, Dock W, Pichler W, et al: Diagnosis of liver trauma: Ultrasound versus computed tomography (English abstract). ROFO 150 : 163-166, 1989.
34. Hadidi A: Sonography of hepatic echinococcal cysts. Radiology 147 : 913-927,1983.
35. Harbin WP, Robert NJ, Ferrucci JF: Diagnosis of cirrhosis based on regional changes in hepatic morphology: Radiological and pathological analysis. Radiology 135 : 273-288, 1980.
36. Heckemann R, Wernecke K: Treatment of intra-abdominal abscesses by ultrasonically guided fine-needle puncture (English abstract). ROFO 138 : 208-213, 1983.
37. Hill MC, Dach JL, Shawker TH: Ultrasonography in portal hypertension. Clin Gastroenterol (England) 14 : 83-104, 1985.
38. Hollinshead WH: Anatomy for Surgeons, vol 2: Thorax, Abdomen and Pelvis, ed 3. New York, Harper & Row, 1982.
39. Hussain S: Diagnostic criteria of hydatid disease on hepatic sonography. J Ultraound Med 4 : 603-607, 1985.
40. Itai Y, Araki T, Furui S, et al: Computed tomography and ultrasound in the diagnosis of intrahepatic calculi. Radiology 136 : 399-412, 1980.
41. Itai Y, Ohtomo K, Araki T, et al: Computed tomography and sonography of cavernous hemangioma of the liver. Am J Roentgenol 141 : 315-322, 1983.
42. Jain AK, Gupta NC, Gupta PD, et al: Sonographic appearance of hepatic hydatid disease. Australas Radiol 33 : 373-375, 1989.
43. Jend HH, Heller M: Caroli's syndrome in ultrasound and CT. Röntgenblatter 34 : 383-386, 1981.
44. Joseph AEA, Dewbury, KC, McGuire PG: Ultrasound detection of chronic liver disease. Br J Radiol 52 : 184-188, 1979.
45. Juttner HU, Jenney JM, Ralls PW, et al: Ultrasound demonstration of porto-systemic collaterals in cirrhosis. Radiology 142 : 459-466, 1982.
46. Kane RA, Katz SG: Spectrum of sonographic findings in portal hypertension. Radiology 142 : 453-458, 1982.
47. Kauzlaric D, Petrovic M, Barmeir E: Sonography of cavernous transformation of the portal vein. Am J Roentgenol 142 : 383-384, 1984.
48. Kuligowska E, Connors SK, Shapiro JH: Liver abscess : Sonography in diagnosis and treatment. Am J Roentgenol 138 : 253-259, 1982.
49. Kuligowska E, Noble J: Sonography of hepatic abscesses. Semin Ultrasound 4 : 102-112, 1983.
50. Kurtz AL, Rubin CS, Cooper HS, et al: Ultrasound findings in hepatitis. Radiology 136 : 717-725, 1980.
51. Lin HH, Changchien CS, Lin DY: Hepatic parenchymal calcifications: Differentiation from intrahepatic stones. JCU 17 : 411-415, 1989.
52. Ljubicic N, Duvnjak M, Rotkvic I, et al: Influence of the degree of liver failure on portal blood flow in patients with liver cirrhosis. Scand J Gastroenterol 25 : 395-400, 1990.
53. Lyons EA: Atlas of Sectional Anatomy. St Louis, CV Mosby, 1978.
54. McGrath P, Mills P: Atlas of Sectional Anatomy. Basel, Karger, 1984.
55. McMinn RMH, Hutchings RT: A Colour Atlas of Human Anatomy. London, Wolfe Medical, 1977.
56. Mathiew D, Bruneton JN, Drouillard J, et al: Hepatic adenomas and focal nodular hyperplasia: Dynamic CT study. Radiology 160 : 53-58, 1986.
57. Mattrey RF, Scheible FW, Gosink BB, et al: Perfluoroctylbromide: A liver/spleen-specific and tumour imaging ultrasound contrast material. Radiology 145 : 759-767, 1982.
58. Mayes GB, Bernardino ME: Role of ultrasound in the evaluation of hepatic neoplasms. Semin Ultrasound 2 : 212-228, 1981.
59. Mittlestaedt CA, Volberg FM, Fischer GJ, et al: Caroli's disease: Sonographic findings. Am J Roentgenol 134 : 585-587, 1980.
60. Mueller PR, Simeone JF: Intra-abdominal abscesses. Diagnosis by sonography and computed tomography. Radiol Clin North Am 21 : 425-443, 1983.
61. Nelson RC, Chezmar JL: Diagnostic approach to hepatic hemangiomas. Radiology 176 : 11-13, 1990.
62. Netter FH: Ciba Collection of Medical Illustrations, vol 3: Digestive Tract, part III, Liver Biliary Tract and Pancreas, ed 2. Summit, NJ, Ciba Geigy, 1964.
63. Nicholas D: Present status of ultrasound tissue characterization, in Kossoff G, Fukuda M (eds), Ultrasonic

Differential Diagnosis of Tumors. New York, Igaku-Shoin, 1984, pp24-37.
64. Niederau C, Sonnenberg A, Muller JE, et al: Sonographic measurements of the normal liver, spleen, pancreas and portal vein. Radiology 149 : 537-540, 1983.
65. Onodera H, Ohta K, Oikawa M, et al: Correlation of the real-time ultrasonographic appearance of hepatic hemangiomas with angiography. JCU 11 : 421-425, 1983.
66. Pamilo M, Sotaniemi EA, Suramo I, et al: Evaluation of liver steatotic and fibrous content by computerized tomography and ultrasound. Scand J Gastroenterol 18 : 743-747, 1983.
67. Pamilo M, Suramo I, Lahde S: Comparison of ultrasound and CT images of liver metastases. Acta Radiol 24 : 139-143, 1983.
68. Ralls PW, Meyers HI, Lapin SA, et al: Grey-scale ultrasonography of hepatic amoebic abscesses. Radiology 132 : 125-137, 1979.
69. Ralls PW, Quinn MF, Boswell WD, et al: Patterns of resolution in successfully treated hepatic amebic abscess: Sonographic evaluation. Radiology 149 : 541-543, 1983.
70. Ralls PW, Quinn MF, Rogers WF, et al: Sonographic anatomy of the hepatic artery. Am J Roentgenol 136 : 1059-1067, 1981.
71. Rapaccini GL, Pompili M, Caturelli E, et al: Focal ultrasound lesions in liver cirrhosis diagnosed as regenerating nodules by fine-needle biopsy. Follow-up of 12 cases. Dig Dis Sci 35 : 422-427, 1990.
72. Rogers JV, Mack LA, Freeny PC, et al: Hepatic focal nodular hyperplasia: Angiography, CT, sonography, and scintigraphy. Am J Roentgenol 137 : 983-991, 1981.
73. Rubinson HA, Isikoff MB, Hill MC: Diagnostic imaging of hepatic abscesses: A retrospective analysis. Am J Roentgenol 135 : 735-740, 1980.
74. Saint-Martin G, Chiesa JC: "Falling snowflakes," an ultrasound sign of hydatid sand. J Ultrasound Med 3 : 257-260, 1984.
75. Sandler MA, Marks DS, Hriçak H, et al: Benign focal diseases of the liver. Semin Ultrasound 2 : 202-225, 1981.
76. Sandler MA, Petrocelli RD, Marks DS, et al: Ultrasound features and radionuclide correlation in liver cell adenoma and focal nodular hyperplasia. Radiology 135 : 393-407, 1980.
77. Schabel SI, Rittenhberg GM, Javid LH, et al: "Bull's-eye" falciform ligament: Sonographic finding of portal hypertension. Radiology 136 : 157-163, 1980.
78. Scheibel W: Diagnostic algorithm for liver masses. Semin Roentgenol 18 : 84-97, 1983.
79. Schneck CD: The anatomical basis of abdomino-pelvic sectional imaging, in Joseph EAE, Cosgrove DO (eds), Ultrasound in Inflammatory Disease (Clinics in Ultrasound, vol 11), New York, Churchill-Livingstone, 1983, pp13-41.
80. Scott WW, Sanders RC, Siegelman SS: Irregular fatty infiltration of the liver. Am J Roentgenol 135 : 67-75, 1980.
81. Sexton CC, Zeman RK: Pictorial essay: Correlation of CT, sonography and gross anatomy of the liver. Am J Roentgenol 141 : 711-724, 1983.
82. Subramanyam BR, Balthazar EJ, Raghavendra BN, et al: Ultrasound analysis of solid-appearing abscesses. Radiology 146 : 487-491, 1983.
83. Taboury J, Porcel A, Tubiana JM, et al: Cavernous hemangiomas of the liver studied by ultrasound. Enhancement posterior to a hyperechoic mass as a sign of hypervascularity. Radiology 149 : 781-785, 1983.
84. Takayasu K, Moriyama N, Shima Y, et al: Sonographic detection of large spontaneous spleno-renal shunts. Br J Radiol 57 : 565-570, 1984.
85. Tanaka H, Sugimoto H, Yoshioka T, et al: Study of blund hepatic injury by ultrasonography (English abstract). Nippon Geka Gakkai Zasshi 90 : 855-862, 1989.
86. Tanaka S, Kitamura T, Fujita M, et al: Color Doppler flow imaging of liver tumors. AJR 154 : 509-514, 1990.
87. Tanaka S, Kitamura T, Imaoka S, et al: Hepatocellular carcinoma: Sonographic and histologic correlations. Am J Roentgenol 140 : 701-710, 1983.
88. Terrier F, Becker CD, Triller JK: Morphologic aspects of hepatic abscesses at computed tomography and ultrasound. Acta Radiol 24 : 129-737, 1983.
89. Toppet V, Souayah H, Delplace O, et al: Lymph node enlargement as a sign of acute hepatitis A in children. Pediatr Radiol 20 : 249-252, 1990.
90. Van Sonnenberg E, Simeone JF, Mueller PR, et al: Sonographic appearance of hematoma in liver, spleen and kidney. Radiology 147 : 507-512, 1983.
91. Viscomi GN, Gonzalez R, Taylor KJW, et al: Ultrasonic evaluation of hepatic and splenic trauma. Arch Surg 115 : 320-331, 1981.

92. Wang SS, Chiang JH, Tsai YT, et al: Focal hepatic fatty infiltration as a cause of pseudotumors: Ultrasonographic patterns and clinical differentiation. JCU 18 : 401-409, 1990.
93. Welch TJ, Sheedy PF II, Jonson CM, et al: Focal nodular hyperplasia and hepatic adenoma: Comparison of angiography, CT, US, and scintigraphy. Radiology 156 : 593-595, 1985.
94. Zoli M, Cordiani MR, Marchesini G, et al: Ultrasonographic follow-up of liver cirrhosis. JCU 18 : 91-96, 1990.

CHAPTER 4

THE GALLBLADDER AND BILE DUCTS

NORMAL ANATOMY

The biliary system, which transports bile from the liver to the duodenum, consists of the bile ducts and the gallbladder (Figure 4-1). Anatomically, the canaliculi join to form interacinar ductules and then successively small and larger bile ducts which run parallel to the portal venous system. They join to form a right and a left hepatic duct; these, in turn, join at the liver hilum to form the common hepatic duct. The cystic duct, draining the gallbladder, joins the common hepatic duct at a variable level to become the common bile duct, a tubular structure 4 to 6 mm in diameter.

The common bile duct passes behind the first portion of the duodenum, parallel to the portal vein, and penetrates the posterior portion of the head of the pancreas to open into the posteromedial wall of the duodenum at the papilla of Vater.

The gallbladder is a pear-shaped, contractile, hollow organ lying in a fossa on the visceral surface of the right lobe of the liver and is usually located anterior to the right kidney. The filled, relaxed gallbladder measures 7 to 10 cm in length and 2 to 4 cm in diameter. Bile is transferred to the duodenum directly from the liver or after storage in the gallbladder. The gallbladder empties its contents, concentrated bile, by contraction after stimulation by food passage through the duodenum or following injection of cholecystokinin or cerulein.[3]

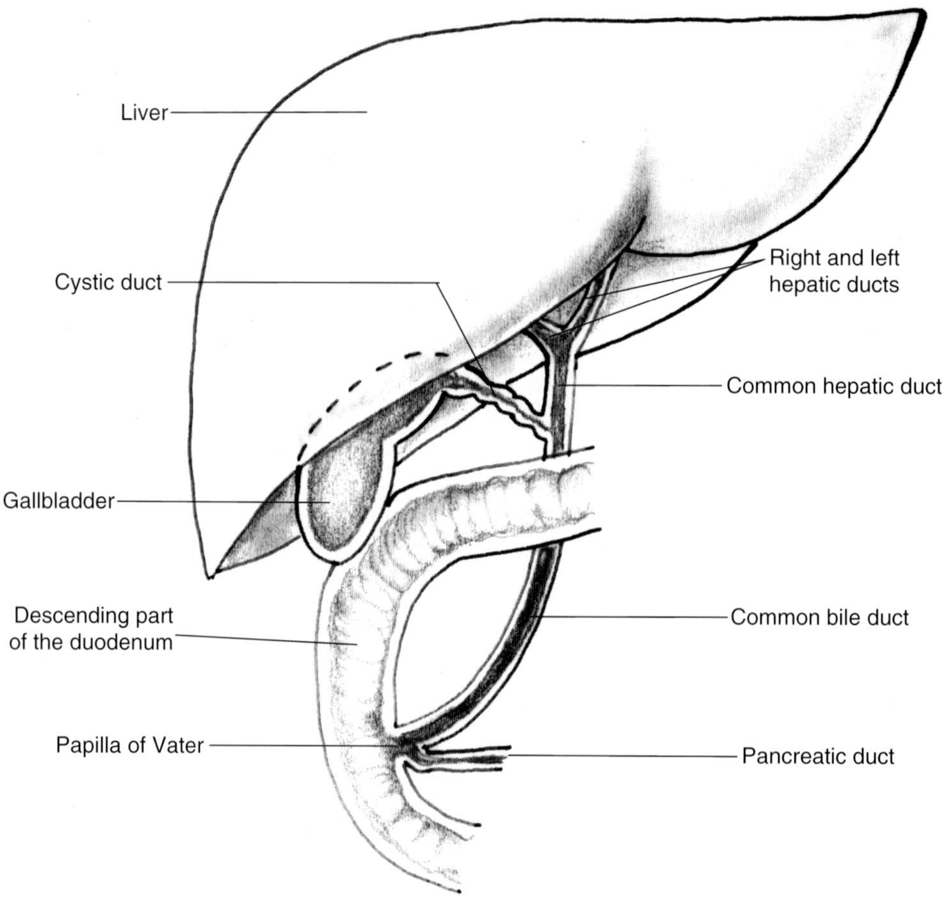

Figure 4-1. Diagram of the normal biliary tree.
Normally, the right and left hepatic ducts join to from the main heptic duct, which becomes the common bile duct below the junction with the cystic duct. Because this junction is difficult to visualize with ultrasound, the system is commonly referred to as the extrahepatic common duct.

ULTRASOUND APPEARANCES

With the improved resolution of modern real-time scanners, the entire biliary system can be imaged relatively easily compared to the limited visualization given by the earlier generation of static contact scanners.

By placing the scanning probe at the right subcostal margin and directing it to superiorly, the right and left hepatic ducts can be imaged as fine channels immediately anterior to the bifurcating right and left branches of the portal vein. By sliding the probe slightly inferiorly, their junction to form the common hepatic duct can readily be observed; it then runs along the anterolateral aspect of the portal vein.

However, the junction of the cystic and common bile ducts is usually difficult to visualize sonographically because of interference by gas in the first part of the duodenum. The common bile duct runs parallel to the portal vein for a short length and then deviates posterolaterally to empty at the duodenal papilla. Scans of the entire length of the common duct can be made either by continuous parallel transverse scans or by sagittal scans in the supine position (Figures 4-2 and 4-3). The right anterior oblique or right coronal scans may be used effectively for this purpose. As shown in Figure 4-4, the entire path of the extrahepatic biliary ducts can be visualized, using right coronal scans with the gallbladder and right lobe of the liver acting as acoustic windows. Adjacent structures—the inferior vena cava, aorta, superior mesenteric vein, and head of the pancreas—can be visualized at the same time.

The caliber of the extrahepatic bile ducts have been variably reported.[6, 18, 24, 51, 65] Recent reports using high-resolution real-time scanners have largely settled the issue. The normal caliber of the common duct lumen is defined as being about 4 mm, at the widest part of the duct in the middle of the extrahepatic bile duct.[72, 74, 92]

The fluid-filled gallbladder appears as a pear-shaped echo-free structure with a clearly defined, echogenic wall. The posterior wall appears more echogenic than the anterior wall because of the low attenuation of bile. The fundus of the gallbladder usually lies closer to the body surface, while the neck lies in a deeper position; there is, however, a great deal of individual variability. The size and shape of the gallbladder are subject to significant anatomical variations and physiological changes. The length of the gallbladder is quite variable and, in particular, is longer in thin asthenic individuals. By contrast, in obese persons, the gallbladder is shortened and situated much closer to the liver; it is often difficult, therefore, to image the whole of the gallbladder adequately by a routine subcostal approach. In the contracted, postprandial state, not only is the gallbladder smaller, but also its wall is thicker.

The thickness of the gallbladder wall in normal subjects rarely exceeds 3 mm. The thickness and echogenicity of the wall change markedly according to its contractile state.

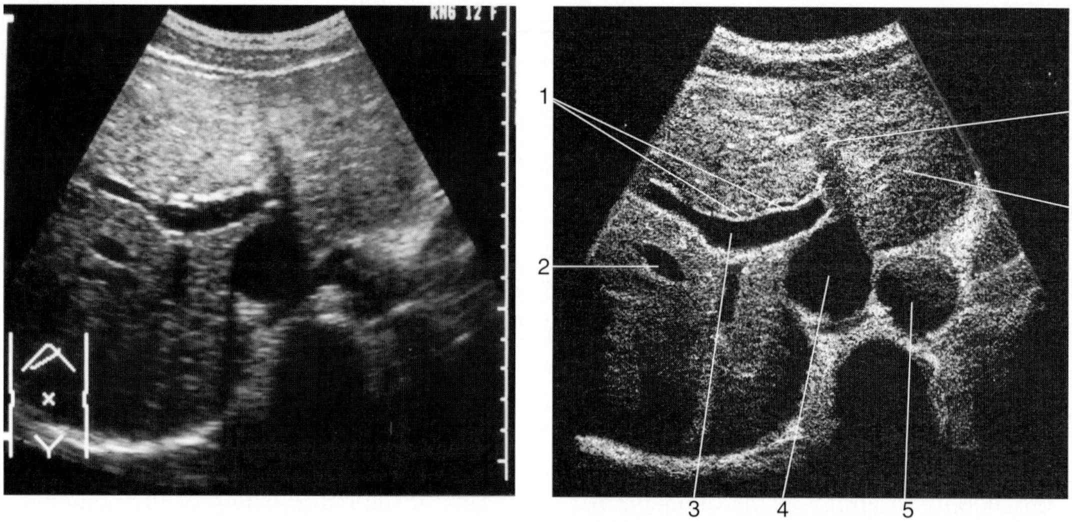

a

1. Right and left hepatic ducts 2. Hepatic vein 3. Portal vein 4. Inferior vena cava 5. Aorta 6. Left lobe of liver 7. Ligamentum teres

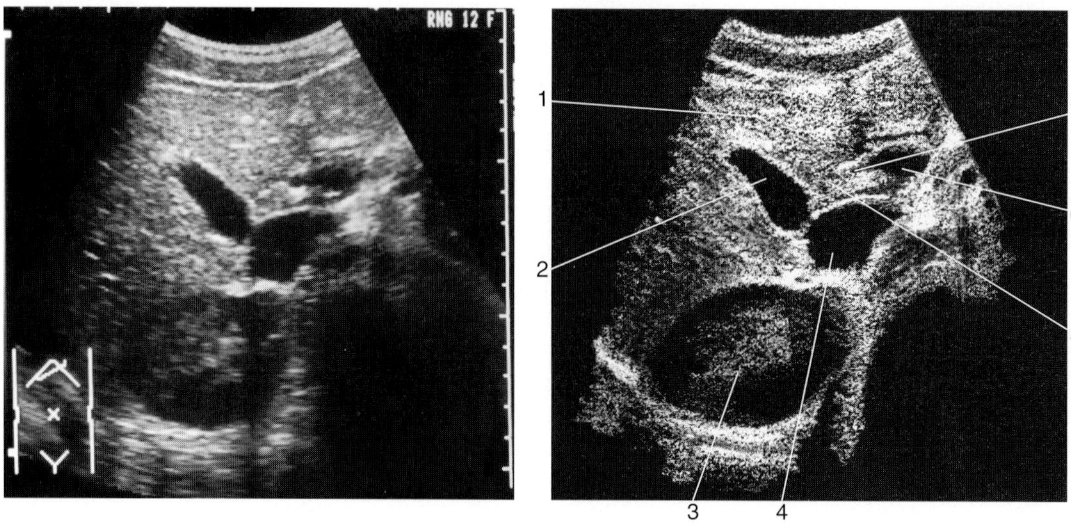

b

1. Liver 2. Gallbladder 3. Right kidney 4. Inferior vena cava 5. Common hepatic duct 6. Portal vein 7. Hepatic artery

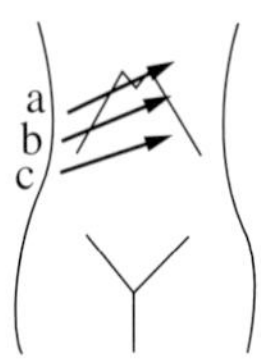

Figure 4-2. The normal biliary system, transverse scan.
Three images of the biliary system were recorded with right subcostal scans in parallel. (a) The right and left hepatic ducts of normal caliber anterior to the main branches of the portal vein. (b) Part of the gallbladder and the inferior vena cava. (c) The normal gallbladder and right kidney.

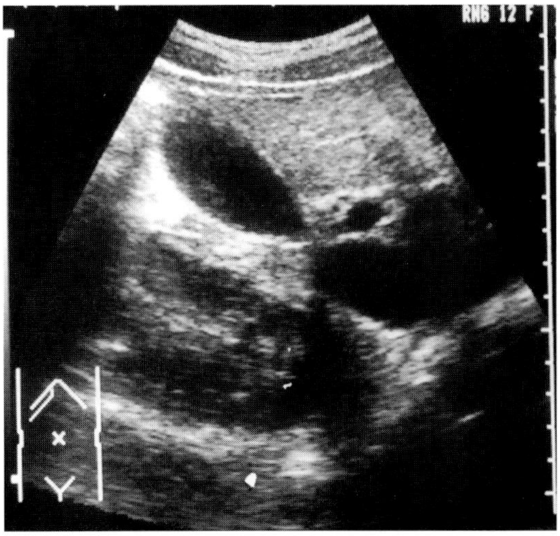

c

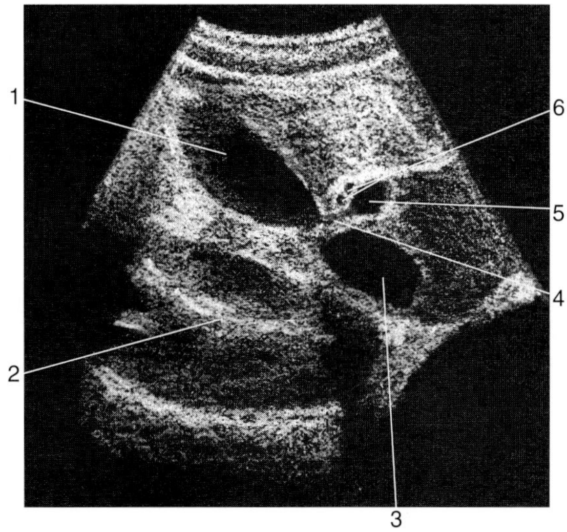

1. Gallbladder 2. Right kidney 3. Inferior vena cava 4. Common bile duct 5. Portal vein 6. Hepatic artery

a

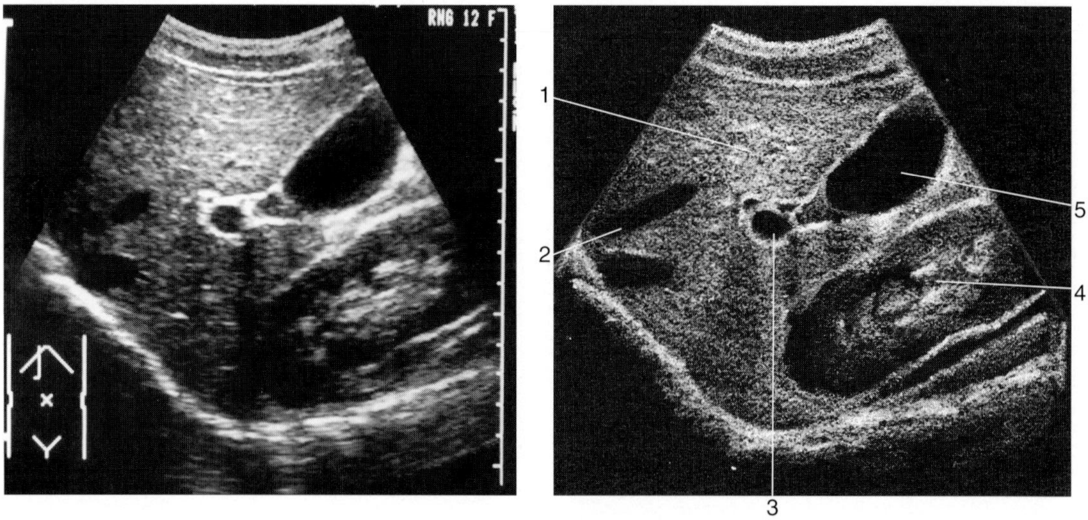

1. Liver 2. Hepatic vein 3. Right portal vein
4. Right kidney 5. Gallbladder

b

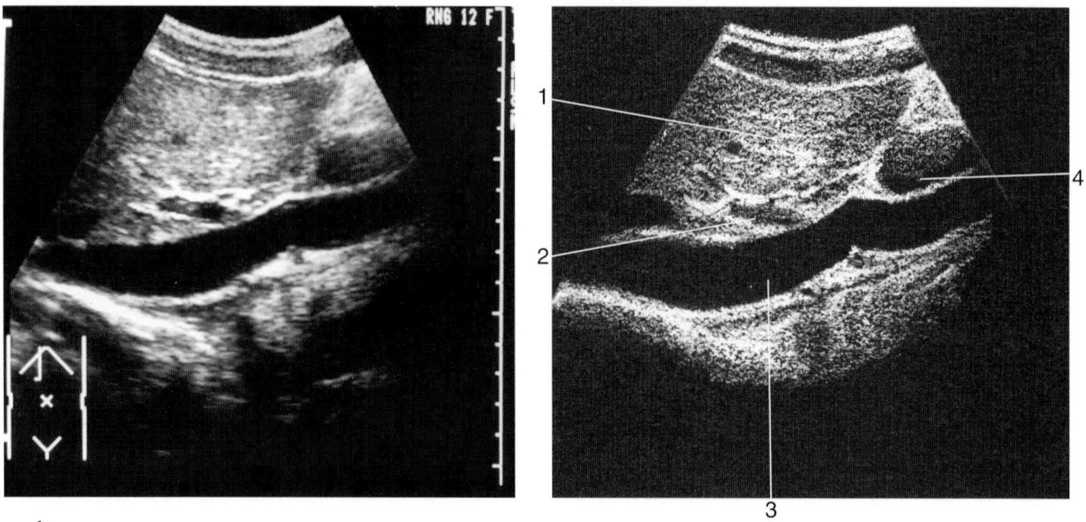

1. Liver 2. Portal vein 3. Inferior vena cava
4. Pancreas

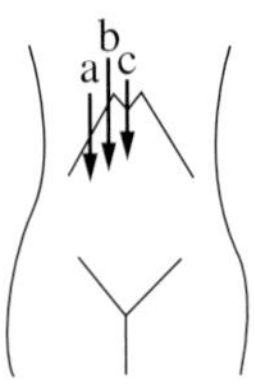

Figure 4-3. The normal biliary system.
Three images of the biliary system are shown, as imaged by parasagittal scans. (a) The normal gallbladder. The small, round structure cephalad to the gallbladder is the right main branch of the portal vein in cross section. (b) Part of the porta hepatis imaged medial to the gallbladder. An oblique section of the portal vein together with the hepatic artery proper and the left hepatic duct have been obtained. (c) A sagittal cross section traversing the pancreatic head. Part of the portal trunk and the common hepatic duct are shown with the inferior vena cava.

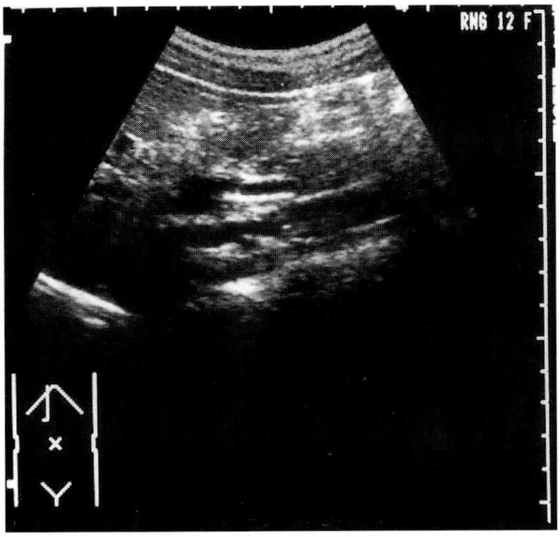

c

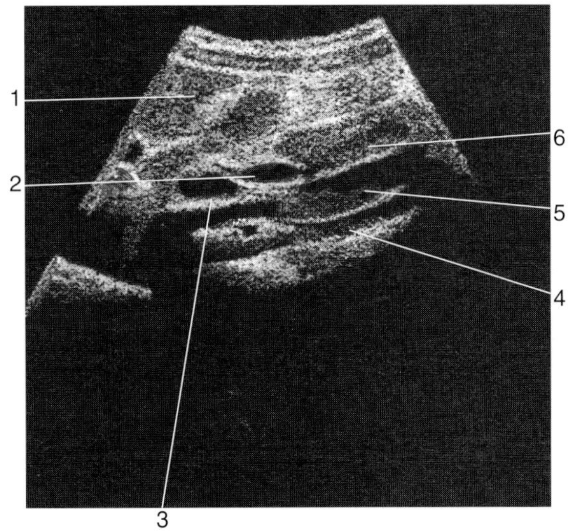

1. Liver 2. Common bile duct 3. Portal vein 4. Diaphragm(Crus media) 5. Inferior vena cava 6. Pancreas

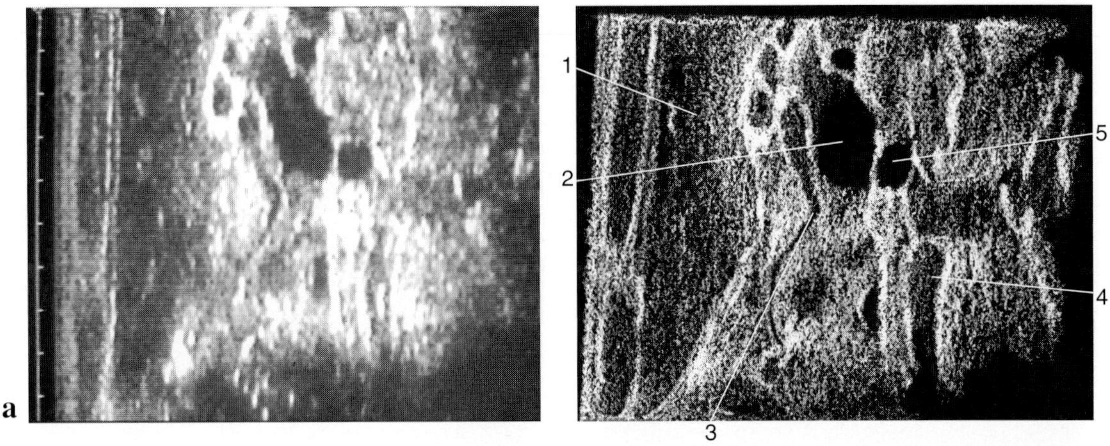

1. Liver 2. Portal vein 3. Common bile duct
4. Superior mesenteric artery 5. Splenic vein

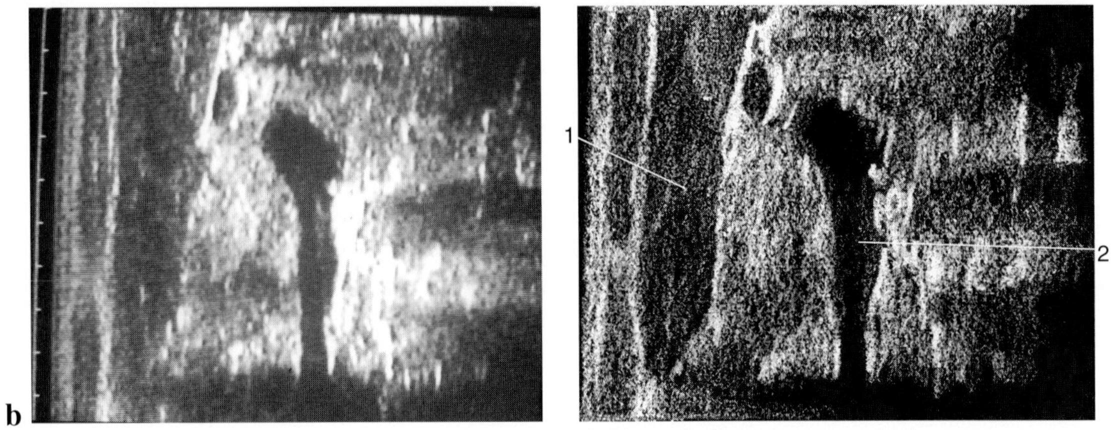

1. Liver 2. Superior mesenteric vein

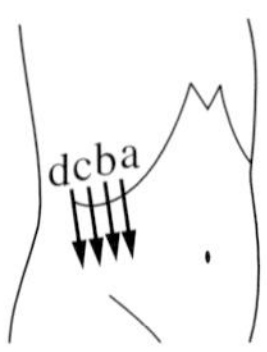

Figure 4-4. Normal biliary system, semicoronal scans.
A series of semicoronal scans of the normal bile duct recorded in the left decubitus position from the posterior to the anterior plane are shown. The normal bile duct is demonstrated lateral to the superior mesenteric vein. The large vessel adjacent to the inferior vena cava is part of the abdominal aorta.

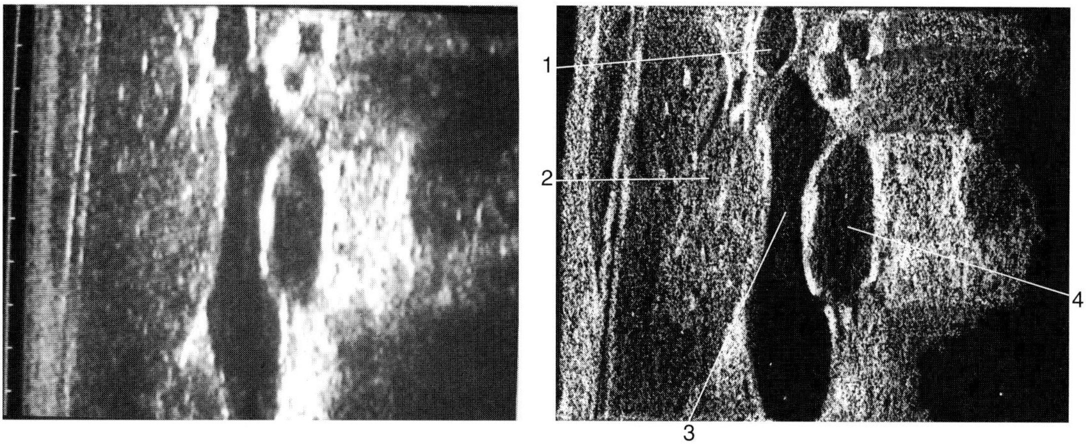

c

1. Renal vein 2. Liver 3. Inferior vena cava 4. Aorta

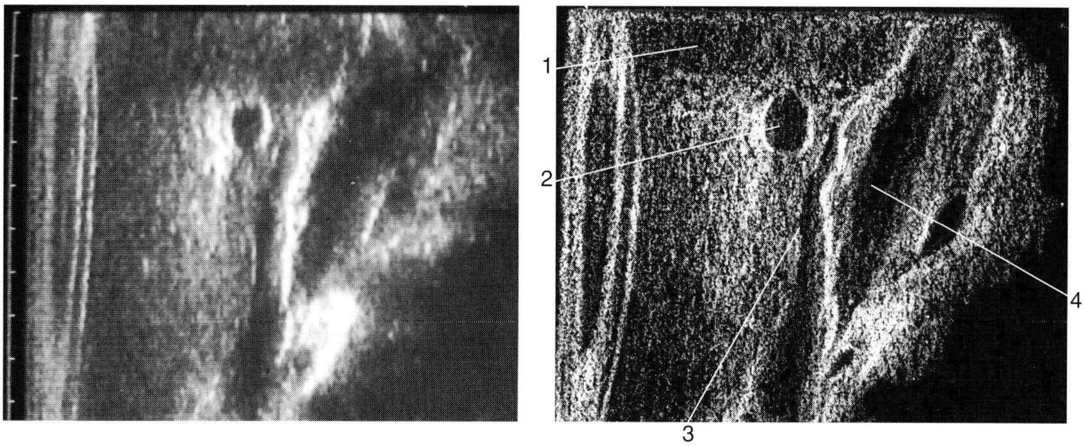

d

1. Liver 2. Portal vein 3. Inferior vena cava 4. Aorta

SCANNING TECHNIQUES

Though the use of a high-resolution real-time scanner greatly facilitates visualization of the biliary system,[92] difficult cases are often encountered. The left decubitus or right anterior oblique positions, which are useful in scanning the extrahepatic bile duct with a static scanner, can be used effectively to image the extrahepatic biliary system by real-time scanning in difficult cases.[6] The right intercostal approach, either in the supine or decubitus position, together with changes in its position with respiration, may also be successful (Figure 4-5).

Another difficulty experienced occasionally is obscuring of the gallbladder image by reverberation echo artifact or by grating or side lobe effects arising from the abdominal wall immediately anterior to the gallbladder. To avoid these problems, scanning via the intercostal spaces is most helpful. In addition, using the left decubitus position and placing the probe below the right costal margin are often beneficial because the right lobe of the liver then creates an acoustic window for the examination.

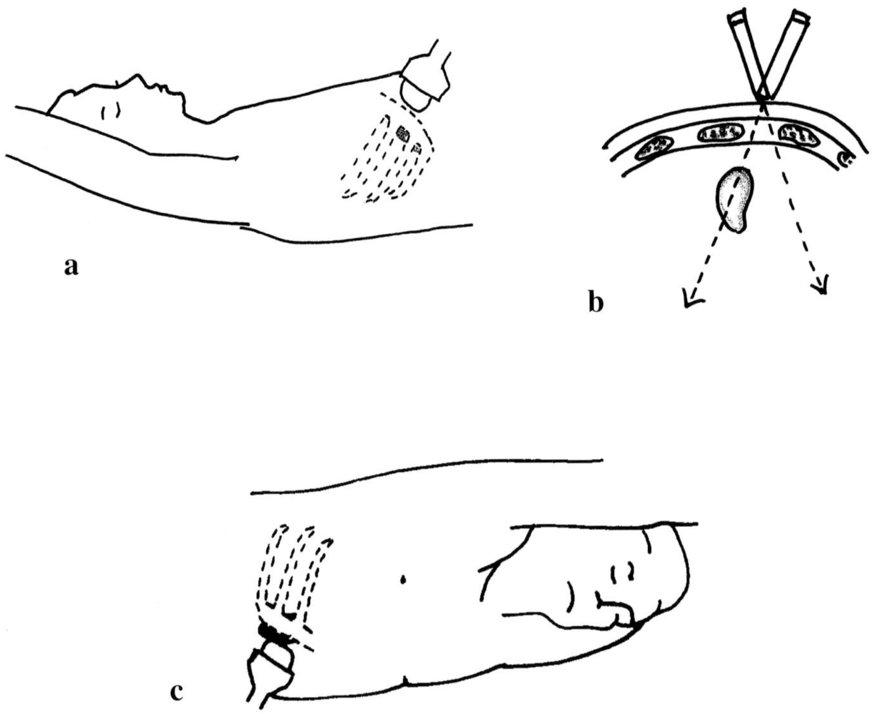

Figure 4-5. Schematic presentation of positioning and placement of a scanning probe. To image the gallbladder in overweight or heavily built patients in whom the direct subcostal approach is difficult (a), an intercostal scan (b) generally is found to be the most suitable to image the entire gallbladder. The right figure (c) indicates the alternative positioning of the probe and the patient in the left decubitus position.

DISEASES OF THE GALLBLADDER

Inflammatory Lesions

Acute inflammation of the gallbladder is characterized by chills, fever and severe right hypochondrial pain, often colicky in nature.[26, 30] The sonographic features vary considerably according to the severity of the disease state; however, the presence of stone(s) in the gallbladder, together with changes in the gallbladder wall such as edematous thickening, the double layer sign, or a diffuse increase in reflectivity and thickening, and accumulation of debris echoes in the lumen are supportive findings [64, 103] (Figure 4-6). Other clinical signs, such as Murphy's sign, tenderness localized over the gallbladder demonstrated by probe pressure, or the presence of pericholecystic fluid, are also supportive findings[30] (Figure 4-7). These acute sonographic changes eventually subside and return to normal following effective antibiotic treatment.

Stones obstructing the cystic duct, the most common cause of acute inflammation of the gallbladder, were rather difficult to visualize with static scanners. However, most of them are readily demonstrated by real-time scanning as shadow-casting, strong echoes at the neck of the gallbladder.

The advantages of sonography in diagnosing acute cholecystitis are its noninvasiveness and the rapidity of the examination.[44, 49] If the gallbladder appears entirely normal sonographically, that is, with a normal shape and wall structure and no internal echoes, then the diagnosis of acute inflammation is highly unlikely. Acalculous cholecystitis is difficult to diagnose.[63a] Wall thickening is suggestive but not invariably present but its value is reduced by the fact that typical patients (postoperative and post-trauma cases) often have other causes for wall thickening such as ascites. One disadvantage of sonography is its inability to differentiate the so-called cystic duct syndrome, a noninflammatory state of the gallbladder, which produces similar symptoms such as right hypochondrial pain, often colicky in nature. An ultrasound examination may reveal a rounded gallbladder due to hyperactivity of the sphincter muscles at the cystic duct of the gallbladder. In these instances, repeated examinations may be necessary to exclude other concomitant disease such as impacted stones in either the cystic or common duct.

The diagnostic criteria for chronic cholecystitis are less well established because of the lack of specific symptoms compared to acute cholecystitis. Chronic cholecystitis is most commonly observed in routine clinical practice as an accompaniment to cholecystolithiasis.[38, 43, 59, 61, 100] Thickening of the wall, together with loss of distensibility of the gallbladder caused by repeated inflammation, can deform the gallbladder wall and simulate tumor. The paucity of the symptoms also makes it difficult to diagnose the disease with confidence, even in the presence of specific signs of inflammation. Dynamic observation of the gallbladder following injection of an agent to induce contraction of the wall or continued observation of the size of the gallbladder over a prolonged period may be useful in assessing the functional integrity of the gallbladder. Acalculous cholecystitis is especially difficult to diagnose when the disease runs a chronic course. [59]

Noninflammatory wall thickening may occur in a number of diseases, including acute hepatitis [27,66] (Figure 4-8), decompensated liver cirrhosis with ascites (Figure 4-9), marked hypoproteinemia,[36] and acute exacerbation of chronic hepatitis, among others.[31, 91] The causes are mostly noninflammatory and are characterized by diffuse thickening of the wall, probably caused by lymphedema. It is well documented that the lymphatic drainage of the gallbladder wall is strongly influenced by the status of lymphatic flow in the liver. The wall thickening disappears rapidly when the liver recovers.

Calculi

Gallstones are common in Western as well as in Oriental populations. They occur in different chemical forms, cholesterol, bilirubin, or pigment stones; the cholesterol types have a higher incidence among urban populations, whereas the other types are found in less affluent populations whose diet contains less fat.[40, 80, 88, 95, 107] Of interest is the fact that the percentage of cholesterol stones in urban populations has shown a steep increase in recent years in Japan.

Sonographically, a gallstone is easily diagnosed as a highly reflective focus in the gallbladder or bile ducts, which casts an acoustic shadow distally[10, 19, 23, 34, 61, 102] (Figures 4-10 through 4-13). Differentiation of the nature of stones by ultrasound imaging is generally considered impossible, because the echo intensity depends mainly upon the acoustic impedance mismatch between the bile and the stone, which is extremely high irrespective of its composition (Figures 4-14 and 4-15). Reflectivity is also strongly governed by physical laws such as the nature of the stone's surface and the angle of the reflecting plane to the ultrasound beam. In pure cholesterol stones, a rounded, diffusely reflective pattern may be experienced because of some penetration of the sound into the stone, as shown in Figure 4-14. This type of stone may be especially amenable to treatment by lithotripsy.

If there is sufficient bile in the lumen, the stones may move with postural changes. Although small stones may lack characteristic shadowing because of diffraction of ultrasound or the relative width of the sound beam compared to the small size of the stone, aggregations of small stones can create clear acoustic shadowing. Stones usually settle on the gallbladder wall; however, floating stones may be found occasionally.[95]

Echoes from debris, most commonly arising from pus, blood clot, or bilirubinate crystals in concentrated bile, frequently occur in acute or chronic inflammation of the gallbladder. In chronic obstruction of the biliary tree, echogenic bile often aggregates into lumps and then may be confused with stones or tumors[17, 28, 50, 85] (Figures 4-16 and 4-17). The distinction from small stones depends on finding acoustic shadowing, which is often possible to demonstrate even with a single tiny stone when the examination is carefully performed with a high-resolution scanner. Debritic echoes in the gallbladder may be physiological in patients during a prolonged fast (e.g., those on parenteral nutrition), in which case the echoes are transient,[59, 87] but otherwise they are abnormal, indicating nonfunction.

The use of modern real-time scanners has greatly reduced false-negative and false-positive results with an accuracy of better than 95 %. The main factor in this improvement is the complete coverage of the gallbladder that can be achieved by a meticulous study with a mobile scan head. The most frequently diagnostic pitfall is an artifact caused by reflective intestinal echoes lying close to the gallbladder, in the colon or the duodenal loop. The gas produces side lobes which often project apparently significant high-level echoes into the gallbladder lumen. Careful scanning is mandatory to exclude artifactual cholecystolithiasis. The same artifact can cause a false-positive diagnosis of stones in the common duct when a gas-containing duodenal diverticulum lies adjacent to the papilla of Vater. Cholesterol polyps and cancer of the gallbladder may mimic the echo appearances of stones. To avoid these diagnostic pitfalls, careful technique is required; scanning from two different directions, observation of positional changes, and a careful search for acoustic shadows are important precautions.

False-negative results, on the other hand, may arise from small stones hidden in the cystic duct and covered by reflective intestinal loops, stones in the folded gallbladder fundus obscured by adjacent gas echoes, and bile duct stones without acoustic shadowing. The use of high-quality real-time scanners has greatly reduced the false-negative rate, however, a careful search by a dedicated specialist is essential for accurate diagnosis of cholelithiasis. Needless to say the sonologist should be aware of the pitfalls in the diagnostic procedures, and whenever possible, sonographic findings should be compared to accurate surgical findings to maintain diagnostic accuracy rates.

Tumors

Benigh tumors

Tumors of the biliary system are generally classified as benign or malignant and may occur in any part of the gallbladder. Among the benign tumors of the gallbladder, small, echogenic, polypoid lesions (cholesterol polyps) are most frequently encountered during routine clinical examinations (Figures 4-18 and 4-19). They may be seen as single or multiple echogenic, polypoid lesions arising from the gallbladder wall, which do not shift with positional changes or in response to external palpation, though the occasional cholesterol polyp with a long pedicle may tend to move, whereas adenomatous or inflammatory polyps are fixed.[7, 13] Even polypoid lesions as large as 5 mm do not cast an acoustic shadow. Cholesterol polyps frequently occur as multiple small lesions seen as homogeneous, echogenic foci; their margins are generally regular. If a polyp is greater than 5 mm in diameter, malignancy should be considered, especially if the surface is irregular or the echo texture heterogeneous; in such case, repeated examinations over monthly or bimonthly intervals are recommended.

Another frequently encountered condition that may be classified as a benign neoplasm of the gallbladder is adenomyomatosis[35, 83, 86, 89] (Figure 4-20). Here the gallbladder wall is either symmetrically or asymmetrically thickened and echogenic, frequently with echo-poor foci corresponding to dilated Rokitansky-Aschoff sinuses that can be visualized with high-resolution equipment (e.g., on endoscopic ultrasound). Calculi forming in the sinuses produce intensely echogenic foci often pathognomonic ring-down or comet-tail artifacts. Careful examination of the gallbladder contours on an intravenous cholecystogram often clinches the diagnosis when taken together with the ultrasound investigation. Cases with minimal focal thickening, however, cause greater difficulty in differentiating adenomyomatosis from cancer of the gallbladder. Focal gallbladder wall changes may also be observed in patients with a previous history of gangrenous cholecystitis, with or without stones. These irregularities correspond to ulcer formation, hemorrhage, or granulation following inflammation.

Malignant tumors

Cancer of the gallbladder is invariably insidious in onset, and is often only discovered after obstructive jaundice appear or by palpation of a hard mass in the right hypochondrium. The slow progression and lack of symptoms make early diagnosis difficult; hence, carcinoma of the gallbladder has a poor outlook compared to other abdominal malignancies. The introduction of high-quality real-time ultrasound offers the promise of its detection at a much earlier stage. At present, this can only occur by chance, but if a high-risk population could be identified, effective screening could be performed by ultrasound. Other diagnostic modalities, such as CT, MRI, or invasive techniques such as angiography or laparoscopy, are only occasionally successful at present.

Due to the lack of symptoms in the early stages, gallbladder cancer is rarely discovered while it is surgically resectable.[57, 58] Early cancers of the gallbladder detected accidentally at cholecystectomy are seen as small polypoid or flat tumors localized in the wall of the gallbladder.

Cholesterol polyps rarely show malignant transformation. However, one personal case is shown in Figure 4-21, in which an early cancer was found on the surface of a polyp. No involvement of the other wall structures was noted on histological examination. Figure 4-22 shows a more typical case of carcinoma of the gallbladder mucosa. The changes are subtle, with only slight thickening of the posterior wall of the gallbladder. Repeated examination, including intraoperative ultrasound, confirmed a reproducible alteration in the mucosal layer, seen as a plaque-like elevation with slightly low echo levels. At surgery, a flat mucosal cancer confined essentially to the mucosal layer was demonstrated, with no dissemination or invasion to the neighboring organs. Another case of gallbladder cancer is shown in Figure 4-23.

Unresectable, advanced cancers are rarely missed by sonography.[15, 76, 82, 104, 111, 113] The sonographic patterns of advanced gallbladder cancer have been classified into 5 categories (Figure 4-24).[113] When a high-resolution real-time scanner is used, advanced gallbladder cancer can be diagnosed accurately based on the findings of focal or diffuse thickening of the gallbladder wall, tumor infiltration into the liver bed, and metastasis to the periportal or retropancreatic lymph nodes (Figures 4-25 through 4-28). Localized ascites may also be demonstrated. Elucidation of the cause of obstructive jaundice often reveals cancer of the gallbladder wall (Figures 4-29 and 4-30). Careful scrutiny of the structure of the gallbladder wall has led to demonstration of a malignant tumor at the stage of invasion into the hepatic hilum with bile duct obstruction (Figure 4-31). It should be emphasized, however, that even in the presence of positive findings by sonography, the final diagnosis in equivocal cases depends on supportive evidence such as positive aspiration cytology or percutaneous transhepatic cholangiography, which can be performed with little risk to the patient.

Metastatic tumor in the gallbladder wall is rare; melanoma is the usual cause (Figure 4-32). The sonographic changes of primary and secondary malignancies are identical.

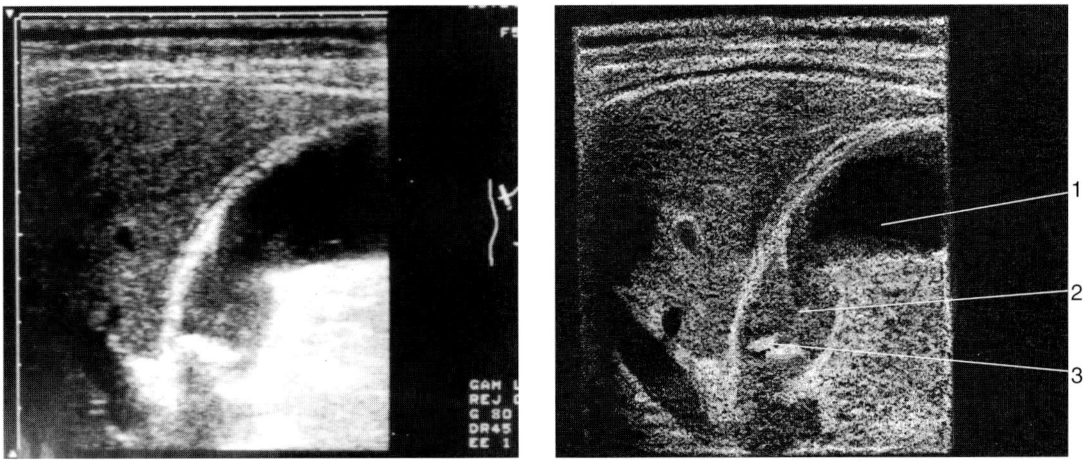

1. Gallbladder 2. Debris 3. Stones

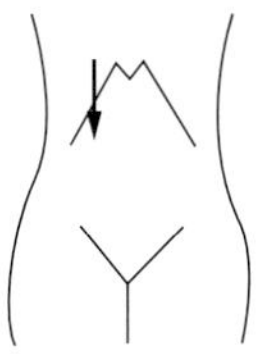

Figure 4-6. Cholecystolithiasis with acute cholecystitis.
Gallstone disease is not infrequently complicated by acute inflammation of the gallbladder. This sonogram demonstrates the enlarged gallbladder containing stones with debris accumulation. A thin, hypoechoic layer of the wall, a characteristic sign of localized edema due to acute cholecystitis, is also demonstrated. The symptoms disappeared completely following intensive medical treatment.

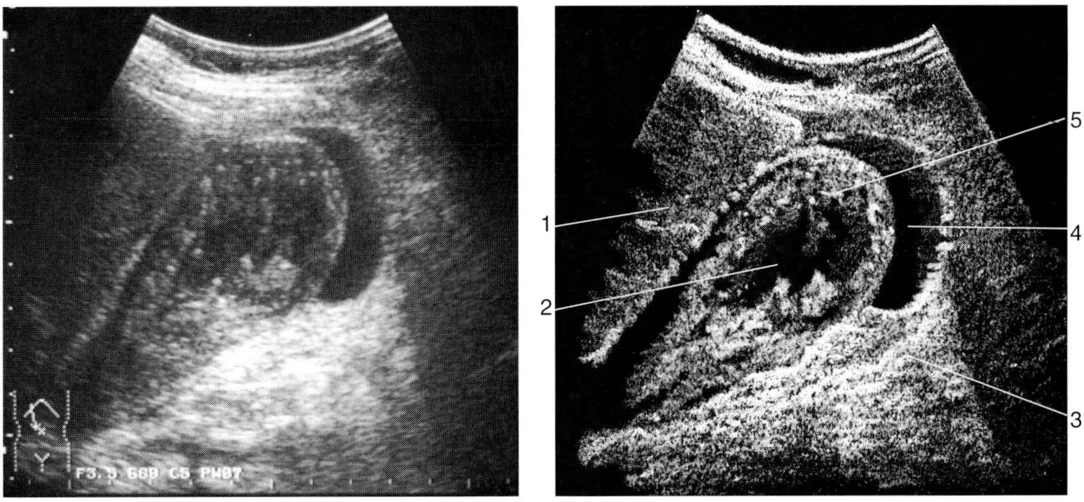

1. Liver 2. Debris 3. Acoustic enhancement
4. Ascites 5. Gallbladder

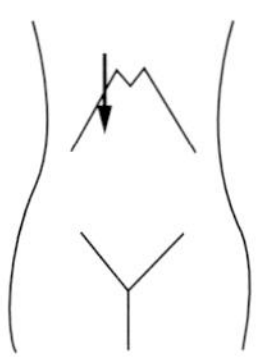

Figure 4-7. Acute cholecystitis with pericystic fluid accumulation.
Acute cholecystitis with severe clinical symptoms produces an accumulation of debritic echoes in the gallbladder lumen and also inflammatory exudate around the body of the gallbladder. Wall thickening is extensive, and multiple, small bright echoes in the debris echoes suggest that the inflammation is a complication of gallstones in the neck of the gallbladder. These changes subsided following intensive antibiotic treatment.

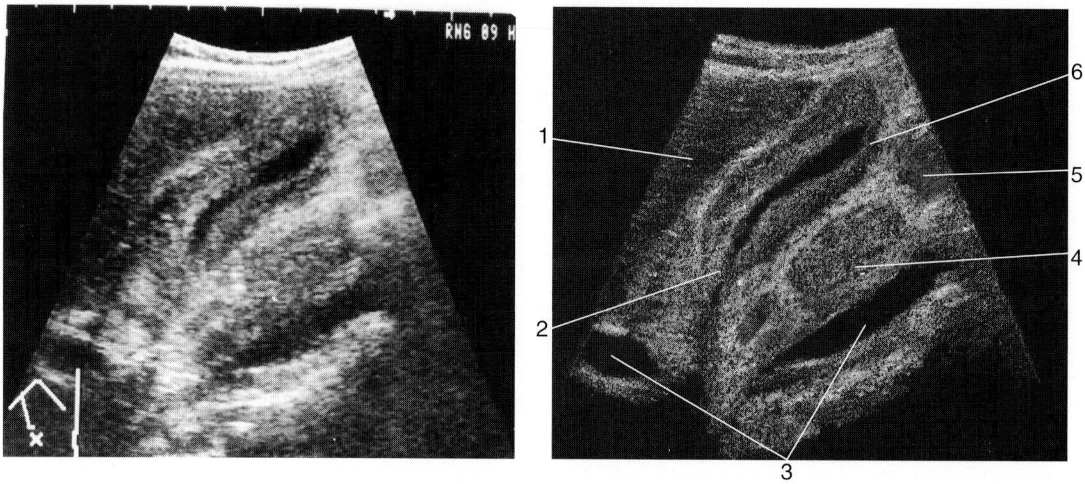

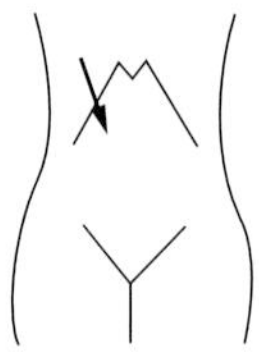

1. Liver 2. Neck of gallbladder 3. Inferior vena cava 4. Head of pancreas 5. Colon 6. Edematous thickened gallbladder wall

Figure 4-8. Thickening of the gallbladder wall in acute hepatitis.
In viral hepatitis, especially during the acute phase, the gallbladder wall is diffusely thickened. The precise etiology is not known; edema of the wall due to lymphatic congestion has been suggested. The changes are reversible and disappear completely upon recovery of liver function.

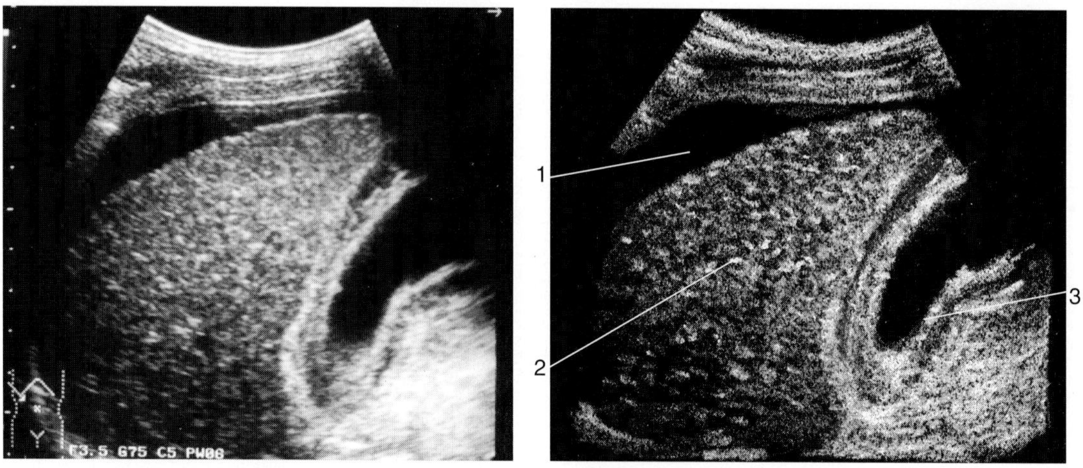

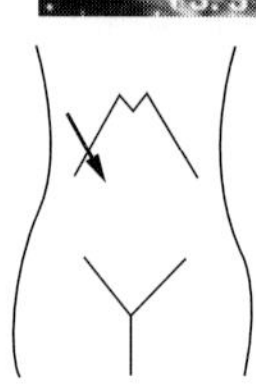

1. Ascites 2. Right lobe of cirrhotic liver 3. Gallbladder wall

Figure 4-9. Liver cirrhosis with edema of the gallbladder.
Edema of the gallbladder is frequently observed in decompensated cirrhosis. Similar changes may occur in a number of clinical states, including hypoproteinemia and chronic hepatitis with or without ascites.

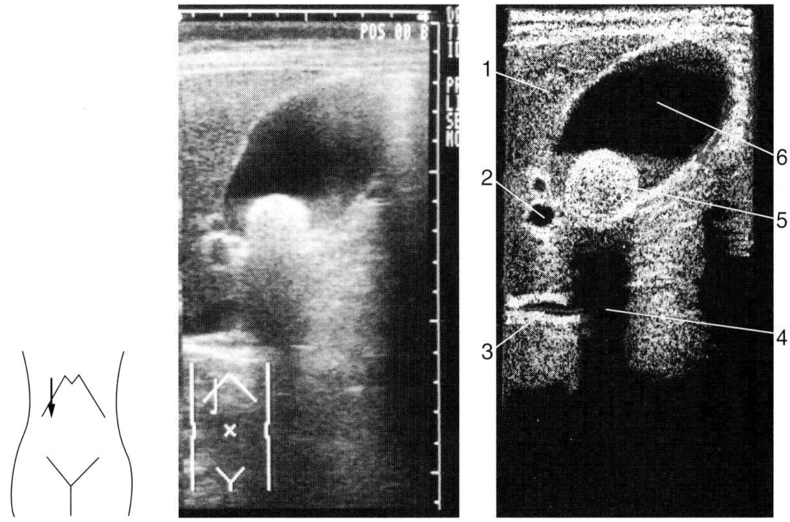

1. Liver 2. Right portal vein 3. Inferior vena cava 4. Acoustic shadow 5. Cholesterol stone 6. Gallbladder

Figure 4-10. Pure cholesterol gallstone.
Gallstones tend to show characteristic echo patterns corresponding to the chemical constituents of the stones. Thus pure cholesterol stones are usually round in shape, with bright echoes indicating some penetration of ultrasound into the stone. This pattern is quite different from that of calcified stones in which no sound penetration occurs.

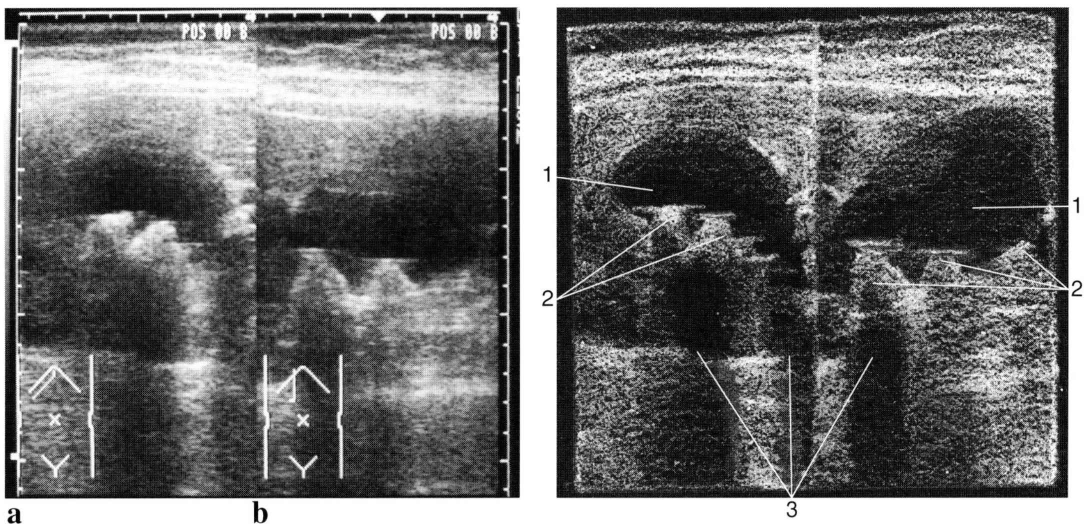

1. Gallbladder 2. Stones 3. Acoustic shadow

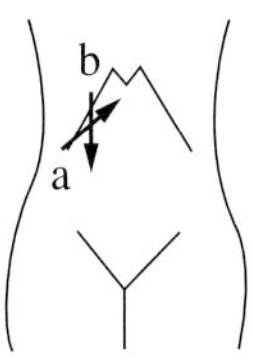

Figure 4-11. Gallstones with side lobe artifact.
Medium-sized gallstones visualized in the gallbladder show a typical artifact of linear echoes extending laterally from the surfaces of the stones. These echoes represent a grating or side lobe artifact exaggerated by the marked impedance mismatch between the calcified stone and surrounding bile.

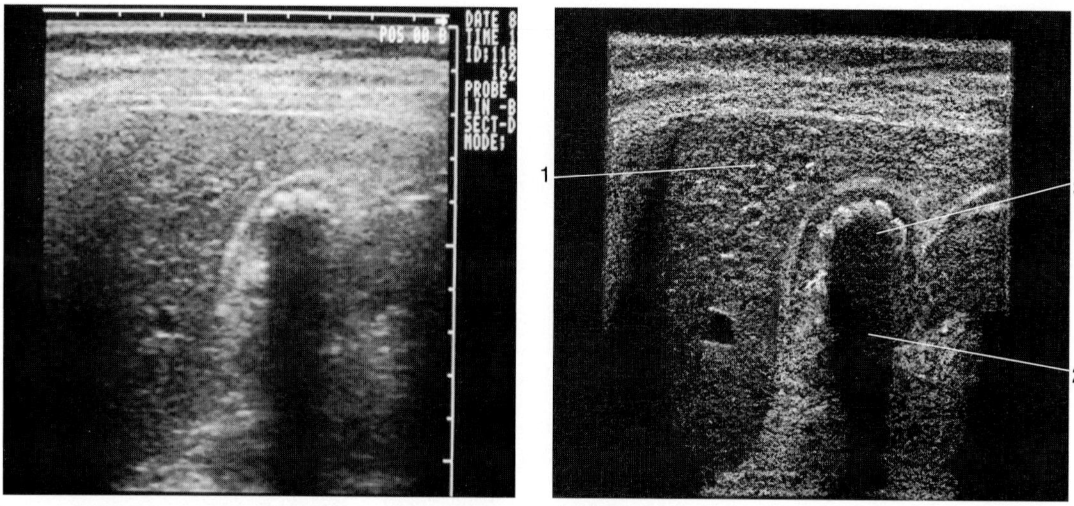

1. Liver 2. Acoustic shadow 3. Stones

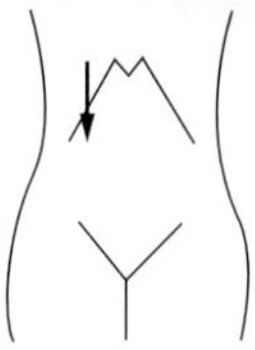

Figure 4-12. Shadow pattern in cholelithiasis.
A sonogram of a "nonvisualized" gallbladder packed with stones which produced the so-called shadow pattern is shown. Absence of a fluid layer with wide acoustic shadowing indicates packing of the gallbladder with multiple stones. However, careful scrutiny is essential to avoid misinterpreting the similar appearance of bowel gas.

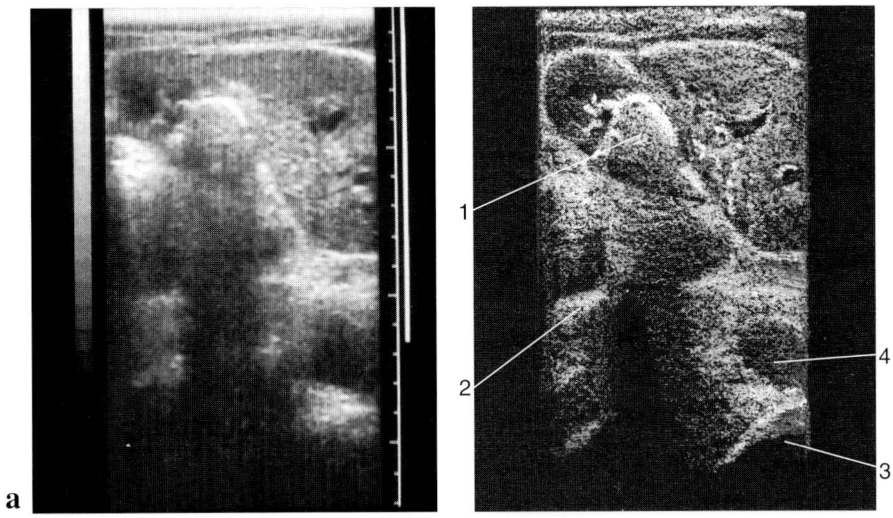

1. Gallbladder stones 2. Right kidney
3. Vertebra 4. Aorta

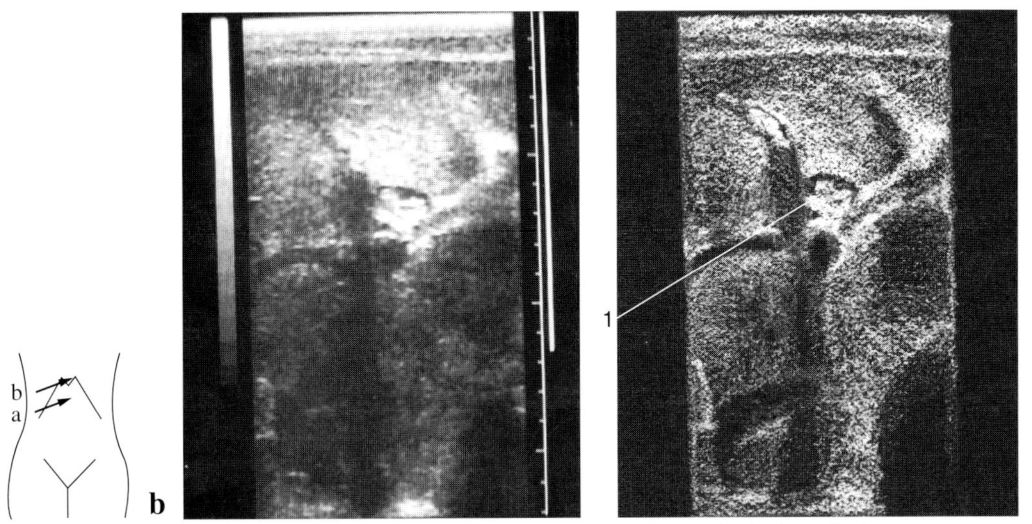

1. Stones in the hepatic ducts

Figure 4-13. Gallstones in the gallbladder and common hepatic duct.
In gallstone disease, stones may appear not only in the gallbladder but also in other parts of the biliary tract. In this case multiple stones were seen in the gallbladder (a) together with small stones packed in the common hepatic duct (b).

a

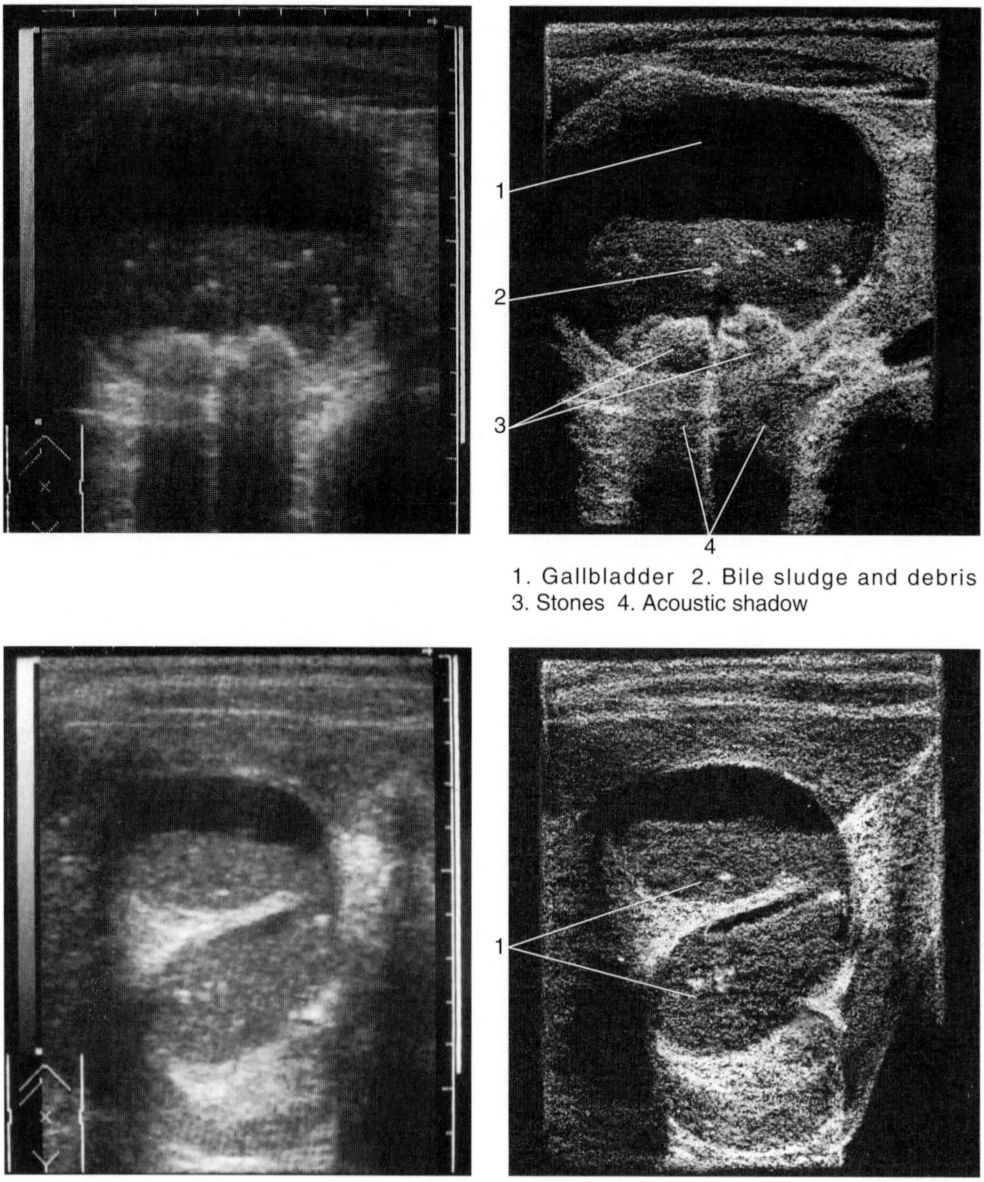

b

1. Gallbladder 2. Bile sludge and debris
3. Stones 4. Acoustic shadow

1. Bile sludge and debris

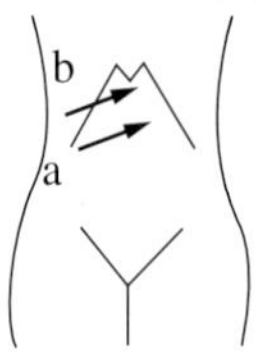

Figure 4-14. Gallstones with debris.
A dilated gallbladder with dependent calculi together with abundant debritic echoes (cholesterol sand) creating a fluid-debris interface is imaged (a). The debritic echoes moved with postural changes of the patient in a manner similar to the appearance of sand in an hourglass (b).

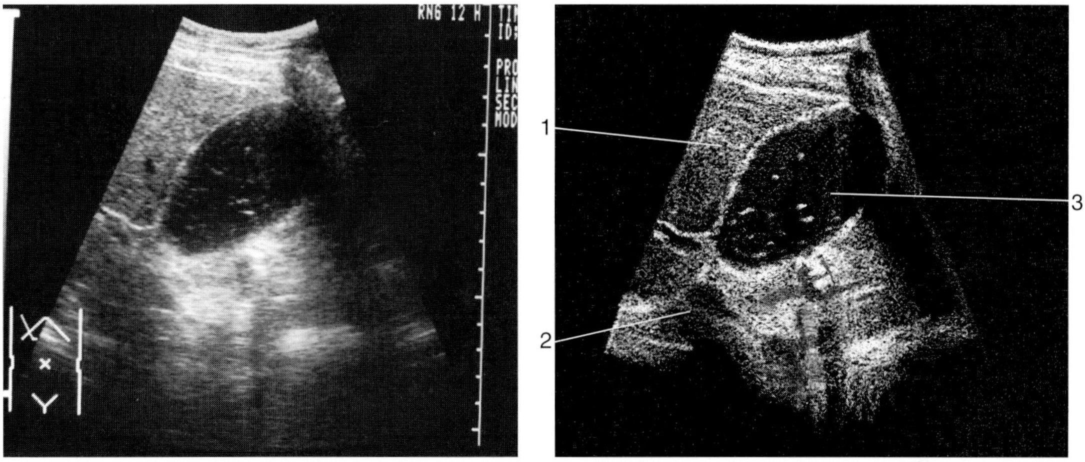

1. Liver 2. Stones 3. Dilated gallbladder

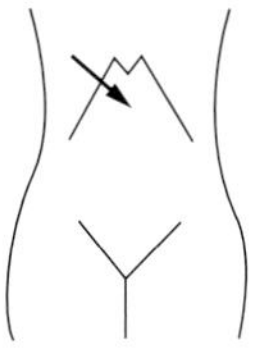

Figure 4-15. Cholecystolithiasis.
A dilated gallbladder with floating bile debris is demonstrated by subcostal and intercostal scanning. The right intercostal scan discloses small shadowing stones in the cystic duct; these presumably caused the obstruction that led to stagnation of bile, causing the sludge.

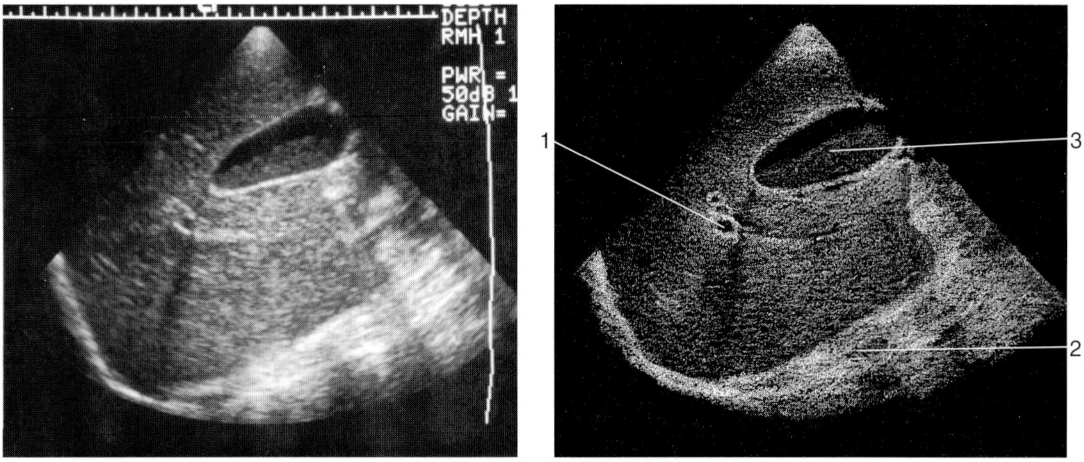

1. Portal vein 2. Sacrospinalis muscle 3. Debris in gallbladder

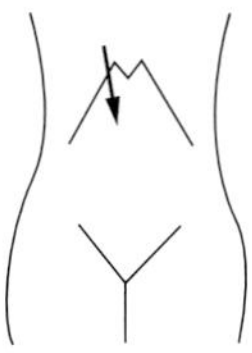

Figure 4-16. Debritic echoes of the gallbladder.
Bilirubin crystals form in the normal gallbladder if it is not emptied, as occurs in a prolonged fast. In this patient on parenteral nutrition, the crystals are seen as an echogenic, dependent layer in the gallbladder. They are of no clinical significance and clear when the gallbladder begins to function again.

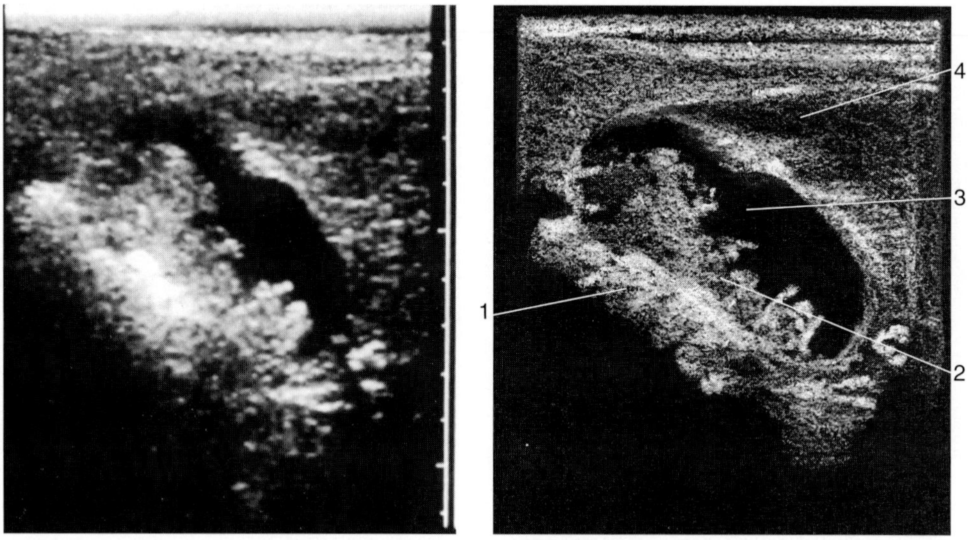

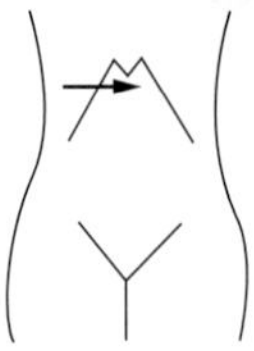

1. Intestinal gas echoes 2. Debris 3. Lumen of gallbladder 4. Liver

Figure 4-17. Debritic echoes in the gallbladder.
Debris in the gallbladder is due either to cholesterol crystals, blood, or pus. This sonogram shows the coarse debris pattern known as lumpy bile. Even a positional change may fail to move such debris. In this case, the appearance was considered suspicious of carcinoma and led to aspiration biopsy, which recovered only lumpy bile. In these instances, examination on another day may disclose definite changes in shape and thus exclude a true mass.

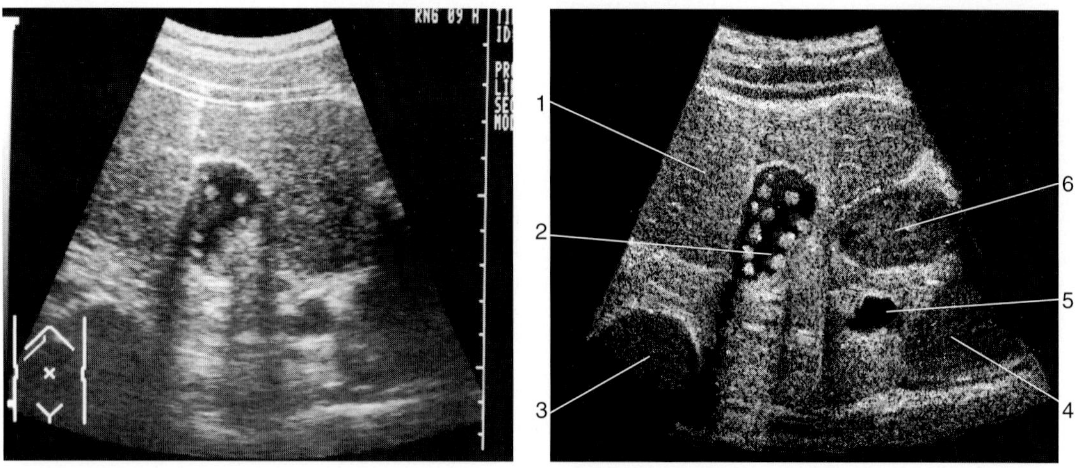

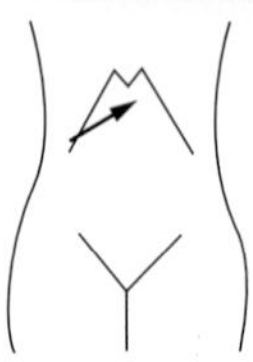

1. Liver 2. Multiple cholesterol polyps 3. Right kidney 4. Pancreas 5. Portal vein 6. Stomach

Figure 4-18. Cholesterol polyps of the gallbladder.
Multiple small, echogenic, polypoid lesions without acoustic shadowing are visualized on the anterior and posterior walls of the gallbladder on subcostal and intercostal scans. Cholesterol polyps usually remain relatively small, and careful scanning frequently reveals a cleft separating the polyp from the wall of the gallbladder.

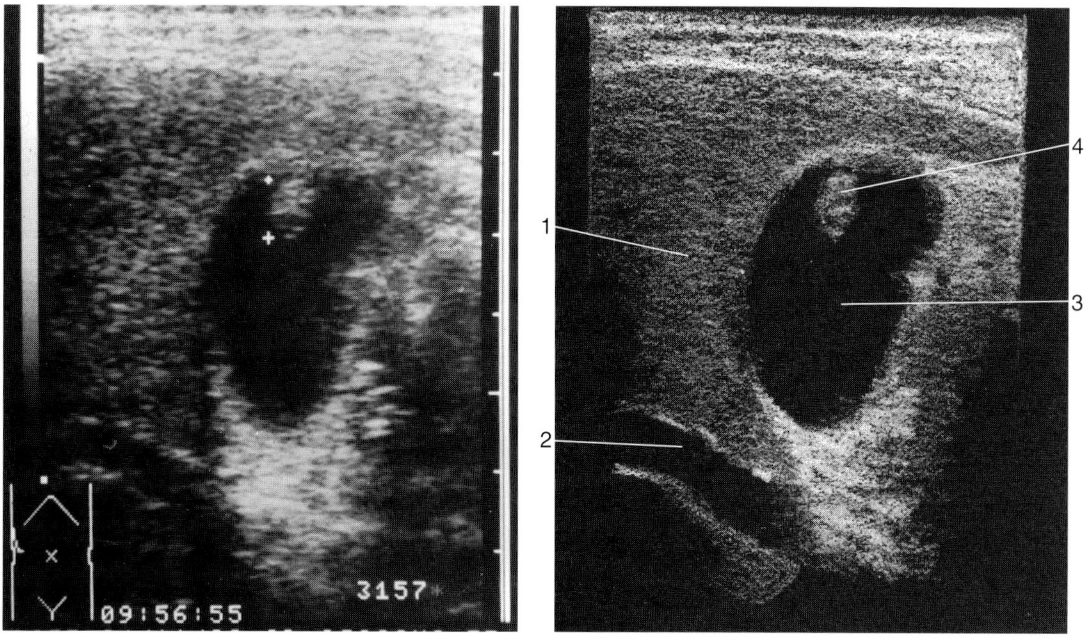

1. Liver 2. Portal vein 3. Gallbladder 4. Adenomatous polyp

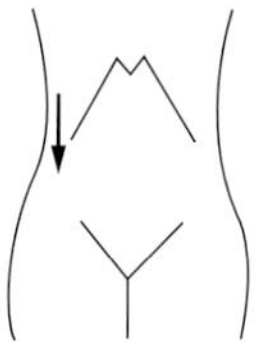

Figure 4-19. Adenomatous polyp of the gallbladder.
Polypoid lesions of the gallbladder may have different etiologies even though they are sonographically identical. This small mass protruding from the gallbladder wall appeared less reflective than a typical cholesterol polyp. Diagnosis can only be confirmed by surgical excision.

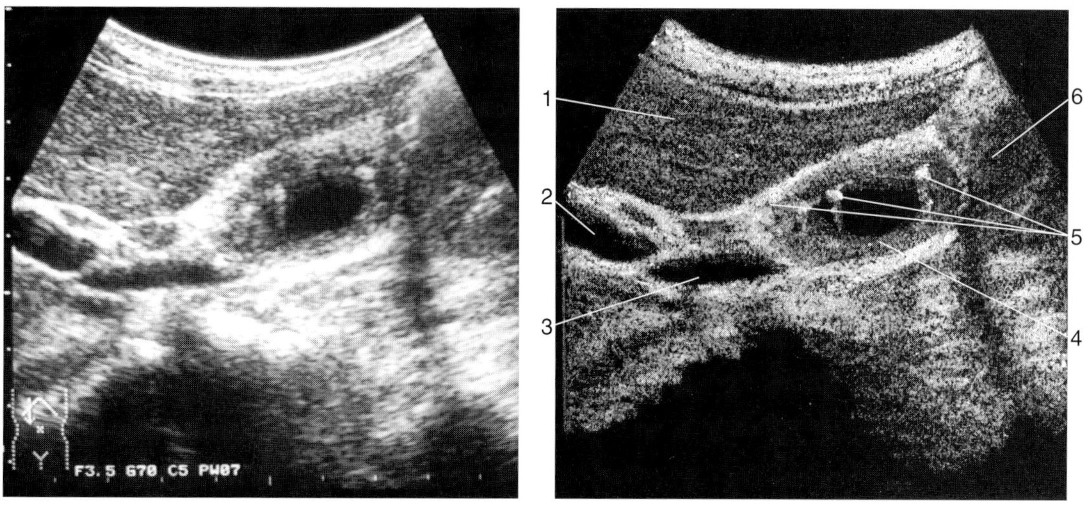

1. Liver 2. Portal vein 3. Inferior vena cava 4. Adenomyomatosis of gallbladder 5. Intramural stones 6. Intestinal gas

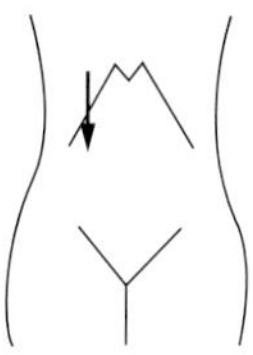

Figure 4-20. Adenomyomatosis of the gallbladder.
A benign condition of the gallbladder, adenomyomatosis is characterized by diffuse or focal thickening of the gallbladder wall, which contains echogenic foci from calcification in the Rokitansky-Aschoff sinuses. The calcium casts acoustic shadows, often with reverberation echo artifact, referred to as the comet tail sign.

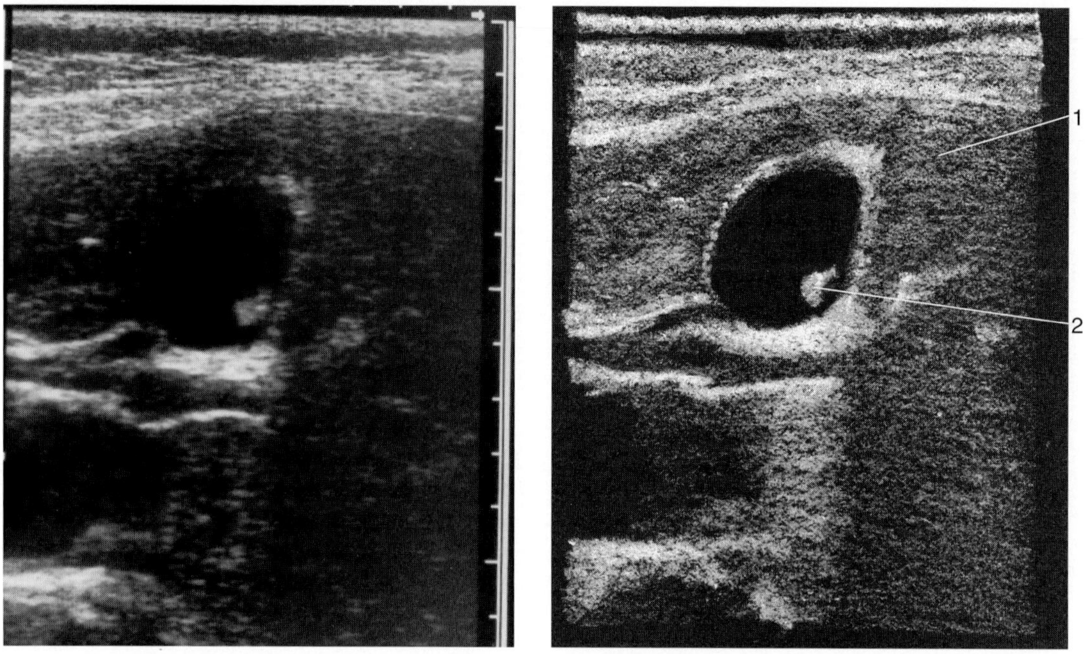

1. Liver 2. Polypoid lesion (cancer on top of a cholesterol polyp)

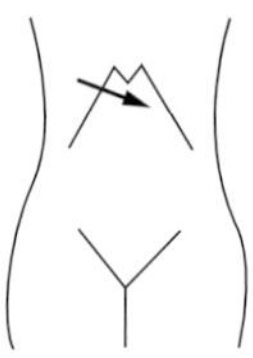

Figure 4-21. A small gallbladder cancer superimposed on a cholesterol polyp of the gallbladder. Cholesterol polyps of the gallbladder are fairly common and seldom if ever undergo malignant transformation. In this case, though the sonographic findings are typical of a cholesterol polyp, a superficial carcinoma was found at the very tip of the polyp at surgery.

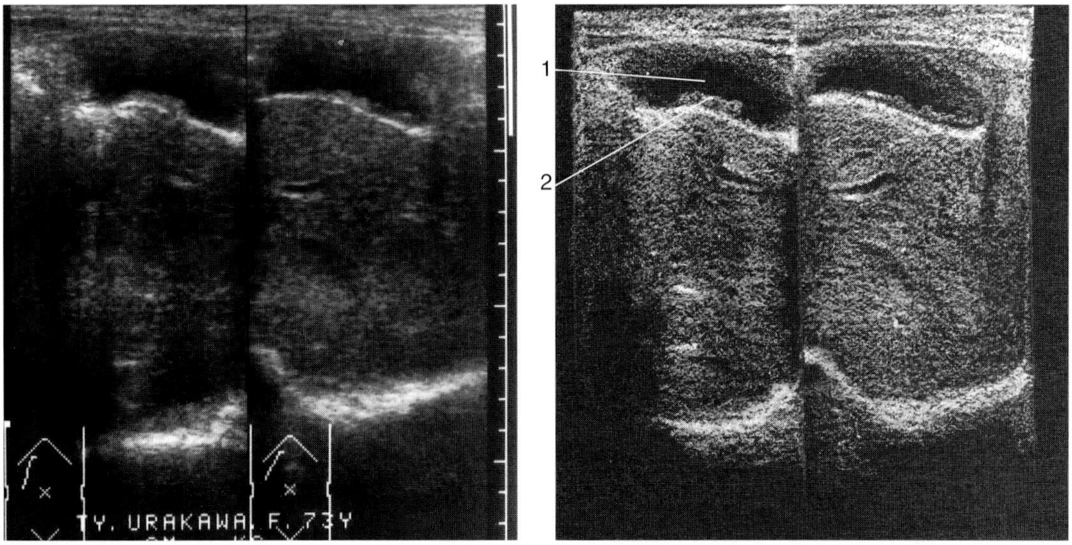

1. Gallbladder 2. Mucosal cancer

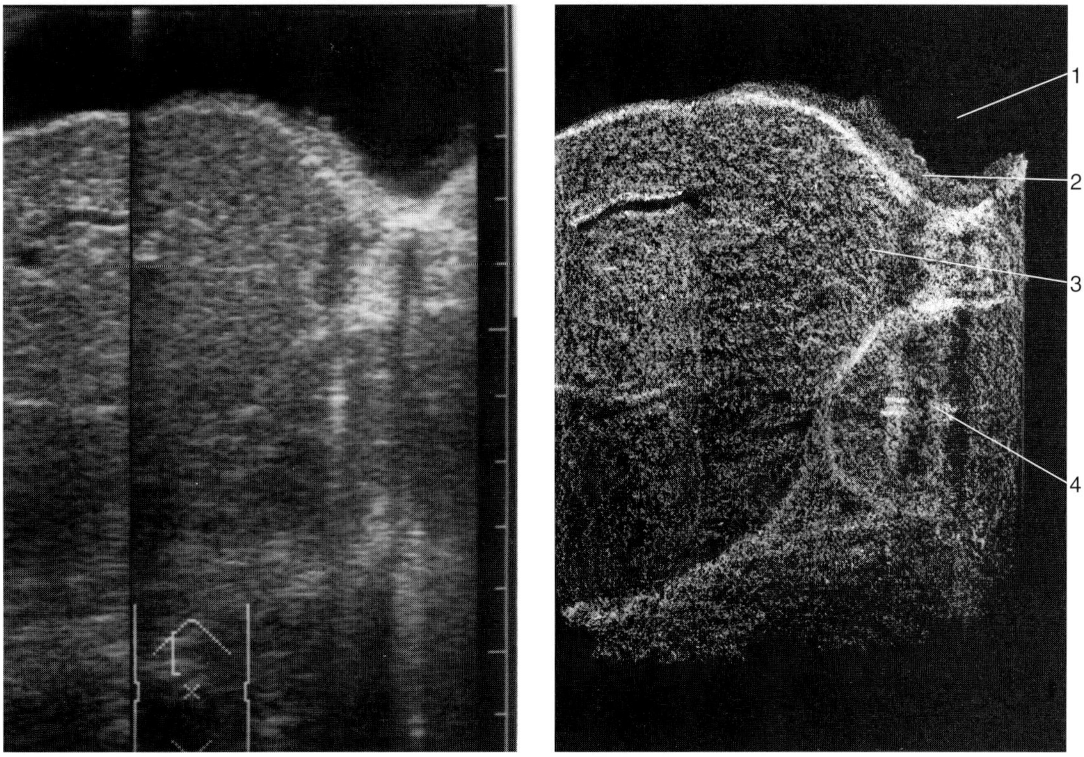

1. Gallbladder 2. Mucosal cancer 3. Liver 4. Right kidney

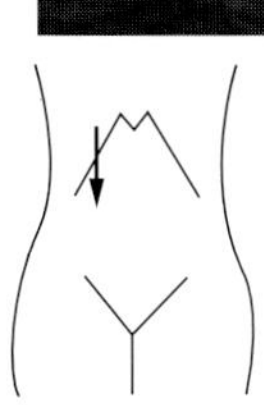

Figure 4-22. Mucosal cancer of the gallbladder.
Gallbladder malignancy is rarely detected at a very early stage because of the lack of symptoms. This 73-year-old female, who was operated on for esophageal varices, was found to have a slight elevation of the posterior wall of the gallbladder on routine ultrasound. Since the lesions persisted for 5 months, cholecystectomy was performed and a small, flat mucosal cancer was discovered. (a) A conventional scan with a 3.5-MHz linear-array scanner. (b) An intraoperative scan with a 5-MHz linear probe. (Courtesy of Dr. H. Fukui, Nagasaki Memorial Hospital, Nagasaki, Japan.)

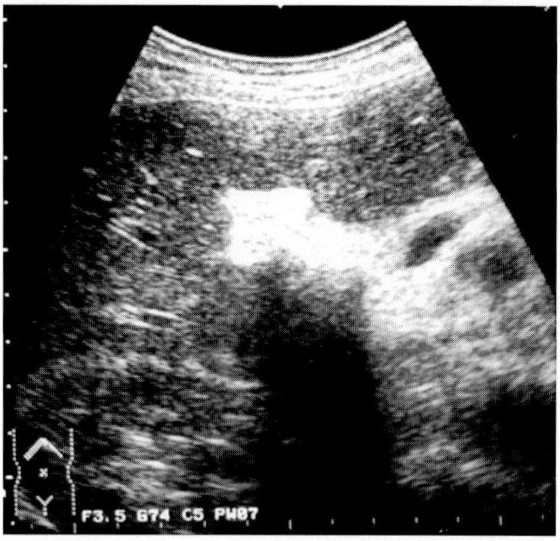

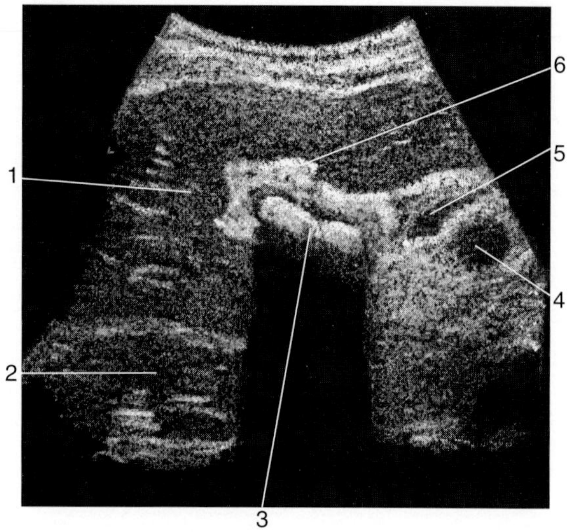

1. Liver 2. Right kidney 3. Stones with acoustic shadow 4. Portal vein 5. Left hepatic duct 6. Gallbladder cancer

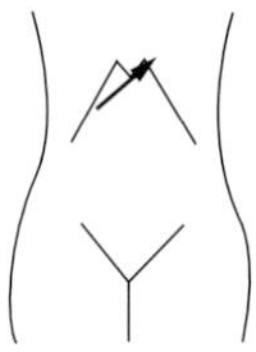

Figure 4-23. Cancer of the gallbladder.
Cancer of the gallbladder produces a variety of echo patterns. This case was found during routine clinical examination as a shrunken gallbladder accompanied by stones. The gallbladder showed an abnormal contour with thickening of the wall suggestive of malignant change. Because of the sonographic abnormalities, exploratory laparotomy was performed and malignancy was found.

Type			No. of Cases
Ⅰa	diffuse weak echoes	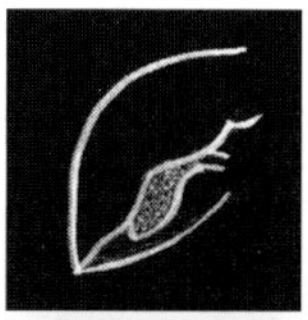	6
Ⅰb	strong central echoes in addition to diffuse weak echoes	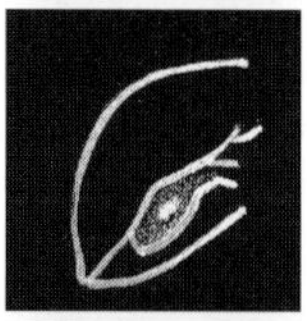	2
Ⅱ	thickened gallbladder wall	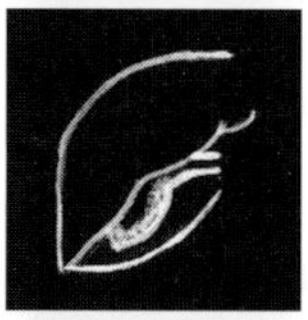	3
Ⅲ	fungating mass	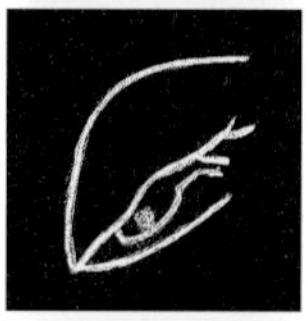	2
Ⅳ	Type Ⅱ and Type Ⅲ	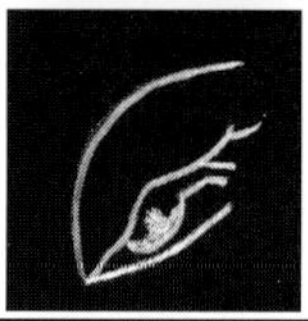	1

Figure 4-24. Sonographic classification of gallbladder cancer.
(From Yeh HC: Ultrasonography and computed tomography of carcinoma of the gallbladder. Radiology 133:167-173, 1979).

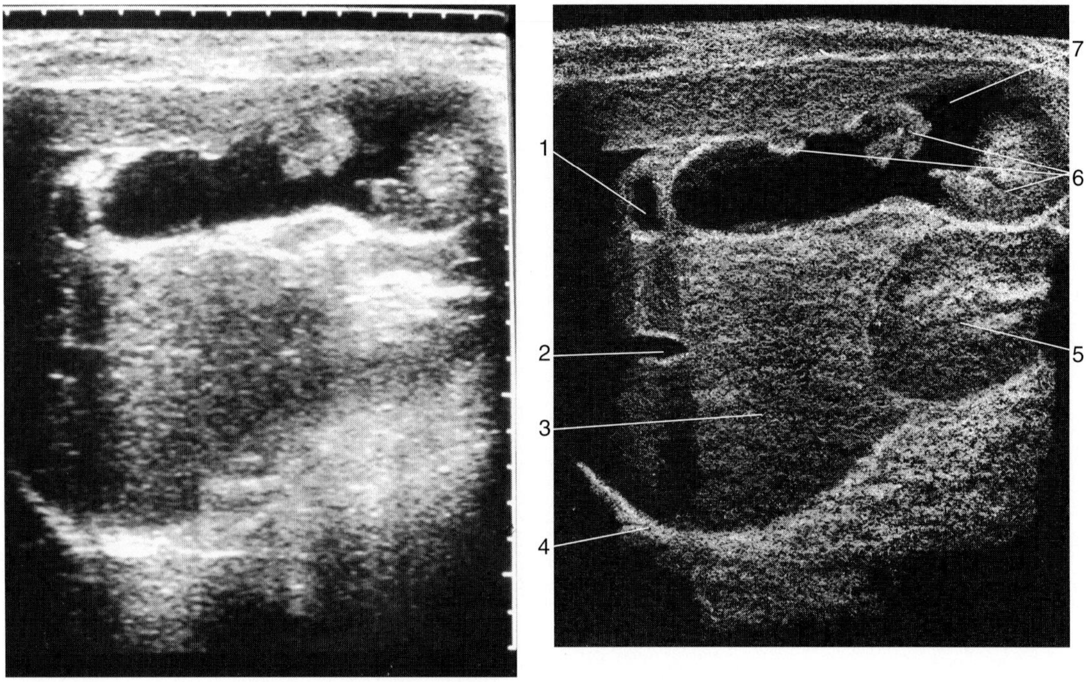

1. Right portal vein 2. Hepatic vein 3. Liver
4. Diaphragm 5. Right kidney 6. Tumor
7. Gallbladder

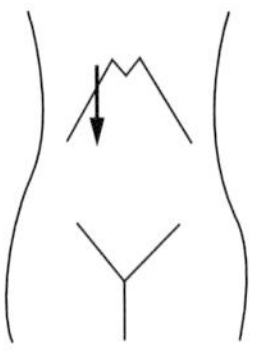

Figure 4-25. Cancer of the gallbladder.
The patient complained of vague discomfort in the right hypochondrium and had minimal weight loss. An upper gastrointestinal series failed to show any abnormality; however, sonographic examination disclosed a small degree of dilatation of the gallbladder, with three irregular, exophytic tumor masses. Fortunately, laparotomy disclosed no distant metastasis, and radical resection of the mass was performed without reccurrence.

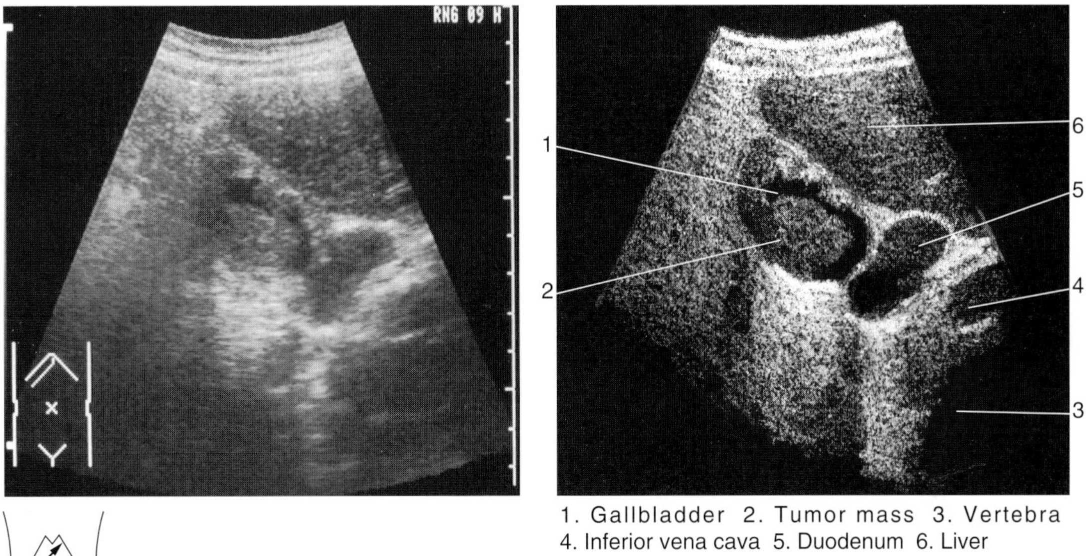

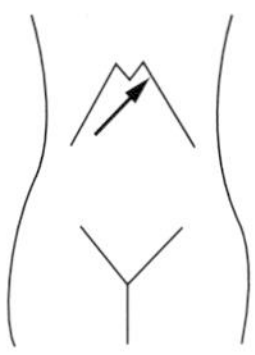

Figure 4-26. Cancer of the gallbladder.
Diffuse, irregular swelling of the gallbladder is a hallmark of advanced primary carcinoma. This sonogram shows the characteristic features of gallbladder carcinoma: echo-poor thickening of the gallbladder wall with irregularly distributed, echogenic foci together with complete disappearance of normal architecture. Posterior acoustic enhancement indicated less attenuation by the tumor than the liver. Although no distant metastasis was found, direct tumor invasion of the liver was suggested.

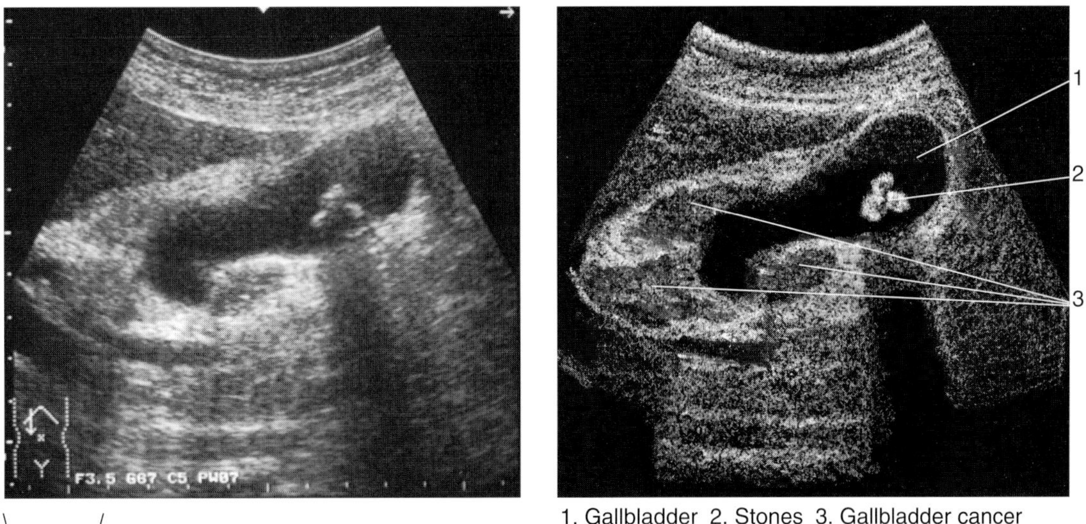

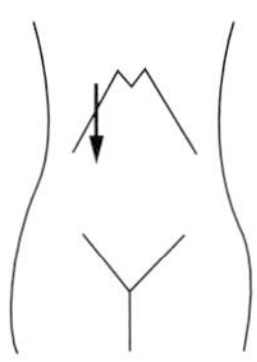

Figure 4-27. Advanced gallbladder cancer with stones.
Gallbladder cancer and gallstones often coexist. On this sagittal scan, an enlarged gallbladder with irregular thickening of the wall caused by the infiltrating tumors was imaged together with stone echoes in the lower third. Lymph node metastases were detected superior to the gallbladder, and there was a large, metastatic nodule in the central portion of the liver.

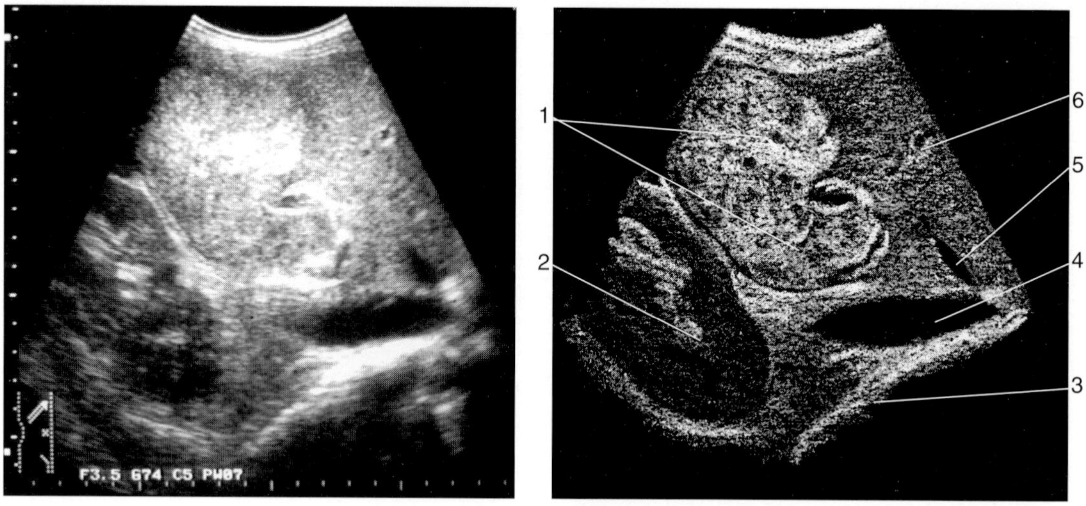

1. Cancer of gallbladder 2. Right kidney 3. Diaphragm 4. Inferior vena cava 5. Right hepatic vein 6. Liver

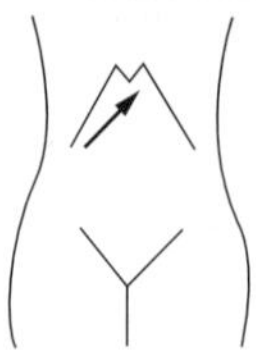

Figure 4-28. Advanced gallbladder cancer.
A subcostal scan disclosed a large tumor between the liver and the right kidney. The gallbladder lumen has disappeared completely, indicating massive growth of the tumor.

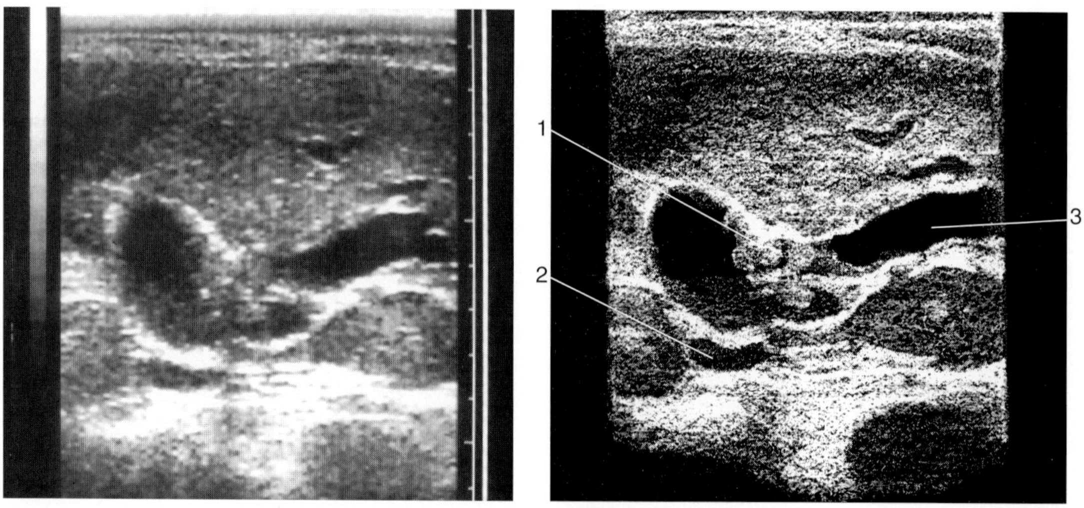

1. Cancer of gallbladder 2. Inferior vena cava 3. Dilated left hepatic duct

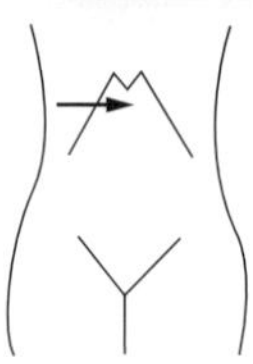

Figure 4-29. Gallbladder cancer with jaundice.
Gallbladder cancer may distort the gallbladder only slightly and yet may extensively infiltrate the surrounding liver. In this case, a small tumor near the cystic duct showed direct extension to and infiltration of the porta hepatis, causing obstructive jaundice. The left hepatic duct is considerably dilatated due to direct invasion by the mass.

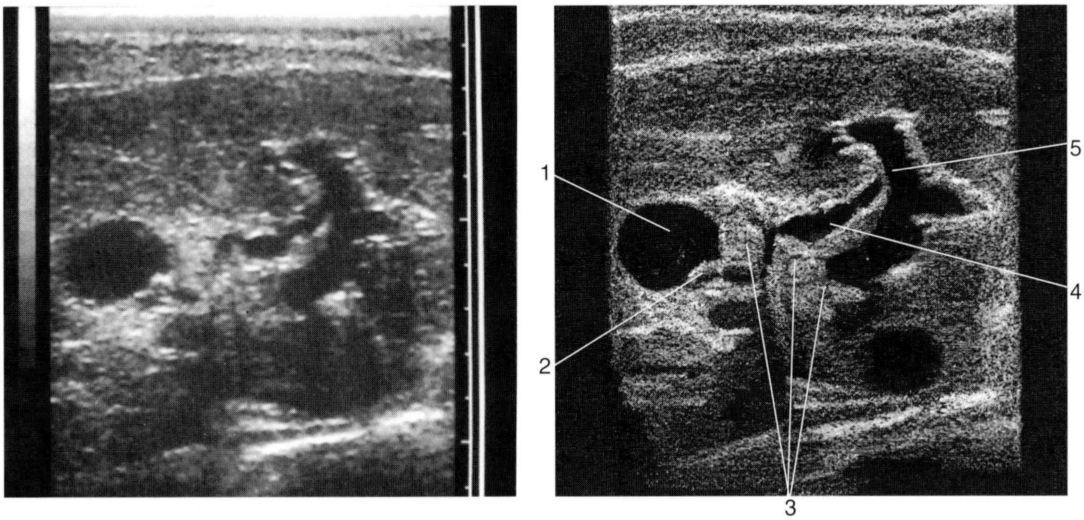

a

1. Gallbladder 2. Gallbladder cancer 3. Infiltrating tumors 4. Dilated hepatic duct 5. Umbilical portion of portal vein

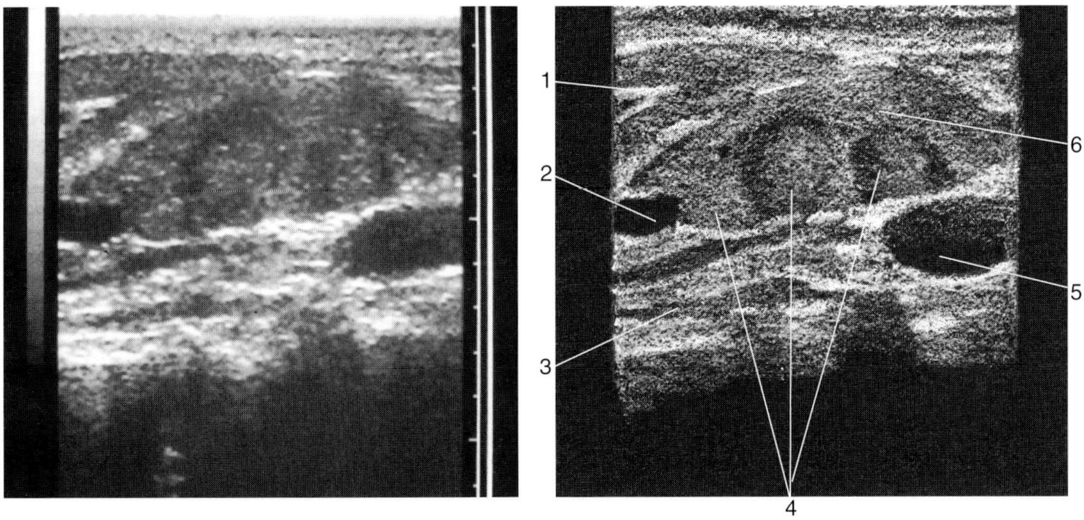

b

1. Liver 2. Portal vein 3. Diaphragm 4. Metastatic lymph node swelling 5. Inferior vena cava 6. Pancreas

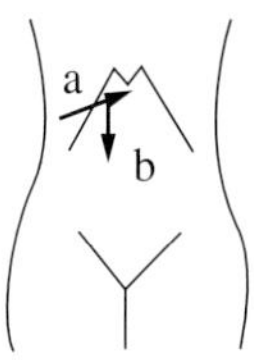

Figure 4-30. Advanced gallbladder cancer.
Extension of gallbladder cancer may occur in multiple directions. (a) Direct invasion of a gallbladder cancer into the porta hepatis, seen as an echogenic, ill-defined mass. Extensive involvement of the retropancreatic lymph nodes was also present, mimicking pancreatic malignancy (b).

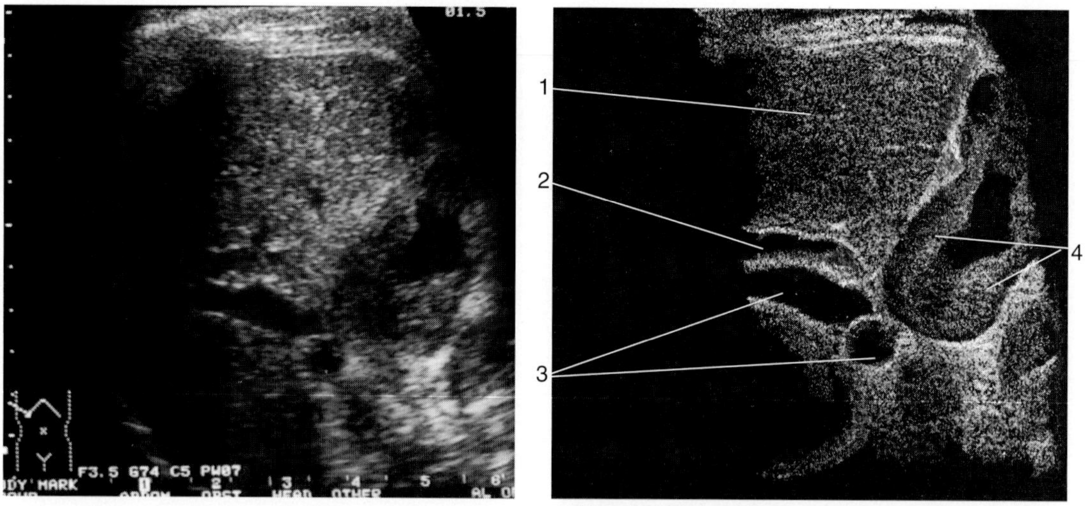

1. Liver 2. Right hepatic duct 3. Portal vein branches 4. Thickened gallbladder wall(cancer)

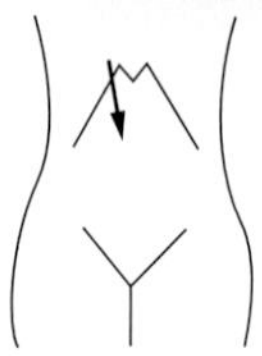

Figure 4-31. Gallbladder cancer mimicking chronic cholecystitis.
In this patient, thickening of the gallbladder wall suggestive of gallbladder carcinoma is especially well demonstrated on the right intercostal scan. Because of the slight dilatation of the intrahepatic bile duct, carcinoma of the gallbladder was strongly suggested despite a negative biopsy. Other modalities, including angiography and x-ray CT, supported the diagnosis of malignancy, which was finally proven by detailed postoperative histological examination.

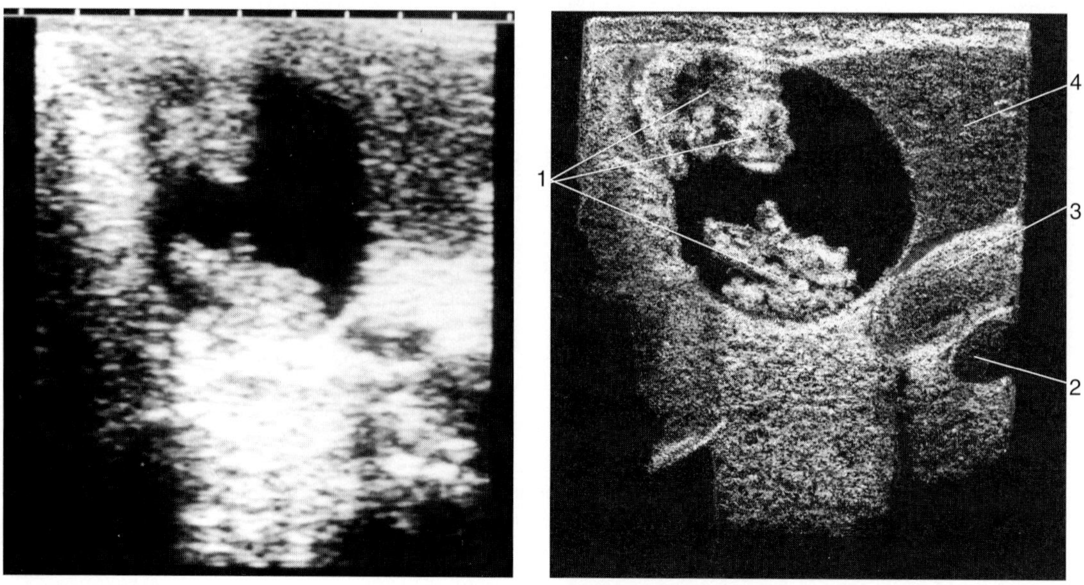

1. Metastatized malignant melanomas 2. Inferior vena cava 3. Head of pancreas 4. Liver

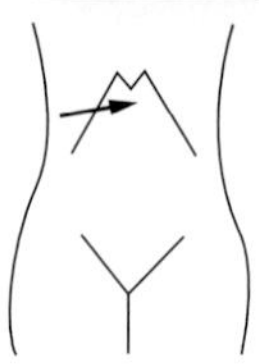

Figure 4-32. Metastasis of malignant melanoma to the gallbladder.
Metastasis of malignant tumors to the gallbladder is relatively rare and is usually encountered with carcinomatosis. This case is a typical example, with widespread dissemination of a malignant melanoma. The tumor has directly invaded both the body and the neck of the gallbladder, producing exophytic, echogenic masses of varied sizes.(Courtesy of Dr. Schmillevitch J, São Paulo, Brazil)

DISEASES OF THE BILE DUCTS

Jaundice

Jaundice, an elevation of the serum bilirubin, is traditionally subdivided into three types, prehepatic, hepatic and posthepatic. In the first group, caused by excessive bilirubin formation (chiefly hemolytic states), ultrasound contributes little beyond detecting the splenomegaly that often accompanies it (see Chapter 6). In the hepatocellular group there are often changes in the liver's size and structure that ultrasound can detect. An example is the echo-poor or "dark" liver that is typically seen in acute viral hepatitis. The changes of cirrhosis (lobulated liver surface, enlarged caudate lobe, B-mode and Doppler features of portal hypertension) can also sometimes be identified. These are discussed in detail in the section on Diffuse Diseases (Chapter 3).

The main role of ultrasound is in detecting the duct dilatation that results from obstruction of the biliary tree and in defining the level and cause of the obstruction. [9, 45, 63, 93, 105] This application was one of the early triumphs of ultrasound. The features of duct dilatation in its intrahepatic and extrahepatic portions can be considered separately.

Dilatation on the intrahepatic tree renders visible the small bile duct radicals that normally are too small to be resolved by ultrasound.[32] Normally only the larger ducts at the porta (the left and right main ducts and the common hepatic duct) can be made out. When the intrahepatic ducts become visible they are seen as a branching tree-like pattern of ducts converging onto the porta hepatis (Figure 4-33). In early cases they are seen as fine tubular structures and, as the lie alongside the branches of the portal vein, form additional channels, two being present where normally only one can be visualized. Seen in sections along their length this produces the "parallel channel" sign,[8] while in sections that cut across their lie the two lumina are seen lying close together as pairs of echo-free rings, the "double-barrelled shotgun" sign. Though detectable in all parts of the liver, the parallel channel sign is often more obvious in the left lobe, perhaps because here the ducts run across the upper abdomen and are more superficial. These configurations are typical and specific, the only problems being the possibility of confusing a pair of portal veins just downstream of a branching point (but usually they diverge quite rapidly rather than running truly parallel) and the occasional difficulty caused by the improved resolution of high quality scanners that offer the possibility of visualizing normal intrahepatic tubular structures (ducts and hepatic artery branches) near to the porta hepatis. True duct dilatation is seen half way or so into the liver from the porta while these normal structure can only be detected closer to it. Obviously this situation means that there is sometimes uncertainty when cases with early jaundice are seen: a rescan in a few days time will generally resolve the difficulty.

As the dilatation becomes more marked, the beaded shape of the ducts becomes obvious as does their arrangement converging on the porta. This produces a characteristic stellate pattern that is very striking. In the periphery of the liver the additional tubular structures give an overall impression of an excessive number of ductal structures (the "too many tubes" sign) though distinguishing dilated biliary from vascular structures is neither easy nor important clinically. Because the attenuation of bile is lower than that of liver parenchyma, bands of acoustic enhancement may be seen deep to larger ducts; this feature helps distinguish them from veins. Doppler, of course, can be used to make the distinction though it is rarely required for this.

Diagnosis of duct dilatation at and below the porta hepatis depends on measuring their calibers, though in gross cases the dilatation may be immediately obvious (Figure 4-34). The normal duct, measures at the porta hepatis and ideally at the point where it crosses the hepatic artery, is only a few millimeters in inner diameter; it is generally accepted that it may increase in caliber slightly with age and so a practical and memorable figure is to allow 1 mm for each decade of life.[93] In this way an upper limit of normal for an adult falls in the 4 to 6 mm range with 7 or 8 mm allowed for the elderly. Lower in the porta the duct is somewhat larger (perhaps because of the additional bile from the gallbladder) and an additional millimeter-or-so must be allowed in defining the limits of normal.

The accuracy of ultrasound in demonstrating duct dilatation is almost 100% though this purely anatomical sign must be used intelligently if its clinical significance is to be dependable. The occasional problem when the ducts have not yet dilated in a case of early obstruction has been mentioned; a repeat study in a few days should resolve the difficulty. The fact that once dilated, ducts may not return completely to normal after relief of the obstruction is a common difficulty. Examples include questions on recurrent obstruction (e.g., post-cholecystectomy pain or jaundice, patent biliary stent) and here only an increase in caliber from a baseline scan obtained after the procedure is truly reliable. Falling this, indirect signs such as the presence of air from gut in the bile ducts[14] or absence of dilatation after a stress meal[22] or cholecystokinin injection can be helpful, but usually an x-ray contrast study or radionuclide(IDA) study is needed to check the patency.[70]

The anatomical level of the obstruction can be inferred more or less precisely from the pattern of changes observed. The commonest site is at the lower end of the duct in the head of the pancreas (e.g., gallstones, pancreatic carcinoma or chronic pancreatitis): in this case the entire biliary tree is dilated, possibly also with dilatation of the pancreatic duct (Figure 4-35). Obstructions above this level can be inferred provided the normal caliber duct below the level of the obstruction can be imaged and this may be difficult. A lesion at the porta hepatis (e.g., Klatskin cholangiocarcinoma) produces dilatation of both right and left main ducts but with a normal caliber common duct.[1] When the lesion is intrahepatic (e.g., liver metastasis) only the ducts in one lobe or liver segment are dilated—in this case the patient is not usually jaundiced because the remaining liver is well able to cope with the entire bilirubin load unless it itself is also damaged. Overall, ultrasound has a success rate of some 80% at defining the level of obstruction.

The cause of biliary obstruction can be determined by observing the obstructing lesion itself (Figure 4-36). Gallstones in the common duct may have the same appearances as those in the gallbladder: echogenic masses with distal enhancement, but in some cases only ill-defined soft tissue mass is seen.[25, 54] This may be because the stone, though typical in consistency, is surrounded by duct wall rather than by fluid or it may be that inspissated bile (akin to the "lumpy bile" encountered in the gallbladder) is responsible. The accuracy of ultrasound in detecting stones in the bile duct is markedly lower than in the gallbladder and the soft tissue type is easily misread as tumor. Extrinsic tumors (most commonly of the pancreatic head but lymphadenopathy is also a cause) produce a tapering pattern to the lower end of the duct and it may be possible to demonstrate the surrounding mass itself.

Cholangiocarcinomas are particularly difficult to visualize on ultrasound, only an ill-defined mass being apparent even in the most favorable cases.[1, 114] This difficulty probably results from the widely infiltrating growth pattern of this tumor. Rarer causes that may be readily defined include choledochal cysts and intraductal ascaris worms.[46, 48, 52, 96] A pitfall is to assume that stones in the gallbladder mean that the obstruction is caused by bile duct stones: cholelithiasis is a very common incidental finding and may not be related to the obstruction. Only demonstrating a stone in the duct itself is diagnostic. Overall the accuracy of ultrasound in defining the cause of obstruction is lower than its ability to define the level or the presence of duct dilatation and is perhaps of the order of 50%, depending somewhat on the population group being studied.

Considering the role of ultrasound in the diagnostic sequence for evaluating jaundice, after blood tests to separate out the patients with hemolysis, it should be the first imaging test. The main question to be addressed is whether or not the ducts are dilated: this separates the "medical" from the "surgical" groups.[105] Any additional information ultrasound can give should be regarded as a bonus; it will usually give a good indication of the level of obstruction and this can be useful to guide any subsequent imaging—a high obstruction may be best persued with a percutaneous transhepatic cholangiogram (PTC) while a lower-end obstruction may be more accessible endoscopically.[70] If ultrasound also demonstrates the cause of the obstruction, it may be possible to dispense with other imaging or to use the ultrasound as a guide to needle biopsy, depending on the findings.

Choledochal Cysts

The diagnosis of idiopathic choledochal dilatation or choledochal cysts is straightforward with real-time ultrasound.[41, 42, 56, 76, 84] It is simple to identify the communication of the cyst with the extrahepatic bile duct (Figure 4-37). The cystic dilatation may extend up to the porta hepatis or be restricted to the retropancreatic space (Figure 4-38). Direct confirmation of the convergence of the bile duct with the pancreatic duct may be difficult and usually requires x-ray studies at endoscopic retrograde cholangiopancreatography (ERCP) or percutaneous transhepatic cholangiography (PTC).[77] Complicating bile duct cancers are difficult to detect even on careful study.[54, 61, 114]

Inflammatory Lesions

Both acute and chronic inflammation of the extrahepatic bile tree occur, either as an isolated phenomenon or as a consequence of biliary lithiasis.[82, 94, 98] Due possibly to its deep localization, the thin walls of the system, and adhesions of adjacent echogenic structures such as intestinal loops, an inflamed bile duct is often difficult to visualize sonographically, particularly in emergency cases with fulminant suppurative cholangitis caused by impacted biliary stones. In one case, direct drainage of the hilar portion of the dilated hepatic duct under ultrasonic guidance yielded purulent bile, and cannulation of the duct followed by surgical intervention saved the life of the patient.

Visualization of the dilated extrahepatic biliary system, especially its upper third, may be achieved relatively easily with modern real-time machines; the lower two-thirds are often difficult to image by the usual abdominal approach. Evaluation of the very thin wall of the bile duct to detect inflammatory changes seemes to be beyond the ability of the instruments available at present. However, in the relatively rare condition of chronic sclerosing cholangitis, the thickened extrahepatic common duct can be demonstrated as a thick, echo-poor, tube-like structure along the whole length of the duct, both in longitudinal and transverse scans (Figure 4-39). Sonography may be the only technique to reveal these characteristic changes[11, 68, 101] and so raise the suspicion when interpreted together with a carefully performed roentgenologic study such as ERCP or PTC. In practice, however, the differential diagnosis between chronic inflammation and infiltrating malignant tumors may be difficult to make even with pathological specimens.

Stones

Stones in the common duct can develop in isolation or in combination with cholecystolithiasis (Figure 4-40). Unlike stones in the gallbladder, choledocholithiasis is difficult to diagnose on ultrasound. In addtion, the accuracy of ultrasound in assessing the number and location of stones still remains low compared to that of direct imaging of the bile duct by x-ray contrast methods.[18, 25, 29, 54, 69, 79, 109] Scanning skill and the condition of the individual patient may play significant roles in determining the success of visualization of the ducts or of stones within them. As described in a previous section, scanning of the upper third of the extrahepatic bile duct is straightforward, whereas the lower two-thirds of the bile duct are often difficult to image because of gas in the first portion of the duodenum.

Diagnostic failures of over 60% are reported in some series, while the best reports described a positive diagnosis in as high as 80% (Table 4-1). The causes of these striking differences in diagnostic accuracy are multiple, but technique and instrumentation, especially the use of high-resolution real-time scanners, may play a significant role.

Dilatation of the common duct is frequently found in choledocholithiasis, without marked dilatation of the intrahepatic bile ducts and usually without jaundice. The reasons are not entirely clear, but stones alone seldom cause total obstruction of the common duct, whereas complete obstruction occurs much more frequently in malignant neoplasms arising from the bile duct or the pancreatic head. A careful search for stones in the common duct may be carried out by the technique described previously, especially using right coronal scans or transverse scans with simultaneous compression by the probe (Figure 4-41). It is often claimed that bile duct stones not infrequently lack the characteristic echo appearance of stones seen in the gallbladder; however, if the sensitivity and scan plane are carefully adjusted, typical sonograms with acoustic shadowing are obtained relatively easily. Difficulties are experienced in patients who have undergone previous surgery and those with adhesions of intestinal loops around the common duct caused by previous inflammation.

Ascaris

Biliary ascariasis occurs in underdeveloped countries (China, Africa, India). It is characterized by colicky pains in the upper abdomen and a typical ultrasonic configuration of a brightly echogenic worm body located in the biliary tract.[21, 44, 47, 51] On the ultrasonogram the ascaris body is visualized as an echogenic band in the bile duct, and on close observation one may identifiy the characteristic worm movement which aggravates the upper abdominal pain (Figure 4-42).

Malignant Tumors

The most prominent sonographic finding in biliary malignancy is dilatation of both extrahepatic and intrahepatic bile ducts.[16, 33, 39, 67, 73, 110] Wide dilatation of the common duct and/or the gallbladder (larger than 10 mm and 4 cm in diameter, respectively) are indicative of malignant obstruction.[75, 88, 92, 105, 106, 113]

The obstructing lesion may lie at any level,[2, 37, 44, 54] the most frequent being cancer at the head of the pancreas though a cancer arising from the body of the pancreas may cause obstruction when the tumor mass extends beyond the midline. Bile duct cancer may affect any part of the extrahepatic biliary tree (Figures 4-43 to 4-45). Tumors arising in the lower third tend to infiltrate into the pancreatic parenchyma, while those arising at a higher level often extend into the liver hilum and parenchyma via the periductal lymphatics. The tumor may take a papillary or infiltrating scirrhous form; each may show characteristic tissue echo patterns. If the tumor mass is located within the bile duct, the probability of biliary cancer is high; if no intraluminal mass is identified, the possibility of an invasive extramural tumor must be considered. The distinction is difficult but important because the polypoid type may be curable, whereas the infiltrating variety has a poorer prognosis because of its late presentation.

Cancer of the papilla of Vater causes extensive dilatation of the common duct and gallbladder and thus may present at an early stage (Figure 4-46). Visualization of the small tumor mass itself is usually impossible. This is partly due to duodenal gas which can be shifted by the peristalsis that follows injection of a pancreatic stimulant such as secretin, thus facilitating imaging of a tumor nodule protruding into the duodenum. Endoscopic sonography improves imaging markedly in these cases.

Other tumors which may compress the common duct include metastatic lymph nodes, such as those originating from cancer of the liver, stomach, breast, lung, gallbladder, and even malignant lymphoma. Lymphoma is especially important to the differential diagnosis since it is amenable to chemotherapy.

In obstructive jaundice, the sonographic parallel channel or shotgun signs are a reliable indication of persistent obstruction of the biliary system (Figure 4-47). It is often difficult to identify the true cause of obstruction by sonography alone because gas in the intestine prevents adequate visualization of the duct. X-ray CT scans, endoscopic retrograde cholangiography (ERCP) or ultrasound-guided puncture with contrast injection into the upper biliary tract percutaneous transhepatic cholangiography (PTC) may be required to establish the diagnosis. Likewise, correct assessment of the extent of extrabiliary infiltration of the malignant tumor to the adjacent tissues may be made difficult by echoes from nearby gas pockets.

Finally, the precise differential diagnosis of chronic inflammatory conditions of the extrahepatic bile ducts such as sclerosing cholangitis, is difficult by conventional ultrasound. However, high-resolution endoscopic ultrasound from within the second part of the duodenum often gives clues in differentiating these difficult cases (Figure 4-48) (cf. Chapter 9).

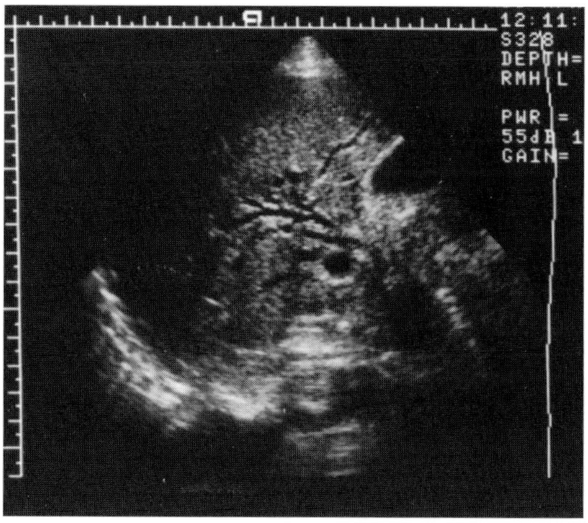

a

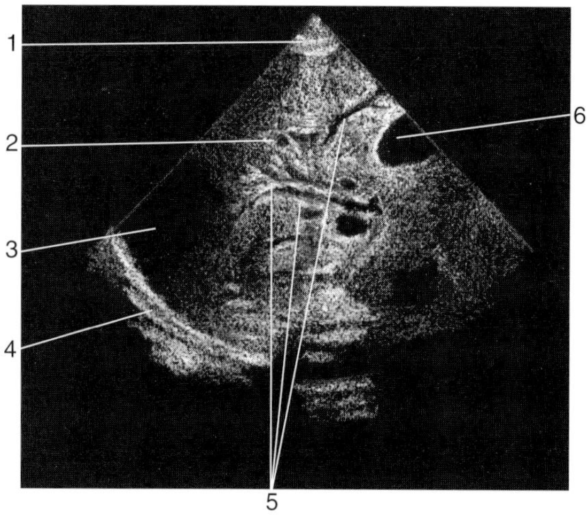

1. Surface of liver 2. Portal vein 3. Right lobe of liver 4. Diaphragm 5. Dilated intrahepatic bile duct 6. Gallbladder

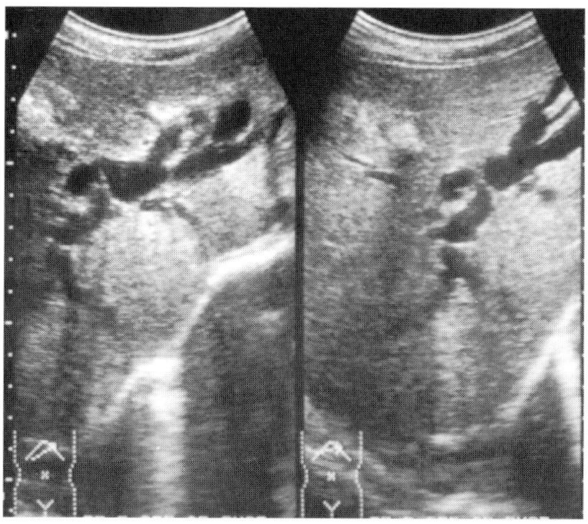

b

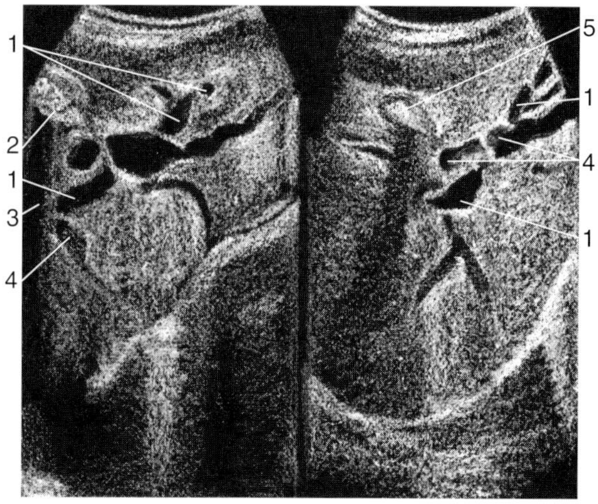

1. Portal vein 2. Stone 3. Shadow 4. Dilated hepatic duct 5. Tumor

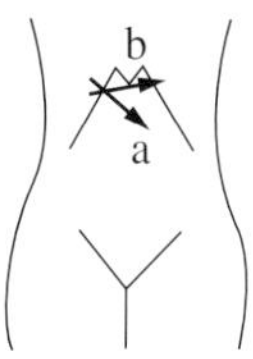

Figure 4-33. Features of intrahepatic bile duct dilatation.
Additional tubular structures forming parallel channels (a) is an early feature of dilatation of the intrahepatic bile ducts. With further dilatation, the stellate pattern and distal acoustic enhancement become obvious. In late stage of intrahepatic ductal dilatation, ductal dilatation reaches to its extreme (b).

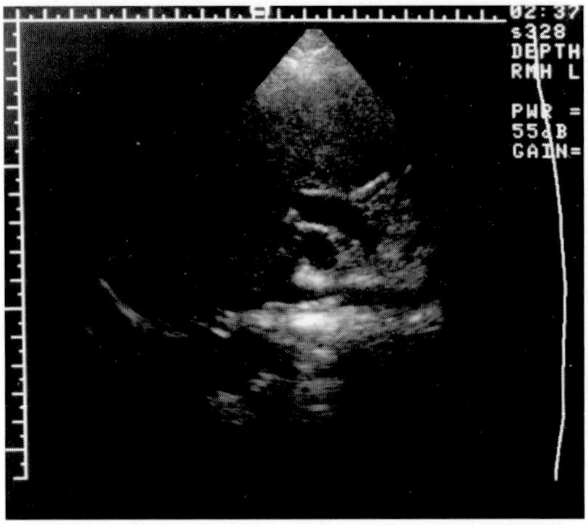

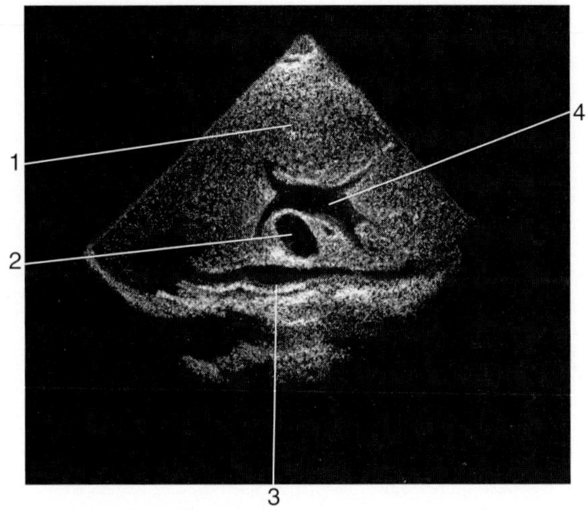

1. Liver 2. Portal vein trunk 3. Inferior vena cava
4. Dilated hepatic duct

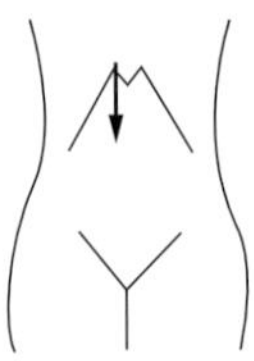

Figure 4-34. Features of extrahepatic bile duct dilatation.
Enlargement of the common duct beyond about 4 mm is characteristic of extrahepatic duct dilatation. The dilated duct seen in the porta is overlying the hepatic artery and portal vein.

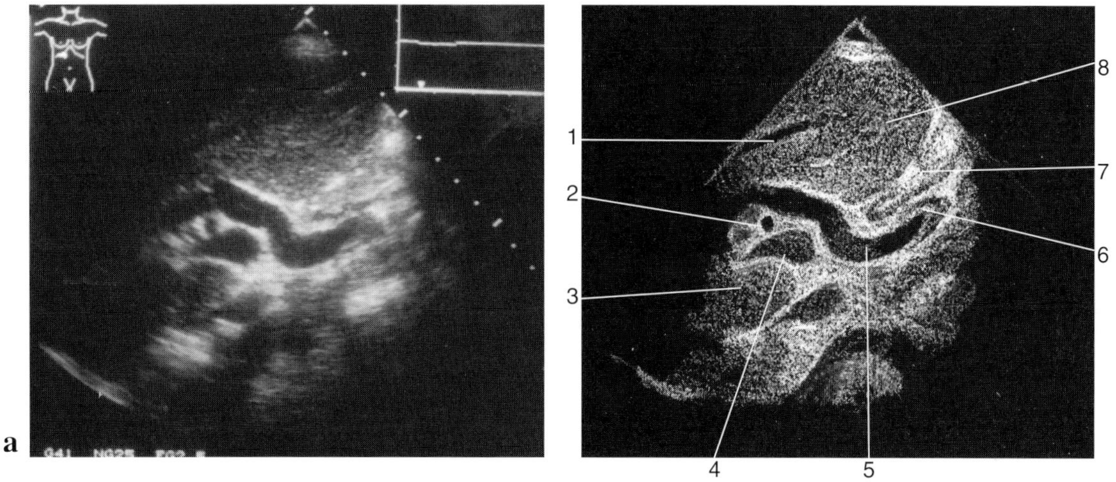

1. Hepatic vein 2. Hepatic artery 3. Liver 4. Portal vein 5. Dilated common bile duct 6. Obstructing tumor (cancer) 7. Duodenum 8. Liver

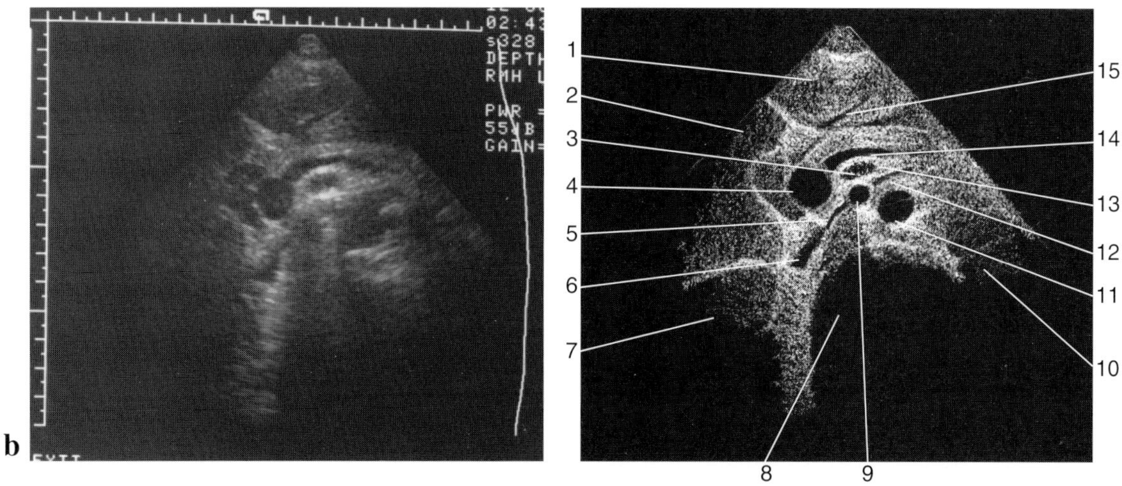

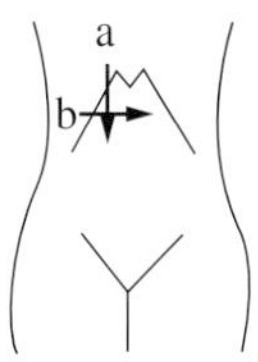

1. Left lobe of liver 2. Right lobe of liver 3. Splenic vein 4. Dilated common bile duct 5. Inferior vena cava 6. Right renal vein 7. Right kidney 8. Vertebra 9. Superior mesenteric vein 10. Left kidney 11. Aorta 12. Left renal vein 13. Dilated pancreatic duct 14. Body of pancreas 15. Left hepatic vein

Figure 4-35. Levels of obstruction.
The common ducts in (a) can be traced down beyond the duodenum suggesting that the obstructing lesion lies at its lower end. In another case (b), the dilated common duct is seen in transverse section lying within the head of the pancreas.

a

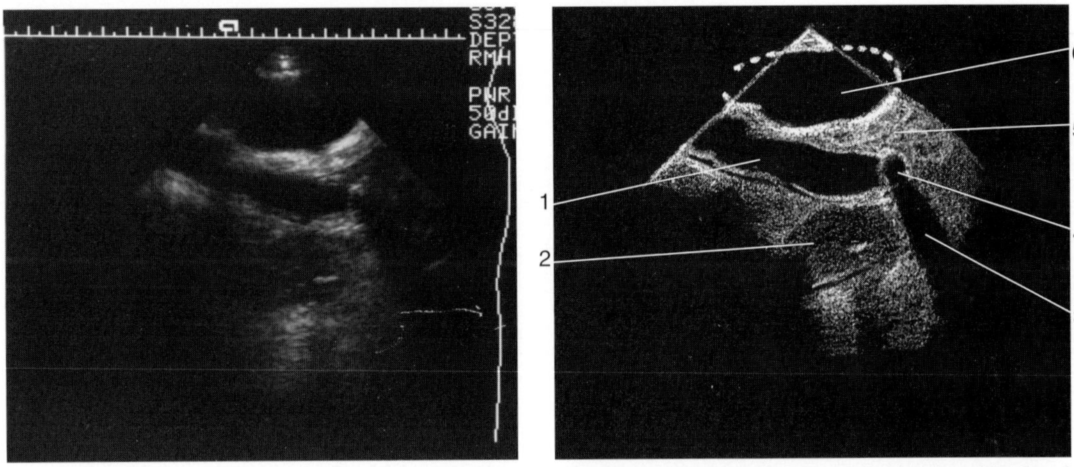

1. Dilated common bile duct 2. Head and body of pancreas 3. Acoustic shadow 4. Stone 5. Duodenum (descending part) 6. Dilated gallbladder

b

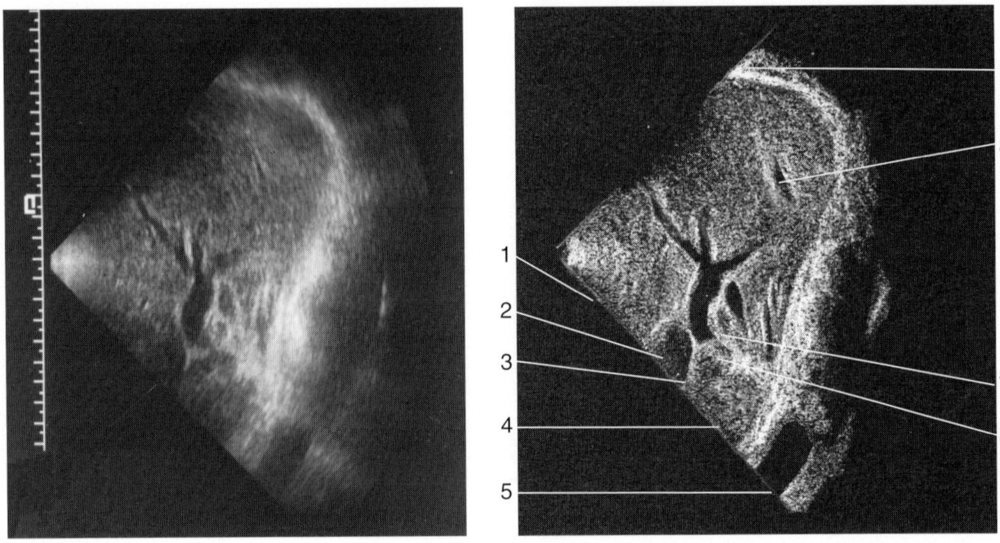

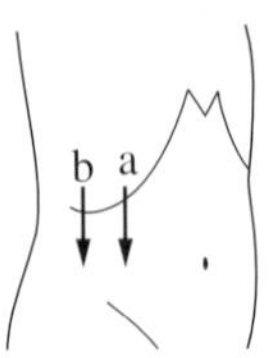

1. Dilated bile duct 2. Part of gallbladder 3. Obstruction 4. Tumor 5. Aorta 6. Hepatic artery 7. Portal vein 8. Hepatic vein 9. Diaphragm

Figure 4-36. Causes of bile duct obstruction.
A stone lying in the lower end of the common duct could be identified in (a) as the cause of the obstruction. In this case, a window was provided by the dilated gallbladder which often provides access in patients with obstructive jaundice. Its value can be maximized by scanning with the patient rotated into the left decubitus position.
The dilated common duct in (b) could be demonstrated ending in a mass of the head of the pancreas; biopsy revealed a pancreatic carcinoma. This was a coronal scan, a projection that maximizes access to the duct by using a retroperitoneal line-of-sight.

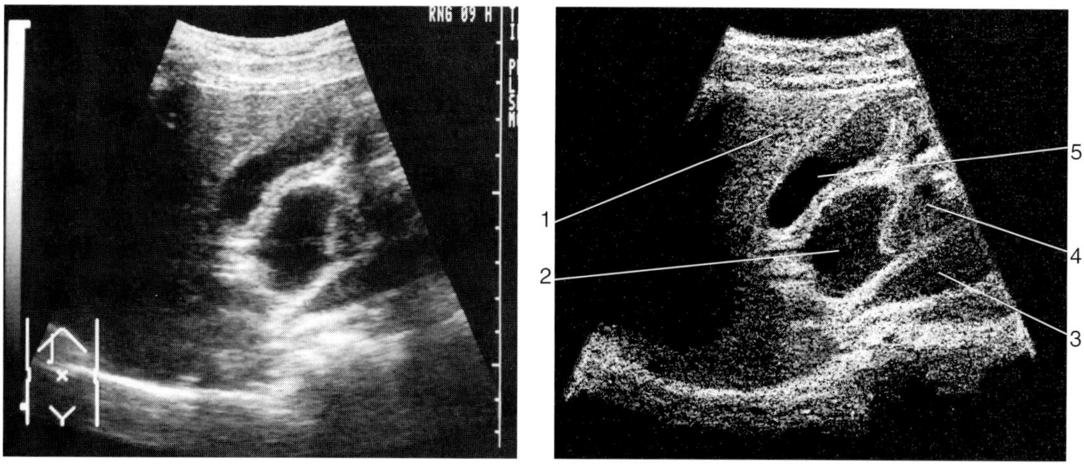

1. Liver 2. Dilated bile duct 3. Inferior vena cava 4. Pancreas 5. Gallbladder

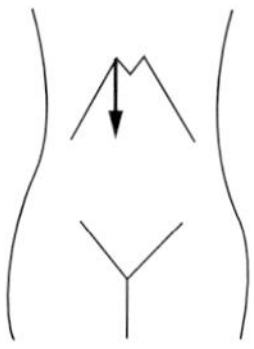

Figure 4-37. Choledochal cyst.
The dilatation of the common bile duct, a congenital anomaly, can be either cystic or fusiform in shape (combinations also occur) and can affect the extrahepatic as well as the intrahepatic bile duct. This sagittal sonogram discloses a round, cystic mass in the midportion of the extrahepatic common bile duct. A normal gallbladder is simultaneously visualized anterior to the dilated common duct.

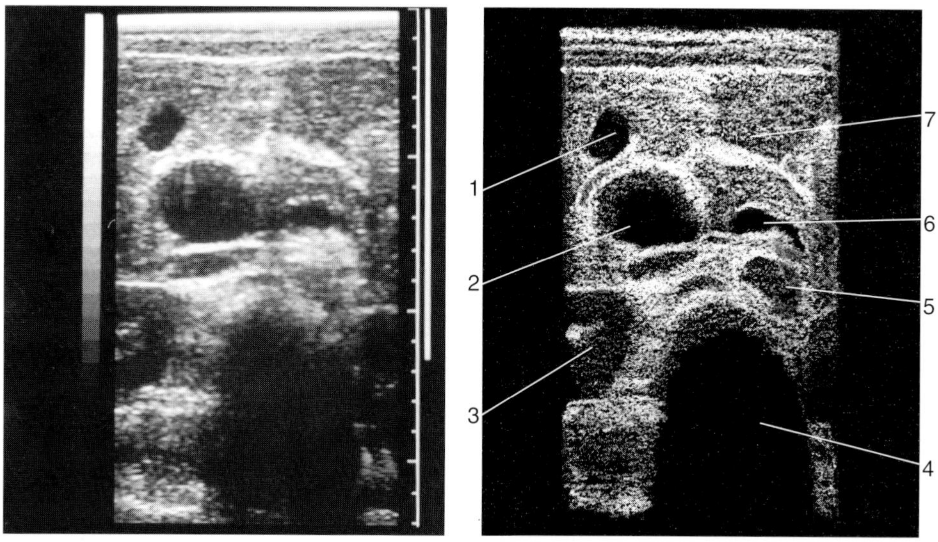

1. Gallbladder 2. Dilated bile duct 3. Right kidney 4. Vertebra 5. Aorta 6. Pancreas 7. Liver

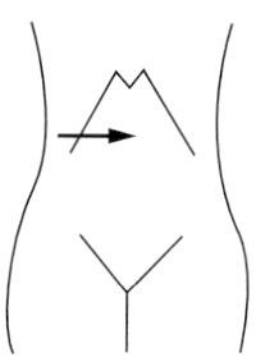

Figure 4-38. Idiopathic choledochocele at the lower end of the duct.
Cystic dilatation of the lower part of the bile duct is visualized as a round, anechoic mass inferior to the head of the pancreas on a transverse scan of the epigastrium. An abnormal junction of the common duct and the pancreatic duct frequently accompanies and this anomaly, as demonstrated on intravenous cholangiography.

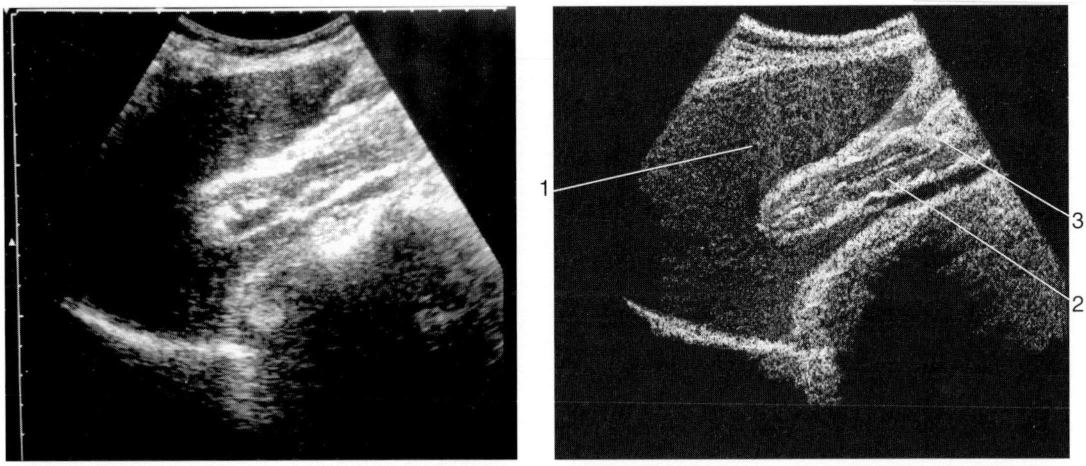

1. Liver 2. Inflamed extrahepatic bile duct 3. Part of pancreas

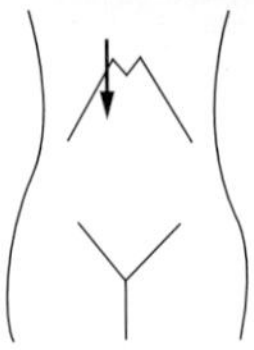

Figure 4-39. Chronic sclerosing cholangitis.
Biliary stagnation can also be caused by chronic inflammation of the bile duct. The longitudinal scan of the extrahepatic bile duct of a patient with fluctuating jaundice clearly reveals the echo-poor, cylindrical thickening of the entire duct system extending to the intrahepatic bile ducts. The change was also evident on x-ray CT. Explorative laparotomy disclosed characteristic changes of chronic sclerosing cholangitis.

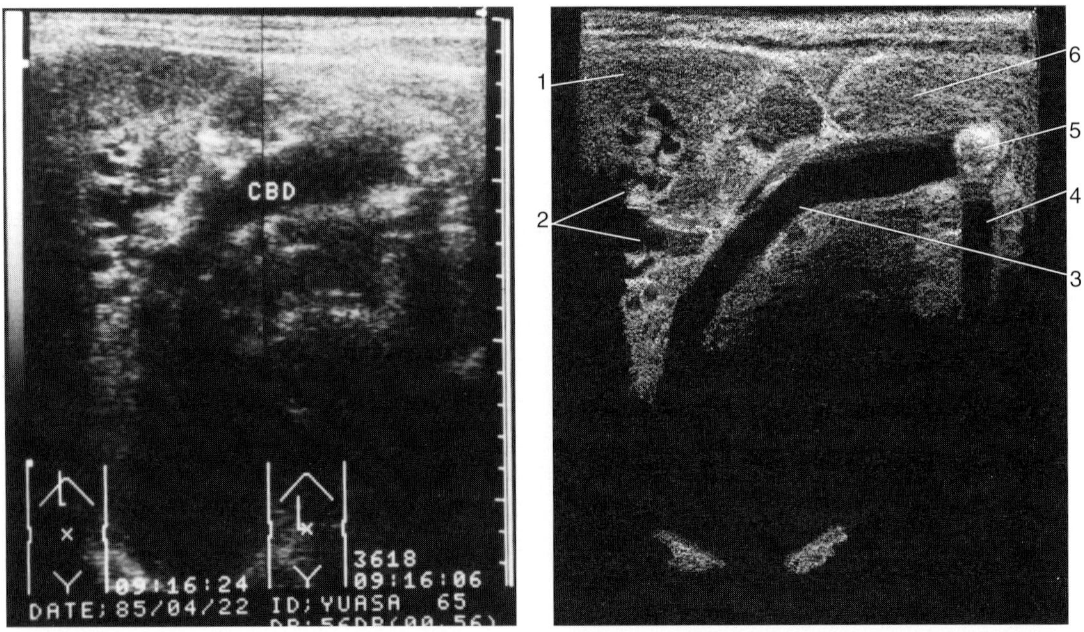

1. Liver 2. Dilated bile ducts 3. Common bile duct 4. Acoustic shadow 5. Stone 6. Pancreas

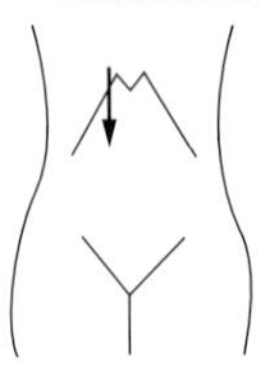

Figure 4-40. Choledochal stone.
Choledocholithiasis occurs either alone or in combination with cholecystolithiasis and usually causes dilatation of the extrahepatic bile duct. An echogenic common duct stone casting an acoustic shadow is demonstrated on a longitudinal scan of the duct. Positive diagnosis of common duct stones is often impeded by gas echoes of the digestive tract, especially the duodenum and stomach. Careful scanning is mandatory to exclude the presence of stone echoes in a slightly dilated bile duct.

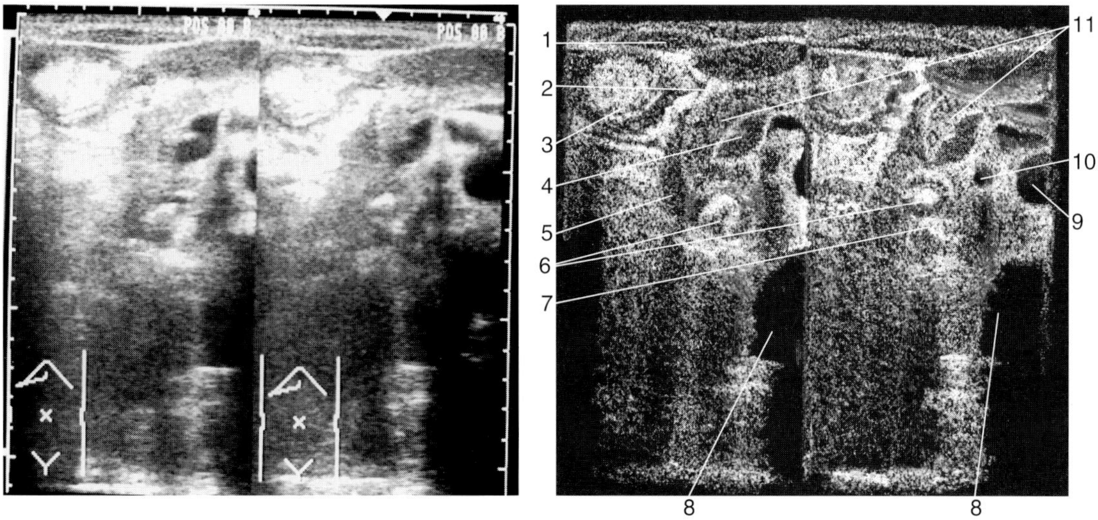

1. Rectus abdominis muscle 2. Gas in the duodenum 3. Intestine 4. Splenic vein 5. Acoustic shadow 6. Stones in common bile duct 7. Acoustic shadow 8. Vertebra 9. Aorta 10. Superior mesenteric artery 11. Head of pancreas

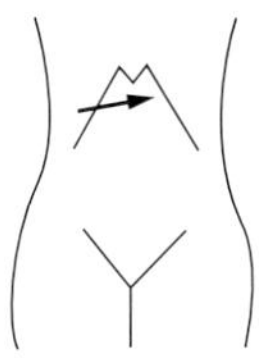

Figure 4-41. Choledochal stone.
Stones in the lower end of the common bile duct are often difficult to image by either longitudinal or transverse scanning. As shown in these two sonograms of semioblique scans, a small, echogenic focus is identified at the lower end of the common duct, with a weak distal shadow in only one sonogram.

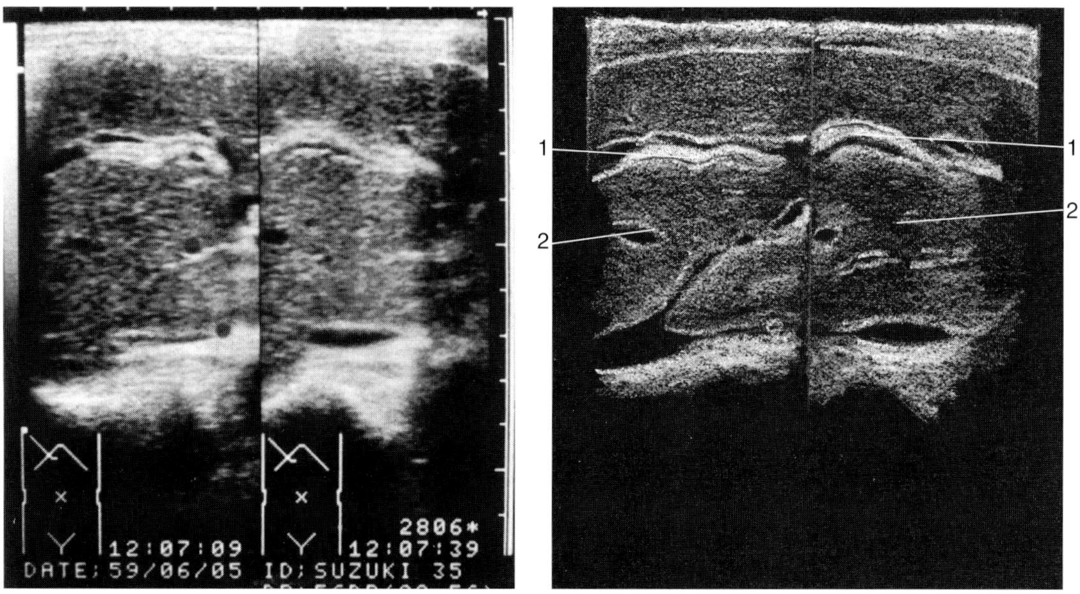

1. Ascaris 2. Liver

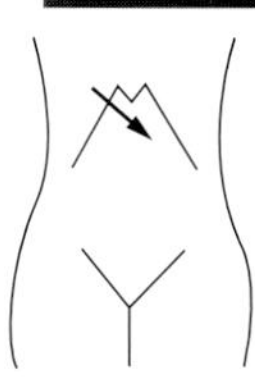

Figure 4-42. Ascaris in the bile tree.
Biliary ascariasis is rather uncommon in urban populations of developed countries. In this woman with a sudden bout of right hypochondrial pain, an echogenic, tubular structure was revealed in the common duct. After a while, the echogenic strand moved to the gallbladder. Her pain was relieved as soon as the worm moved from the common duct.

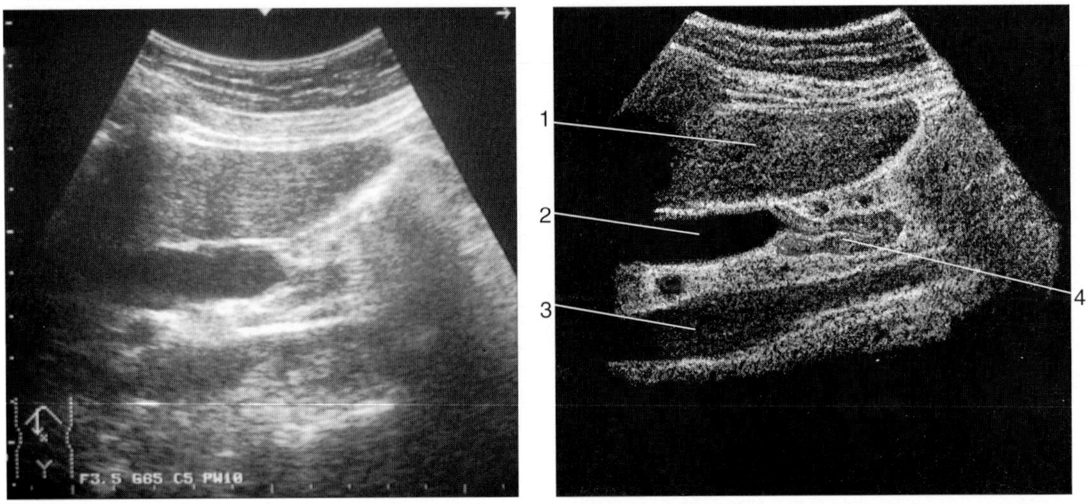

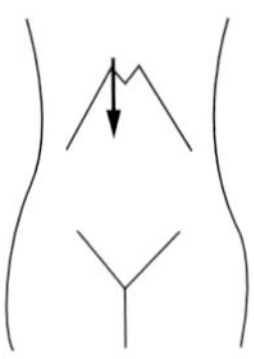

1. Liver 2. Dilated common bile duct 3. Inferior vena cava 4. Bile duct cancer

Figure 4-43. Cancer of the common bile duct.
On real-time ultrasound scans, choledochal carcinoma is often suspected in the presence of persistent obstructive jaundice accompanied by a dilated common duct system. The difficulty of visualizing the lower third of the duct in the supine position may be overcome by scanning in the left semirecumbent position, as shown in this case. The dilated common duct is obstructed by a tumor mass fillig the lumen. No acoustic shadowing is observed.

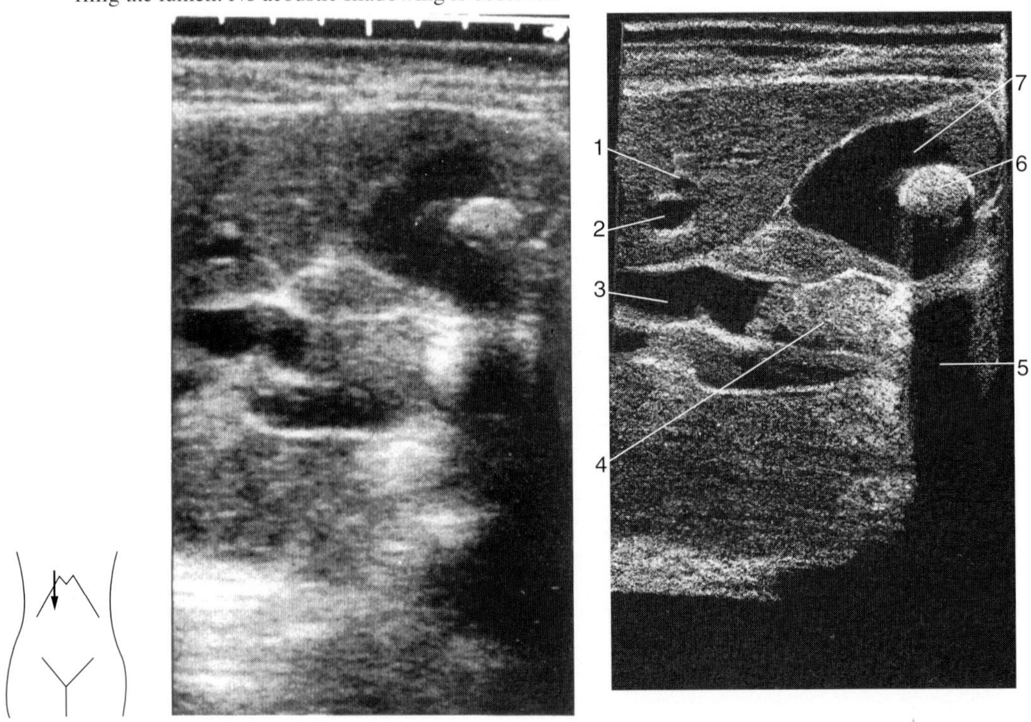

1. Liver 2. Portal vein 3. Dilated common bile duct 4. Tumor mass 5. Acoustic shadow 6. Stone 7. Gallbladder

Figure 4-44. Carcinoma of the lower choledochus.
This patient presented with painless jaundice. Real-time ultrasound scanning with a linear probe disclosed a markedly dilated common duct that terminated suddenly in a hypoechoic mass which filled the lumen of the bile duct.

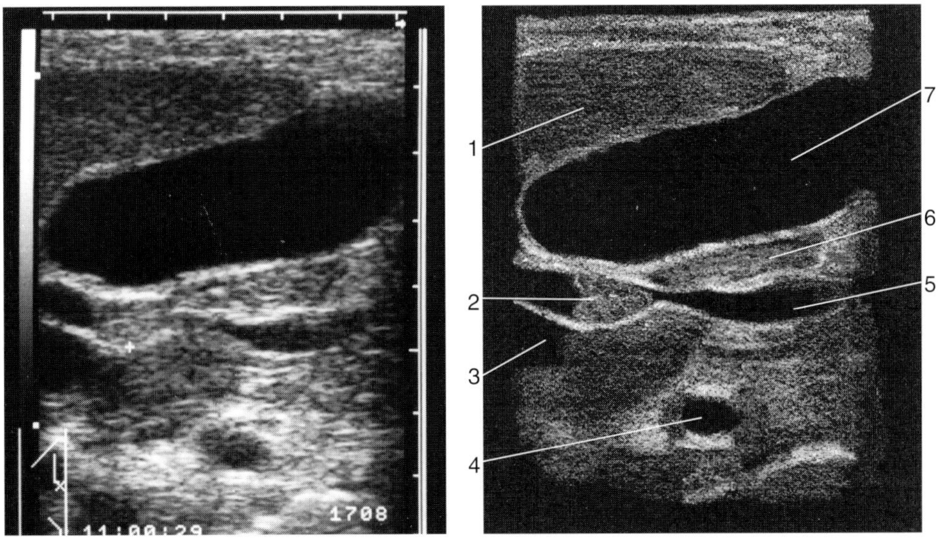

1. Liver 2. Tumor 3. Portal vein 4. Right renal vein 5. Common bile duct 6. Duodenum 7. Gallbladder

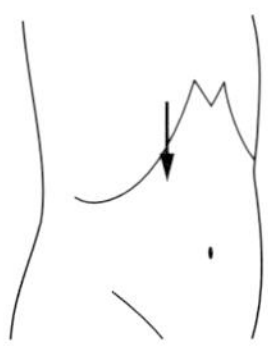

Figure 4-45. Marked dilatation of the intrahepatic bile ducts in a case of cholangiocarcinoma of the common hepatic duct.
Subcostal scanning along the right costal margin showed marked dilatation of the intrahepatic bile duct system. Unlike the curvilinear portal veins, the abnormally dilated intrahepatic bile ducts create rather tortuous, bizarre-shaped tubular structures around the hepatic hilum. A small carcinoma was found infiltrating the common hepatic duct.

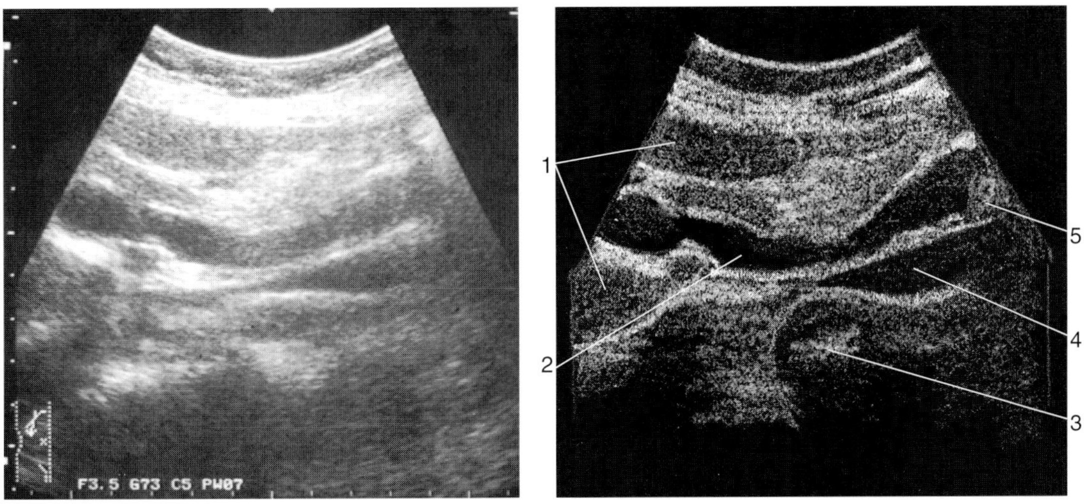

1. Liver 2. Common bile duct 3. Part of right kidney 4. Inferior vena cava 5. Tumor

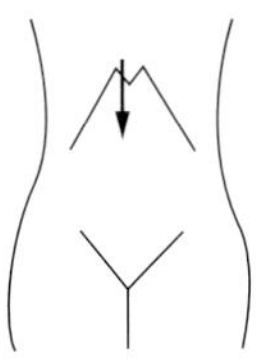

Figure 4-46. Cancer at the duodenal papilla.
Because of the typical course of the extrahepatic common duct with angulation at the knee portion, a small tumor at the papilla of Vater is often difficult to demonstrate on a single sonogram together with the dilated choledochus. In this case, a small tumor mass was found at the lower end of the common duct.

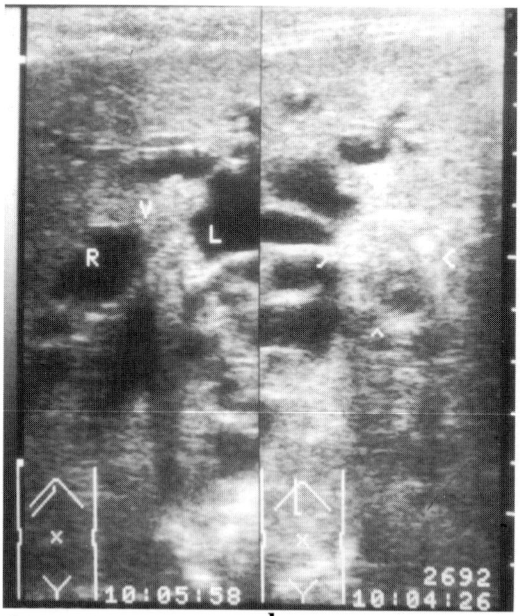

a b

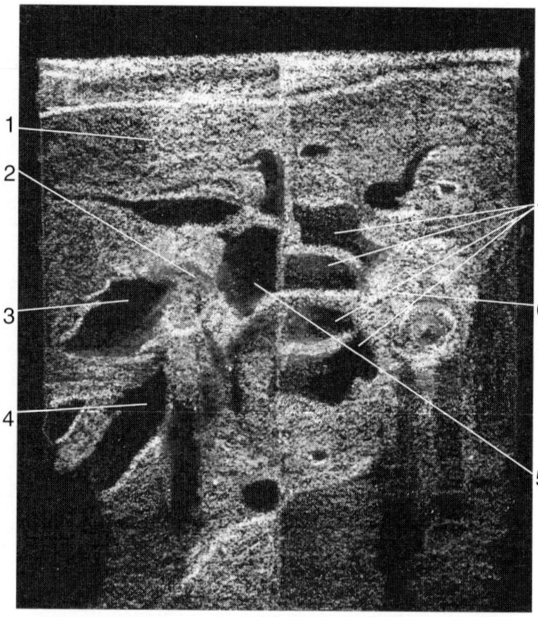

1. Liver 2. Tumor 3. Right hepatic duct 4. Dilated hepatic duct 5. Left hepatic duct 6. Tumor 7. Dilated intrahepatic duct

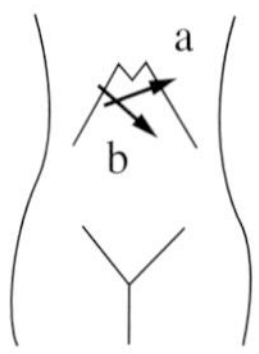

Figure 4-47. Carcinoma of the common duct demonstrated by transduodenal endoscopic sonography.
In examining patients with suspected choledochal tumors, endoscopic ultrasound appears to be the most sensitive method. As shown in this sonogram recorded by transduodenal scanning, the tumor mass obstructing the entire lumen was clearly demonstrated in the common duct. The internal echo texture is much better visualized because of the high resolution of the transducer used.

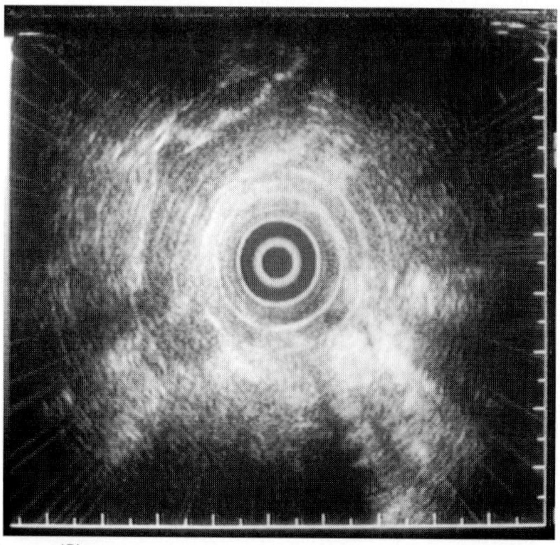

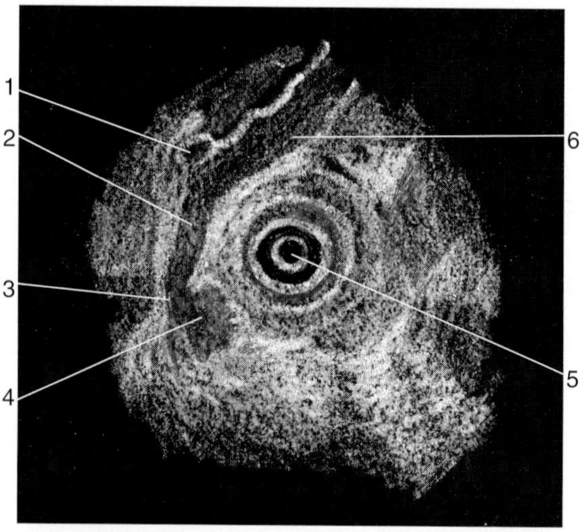

1. Cystic duct 2. Common bile duct 3. Stenosis
4. Bile duct cancer 5. Scanhead in duodenal lumen
6. Common hepatic duct

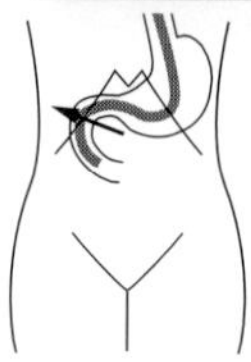

Figure 4-48. Endoscopic ultrasound scan of bile duct cancer.
Intraduodenal scanning of a case of suspected choledochal cancer by endoscopic ultrasound. The mechanical radial scanning method has disclosed a hypoechoic, small tumor mass at the lower part of the choledochus together with a small degree of ductal dilation. The tumor mass not only protruded into the lumen but also infiltrated the surrounding tissue.

REFERENCES

1. Adams A, Benjamin IS: The staging of cholangiocarcinoma. Clin Rad 46 : 299-203, 1992.
2. Armstrong CP, Dixon JM, Taylor TV, et al: Surgical experience of deeply jaundiced patients with bile duct obstruction. Br J Surg 71 : 234-238, 1984.
3. Atkins HL, Oster ZH: Asymmetric gallbladder contraction following cholecystokinin hepatobiliary imaging. Clin Nucl Med 14 : 82-86, 1989.
4. Bartrum RG Jr, Crow HC, Foote SR: Ultrasonic and radiographic cholecystography. N Engl J Med 296 : 538-541, 1977.
5. Becker CD, Hassler H, Terrier F: Preoperative diagnosis of the Mirizzi syndrome: Limitations of sonography and computed tomography. AJR 143 : 591-596, 1984.
6. Behan M, Kazam E: Sonography of the common bile duct: Value of the right anterior oblique view. AJR 130 : 701-709, 1978.
7. Berk RN, Van Der Vegt JH, Lichtenstein JE: The hyperplastic cholecystoses: Cholesterolosis and adenomyomatosis. Radiology 146 : 593-601, 1983.
8. Bressler EL, Rubin JM, McCracken S: Sonographic parallel channel sign: A reappraisal. Radiology 164 : 343-346, 1987.
9. Burrell MI, Zeman RK, Simeone JF, et al: The biliary tract: Imaging for 1990s. AJR 157 : 223-233, 1991.
10. Carroll BA: Gallstones: In vitro comparison of physical, radiographic, and ultrasonic characteristics. AJR 131 : 223-226, 1978.
11. Carroll BA, Oppenheimer D: Sclerosing cholangitis: Sonographic demonstration of bile duct wall thickening. AJR 130 : 279-286, 1982.
12. Carter SJ, Rutledge J, Hirsch JH, et al: Papillary adenoma of the gall bladder: Ultrasonic demonstration. JCU 6 : 433-435, 1978.
13. Chang MH, Wang TH, Chen CC, et al: Congenital bile duct dilatation in children. J Pediatr Surg 21 : 112-117, 1986.
14. Chu J, Husband J, Cosgrove DO, et al: The B-scan appearance of gas in the biliary tree. Br J Radiol 51 : 728-730, 1978.
15. Coelho JC, Wallback A, Kasting G, et al: Ultrasonic diagnosis of primary sarcoma of the gallbladder. JCU 12 : 168-170, 1984.
16. Conrad MR, Landay MJ, Janes JO: Sonographic "parallel channel" sign of biliary tree enlargement in mild to moderate obstructive jaundice. AJR 130 : 279-286, 1978.
17. Conrad MR, Janes JO, Dietchy J: Significance of low level echoes within the gallbladder. AJR 132 : 967-972, 1978.
18. Cooperberg PL: High resolution real-time ultrasound in the evaluation of the normal and obstructive biliary tract. Radiology 129 : 477-480, 1978.
19. Cooperberg PL, Burhenne HJ: Real-time ultrasonography: Diagnostic technique of choice in calculous gallbladder disease. N Engl J Med 302 : 1277-1279, 1980.
20. Crade M, Taylor KJW, Rosenfield AT, et al: Surgical and pathologic correlation of cholecystosonography and cholecystography. AJR 131 : 227-229, 1978.
21. Cremin BJ: Biliary ascariasis: Better detected by real-time versus static B-mode sonography [letter]. AJR 140 : 174, 1983.
22. Darweesh RMA, Dodds WJ, Hogan WJ, et al: Fatty meal sonography for evaluating patients with suspected partial common duct obstruction. AJR 51 : 63-68, 1988.
23. Dempsey PJ, Phillips JF, Warren DL, et al: Cholecystosonography for the diagnosis of cholecystolithiasis. Ann Surg 187 : 465-472, 1978.
24. Dewbeury KC: Visualization of normal biliary tract with ultrasound. Br J Radiol 53 : 774-780, 1980.
25. Dewbeury KC, Smith CL: The misdiagnosis of common bile duct stones with ultrasound. Br J Radiol 56 : 625-630, 1983.
26. Dillon E, Parkin GJS: The role of upper abdominal ultrasonography in suspected acute cholecystitis. Clin Radiol 31 : 175-179, 1980.
27. Eberle F, Pfeilsticker D, Rettenmaier G: The size of the gallbladder in acute viral hepatitis. Ultraschall Med 5 : 108-110, 1984.
28. Eberle F, Rettenmaier G: Gallbladder sludge: A sonographically recognizable stage of lithogenesis. Z Gastroenterol 22 : 82-87, 1984.
29. Einstein DM, Lapin SA, Ralls PW, et al: The insensitivity of sonography in the detection of choledocholithiasis. AJR 142 : 725-728, 1984.

30. Elyaderani MK, Gabriele OF: Cholecystosonography in detection of acute cholecystitis: The halo sign, a significant sonographic finding. South Med J 76 : 174-180, 1983.
31. Engel JM, Deitch EA, Sikkema W: Gallbladder wall thickness: sonographic accuracy and relation to disease. AJR 134 : 907-909, 1980.
32. Fried AM, Bell RM, Bivins BA: Biliary obstruction in canine model: Sequential study of the sonographic threshold. Invest Radiol 16 : 317-319, 1981.
33. Ferrucci JT, Adson MA, Mueller PR, et al: Advances in the radiology of jaundice: A symposium and review. AJR 141 : 1-20, 1983.
34. Filly RA, Moss AA, Way LW: In vitro investigation of gallstone shadowing with ultrasound tomography. JCU 7 : 255-262, 1979.
35. Fiske CE, Laing FC, Brown TW: Ultrasonographic evidence of gallbladder wall thickening in association with hypoalbuminemia. Radiology 135 : 713-716, 1980.
36. Fowler RC, Reid WA: Ultrasound diagnosis of adenomyomatosis of the gallbladder: Ultrasonic and pathological correlation. Clin Radiol 39 : 402-406, 1988.
37. Gibson R, Yeung E, Thompson J, et al: Bile duct obstruction: Radiologic evaluation of level, cause and tumor resectability. Radiology 160 : 43-47, 1986.
38. Goldberg BB, Harris K, Broocker W: Ultrasonic and radiographic cholecystography. Radiology 111 : 405-509, 1974.
39. Goldberg BB: Ultrasonic cholangiography. Radiology 118 : 401-404, 1976.
40. Good LI, Edell SL, Soloway RD, et al: Ultrasonic properties of gallstones: Effect of stones size and composition. Gastroenterology 77 : 258-263, 1979.
41. Hadidi A: Types I and III choledochal cyst. Preoperative diagnosis by ultrasound. Am J Dis Child 137 : 663-665, 1983.
42. Heikkinen ES, Salminen PM: Congenital choledochal cyst opening into the intraduodenal part of the common bile duct and complicated by cystolithiasis and acute pancreatitis. Acta Chir Scand 150 : 183-185, 1984.
43. Harbin WP, Ferrucci JT, Wittenberg J, et al: Nonvisualized gallbladder by cholecystosonography. AJR 132 : 727-728, 1979.
44. Hess ML, Cunningham JJ: Effect of examination time of day on the quality of real-time cholesonograms. AJR 143 : 251-253, 1984.
45. Irving H: The biliary tree (Chap 13), in Cosgrove DO, Meire HB, Dewburry KC (eds), Clinical Ultrasound. London, Churchill Livingstone, 1993.
46. Jessen K, Al Mofleh I, Al Mofarreh M: Endoscopic treatment of ascariasis causing acute obstructive cholangitis. Hepatogastroenterology 33 : 275-277, 1986.
47. Jones TB, Dubuisson RL, Hughes JJ, et al: Abrupt termination of the common bile duct: A sign of malignancy identified by high-resolution real-time sonography. J Ultrasound Med 2 : 345-348, 1983.
48. Kamath PS, Joseph DC, Chandran R, Rao SR, et al: Biliary ascariasis: Ultrasonography, endosocpic retrograde cholangiopancreatography, and biliary drainage. Gastroenterology 91 : 730-732, 1986.
49. Kane RA: Ultrasonographic diagnosis of gangerenous cholecystitis and empyma of the gallbladder. Radiology 134 : 191-194, 1980.
50. Kane RA, Jacobs R, Katz J, et al: Porcelain gallbladder: Ultrasound and CT appearance. Radiology 152 : 137-141, 1984.
51. Kaude JV: The width of the common bile duct in relation to age and stone disease. An ultrasonographic study. Eur J Radiol 3 : 115-117, 1983.
52. Khuroo MS, Zargar SA, Mahajan R, et al: Sonographic appearances in biliary ascariasis. Gastroenterology 93 : 267-272, 1987.
53. Kurol M, Forsberg L: Ultrasonography in the diagnosis of acute cholecystitis. Acta Radiol [Diagn] 25 : 379-383, 1984.
54. Laing FC, Jeffrey RB Jr: Choledocholithiasis and cystic duct obstruction: difficult ultrasonographic diagnosis. Radiology 146 : 475-479, 1983.
55. Laing FC, Jeffrey RB Jr, Wing VW, et al: Biliary dilatation: defining the level and cause by real-time US. Radiology 160 : 39-42, 1986.
56. Lammer J, Fotter R, Becker H: Congenital bile duct dilatation (Caroli's disease-Grumbach's disease). Eur J Radiol 4 : 198-201, 1984.
57. Lampmann LE, Meijer JG, Stroucken AA: Sonographic detection of early gallbladder cancer. Clin Med 53 : 99-103, 1984.
58. Lawson TL: Gray scale cholecystosonography: Diagnostic criteria and accuracy. Radiology 122 : 247-251, 1977.

59. Lee AW, Proudfoot WH, Griffen WO Jr: Acalculous cholecystitis. Surg Gynecol Obstet 159 : 33-35, 1984.
60. Lee SP, Maher K, Nicholls JF: Origin and fate of biliary sludge. Gastroenterology 94 : 170-176, 1988.
61. Leopold GR, Amberg J, Gosink BB, et al: Gray scale ultrasonic cholecystography: A comparison with conventional radiographic techniques. Radiology 121 : 445-448, 1976.
62. Lokich JJ, Kane RA, Harrison DA, et al: Biliary tract obstruction secondary to cancer: Management guidelines and selected literature review. J Clin Oncol 5 : 969-981, 1987.
63. Lunderquist A: The radiology of jaundice. Clin Gastroenterology 3 : 387-406, 1989.
63a. Madl C, Grimm G, Mallek R, et al: Diagnosis of gallbladder perforation in acute acalculous cholecystitis in critically ill patients. Intensive Care Med 18 : 245-246, 1992.
64. Marchal GJF, Casaer M, Baert AL, et al: Gallbaldder wall sonolucency in aute cholecystitis. Radiology 133 : 439-443, 1979.
65. Mahour GH, Wakim KG, Ferris DO: The common bile duct in man: Its diameter and circumference. Ann Surg 165 : 415-419, 1967.
66. Maresca G, De Gaetano AM, Mirk P, et al: Sonographic patterns of the gallbladder in acute viral hepatitis. JCU 12 : 141-146, 1984.
67. Meyer DG, Weinstein BJ: Klatskin tumors of the bile ducts: Sonographic appearance. Radiology 148 : 803-804, 1983.
68. Meire HB: Ultrasound in gastroenterology. Clin Gastroenterol 13 : 183-203, 1984.
69. Mitchell SE, Clark RA: A comparison of computed tomography and sonography in choledocholithiasis. AJR 142 : 729-733, 1984.
70. Mueller PR, Ferrucci JT, Simeone JF, et al: Postcholecystectomy bile duct dilatation: Myth of reality? AJR 136 : 355-358, 1981.
71. Mueller PR: Jaundice, in Simeone J (ed), Coordinated Diagnostic Imaging (Clinics in Diagnostic Ultrasound, Vol 14). New York, Churchill Livingstone, 1984.
72. Niederau C, Muller J, Sonnenberg A, et al: Extrahepatic bile ducts in healthy subjects, in patients with cholelithiasis, and in postcholecystectomy patients: A prospective ultrasonic study. JCU 11 : 23-27, 1983.
73. Nix GA, Wilson JH, Schmitz PI, et al: Carcinoma of the ampulla and papilla of Vater. ROFO 138 : 531-535, 1983.
74. O'Connor HJ, Bartlett RJ, Hamilton I, et al: Bile duct calibre : The discrepancy between ultrasonic and retrograde cholangiographic measurement in the post-cholecystectomy patient. Clin Radiol 36 : 507-510, 1985.
75. Okuda K, Tsuchiya Y, Saotome N, et al: How to investigate cholestasis: Utility of ultrasound as the first imaging study. Semin Liver Dis 3 : 308-317, 1983.
76. Olken SM, Bledsoe R, Newmark H: The ultrasonic diagnosis of primary carcinoma of the gallbladder. Radiology 129 : 481-482, 1978.
77. Paivansalo M, Merikanto J, Lahde S, et al: Radiographic diagnsois of bile duct cysts: Retrospective analysis of thirteen cases. Acta Radiol 29 : 657-660, 1988.
78. Parulekar SG: Sonography of the distal cystic duct. J Ultrasound Med 8 : 367-373, 1989.
79. Parulekar SG, Mcnamara MP Jr: Ultrasonography of choledocholithiasis. J Ultrasound Med 2 : 395-400, 1983.
80. Parulekar SG: Ultrasonic detection of calcification in gallstones: "The reverberation shadow." J Ultrasound Med 3 : 123-129, 1984.
81. Plillay SP, Hardue IR: Acute obstructive suppurative cholangitis. Med J Aust 140 : 332-336, 1984.
82. Raghavendra BN: Ultrasonographic features of primary carcinoma of the gallbladder: Report of five cases. Gastrointest Radiol 5 : 239-244, 1980.
83. Raghavendra BN, Subramanyam BR, Balthazar EJ, et al: Sonography of adenomyomatosis of the gallbladder: Radiologic-pathologic correlation. Radiology 146 : 747-752, 1983.
84. Rattner DW, Schapiro RH, Warshaw AL: Abnormalities of the pancreatic and biliary ducts in adult patients with choledochal cysts. Arch Surg 118 : 1068-1073, 1983.
85. Reinig JW, Stanley JH: Sonographic hepatization of the gallbladder: A cause of nonvisualization of the gallbladder by cholecystosonography. JCU 12 : 234-236, 1987.
86. Rice J, Sauerbrei EE, Semogas P, et al: The sonographic appearance of adenomyomatosis of the gallbladder. JCU 9 : 336-337, 1981.
87. Roslyn JJ, Pitt HA, Mann L, et al: Parenteral nutrition induced gallbladder disease: A reason for early cholecystectomy. Am J Surg 148 : 58-63, 1984.
88. Rubaltelli L, Talenti E, Rizzatto G, et al: Gas-containing gallstones: Their influence on ultrasound

images. JCU 12 : 279-282, 1984.
89. Sagar G, Naik DR: Ultrasound diagnosis of adenomyomatosis of the gallbladder. Br J Radiol 57 : 432-435, 1984.
90. Sample WF, Sarti DA, Goldstein LI, et al: Gray scale ultrasonography of jaundiced patient. Radiology 128 : 719-725, 1978.
91. Sanders RC: The significance of sonographic gallbladder wall thickening. JCU 8 : 143-146, 1980.
92. Sauerbrei EE, Cooperberg PL, Gordon P, et al: The discrepancy between radiographic and sonographic bile duct measurements. Radiology 137 : 751-755, 1980.
93. Sauerbrei EE: Ultrasound of the common bile duct, in Sanders RC, Hill M (ed), Ultrasound Annual 1983. New York, Raven Press, 1983, pp1-46.
94. Scharschmidt BF, Goldberg HI, Schmid R: Current concepts in diagnosis. Approach to the patient with cholestatic jaundice. N Engl J Med 308 : 1515-1519, 1983.
95. Scheske GS, Cooperberg PL, Cohen MM: Floating gallstones: The role of contrast material. JCU 8 : 227-231, 1980.
96. Schulman A: Non-western patterns of biliary stones and the role of ascariasis. Radiology 162 : 425-430, 1987.
97. Senecail B, Jestin Y, Meunier P: Echographic aspects of biliary lithiasis and its complications. J Radiol 64 : 299-306, 1983.
98. Shah KK, Shah KK, Fink-Bennett D, et al: Extrahepatic biliary obstruction versus intrahepatic disorder. Differentiation with hepatobiliary scintigraphy and ultrasonography. J Clin Gastroenterol 10 : 191-196, 1988.
99. Shea JA: Preoperative evaluation of the biliary tract. Surg Clin North Am 65 : 47-58, 1985.
100. Shlaer WJ, Leopold GR, Scheible FW: Sonography of the thickened gallbladder wall: A nonspecific finding. AJR 136 : 337-339, 1981.
101. Sigel B, Machi J, Beitler JC, Donahue PE, et al: Comparative accuracy of operative ultrasonography and colangiography in detecting common duct calculi. Surgery 94 : 715-720, 1983.
102. Sommer FG, Taylor KJW: Differentiation of acoustic shadowing due to calculi and gas collections. Radiology 135 : 399-403, 1980.
103. Stoller JL, Cooperberg PL, Simpson WM: Diagnostic ultrasonography in acute cholecystitis. Can J Surg 22 : 374-376, 1979.
104. Suramo I, Paivansalo M, Myllyla V, et al: Ultrasonography of carcinoma of the gallbladder. The images and differential diagnostic problems. ROFO 139 : 680-683, 1983.
105. Taylor KJW, Rosenfield AT: Gray-scale ultrasonography in the differential diagnosis of jaundice. Arch Surg 112 : 820-825, 1977.
106. Taylor KJW, Rosenfield AT, Spiro HM: Diagnostic accuracy of gray scale ultrasonography for the jaundiced patient: A report of 275 cases. Arch Intern Med 139 : 60-63, 1979.
107. Taylor KJW, Jacobson P, Jaffe CC: Lack of an acoustic shadow on scans of gallstones: A possible artifact. Radiology 131 : 463-464, 1979.
108. Van Gansbeke DE, Toeuf J, Cremer M, et al: Suprahepatic gallbladder: A rare congenital anomaly. Gastrointest Radiol 9 : 341-343, 1984.
109. Vennes JA: Management of calculi in the common duct. Semin Liver Dis 3 : 162-171, 1983.
110. Weill F, Eisencher A, Zeltner F: Ultrasonic study of the normal and dilated biliary tree. Radiology 127 : 221-224, 1978.
111. Weiner SN, Koenigsberg M, Morehouse H, et al: Sonography and computed tomography in the diagnosis of carcinoma of the gallbladder. AJR 142 : 735-739, 1984.
112. Williamson SL, Williamson MR: Cholecystosonography in pregnancy. J Ultrasound Med 3 : 329-331, 1984.
113. Yeh H-C: Ultrasonography and computed tomography of carcinoma of the gallbladder. Radiology 133 : 167-173, 1979.
114. Yeung EY, McCarthy P, Gompertz RH, et al: The ultrasonic appearances of hilar cholangiocarcinoma (Klatskin tumours). Br J Radiol 61 : 991-996, 1988.
115. Yoshida H, Itai Y, Minami K, Kokubo T, et al: Biliary malignancies occurring in choledochal cysts. Radiology 173 : 389-332, 1989.
116. Yum HY, Fink AH: Sonographic findings in primary carcinoma of the gallbladder. Radiology 134 : 693-696, 1987.

CHAPTER 5

THE PANCREAS

NORMAL ANATOMY

The pancreas lies transversely or obliquely in the upper abdomen, with the head inferior to the body of the organ. In the midline, the pancreas lies markedly anteriorly as it curves across the vertebral bodies. The head of the pancreas is usually larger than the rest of the organ and lies immediately medial to the second part of the duodenum. The inferior vena cava lies posterior to the head (Figure 5-1).

The superior mesenteric vein lies behind the neck of the pancreas and in front of the uncinate process. The tail of the pancreas crosses over the left kidney and extends to the splenic hilum.[17, 19, 29, 77] Visualization of this portion of the pancreas is ordinarily hindered by gas in the stomach, and it is often necessary to perform the scan with the patient standing to create an acoustic window for adequate imaging. Alternatively, scanning of the tail of the pancreas by left coronal viewing via the spleen may give a satisfactory result.[13, 77]

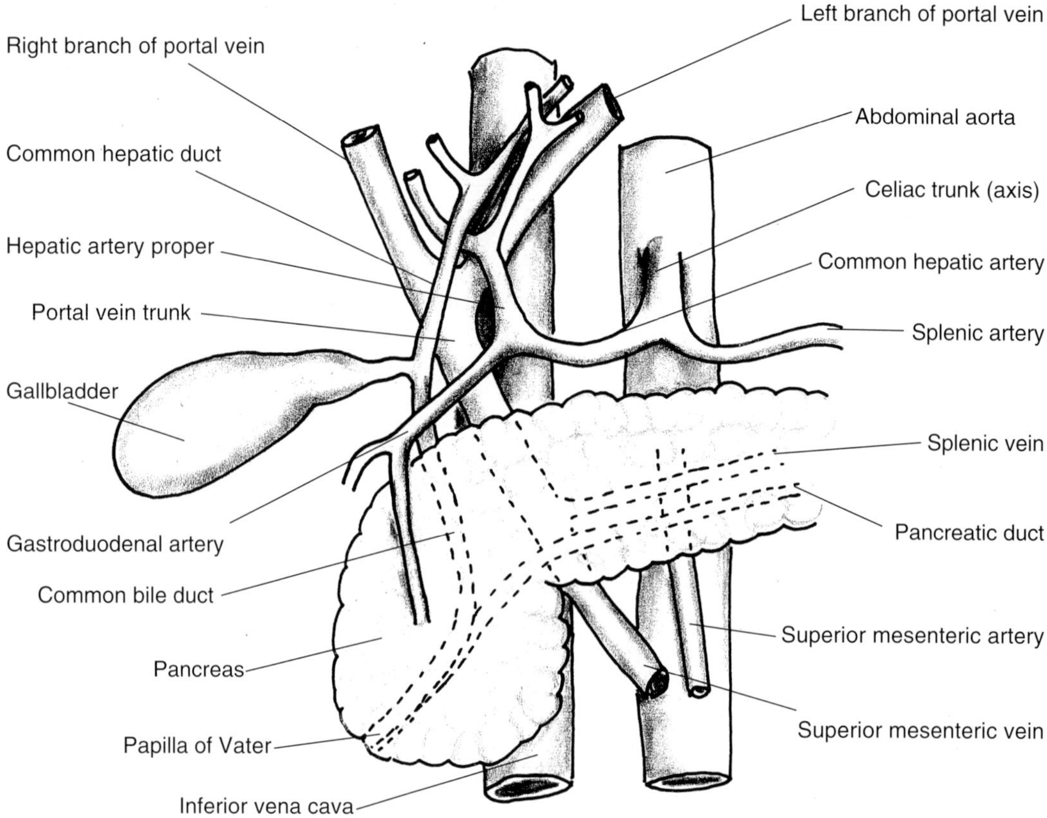

Figure 5-1. The pancreas.
Schematic diagram of the anatomy of the pancreas and surrounding landmarks, especially the major vessels and biliary tract, which are useful in identifying the pancreas.

ULTRASONIC APPEARANCES

The pancreas has numerous fine blood vessels, ducts, and a lobular architecture.[26, 50] Together with the fatty tissues in the interacinar spaces, these multiple interfaces tend to produce strong echoes of variable intensity.[47, 52, 59, 92] The echogenicity of the normal pancreas of younger subjects is similar to that of the liver, and reflectivity increases with increasing age. This increase in reflectivity is mostly attributable to the increase in the fat content of the parenchyma, as shown in x-ray CT scans.[47, 59]

Echographically, the margins of the pancreas are not clearly demarcated due to the normal irregularity of the organ and the absence of a well-defined capsule.[17, 19, 24]

Various landmarks are important in imaging the pancreas.[19, 31, 77] A series of transverse sonograms at various levels (Figures 5-2 and 5-3) demonstrate the important landmarks including the main pancreatic duct, the abdominal aorta, the inferior vena cava, the splenic vein, the celiac trunk and its branches, as well as the superior mesenteric artery and vein, which serve as landmarks for locating the pancreas.

The main pancreatic duct, with a caliber of 1 to 2 mm and positioned in the central portion of the parenchyma, is recognized by its echogenic borders. The main pancreatic duct and the common bile duct are important indices of pancreatic disease (Figure 5-3).[31, 58, 61, 77, 87]

Sagittal sonograms of the pancreas (Figure 5-4) depict landmarks which are important in assessing the position and margins of the pancreas because adjacent organs such as the duodenojejunal flexure, the stomach wall, and the small intestine can easily be mistaken.[5, 8] To avoid this problem, it is important to scan the area in at least two different planes, sagittal and transverse.

In sagittal section, the body of the pancreas is demonstrated as a rhomboid shape lying between the left lobe of the liver and the abdominal aorta, with a slightly echogenic parenchyma, with the splenic vein and superior mesenteric artery lying posterior to it (Figure 5-4b). The celiac axis should also be identified superior to the pancreatic body on transverse (Figure 5-2a) and sagittal scans (Figure 5-4a). At the neck and head portions of the pancreas, the anatomical landmarks of the gastroduodenal artery, common bile duct, descending duodenum, gallbladder, and portal vein at the confluence of the splenic and superior mesenteric veins should be identified.[31, 57, 58, 61, 77]

Measurements of the sizes of the pancreas (Table 5-1) are sometimes used for quantitative assessment of disease. However, individual variations limit their value and features such as the shape and contour of the organ and the echogenicity of the parenchyma are often more informative.[36, 57, 84]

Table 5-1. Sonographic determiantion of the nomal pancreas.

	Arger	de Graaff	Haber	Lawson	Weill	Kataoka*
Head (mm)	18+1.2	21+8	27±7	20−25	11−30	13−19
Body	17.5+1.4	11+6	22±7	15−20	4−21	9−13
Tail	17.5+1.1		24±4	10−15	7−28	9−14

Addendum: Values are given as the median value, however, the sizes of the pancreas changes accoding to the age group and younger generation has the largest value and decrease accordingly.

*Kataoka K, Kashima K, Horii Y, et al: Effect of age on pancreatic ultrasonography. Proc JSUM 40 : 433-434, 1982.

a

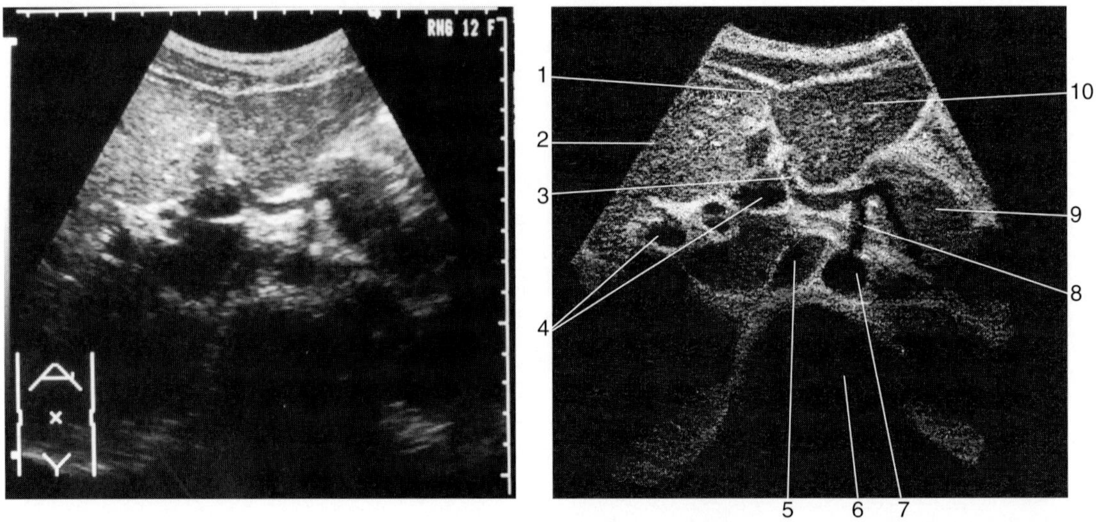

1. Falciform ligament 2. Liver 3. Proper hepatic artery 4. Portal vein 5. Inferior vena cava 6. Spine 7. Aorta 8. Celiac trunk 9. Tail of pancreas 10. Left lobe of liver

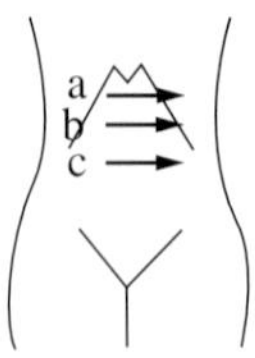

Figure 5-2. The normal pancreas, transverse scans.
The normal pancreas demonstrates a certain degree of individual variations. Therefore, a basic anatomical understanding of these variations is crucial to identification of the pancreas, especially when the quality of the image is poor. A transverse scan at the upper border of the pancreas (a) reveals the celiac trunk, aorta, inferior vena cava, portal vein, and common hepatic duct. (b) Part of the body of the pancreas, the gallbladder, the splenic vein and other large vessels in a transverse scan slightly inferior and parallel to (a). (c) A transverse scan of the pancreatic body showing the normal main pancreatic duct running parallel to the splenic vein.

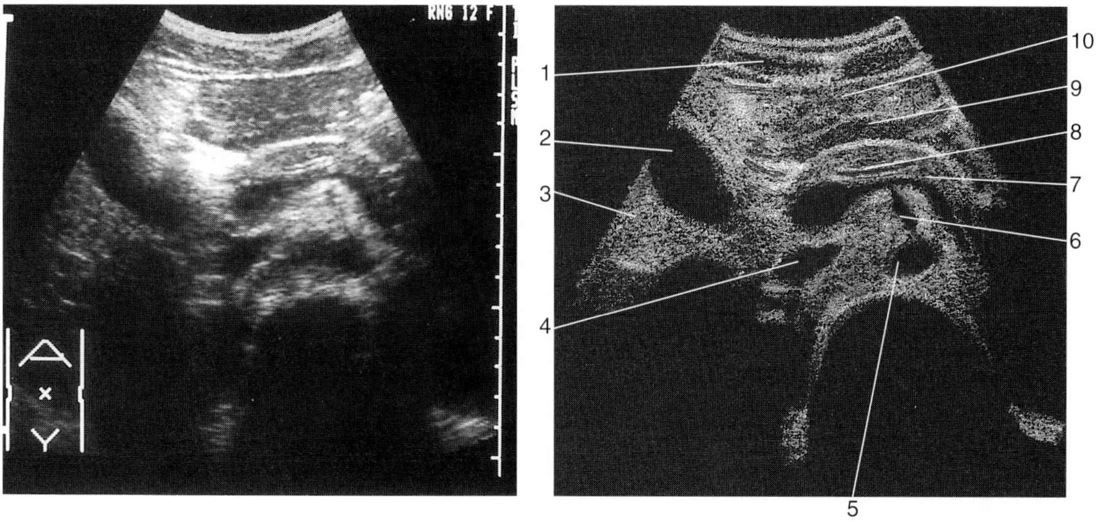

b

1. Rectus abdominis muscle 2. Gallbladder 3. Right lobe of liver 4. Inferior vena cava 5. Aorta 6. Superior mesenteric artery 7. Pancreas 8. Pancreatic duct (Wirsung's duct) 9. Gastric antrum 10. Left lobe of liver

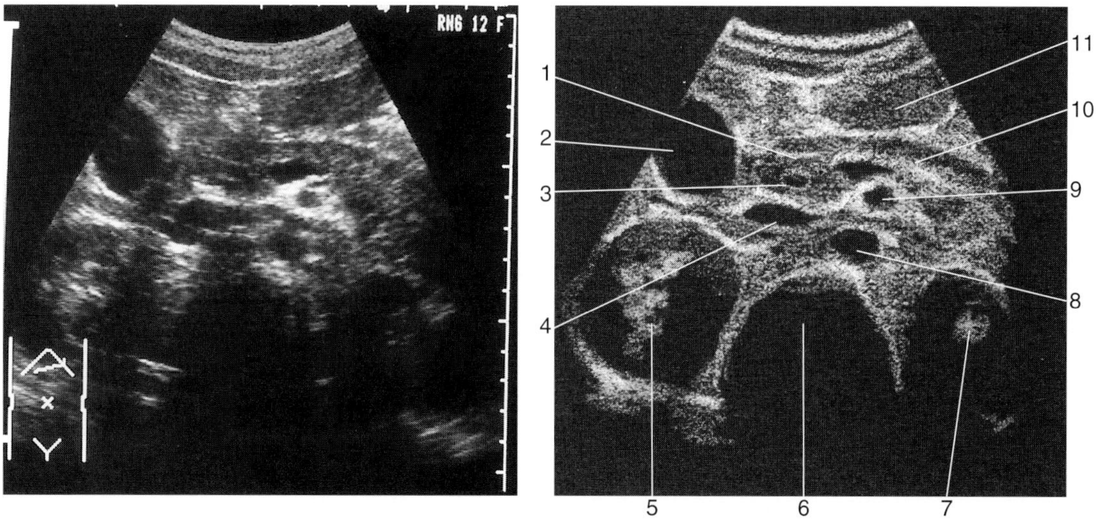

c

1. Santorini's duct 2. Gallbladder 3. Common bile duct 4. Inferior vena cava 5. Right kidney 6. Spine 7. Left kidney 8. Aorta 9. Superior mesenteric artery 10. Tail of pancreas 11. Left lobe of liver

a

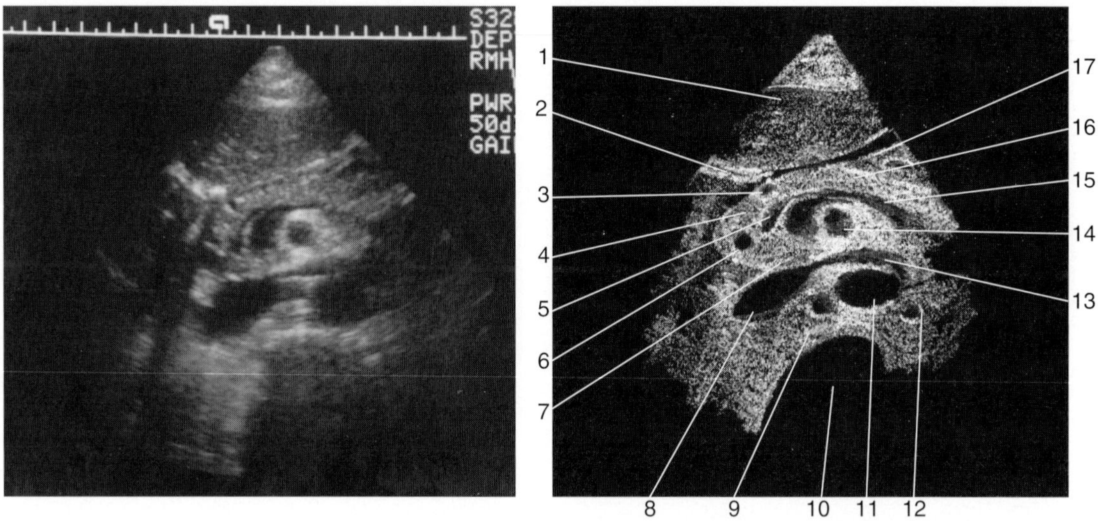

1. Liver 2. Duodenum 3. Gastroduodenal artery 4. Head of pancreas 5. Pancreatic duct 6. Common bile duct 7. Uncinate process 8. Inferior vena cava 9. Crus of diaphragm 10. Spine 11. Aorta 12. Crus of diaphragm 13. Left renal vein 14. Superior mesenteric artery 15. Splenic vein 16. Pancreas 17. Stomach

b

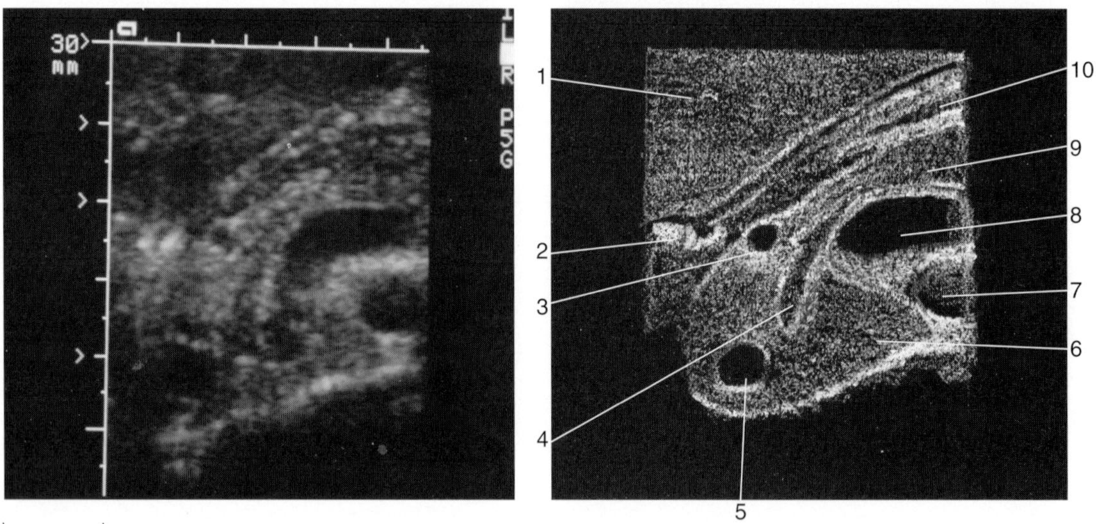

1. Liver 2. Duodenum 3. Gastroduodenal artery 4. Pancreatic duct 5. Common bile duct 6. Uncinate process 7. Superior mesenteric artery 8. Superior mesenteric vein 9. Pancreas (neck) 10. Antrum of stomach

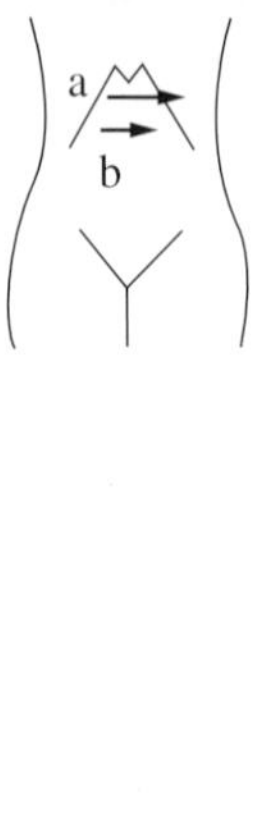

Figure 5-3. The normal pancreas transverse scan.
In subjects who give good ultrasound images ("glass subjects"), exquisite detail can be obtained. The neck, head and uncinate process of the pancreas are well delineated in this example, as well as the lower end of the common bile duct and the gastroduodenal artery. The pancreatic duct can be discerned as it curves posteriorly in the head of the pancreas.

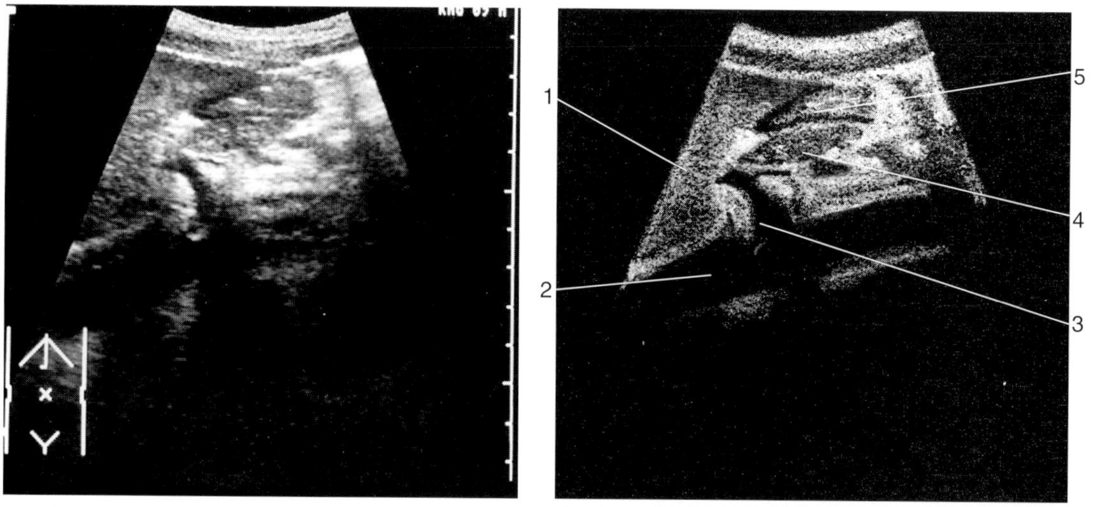

a

1. Liver 2. Aorta 3. Celiac axis 4. Body of pancreas 5. Antrum of stomach

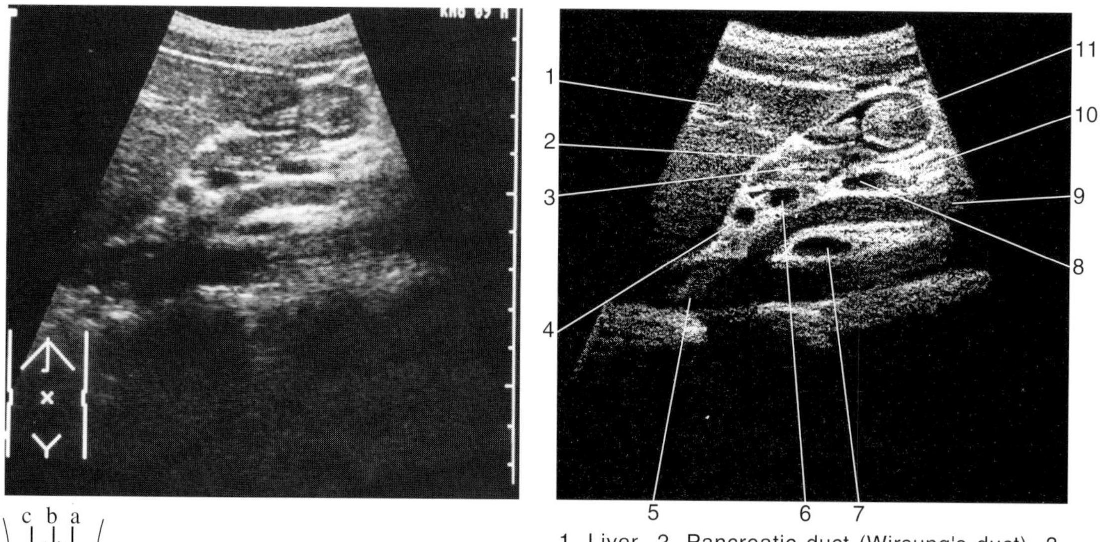

b

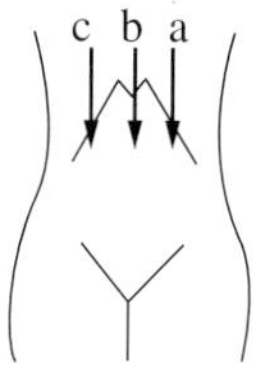

1. Liver 2. Pancreatic duct (Wirsung's duct) 3. Body of pancreas 4. Common hepatic artery 5. Aorta 6. Splenic vein 7. Left renal vein 8. Inferior mesenteric vein 9. Superior mesenteric artery 10. Splenic vein 11. Antrum of stomach

Figure 5-4. The normal pancreas, sagittal scans.
(a) A left parasagittal scan traversing the abdominal aorta and celiac axis. Part of the left lobe of the liver and the stomach are demonstrated. The body of the pancreas lies directly behind the gastric antrum. (b) A midline sagittal scan showing (from anterior to posterior) the left lobe of the liver, gastric antrum, pancreatic body, splenic vein and superior mesenteric artery, left renal vein, and the aorta. (c) This figure, taken just to the right of the midline, shows part of the pancreatic head, the main portal trunk, and the inferior vena cava. A cross section of the common duct and part of the liver are seen. The dark zone posterior to the cava is the right psoas muscle.

c

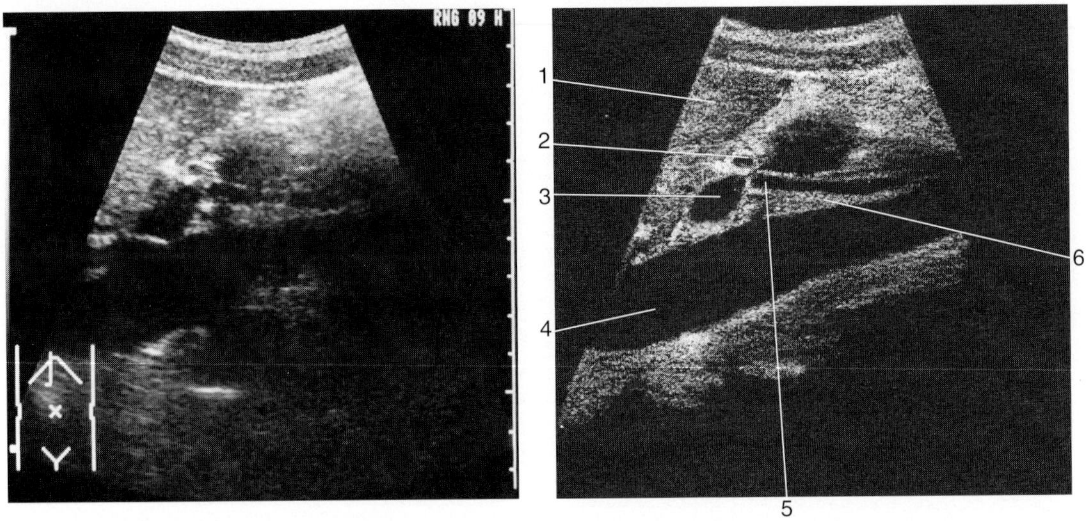

1. Liver 2. Common hepatic artery 3. Portal vein
4. Inferior vena cava 5. Common hepatic duct
6. Uncinate lobe

Figure 5-4.

SCANNING TECHNIQUES

The pancreas lies obliquely across the upper abdomen, with the splenic vein running immediately posteriorly. In thin patients, scanning may be performed relatively easily, but it is more difficult to image the pancreas in a heavily built or obese patient. To provide a window to visualize the pancreas, a deep inspiration to displace the left lobe of the liver downward is often helpful. Pressure by the scanning head on the relaxed abdominal wall while the patient is standing or a scanning through a water-filled stomach may be most helpful in imaging the pancreas under difficult circumstances.[13, 43, 52, 81]

Scanning usually begins at the midline, identifying first the cross section of the body of the pancreas. Then the transducer is turned to the transverse direction to image the length of the organ, including the surrounding landmarks. Because of poor penetration of the ultrasound beam in unfavorable subjects, a lower-frequency transducer may give better images. Every possible technique should be employed before abandoning the scan.

In the fluid-filled stomach technique, after an overnight fast the patient drinks 500 to 700 ml of water and lies in the left decubitus position to allow the air bubbles in the stomach to escape through the pyloric canal. When these bubbles have cleared, the patient is placed in the right semidecubitus position for scanning.[13, 43, 81] Usually the entire pancreas is covered by the stomach, permitting good visualization with the probe on the epigastrium. It is often necessary to reduce the gain setting approximately 10 dB to compensate for the increased reflectivity of the pancreatic parenchyma due to the lack of attenuation in the stomach water.

Figure 5-5 shows the sonographic appearance of the normal pancreas obtained by this method. The pancreatic parenchyma is surrounded by the echogenic gastric wall, and the remainder of the pancreas is covered either by the second part of the duodenum or by the echogenic retropancreatic fat pad. If the pancreas is not well demonstrated, the patient is asked to sit or to lie in the left decubitus position to improve imaging.

The tail of the pancreas can be usually imaged without difficulty by this procedure using real-time equipment. The landmarks for its identification are the splenic vein and artery, the spleen itself, and the left kidney. The procedure also allows identification of the duodenojejunal flexure, located directly inferior to the junction of the body and tail of the pancreas. The flexure may be distinguished from a tumor or cyst at the tail of the pancreas by the movement of air bubbles or by the intraluminal contents.[5, 8]

All of these method may fail, however, in patients with anatomical disturbances such as severe postpancreatitic adhesions, in patients after the upper abdominal surgery, or in those with excessive fecal loading. In such cases, x-ray CT scanning is the method of choice.

a

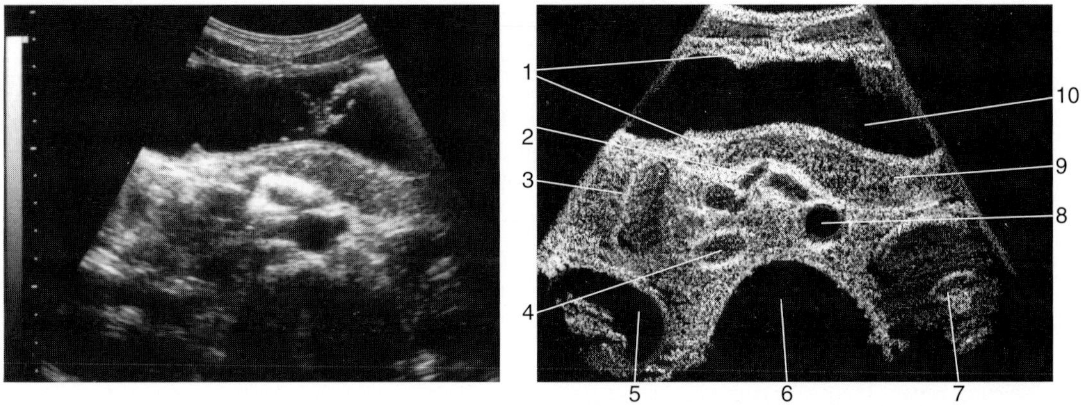

1. Gastric wall 2. Common hepatic artery 3. Duodenum 4. Inferior vena cava 5. Right kidney 6. Spine 7. Left kidney 8. Aorta 9. Tail of pancreas 10. Stomach

b

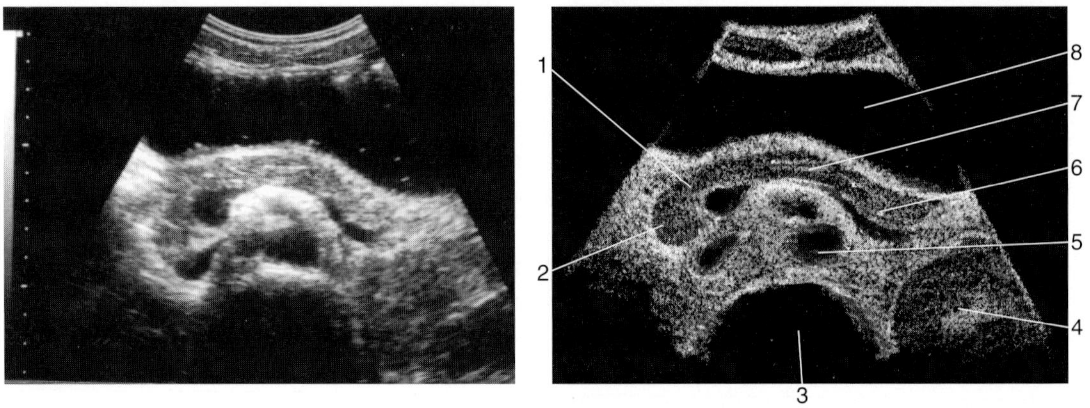

1. Gastroduodenal artery 2. Head of pancreas 3. Spine 4. Left kidney 5. Aorta 6. Tail of pancreas 7. Pancreatic duct 8. Stomach

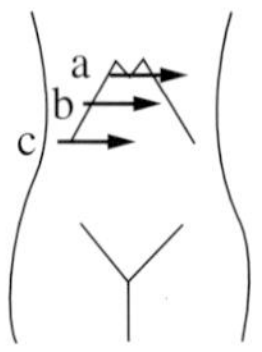

Figure 5-5. A series of transverse scans of the normal pancreas visualized via the water-filled stomach.
An acoustic window produced by the fluid-filled stomach following ingestion of an adequate amount of water, together with appropriate positioning of the patient, allows imaging of the entire pancreas at various levels: (a) the pancreatic body, (b) the head and body of the pancreas, and (c) the head and uncinate process of the pancreas.

c

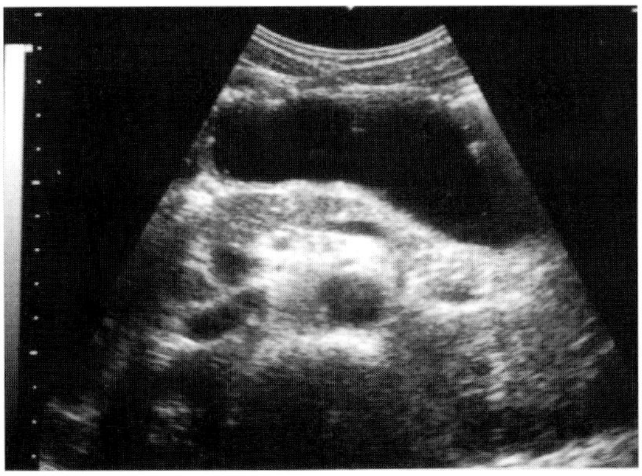

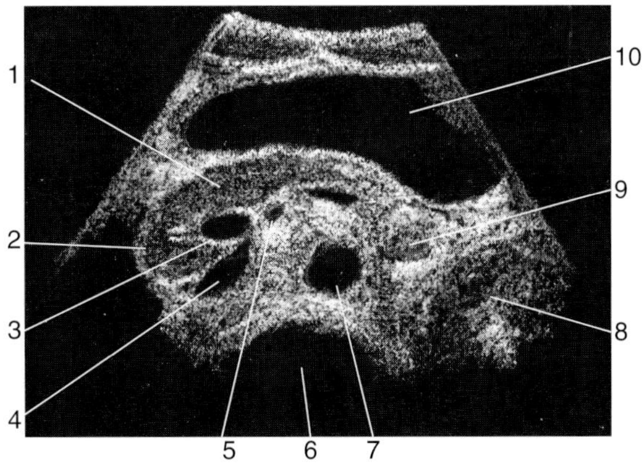

1. Body of pancreas 2. Head of pancreas 3. Superior mesenteric vein 4. Inferior vena cava 5. Superior mesenteric artery 6. Spine 7. Aorta 8. Left kidney 9. Duodenojejunal flexure 10. Stomach

INFLAMMATORY LESIONS

Pancreatitis

Sonography is extremely helpful in patients with suspected acute pancreatitis, providing accurate diagnostic findings swiftly and economically. The signs of edema in the pancreatic area on ultrasound can confirm the suspicion of pancreatitis in a patient with nonspecific symptoms of an acute abdomen.[11, 17, 38, 49, 56, 70] However, in some cases, the examination may not be contributory because of excessive gas around the pancreatic region due to the localized ileus that often follows the acute inflammatory process. In this situation, x-ray CT is the method of choice.[38, 56, 70]

The sonographic characteristics of acute pancreatitis are diffuse swelling of the pancreas,with uniformly decreased echo levels (Figures 5-6 and 5-7) reflecting profuse edema of the parenchyma. The main pancreatic duct is usually almost normal in caliber, except in the acute stages of chronic recurrent pancreatitis, in which irregularity and dilatation of the main pancreatic duct are common. In combination with the swelling of the organ, peripancreatic fluid collections can be visualized. The fluid collections may occur in the vicinity of the pancreas (Figure 5-8) but often accumulate in distant abdominal recesses, for example, behind the urinary bladder.[16, 28, 85] Repeated observations through the course of the illness may disclose tracking of the fluid. It may also reveal pseudocysts of the pancreas, the most common sequela of acute pancreatitis.

Acute severe pancreatitis may progress to hemorrhagic necrosis of the pancreatic parenchyma; this may lead to a pancreatic abscess or a pancreatic phlegmon, in which bacterial contamination of a severely inflamed pancreas produces multiple small abscesses with severe or even fatal multiple organ failure. At this stage, x-ray CT scanning is again the method of choice because it provides clearer images revealing a swollen pancreas with an irregular distribution of low-density areas in the parenchyma together with fluid around the organ.

In chronic pancreatitis, on the other hand, swelling of the pancreas is usually minimal and parenchymal atrophy may be present (Figures 5-9 to 5-11). In a small proportion of cases, recurrent inflammation can cause localized swelling of the organ, often mimicking a malignant tumor (Figure 5-12). The swollen head of the pancreas may precipitate obstructive jaundice or dilatation of the main pancreatic duct, further simulating cancer at the head of the pancreas (Figure 5-13).

Pancreatolithiasis

In chronic recurrent pancreatitis, which is mostly caused by prolonged abuse of alcohol [1, 38] or, in lesser degrees, by chronic biliary tract infections complicating choledocholithiasis, stones and dilatation of the main pancreatic duct may occur concurrently (Figure 5-14).[16, 17, 31, 87, 50, 88] Stones in the duct cast strong acoustic shadows distally (Figure 5-15). Dilatation of the main pancreatic duct is usually easy to detect, but the mucous plugs that may occur are often indistinguishable from the more common genuine stones. Some authors have linked carcinoma to pancreatic stones.[39] Such tumors are difficult to diagnose until a late stage because of the paucity of symptoms and signs of malignant transformation. The differentiation of complicating carcinoma from benign inflammation with marked degrees of fibrosis is extremely difficult because of the sonographic similarity of the two conditions. In particular, chronic relapsing pancreatitis accompanied by focal swelling of the head or body of the pancreas is extremely difficult to distinguish from pancreatic carcinoma even in combination with the other imaging methods.[62-64, 86] Rinnen pancreatitis or a duodenal wall diverticulum may sometimes cause a specific form of focal pancreatitis which is difficult to distinguish from a carcinoma of the head of the pancreas.[73] Except for this rather rare condition, focal swelling of the pancreas tends to subside over time, and careful observation at frequent intervals may demonstrate gradual regression of the swelling. However, not infrequently, ultrasound-guided puncture is necessary to establish the true diagnosis.[27, 33, 37, 42, 67, 78]

Pancreatic Pseudocyst

Another frequent sequela of chronic pancreatitis is the formation of a pancreatic pseudocyst.[4, 18, 28, 32, 40] Cysts of varying sizes frequently occur in the tail of the pancreas (Figures 5-16 and 5-17). However, they may also occur in the pancreatic head (Figure 5-18). The cyst may be observed within the pancreatic parenchyma or in the area surrounding the pancreatic tissue. Pseudocysts are usually smooth and round with no wall irregularity. The interior of the cyst is typically anechoic, with acoustic enhancement distal to the cyst. However, it is not uncommon to find membranous septations, strand-like structures or debritic echoes within the cyst [2, 14, 28, 49] (Figure 5-17). Pseudocysts may occur in the spleen,[18] the liver, [40] and even the mediastinum.[85]

Pseudocysts may also follow blunt abdominal trauma due to laceration or even transsection of the pancreatic body.[20, 44, 66] Leakage of digestive enzymes in the pancreatic juice causes pseudocyst formation. These pseudocyst may regress by spontaneous drainage of their contents into the duodenum or the stomach cavity, but often they require surgical intervention for drainage, using real-time ultrasound to guide needle insertion. Careful follow-up of progress by sonography or CT is mandatory.[70]

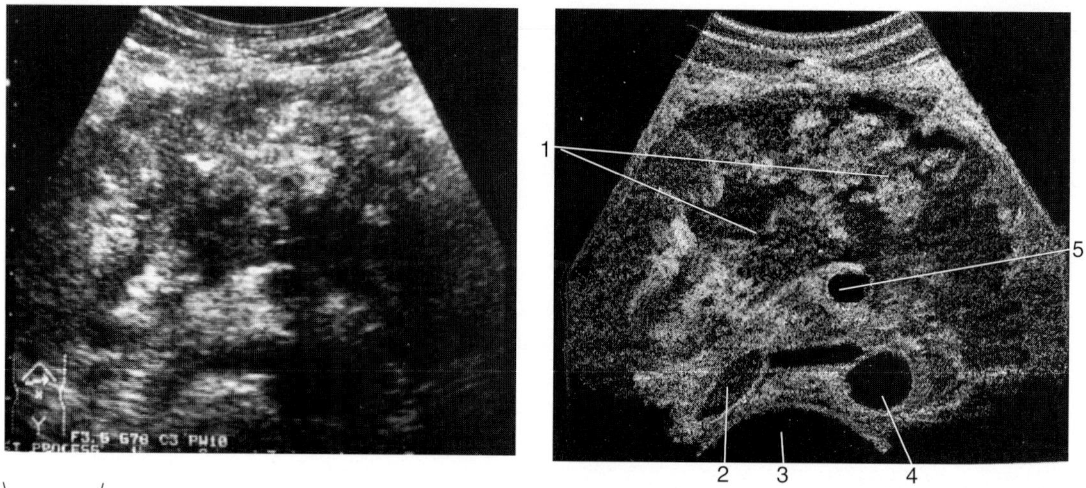

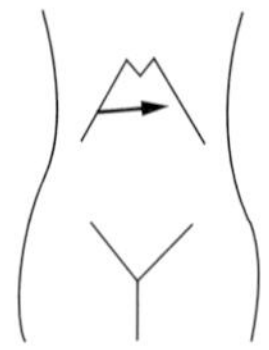

1. Pancreas (excessive swelling with edema) 2. Inferior vena cava 3. Spine 4. Aorta 5. Superior mesenteric artery

Figure 5-6. Acute pancreatitis with marked swelling.
A typical sonogram of acute pancreatitis with diffuse swelling of the whole pancreas. The echogenicity is low, and the texture of the pancreas irregular throughout, reflecting the edematous changes due to massive inflammation. Although such extreme swelling of the whole pancreas is not frequently encountered, it is diagnostic, no other condition producing this pattern.

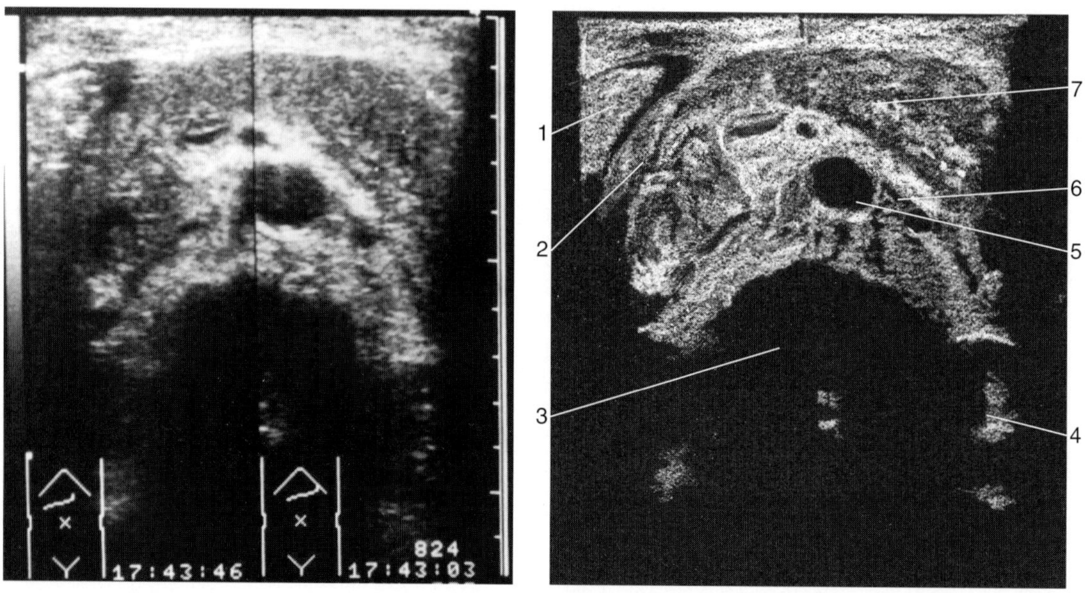

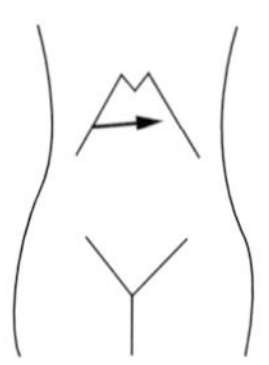

1. Colon 2. Head of pancreas 3. Vertebra 4. Left kidney 5. Aorta 6. Left renal vein 7. Swollen pancreas

Figure 5-7. Acute pancreatitis, transverse scan.
Another case of acute pancreatitis caused by common bile duct stones. The size, shape, and echo texture of the pancreas are quite similar to those of Figure 5-6, except for the presence of packed stones in the lower end of the dilated common duct. Although surgery is rarely indicated in acute pancreatitis, this type is an exception. Prompt surgery is required to remove the obstructing stones which have caused the pancreatitis.

a

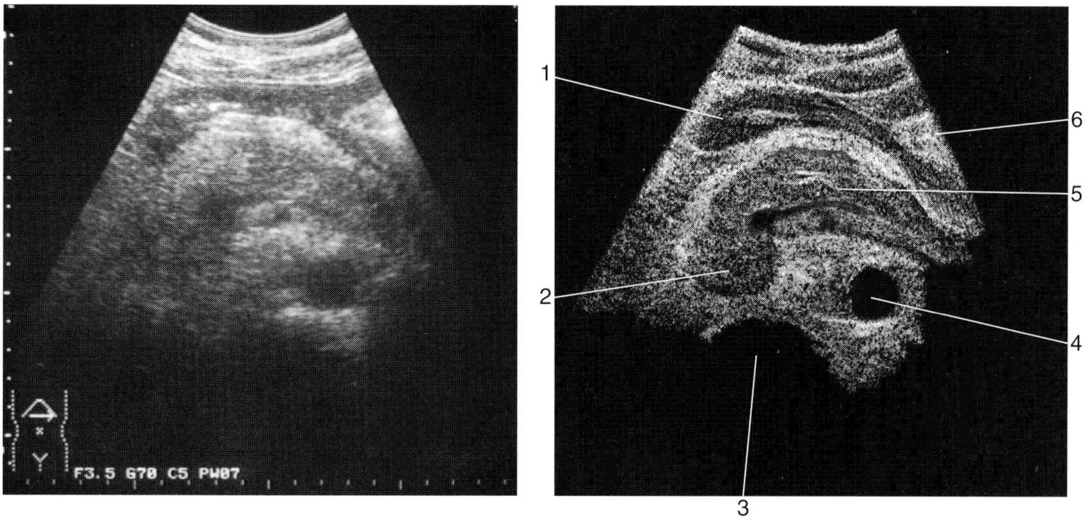

1. Stomach 2. Head of pancreas (swollen) 3. Vertebra 4. Aorta 5. Body of pancreas (swollen) 6. Left lobe of liver

b

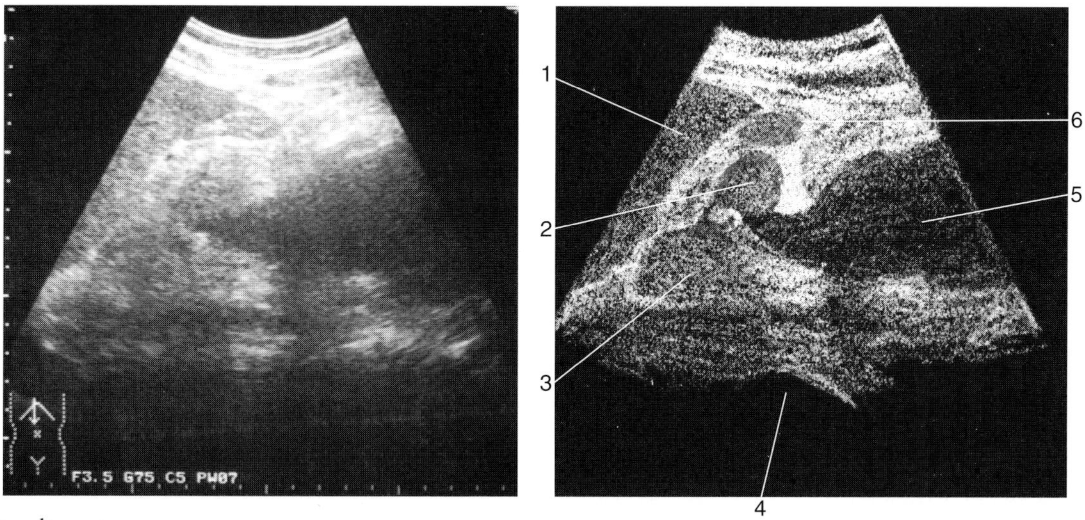

1. Left lobe of liver 2. Body of pancreas 3. Part of head of pancreas 4. Vertebrae 5. Ascites 6. Antrum of stomach

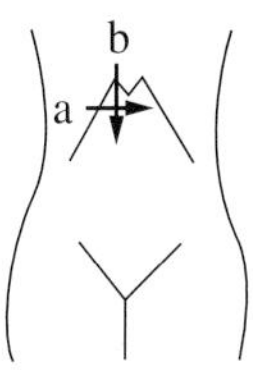

Figure 5-8. Acute pancreatitis.

This patient suffered from epigastric pain, nausea and vomiting. Sonographic examination revealed a swollen pancreas with loss of contours and accumulation of exudate caudal to the body of the pancreas. It also showed an accumulation of ascitic fluid in the lower abdomen, the retrovesical fossa.

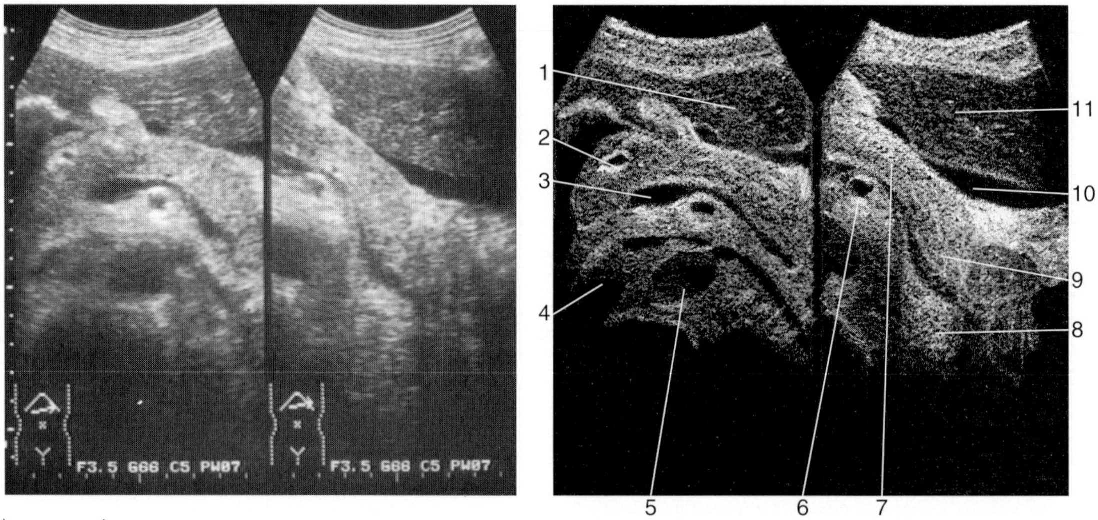

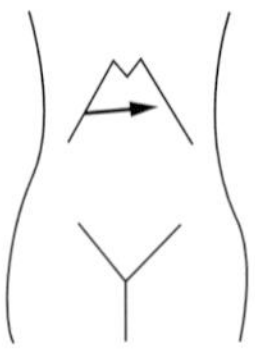

1. Liver 2. Head of pancreas 3. Splenic vein 4. Inferior vena cava 5. Aorta 6. Superior mesenteric artery 7. Duodenojejunal flexure 8. Tail of pancreas (inflamed) 9. Body of pancreas 10. Ascites 11. Left lobe of liver

Figure 5-9. Acute exacerbation of chronic pancreatitis.
Differentiation between an acute episode of chronic relapsing pancreatitis and primary acute pancreatitis is difficult both clinically and sonographically. This case revealed a slightly swollen pancreas with diffusely increased parenchymal echoes accompanied by a peripancreatic accumulation of ascitic fluid. Pancreatolithiasis was not identified. Clinically, it was diagnosed as an acute exacerbation based on the sonograhic findings and the patient's history of prolonged alcohol abuse.

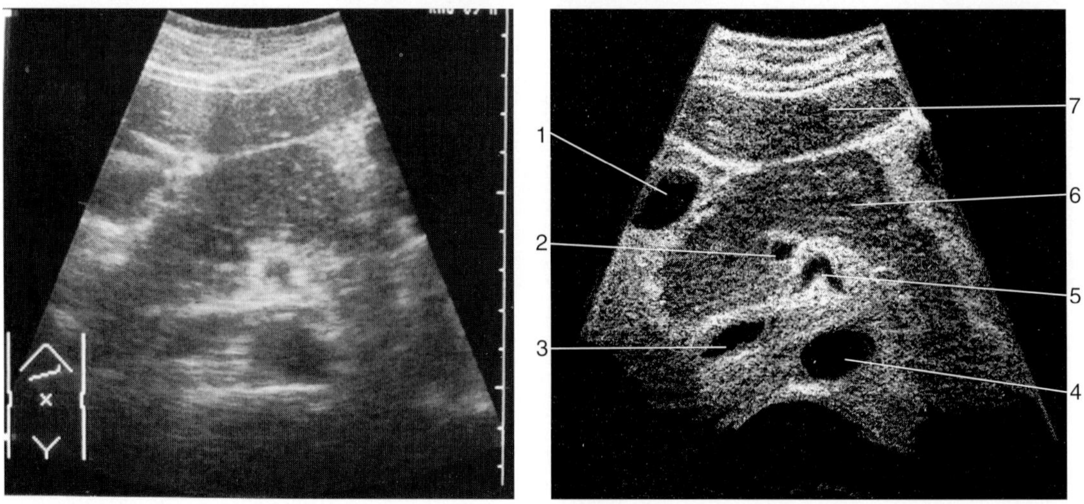

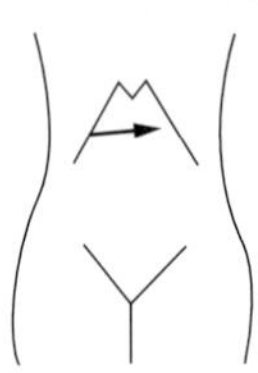

1. Gallbladder 2. Portal vein 3. Inferior vena cava 4. Aorta 5. Superior mesenteric artery 6. Pancreas 7. Liver

Figure 5-10. Chronic pancreatitis mainly affecting the body of the pancreas.
Chronic pancreatitis may also produce localized swelling in any part of the pancreas. Sonographic examination revealed relatively localized swelling of the body, with decreased echo levels containing minute echogenic foci. The patient had complained of upper abdominal pain for several months. He also had a history of alcoholic abuse.

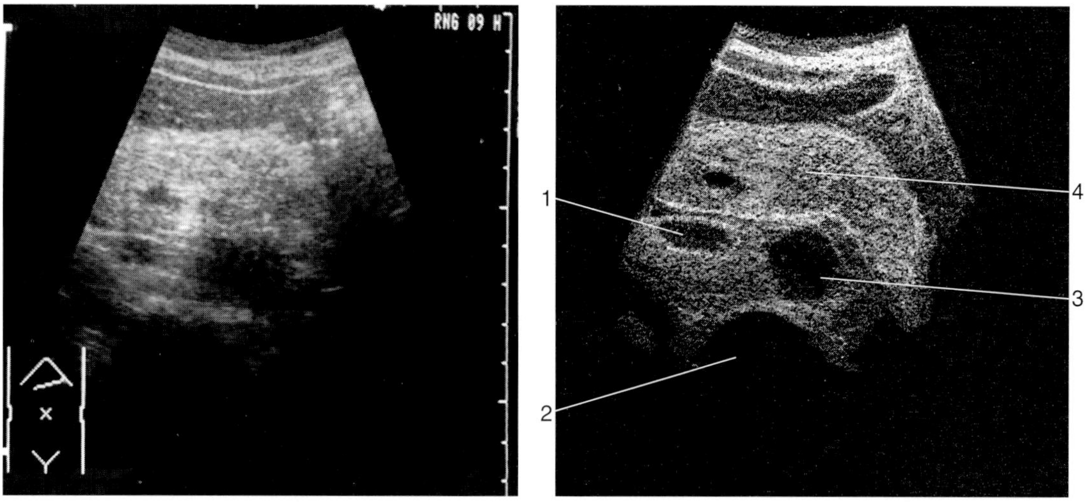

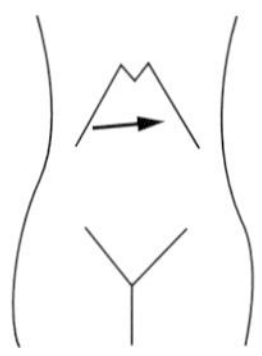

1. Inferior vena cava 2. Vertebra 3. Aorta
4. Swollen and echogenic body of pancreas

Figure 5-11. Chronic pancreatitis, diffusely echogenic type.
The patient suffered from long-standing epigastric pain and weight loss. Sonographic examination revealed a diffusely swollen pancreas with considerably increased parenchymal echogenicity. The caliber of the main pancreatic duct was normal throughout its course, and no stones were found.

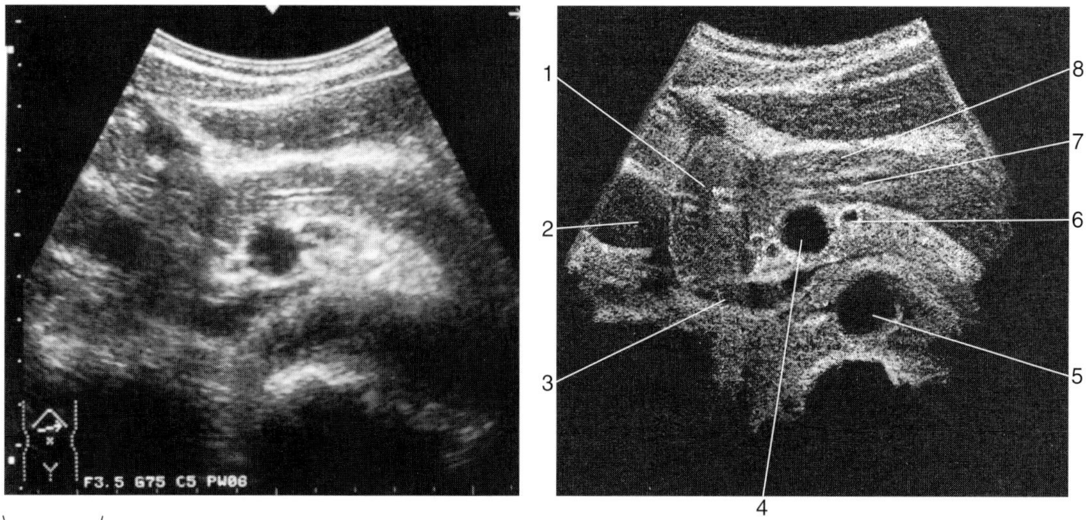

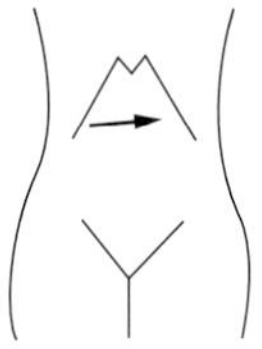

1. Localized enlargement 2. Gallbladder 3. Inferior vena cava 4. Superior mesenteric vein 5. Aorta 6. Superior mesenteric artery 7. Pancreatic duct 8. Pancreas

Figure 5-12. Focal chronic pancreatitis with pseudotumor formation of the head.
Chronic pancreatitis with localized tumor formation poses difficult differential diagnostic problems. The sonogram obtained from a male with long-standing epigastric pain showed localized swelling of the pancreatic head next to the second part of the duodenum. Atrophy of the pancreatic body and the tail together with fine irregularity in contour were found throughout, but there was no dilatation of the pancreatic duct. The absence of altered echogenicity in the swollen part of the pancreas and the gradual diminution of the swelling over a prolonged period of observation support the diagnosis of chronic pancreatitis.

a

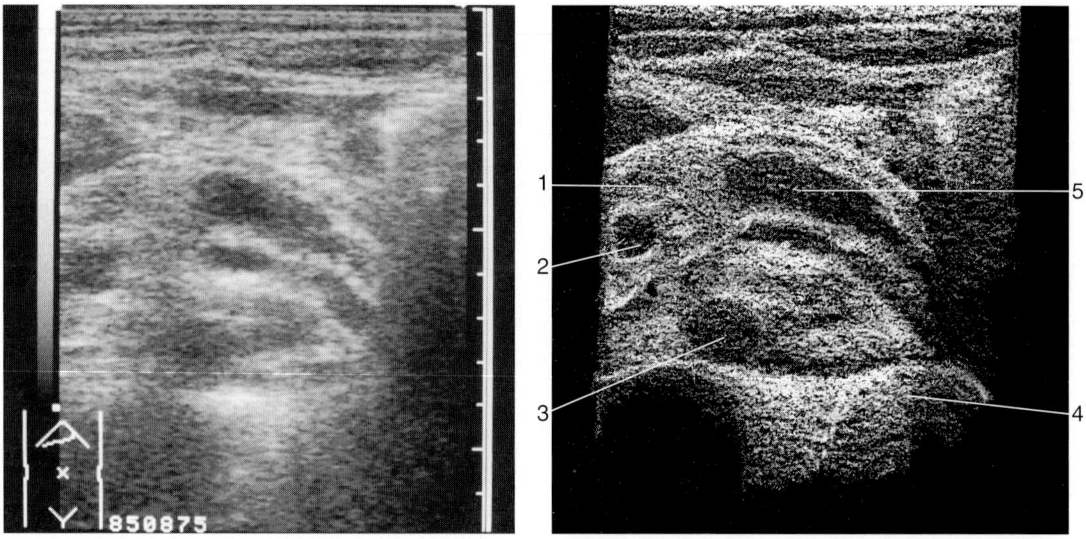

1. Body of pancreas 2. Superior mesenteric vein 3. Aorta 4. Left kidney 5. Dilated Wirsung's duct

b

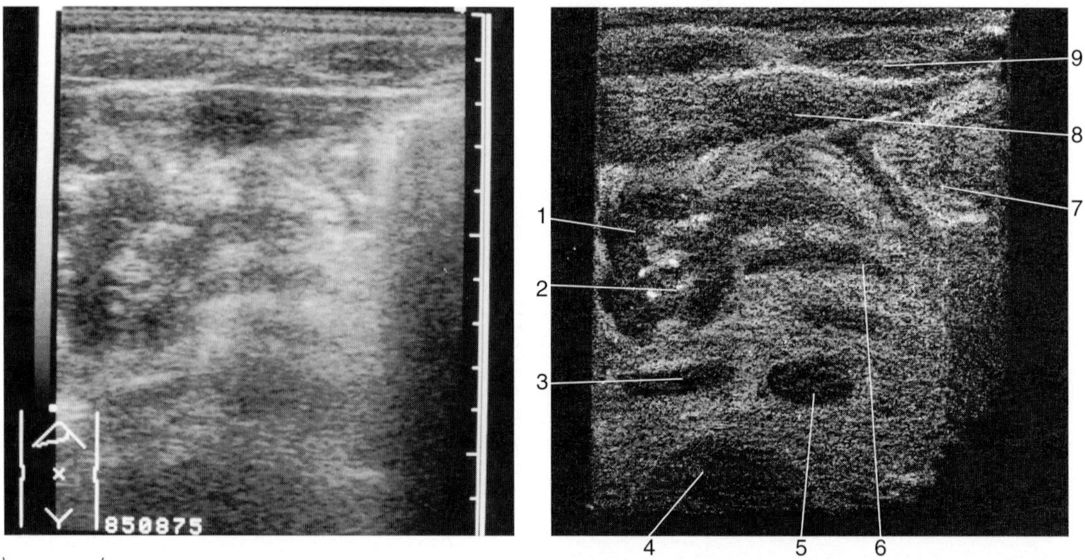

1. Inflamed head of pancreas 2. Pancreatic stones 3. Inferior vena cava 4. Vertebra 5. Aorta 6. Pancreatic duct 7. Stomach 8. Left lobe of liver 9. Rectus abdominis muscle

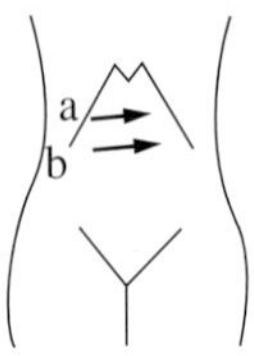

Figure 5-13. Pancreatolithiasis.

Pancreatic stones are frequently found in patients with a long history of chronic alcoholic pancreatitis. The total amount of alcohol consumed is highly correlated with the occurrence of this condition. A transverse scan of the pancreas demonstrates marked dilatation of the main pancreatic duct and clusters of stones casting significant acoustic shadows.

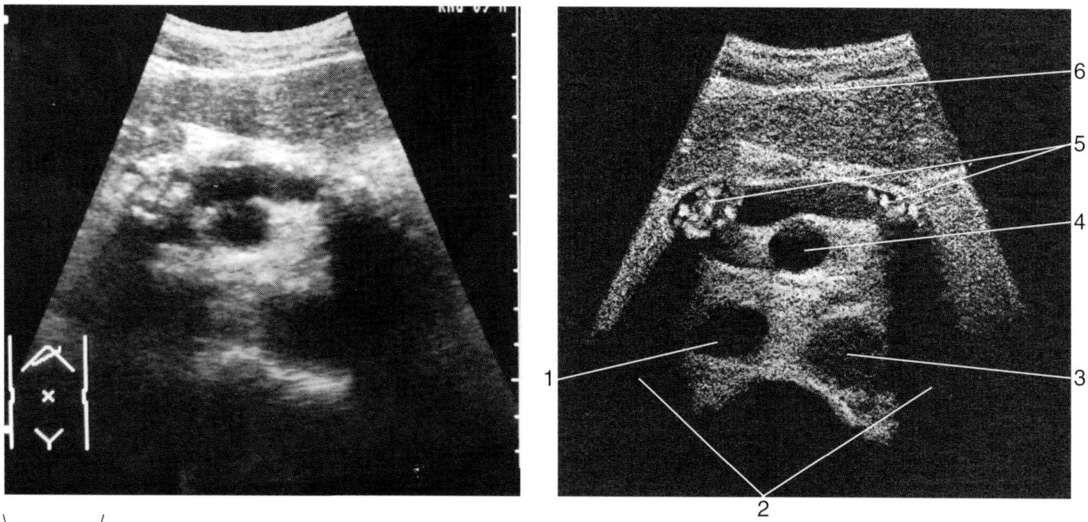

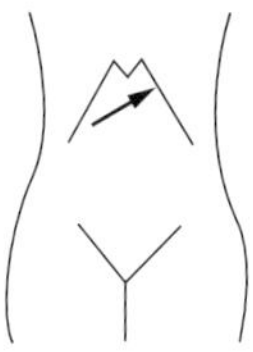

1. Inferior vena cava 2. Acoustic shadows 3. Aorta 4. Superior mesenteric vein 5. Pancreatic stones 6. Left lobe of liver

Figure 5-14. Pancreatolithiasis.
Pancreatic stones, if small, may fail to show discrete acoustic shadowing due to sound diffraction, as shown in this case. Transverse scanning of the pancreas demonstrated marked dilatation of the pancreatic duct. Scanning at a slightly lower level demonstrated small stones together with a localized inflammatory mass of decreased echo intensity showing rather irregular boundaries.

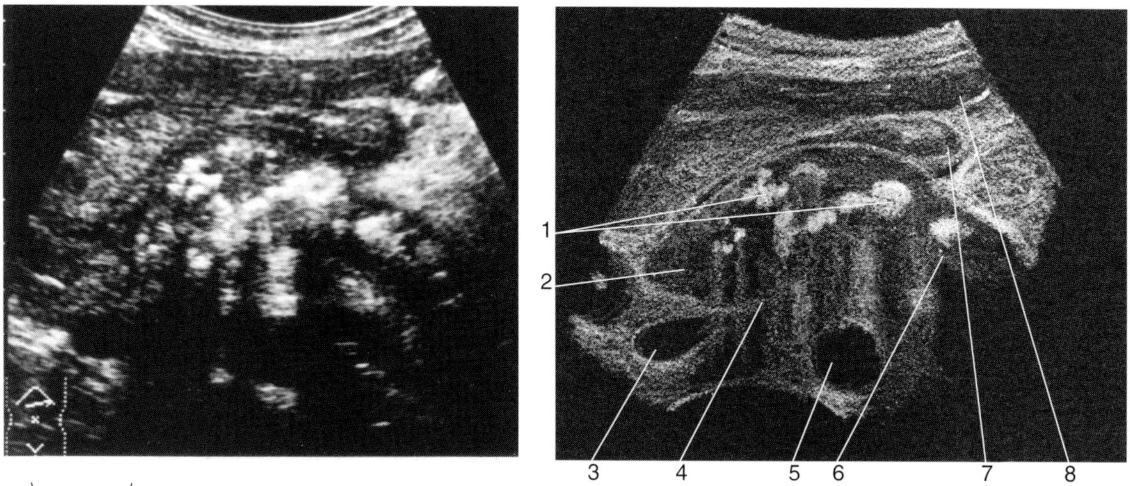

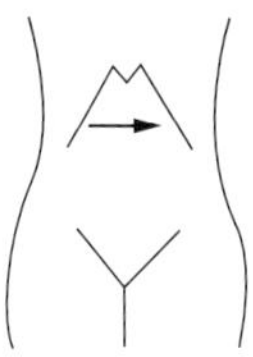

1. Stones 2. Head of pancreas 3. Inferior vena cava 4. Acoustic shadows 5. Aorta 6. Tail of pancreas 7. Antrum of stomach 8. Left lobe of liver

Figure 5-15. Pancreatolithiasis.
This sonogram is a transverse scan of a patient with pancreatolithiasis. Multiple echogenic stones are visualized in the pancreatic parenchyma; however, dilatation of the main pancreatic duct is not apparent on the sonogram because of the extensive acoustic shadows cast by the stones.

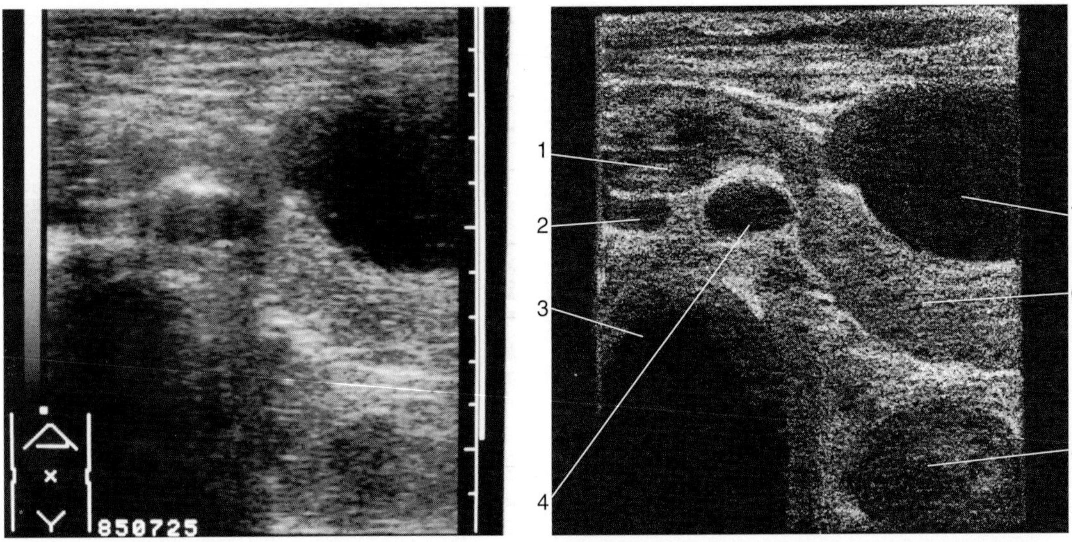

1. Head of pancreas 2. Inferior vena cava 3. Vertebra 4. Aorta 5. Left kidney 6. Tail of pancreas 7. Pseudocyst

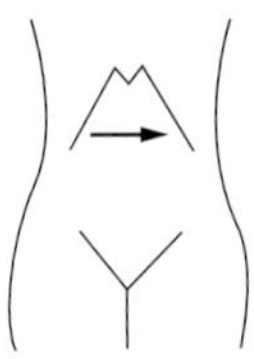

Figure 5-16. Pancreatic pseudocyst.
A large cystic mass was demonstrated on this transverse scan of the tail portion of the pancreas, with distinct acoustic enhancement. The contour of the cyst is smooth and no solid mass was found. The patient had a long history of alcoholic dependency, with frequent episodes of epigastric distress. After drainage of the cyst under ultrasonic guidance, the patient made a complete recovery.

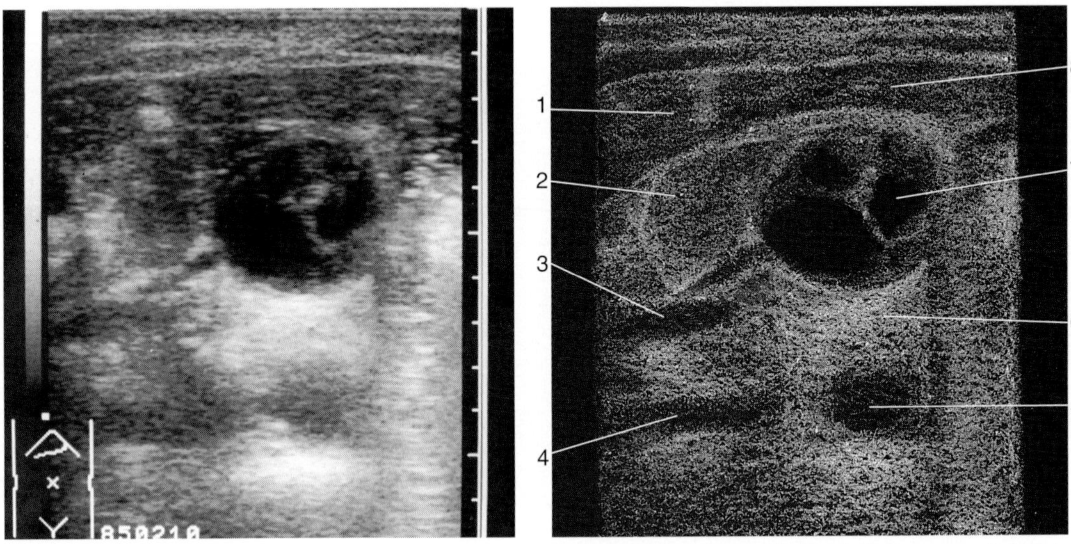

1. Ligamentum teres 2. Head of pancreas 3. Inferior vena cava 4. Right renal artery 5. Aorta 6. Acoustic enhancement 7. Pseudocyst 8. Left lobe of liver

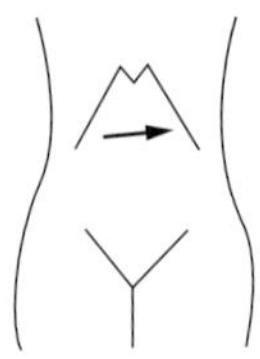

Figure 5-17. Pancreatic pseudocyst.
A round, well-demarcated cystic mass of the body of the pancreas was demonstrated on both transverse and sagittal scans. Some strand-like structures and debritic echoes were found in the cystic mass, however, no solid mass could be seen. Surgical drainage and extirpation of the rest of the organ was performed. Histopathological examination confirmed the diagnosis of pancreatic pseudocyst.

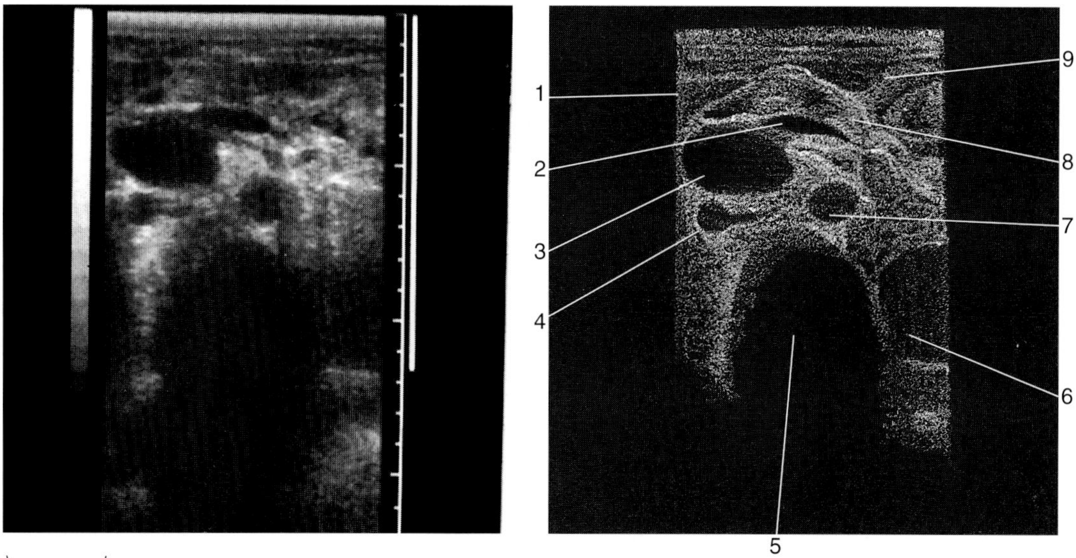

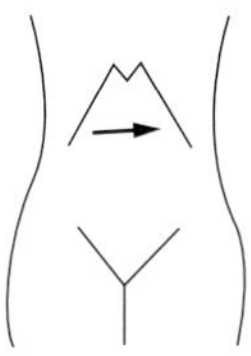

1. Right lobe of liver 2. Splenic vein 3. Pseudocyst 4. Inferior vena cava 5. Vertebra 6. Left kidney 7. Aorta 8. Body of pancreas 9. Stomach

Figure 5-18. Pancreatic pseudocyst (head).
As a sequela of acute inflammation of the pancreas, pseudocysts may form at various sites in and around the pancreas. This patient, with a long history of alcohol abuse, had a small pseudocyst in the head and body of the pancreas. The contour of the pseudocyst was smooth, and no solid mass was found in the vicinity of the cystic changes.

TUMORS

Benign tumors

Benign tumors of the pancreas are rare, apart from the masses encountered in localized chronic pancreatitis. Among them are simple adenomas or cystadenomas together with a number of rare endocrine pancreatic tumors (insulinoma, VIPoma, glucagonoma). [15, 21, 25, 35, 41, 46, 51, 65, 68, 89, 91] With the exception of cystadenoma, these tumors cannot be differentiated by sonography alone. [15, 68]

Cystadenoma of the pancreas, which occurs at any location within the organ, is found in two forms. One is the multilocular type, characterized by multiple small, cystic spaces that produce an intensely echogenic pattern (Figure 5-19). The other, the macrocystic type, has larger cysts (Figure 5-20), and is difficult to differentiate from malignant cystadenocarcinoma, except for the larger size of the malignant lesion.[9, 10]

Endocrine tumors, except benign beta-cell adenomas, and insulinomas, are usually malignant, despite retention of their endocrine function. Sonographically, all are solid lesions indistinguishable from each other, differentiated only by their specific endocrine functions (Figure 5-21). Insulinomas are characterized clinically by acute hypoglycemic attacks which cause sudden disturbances of consciousness, often mistaken for psychiatric disorders. The tumor, a small, encapsulated, round lesion of identical in echogenicity to normal pancreatic parenchyma, is frequently found in the tail or body portion of the organ. [35, 41, 46, 68] It may not show a discrete pattern on conventional ultrasound. Confirmatory evidence is obtained only after assay of immunoreactive insulin in plasma or portal blood sampled during portal vein cannulation.

The endosonographic approach, using a 7.5-MHz transducer via the gastric wall, may succeed in showing a poorly marginated, round tumor mass in the pancreas (Figure 5-22). Confirmation that the lesion is benign is difficult when it is small. Careful follow-up observation and biochemical assessment of its function are needed. If the diagnosis is difficult to establish, ultrasound-guided aspiration cytology or biopsy with a Tru-Cut needle will help to achieve a final diagnosis.

Benign nonfunctioning islet cell tumors also occur (Figure 5-23). Usually the diagnosis is established only by histology and the appearance is indistinguishable from those of insulinomas.

Malignant tumors

Pancreatic carcinoma

The most common pancreatic malignancy is adenocarcinoma, which arises from the exocrine glandular tissue of the organ. It occurs more frequently in the head or body than in the tail of the pancreas. In general, pancreatic carcinoma spreads by local infiltration through and beyond the pancreas; seeding of tumor cells via the main pancreatic duct also occurs. Metastasis to adjacent organs is frequent, and widespread dissemination may take place via the lymphatics or by direct spread to the peritoneal surface to produce carcinomatous peritonitis. The multitude of metastasis and the relative paucity of symptoms or signs of early disease make it extremely difficult to diagnose pancreatic carcinoma at a stage when radical resection can be performed, unless it is complicated by obvious symptoms such as sudden onset of jaundice or rapid emaciation.[3, 9, 12, 22, 62, 64]

The most conspicuous sonographic features of pancreatic carcinoma are a hypoechoic, localized mass with an irregular boundary in the pancreas, often with secondary effects such as compression or obstruction of the ductal systems draining the pancreatic parenchyma, causing dilatation of the pancreatic or common bile ducts [22, 48, 62, 71, 75, 77, 86] (Table 5-2, Figures 5-24 to 5-28). Similar effects may be observed in major blood vessels if the tumor infiltrates into the peripancreatic tissues, distorting or invading adjacent vessels (Figures 5-29 to 5-32). Vessel invasion, however, is often difficult to identify precisely because of the variable and complex arrangement of the tissues around the pancreas. Furthermore, side lobe artifacts produced by intestinal gas or peripancreatic fat may cause blurring of the sonographic images. Peripancreatic lymph node metastasis may occur as solitary or multiple conglomerated masses in the vicinity of the pancreas or remote from it.

The internal reflectivity of pancreatic tumors varies, depending on the size of the tumor and its tissue composition, such as the degree of necrosis, hemorrhage, and connective tissue reaction (Figure 5-33).[22, 86, 90] The histological type of pancreatic carcinoma may also be responsible for some variations in sonographic characteristics, (e.g., adenocarcinoma as a more or less poorly marginated, hypoechoic tumor mass, cystadenocarcinoma, showing the most heterogeneous texture of mixed pattern arrangement). The degrees of cystic change within the tumor mass greatly influences its sonographic appearance.

Carcinoma of the ampulla of Vater is often difficult to assess because of its small size and location close to the duodenum; frequently, the pronounced ductal dilatation of the main pancreatic duct or choledochus is the sole finding. Malignant insulinoma, on the other hand, may reach a considerable size, and is seen as an uniformly isoechoic mass with a rounded appearance. Other tumors are difficult to distinguish by their sonographic appearances alone.

The detectability of malignant tumors also varies greatly, depending on the size, location, and nature of the lesion and on factors such as the obesity of the patient and the amount of gas in the stomach and intestine. Tumors at the head of the pancreas are discovered earliest because they usually obstruct the common bile duct, causing jaundice (Figures 5-34 and 5-35). Other signs such as rapid weight loss, piercing or persistent dull back pain, anorexia, and raised serum amylase may arouse suspicion.

By contrast, carcinoma of the tail or body of the pancreas is usually not detected until late in its course because of the lack of characteristic signs (Figure 5-36). Even an ultrasound examination may fail to demonstrate the lesion because of interference by gas in the stomach or colon.

The sonographic differentiation of malignant neoplasms from benign inflammatory masses is the subject of ongoing controversy. Though a differential diagnosis is sometimes possible, in most cases it is difficult, especially in cases with extensive fibrosis in the pancreatic parenchyma. Certain sonographic signs such as the "penetrating duct sign", are claimed to be useful but are by no means infallible.

Table 5-2. Echo pattern characteristics of pancreatic mass.

The Solid Mass Legion

Tumors	Boundary	Echo texture	Pancreatic duct
Pancreatic carcinoma*	Indistinct boundary smooth to irregular	Echo-poor with internal echo spots	Dilatation smooth in rosary shape
Islet cell carcinoma	Smooth and distinct border	Iso- to hypoechoic mixed pattern in large mass	No duct invasion
Tumor-forming pancreatitis	Less distinct	Iso- to slightly hypoechoic	Partial obstruction, if present

* Invasion to biliary tract, pancreatic duct and surrounding vessels are characteristic features in advanced stage of carcinoma not present in other two conditions. 2-D color flow imaging is useful delineating tumor invasion to vessels.

The Cystic Mass Lesion

Tumors	Boundary	Echo pattern characteristics	Pancreatic duct
Mucinous cystadenoma or adenoca*	Smooth and distinct	Multicystic and variable in size Thick cyst wall with solid masses	No dilatation
Branch type MPT**	Smooth and sharp	Multicystic small to moderate size with thin cystic wall	Mostly marked dilatation
Pseudocyst***	Smooth and sharp	Single cyst with internal debris or strand structure of variable size	Slight to marked with stones

*Serous cystadenoma or adenocarcinoma more or less appears as solid mass lesions with echo-poor or hyperechoic patterns.

**Mucin-producing tumor.

***Pseudocyst formation is one of the sequelae of chronic relapsing pancreatitis, and is often accompanied changes compatible with chronic inflammation of the pancreas.

Not infrequently solid tumors undergo necrotic changes producing central liquefaction. However, it is generally accompnied by thick mass lesion surrounding cystic changes.

(Adapted from Jpn J Med Ultrasonics 19 : 556-557, 1992.)

Ultrasonic pattern recognition

The sonographic characteristics of pancreatic cancer have been extensively described by a number of investigators. The difficulty is that ultrasonic visualization of the pancreas as a whole is not easy if the patient is heavily built or gassy. The sonographic features of pancreatic carcinoma (summarized in Table 5-2) should be evaluated carefully when malignancy is suspected.

The normal pancreas has a smooth outline, whereas a carcinoma produces distortion with a bulge of part of the pancreas. This may be inapparent with lesions in the head of the pancreas. By contrast, tumors in the body or tail show this sign even when relatively small (less than 2 cm in diameter). This sign, however, should be carefully confirmed by scanning in at least two planes to avoid misinterpretation of apparent contour changes not due to the pancreas.

The overall echogenicity of the normal pancreatic parenchyma varies considerably according to the extent of fat deposition, so that internal comparison of the reflectivity on a regional basis is necessary. Careful scanning may reveal an anechoic or hypoechoic area with an irregular boundary, the hallmark of a pancreatic tumor (Figure 5-37). It is important, therefore, to visualize the whole parenchyma to ensure that a lesion is not obscured by shadowing due to intestinal gas. The importance of this procedure is strongly supported by the success of endoscopic sonography, which achieves high diagnostic accuracy in diagnosing cancer of the pancreas because of clearer images without distortion by intervening gas or tissues.

Besides the echogenicity of the parenchyma, ultrasound attenuation by the pancreatic mass is often helpful in detecting malignant changes. In the relatively uncommon situation when the tumor tissue is heavily fibrosed (scirrhous carcinoma), attenuation is high and produces posterior shadowing (Figure 5-37). In most cases, attenuation is minimal and enhancement of posterior echoes may be observed (Figure 5-38).

The distribution of fine echo spots throughout the parenchyma is also a reliable index of the normalcy of the pancreas. Especially in large pancreatic malignancies, the internal echo distribution is very irregular. A nonuniform distribution of coarse echoes is a characteristic finding together with a central hypoechoic pattern suggesting liquefaction of the tumor parenchyma due to autolysis, bleeding, or necrosis. Beside the presence of the tumor mass in the pancreatic parenchyma, it is important to check the peripancreatic lymph nodes carefully for metastasis.

Diagnostic pitfalls in primary pancreatic carcinoma

Pancreatic carcinoma carries a grave prognosis. The only hope of improving survival lies in the detection and diagnosis of the tumors at a resectable stage; ultrasound is the best hope in this quest, other modalities having proved disappointing.[64, 79, 80, 82] However, difficult diagnostic problems still exist, such as the paucity of symptoms and signs in pancreatic carcinoma and the absence of clear-cut diagnostic criteria for differentiating carcinoma from chronic mass-forming inflammation of the pancreas, in which the swelling may reach a considerable size. The mass often has a very similar sonographic appearance to an advanced pancreatic carcinoma, (i.e., an echo-poor mass with biliary obstruction). These diagnostic difficulties were demonstrated by studies of diagnostic accuracy on ROC

(Receiver Operating Characteristics) studies in Japan.[23] This multicenter study, which attempted to evaluate the image-reading accuracy of ultrasound and x-ray CT scans on a number of organs, revealed that the sensitivity of real-time ultrasound in assessing pancreatic tumors was consistently high. By contrast, it was rather low in differentiating nonmalignant, chronic focal pancreatitis from carcinoma; this was also true of x-ray CT.

Another cause of diagnostic failure is the complex structure of pancreatic malignancies. Metastatic carcinoma of the pancreas, even though it is rare, must be distinguished from primary cancer of the pancreas. Lymph node metastasis to the retropancreatic region can simulate the changes of carcinoma of the pancreatic head. The anatomical complexity of the pancreas poses still other problems, such as misinterpretation of the duodenojejunal flexure located high in the postpancreatic region as a cystic mass, or a low-lying elongation of the caudate lobe of the liver as a solid mass. Though these problems sometimes occur with real-time equipment, they are mostly avoidable if the fluid-filled stomach method is employed (see Figure 8-5). In addition, the pancreas is traversed by large vessels, which sometimes contain tumor thrombi originating from hepatocellular or renal carcinoma (Figure 5-39). Malignant left renal or adrenal tumors may sometimes simulate pancreatic carcinoma. Further complicating the situation is the fact that metastasis to the pancreas from tumors of other organs can occur, simulating a primary pancreatic carcinoma (Figures 5-40 to 5-42).

In these difficult cases, the combined use of other imaging modalities including endoscopic ultrasound and dynamic CT plus organ biopsy is mandatory to avoid serious diagnostic errors.

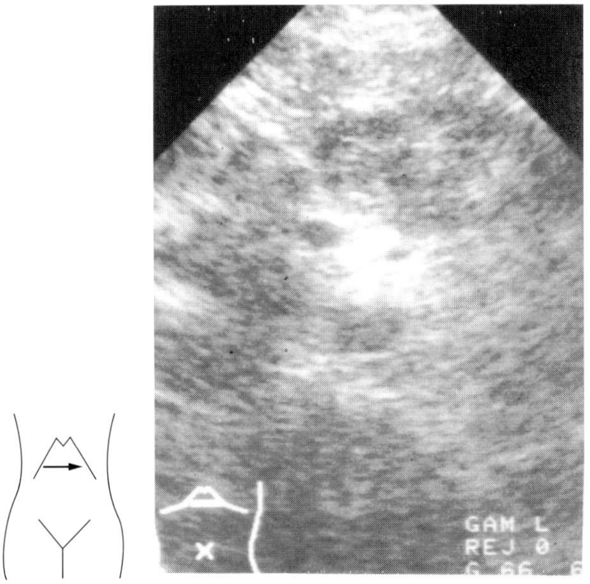

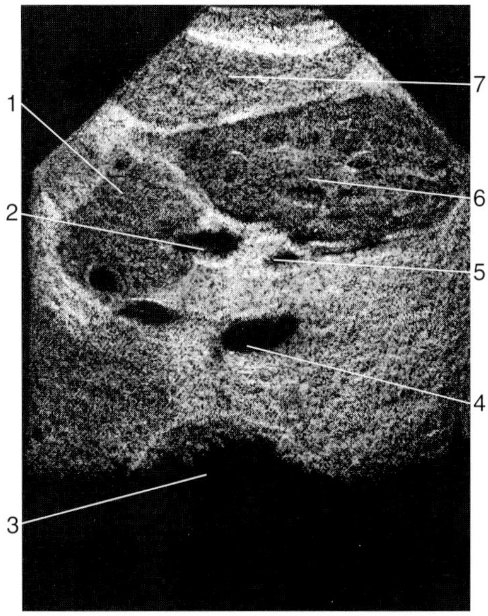

1. Head of pancreas 2. Superior mesenteric vein 3. Vertebra 4. Aorta 5. Superior mesenteric artery 6. Cystadenoma 7. Left lobe of liver

Figure 5-19. Cystadenoma of the pancreas.
Cystadenoma of the pancreas, a rare benign tumor, shows two distinct echo patterns related to the histopathological findings. An echo-poor mass is typical of the macrocystic type and an echogenic mass of the microcystic type. This sonogram demonstrated an oval-shaped echo-poor mass 2 cm in diameter in the body of the pancreas. The texture pattern suggested nesting of multiple small cysts, and acoustic enhancement was found distal to the mass. Histological examination of the excised mass revealed a macrocystic serous cystadenoma without malignant transformation. (Courtesy of Dr. Matsui, Kanazawa University Medical School)

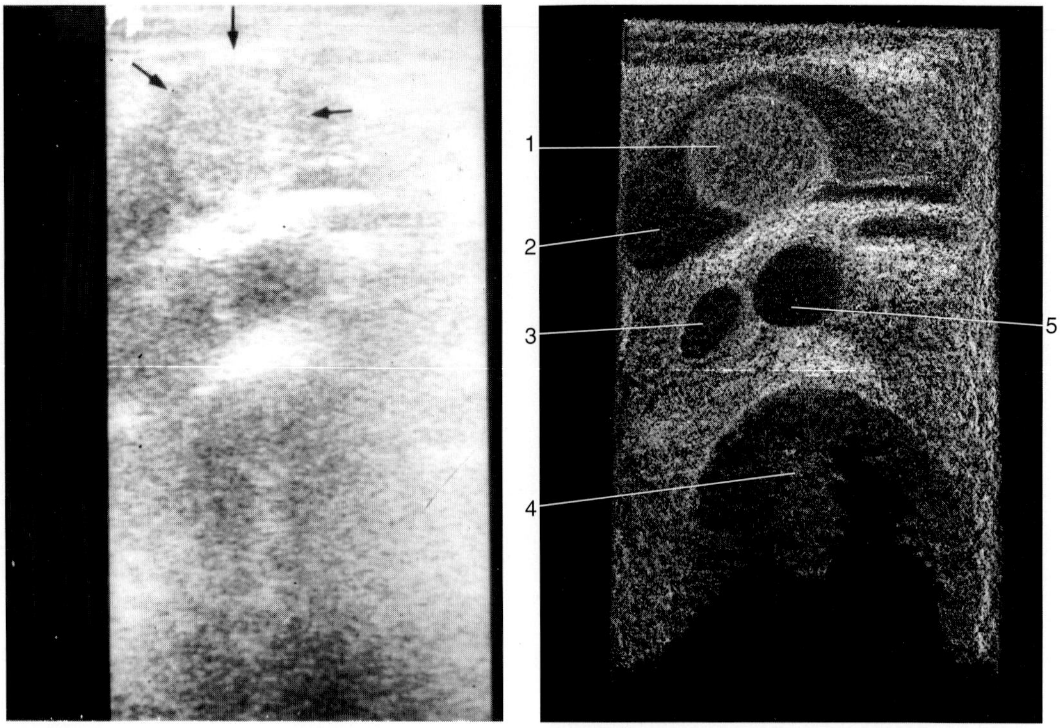

1. Cystadenoma (echogenic type) 2. Pancreas
3. Inferior vena cava 4. Vertebra 5. Aorta

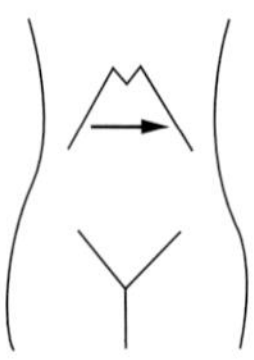

Figure 5-20. Cystadenoma of the pancreas, echogenic type.
A transverse sonogram of the pancreatic body disclosed a round, well-circumscribed tumor mass with increased echogenicity. In spite of its size (over 2 cm in diameter), no signs of compression of the surrounding tissues were observed and the posterior echo enhancement is rather weak. The histopathological diagnosis of the resected mass was microcystic cystadenoma of the pancreas. (Courtesy of Dr. Matsui, Kanazawa University Medical School)

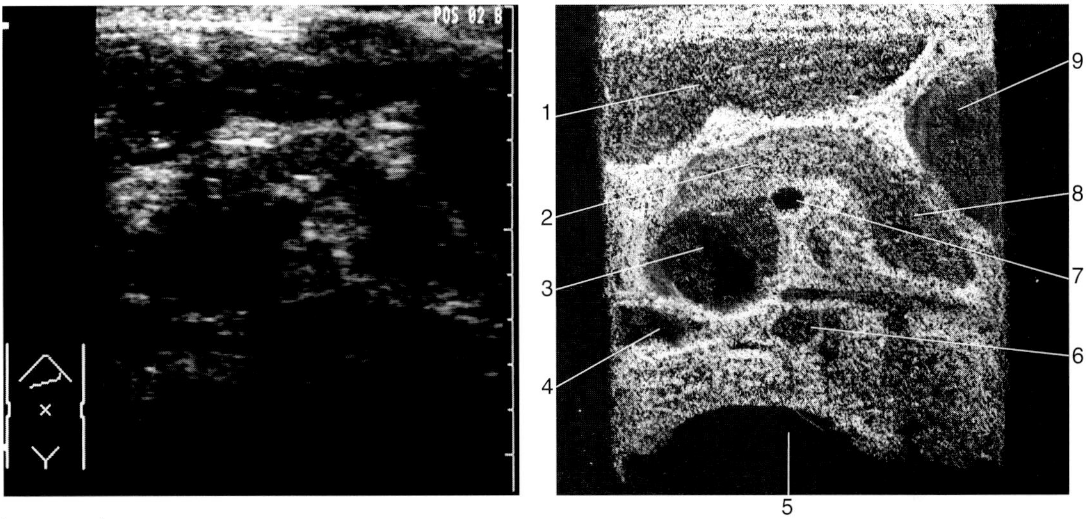

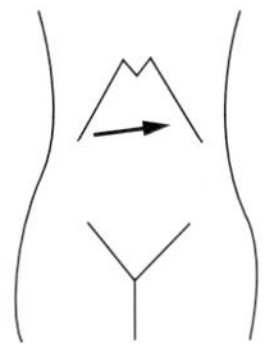

1. Left lobe of liver 2. Body of pancreas 3. VIPoma 4. Inferior vena cava 5. Vertebra 6. Aorta 7. Superior mesenteric artery 8. Tail of pancreas 9. Stomach

Figure 5-21. Endocrine pancreatic tumor, VIPoma.
A medium-sized, hypoechoic mass was demonstrated on a transverse scan of the head of the pancreas. In spite of the size of the mass, which showed features of pancreatic malignancy, neither invasion nor metastases to the regional lymph node were observed. After treatment with an antihormone agent, the tumor decreased in size and the mass was removed by surgery.

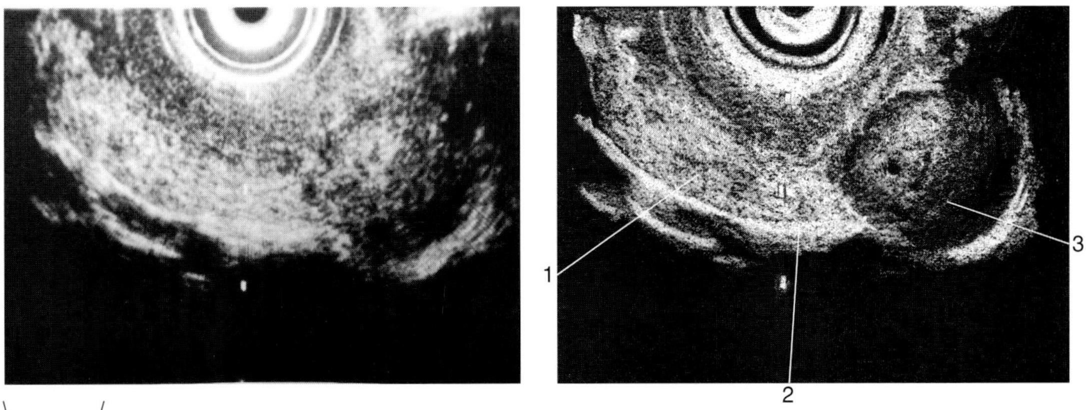

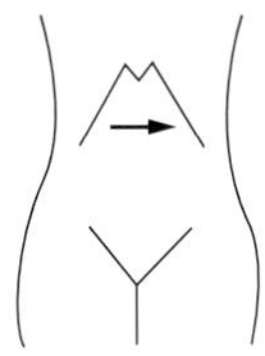

1. Body of pancreas 2. Tail of pancreas 3. Insulinoma

Figure 5-22. Beta-cell insulinoma of the pancreas.
Insulinoma, is a rather common endocrine pancreatic tumor, is characterized clinically by recurrent episodes of hypoglycemia. Due to their small size and isoechogenicity, these tumors are often difficult to identify by ordinary sonography. This tumor was also confirmed on endoscopic sonography and was surgically resected following portal vein sampling which demonstrated increased levels of immunoreactive insulin in the blood.

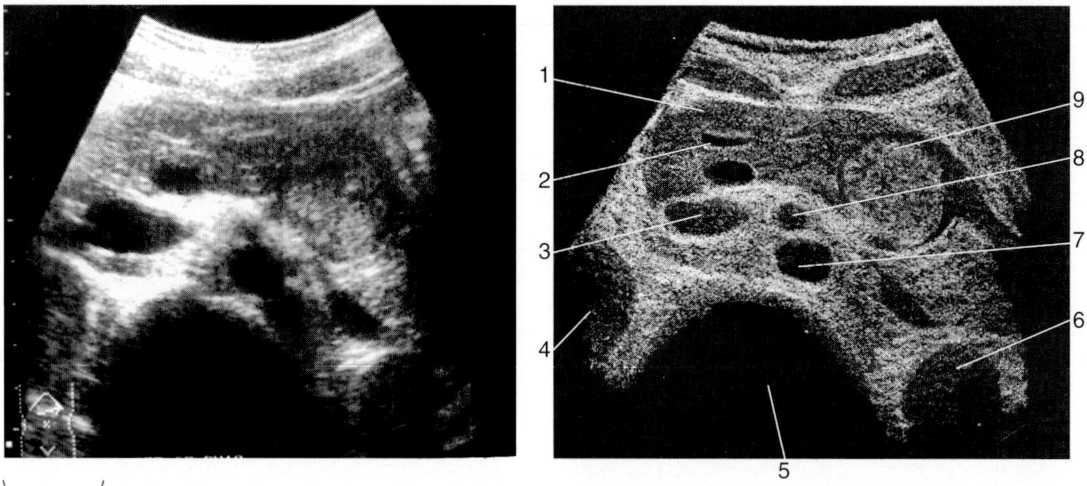

1. Body of pancreas 2. Pancreatic duct 3. Inferior vena cava 4. Right kidney 5. Vertebral body 6. Left kidney 7. Aorta 8. Superior mesenteric artery 9. Islet adenoma

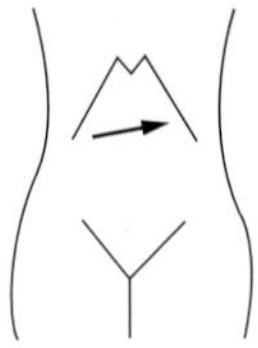

Figure 5-23. Nonfunctioning islet cell tumor.
A medium-sized, round tumor was identified at the body-tail junction of the pancreas. It was diagnosed accidentally during a routine ultrasound survey. The isoechoic mass was diagnosed as a benign, nonfunctional islet cell tumor by ultrasound-guided biopsy and confirmed after surgical resection.

a

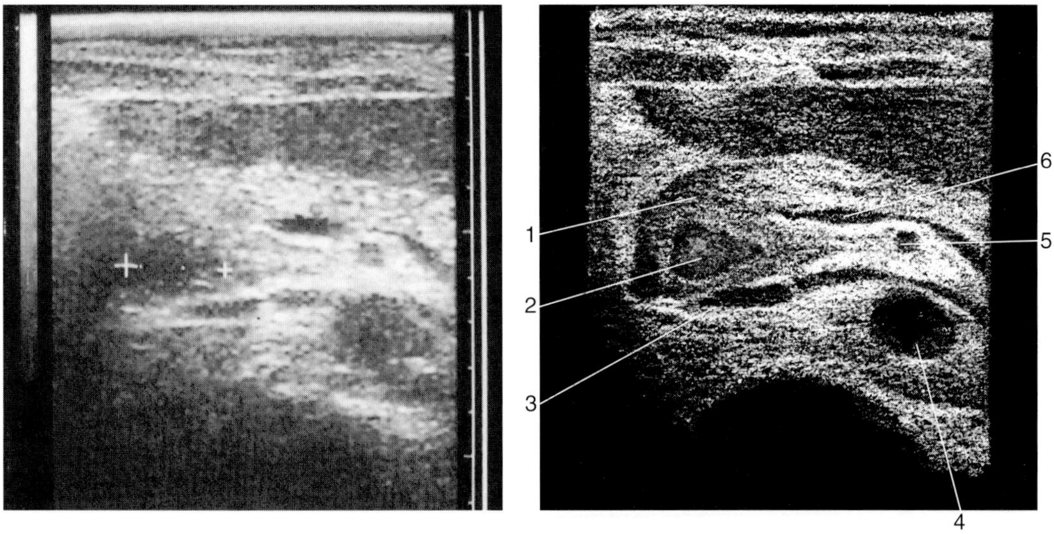

1. Head of pancreas 2. Small hypoechoic mass 3. Inferior vena cava 4. Aorta 5. Superior mesenteric artery 6. Splenic vein

b

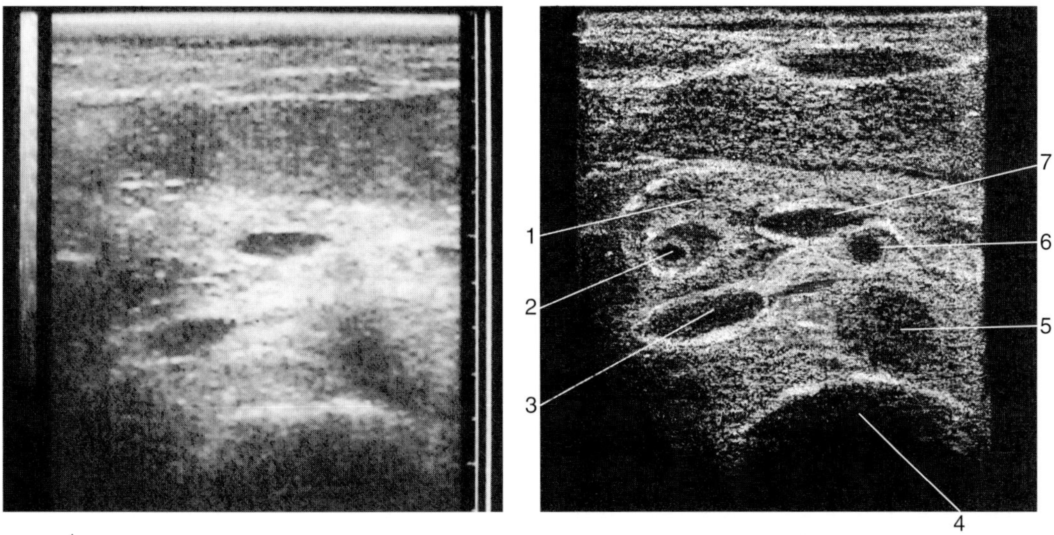

1. Pancreas 2. Hypoechoic mass with dilated common bile duct 3. Inferior vena cava 4. Vertebra 5. Aorta 6. Superior mesenteric artery 7. Splenic vein

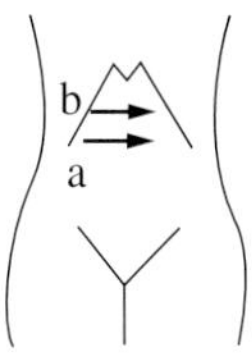

Figure 5-24. Small pancreatic carcinoma.
This patient presented with mild jaundice and emaciation, with no abdominal pain. The sonographic study demonstrated a round echo-poor mass at the lower portion of the head of the pancreas. Although the common bile duct was dilated, stenosis of the pancreatic duct was minimal. Surgery revealed a small adenocarcinoma at the head of the pancreas.

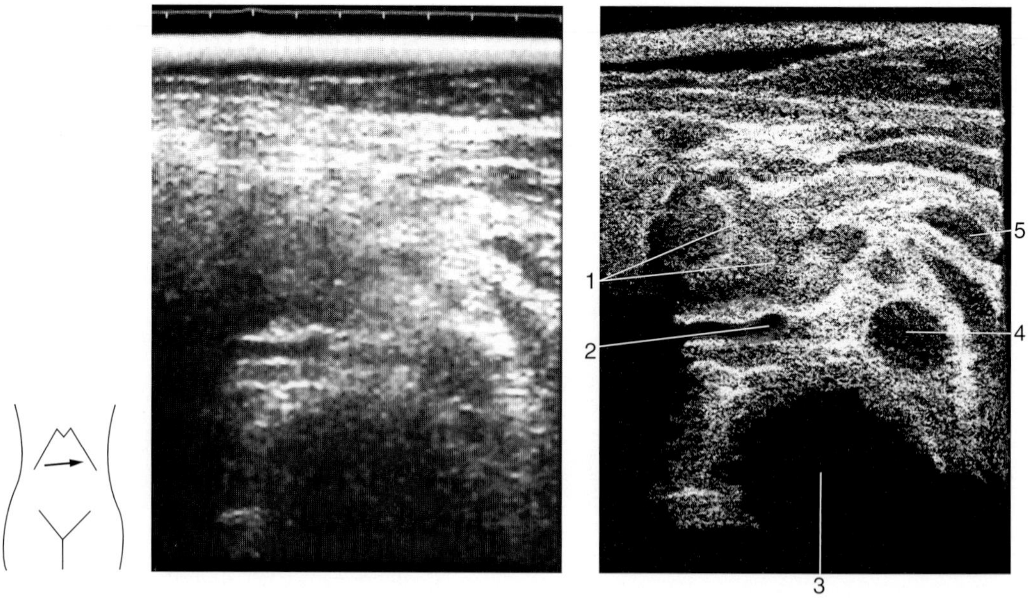

1. Tumor 2. Inferior vena cava 3. Vertebra 4. Aorta 5. Pancreatic duct

Figure 5-25. Carcinoma of the pancreas, head.
This figure shows the typical appearance of pancreatic carcinoma: a hypoechoic mass with an irregular boundary. Although the internal reflection is low, the texture is quite heterogeneous. Dilatation of the main pancreatic duct is demonstrated.

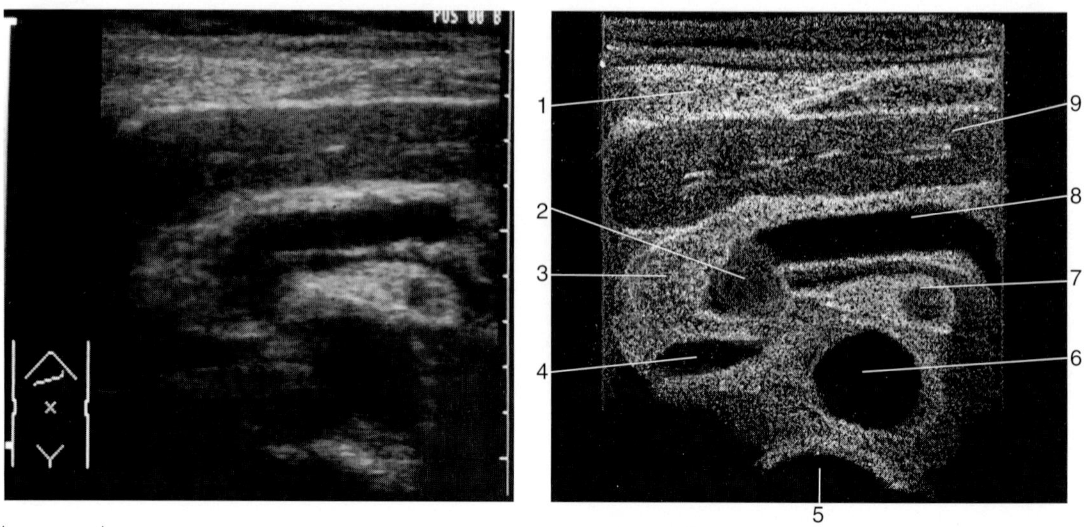

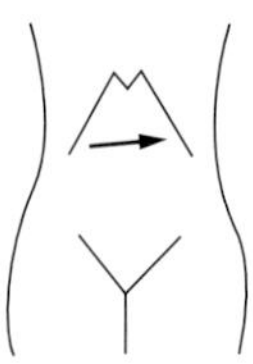

1. Rectus abdominis muscle 2. Tumor 3. Head of pancreas 4. Inferior vena cava 5. Vertebra 6. Aorta 7. Superior mesenteric artery 8. Pancreatic duct 9. Left lobe of liver

Figure 5-26. Marked dilatation of the main pancreatic duct caused by carcinoma of the head of the pancreas.
Although a dilated pancreatic duct is visualized, often no mass is apparent in the sonogram of pancreatic head carcinoma. In this case, a small, echo-poor mass was demonstrated at the head of the pancreas.

a

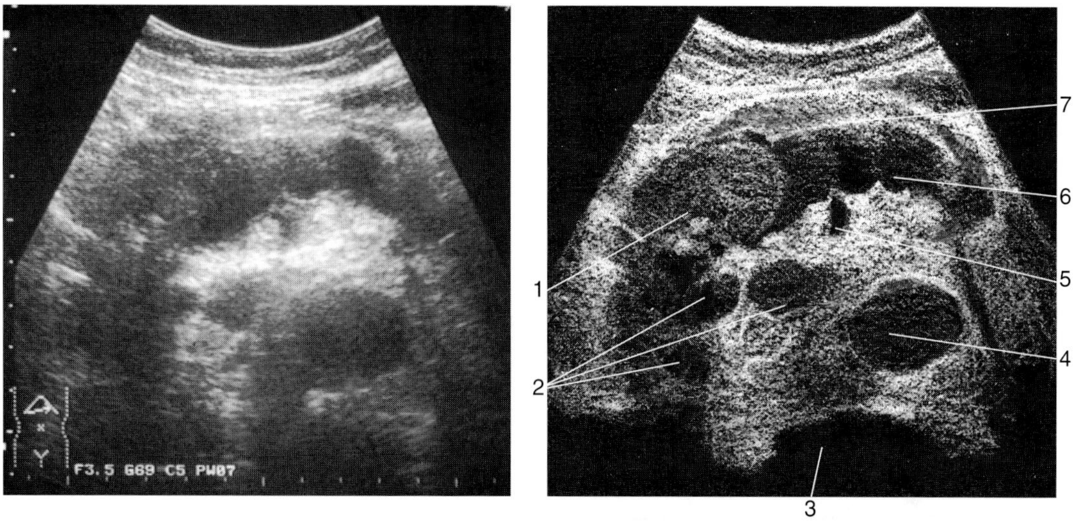

1. Tumor 2. Lymph nodes 3. Vertebra 4. Aorta 5. Superior mesenteric artery 6. Dilated main pancreatic duct 7. Pancreas

b

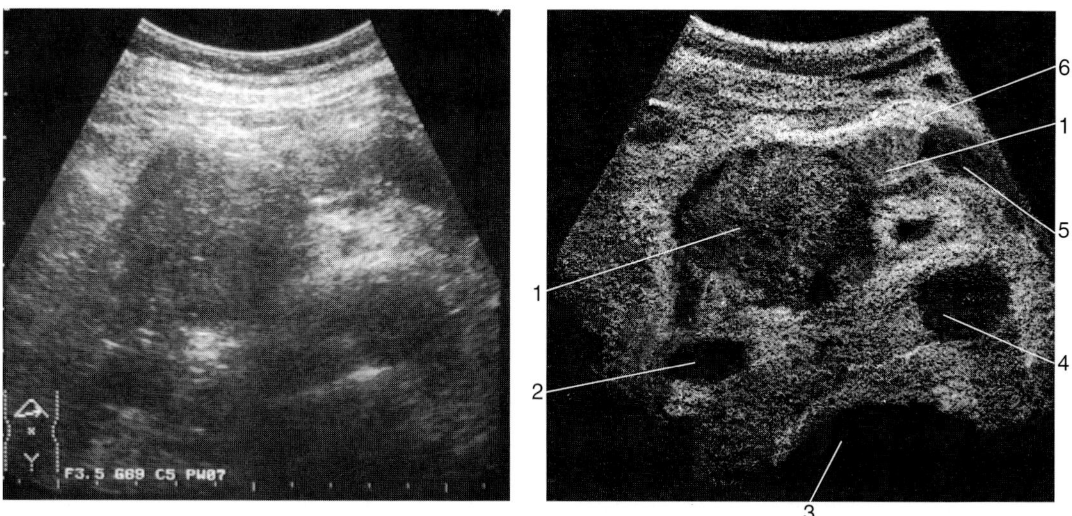

1. Tumor 2. Inferior vena cava 3. Vertebra 4. Aorta 5. Dilated pancreatic duct 6. Pancreas

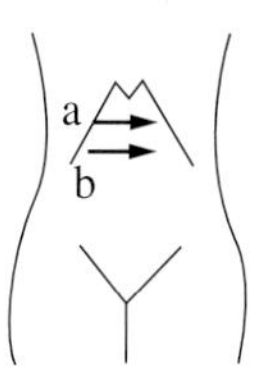

Figure 5-27. Large carcinoma of the head of the pancreas with extensive dilatation of the main pancreatic duct.

(a) Extensive dilated pancreatic duct caused by a pancreatic head cancer. An approximately 4×4 cm hypoechoic mass is demostrated in (b). The patient also had severe obstructive jaundice.

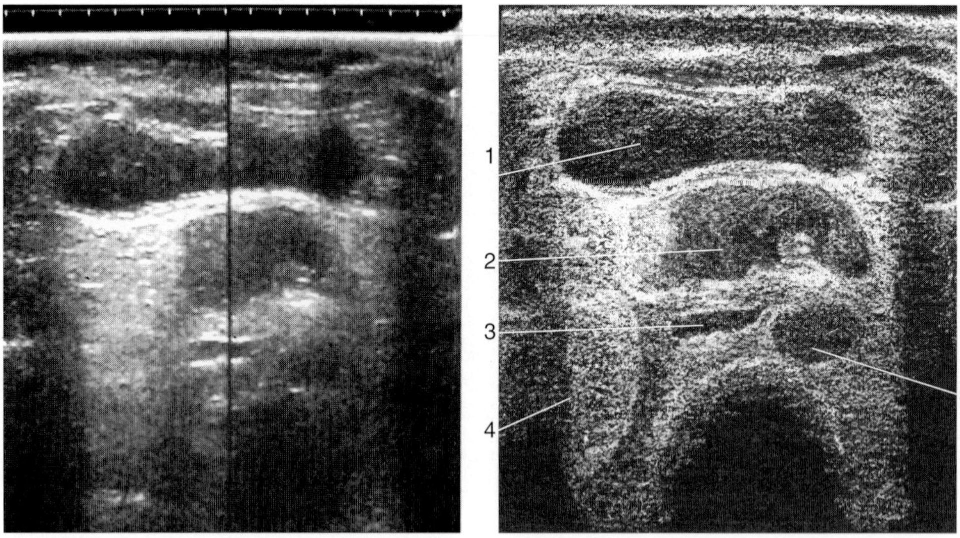

1. Stomach 2. Tumor 3. Inferior vena cava
4. Right kidney 5. Aorta

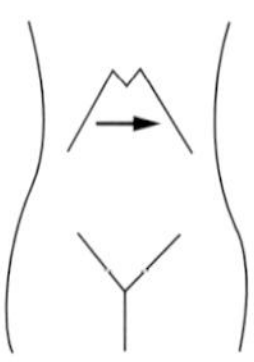

Figure 5-28. Carcinoma of the pancreas, body.
In this 54-year-old female with no significant symptoms except a vague oppressive feeling in the epigastrium, transverse scanning of the pancreas through the fluid-filled stomach revealed a large, hypoechoic mass extending from the neck to the body-tail junction of the pancreas. The contour of the mass was irregular and without attenuation. Dilatation of the main pancreatic duct was also observed.

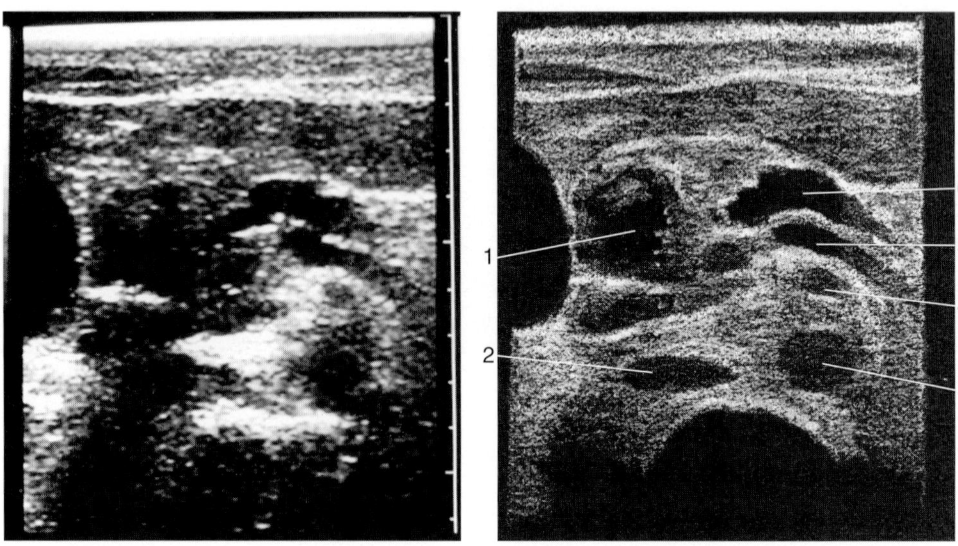

1. Mass 2. Inferior vena cava 3. Aorta
4. Superior mesenteric artery 5. Splenic vein
6. Dilated pancreatic duct

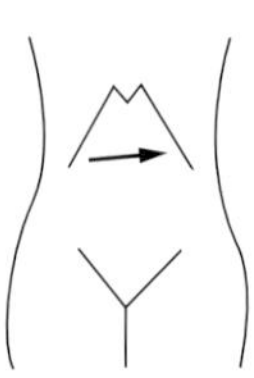

Figure 5-29. Carcinoma of the pancreas, head.
A 49-year-old male with marked jaundice and emaciation was referred for examination. A large, echo-poor mass with irregular boundaries was demonstrated in the pancreatic head together with dilatation of the main pancreatic duct and the biliary system. Extensive infiltration of the tumor mass ruled out the possibility of radical surgery.

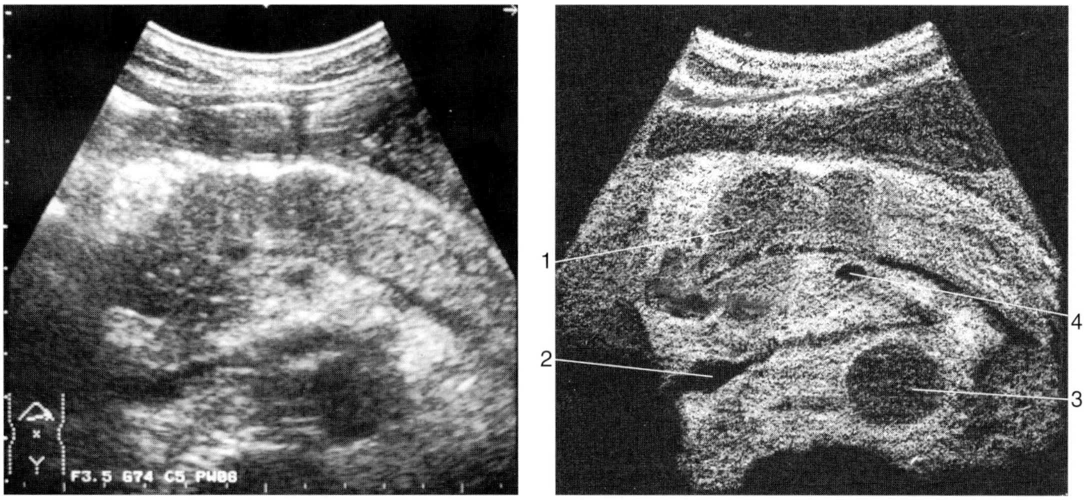

1. Cancer of pancreas 2. Inferior vena cava
3. Aorta 4. Superior mesenteric artery

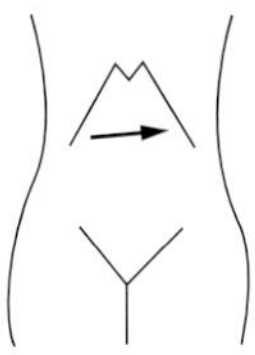

Figure 5-30. Carcinoma of the pancreatic head and body.
Carcinoma of the pancreas does not necessarily form a discrete mass. This patient was referred because of jaundice and emaciation within of relatively short duration. Sonographic examination revealed only slight swelling of the pancreatic head and body. However, there was dilatation of the extrahepatic biliary tract, changes in the parenchymal echo pattern, a hypoechoic texture with irregular distribution of echogenic foci, and gross changes in the organ contour confined to the part of the pancreas.
The dilatation of the main pancreatic duct was minimal. At exploratory laparotomy, an unresectable, diffusely infiltrating carcinoma was found occupying the head and body of the pancreas together with severe biliary tree obstruction by the carcinoma.

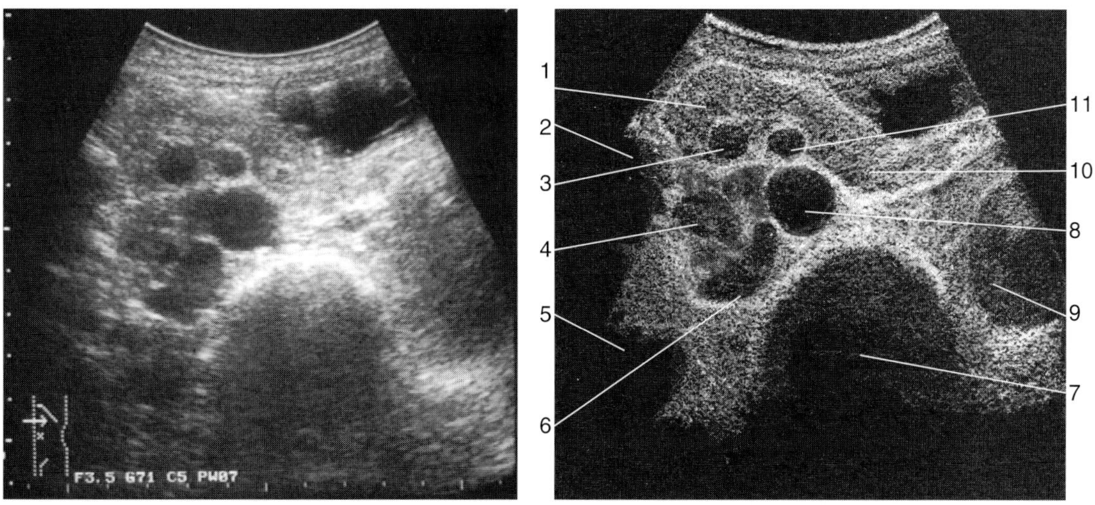

1. Head of pancreas 2. Gas in duodenum 3. Superior mesenteric vein 4. Cancer of pancreas
5. Right kidney 6. Inferior vena cava 7. Vertebra
8. Aorta 9. Left kidney 10. Tail of pancreas
11. Superior mesenteric artery

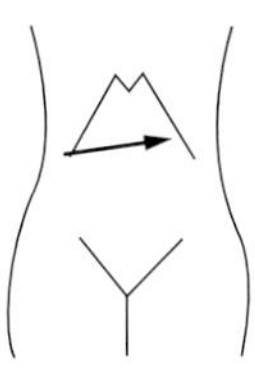

Figure 5-31. Small pancreatic head carcinoma invading vessels and bile duct.
Transverse scanning across the lower end of the pancreatic head disclosed a relatively hypoechoic tumor mass invading the inferior vena cava and common duct. The remainder of the examination was entirely normal, except for mild common duct dilatation.

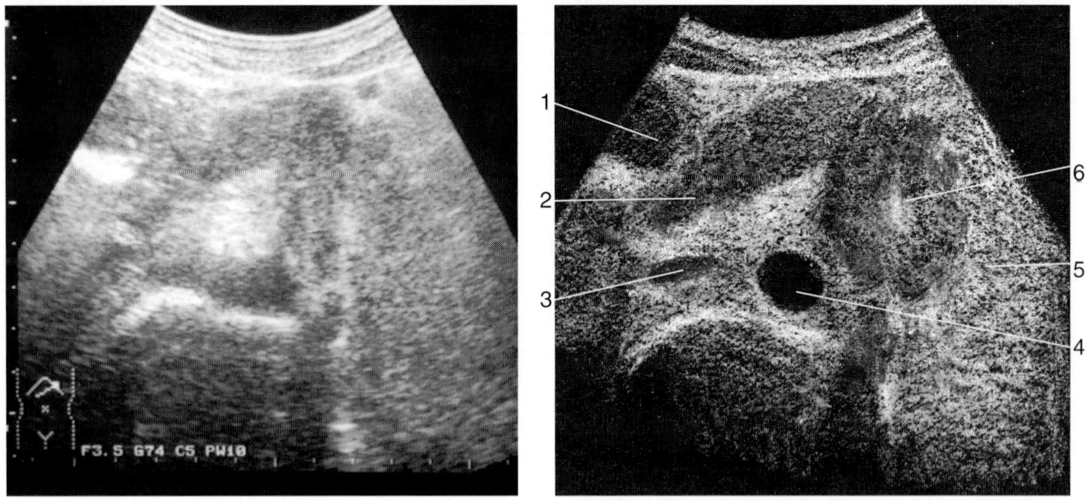

a

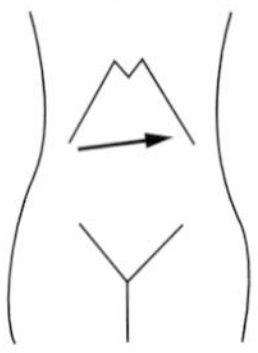

1. Gallbladder 2. Head of pancreas 3. Inferior vena cava 4. Aorta 5. Gas 6. Cancer of body and tail of pancreas

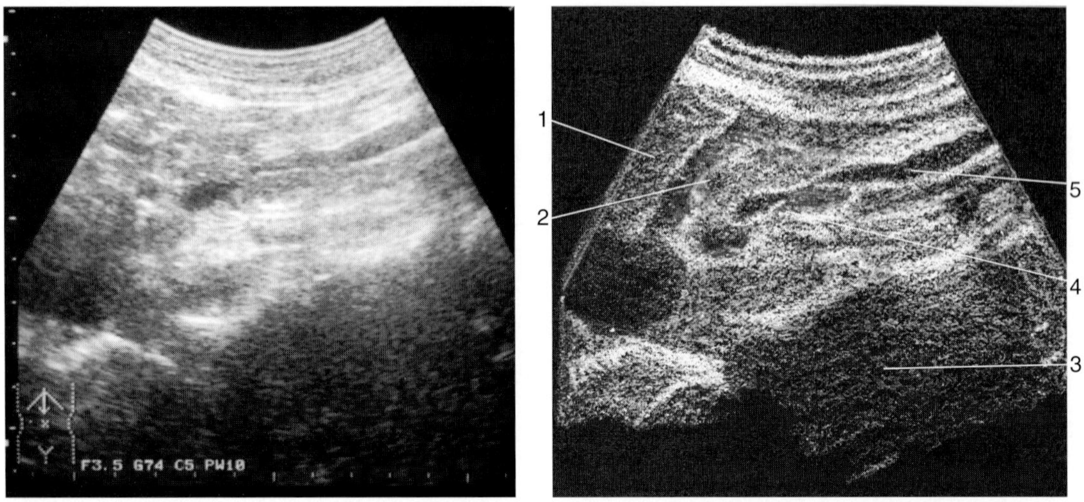

b

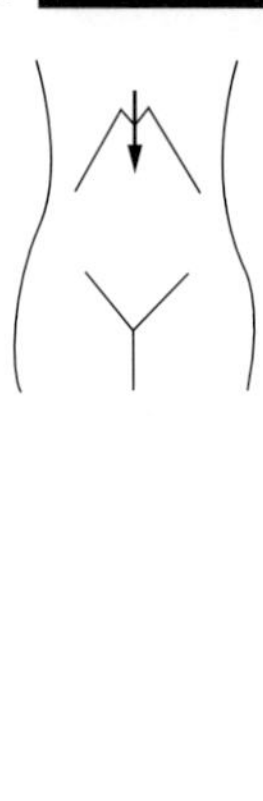

1. Liver 2. Body of pancreas 3. Vertebrae 4. Compression by tumor 5. Superior mesenteric vein

Figure 5-32. Advanced carcinoma of the pancreatic body causing stagnation of flow in the superior mesenteric vein.
A transverse sonogram revealed diffuse swelling of the pancreatic body suggestive of malignancy. The parenchymal echogenicity was normal, but constriction of the superior mesenteric vein by infiltrating carcinoma was apparent on the sagittal scan. Angiography and Doppler analysis clearly demonstrated the abnormality to be a carcinoma.

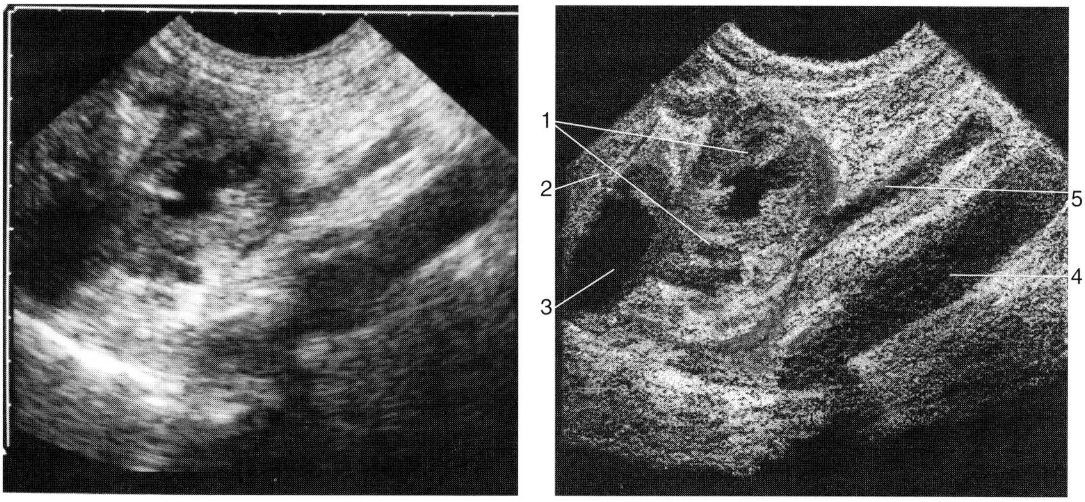

1. Tumor 2. Left lobe of liver 3. Ascites 4. Aorta 5. Superior mesenteric artery

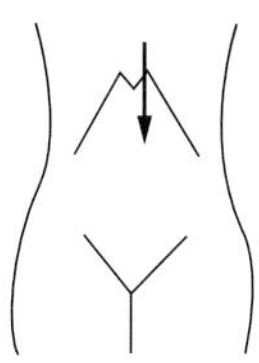

Figure 5-33. Large carcinoma of the body of the pancreas.
A sagittal sector scanning clearly demonstrated a well-demarcated, partially necrotic, large tumor mass in the body of the pancreas. The main tumor apparently compressed the superior mesenteric artery.

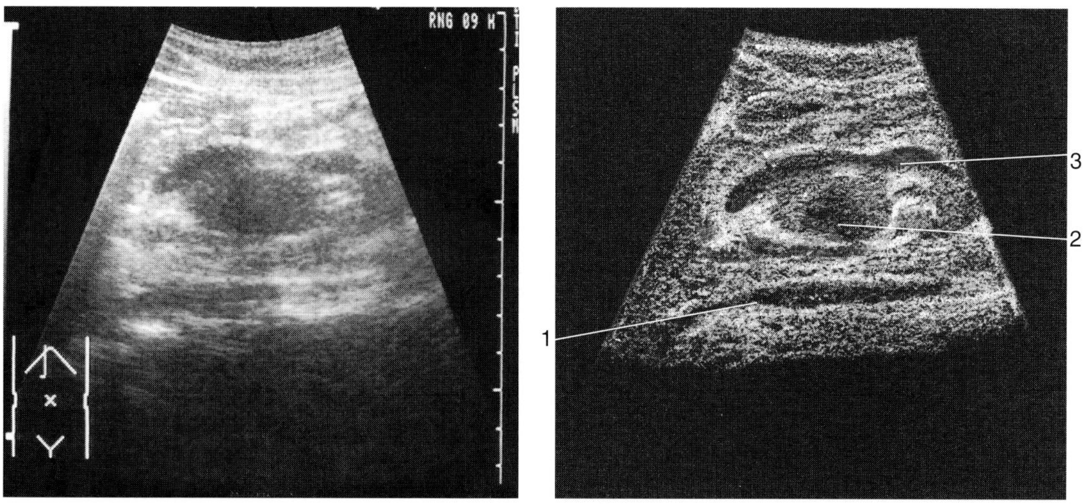

1. Inferior vena cava 2. Tumor 3. Superior mesenteric vein

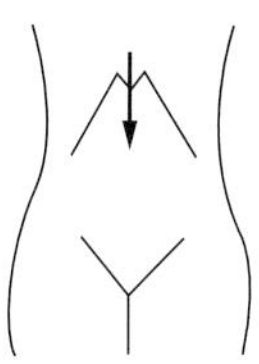

Figure 5-34. Carcinoma of the pancreas, uncinate process.
A malignant tumor located at the uncinate process is often difficult to diagnose because of the paucity of symptoms. A 2×3.5 cm hypoechoic mass with an irregular border was found in the uncinate portion of the pancreas in this 37-years-old male, who presented with mild weight loss but no signs of hepatic dysfunction. Invasion of the superior mesenteric vein was found together with local lymph node metastases.

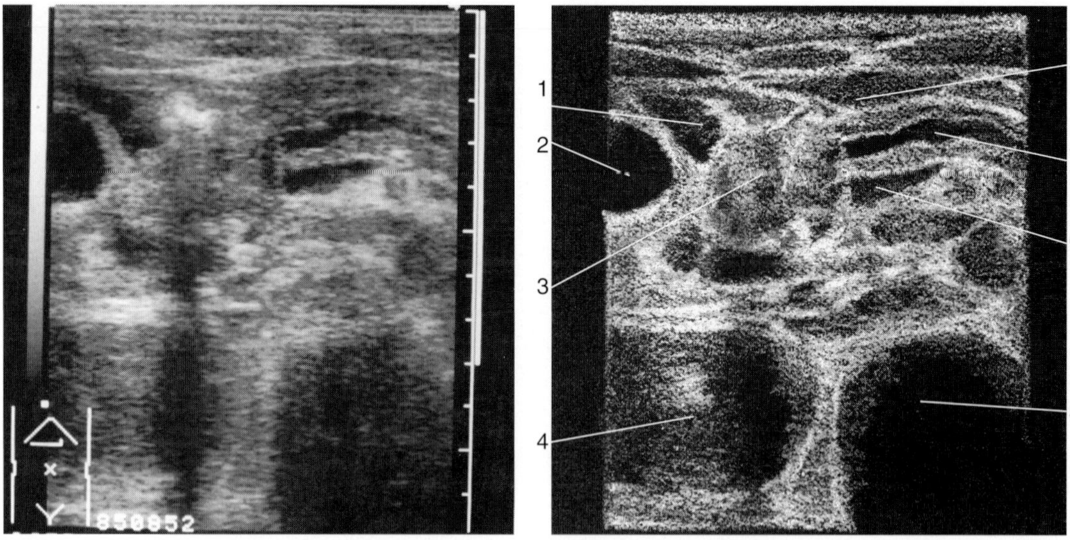

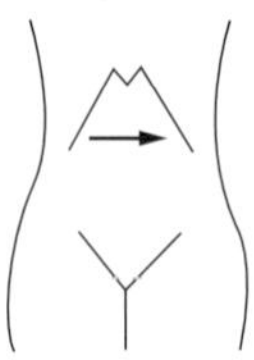

1. Duodenum 2. Gallbladder 3. Cancer of pancreas 4. Right kidney 5. Vertebra 6. Splenic vein 7. Pancreatic duct 8. Left lobe of liver

Figure 5-35. Carcinoma of the pancreas, head.
The echo intensity of malignant pancreatic tumors largely depends on their tissue architecture. The mass in this case is isoechoic with the pancreas. Obstruction of both pancreatic and common ducts by the tumor indicated its malignant nature.

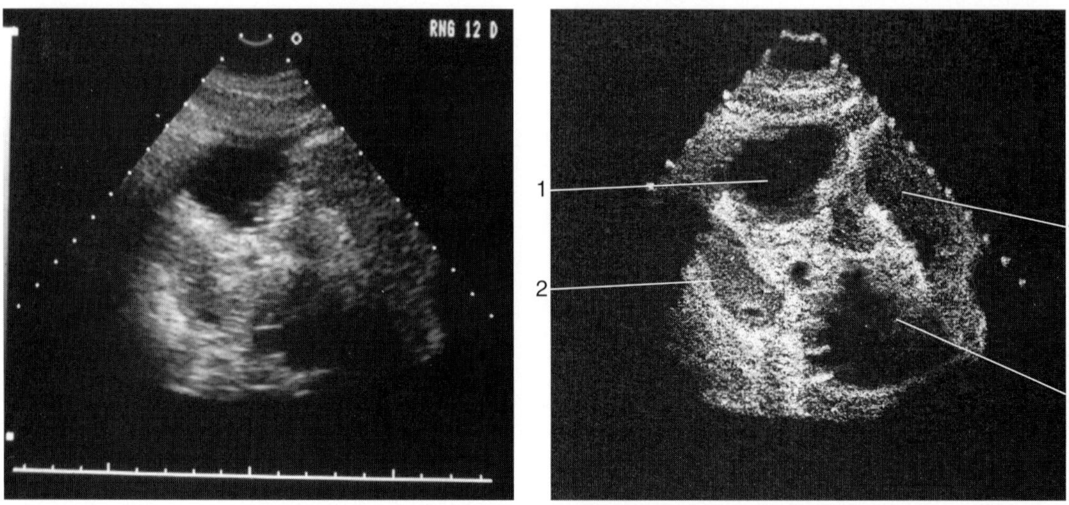

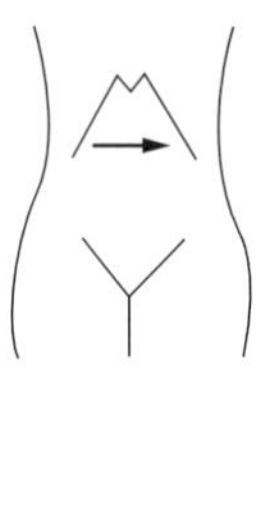

1. Stomach 2. Tail of pancreas 3. Large pancreatic cancer with multiple cystic degeneration 4. Spleen

Figure 5-36. Carcinoma of the pancreas, tail.
Sector scanning of the pancreatic tail through the fluid-filled stomach showed an irregularly shaped, solid mass with a necrotic internal portion. Mild splenomegaly was evident. Aspiration cytology recovered class V malignant cells suggesting adenocarcinoma.

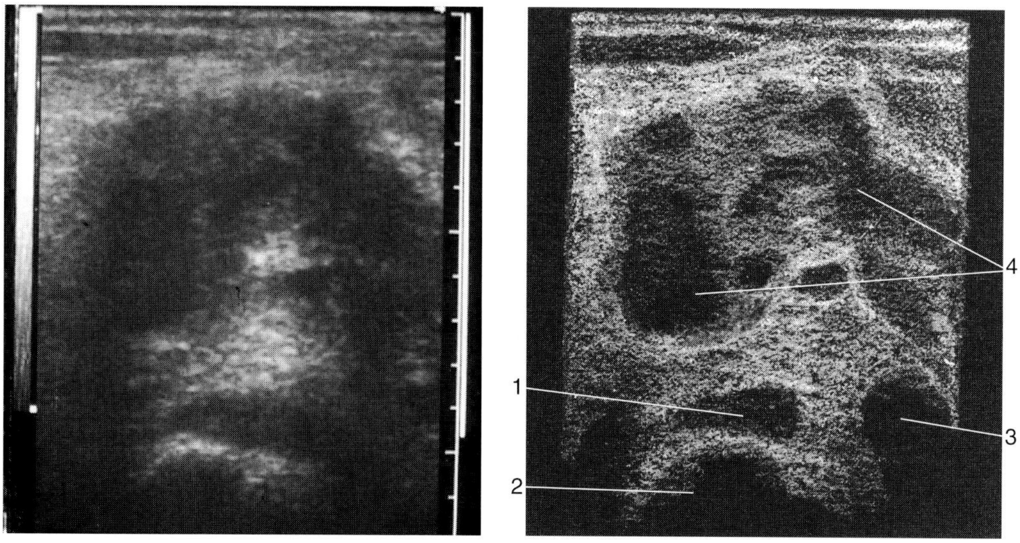

1. Inferior vena cava 2. Vertebra 3. Aorta
4. Diffuse carcinoma of pancreas

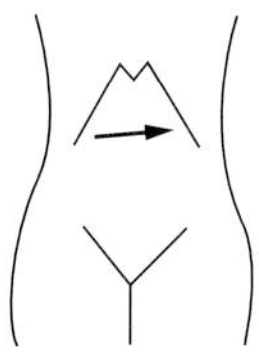

Figure 5-37. Carcinoma of the pancreas, diffuse type.
Transverse scanning at the epigastrium demonstrated a diffusely enlarged pancreas with an irregular, coarse texture and grossly uneven contours.

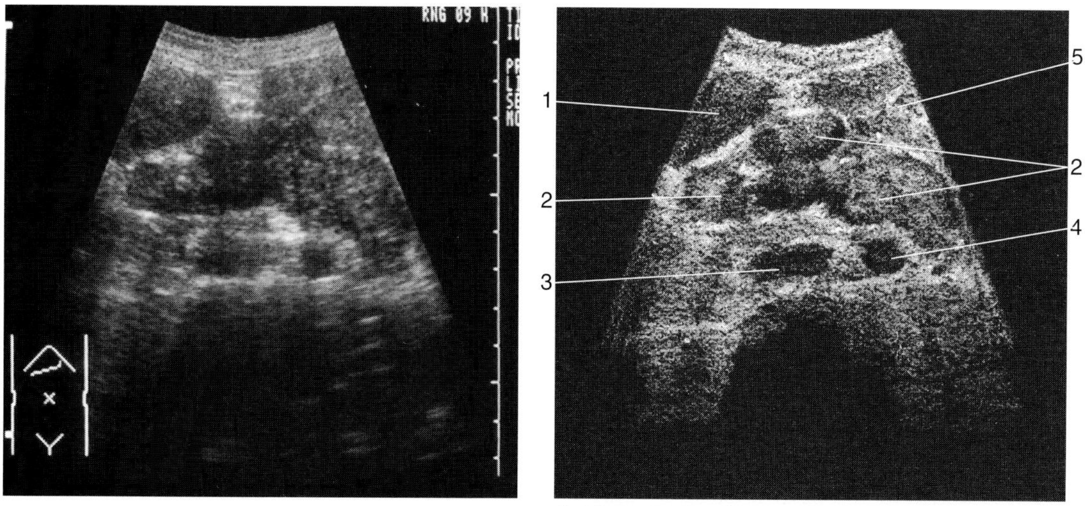

1. Liver 2. Carcinoma of pancreas, diffuse type
3. Inferior vena cava 4. Aorta 5. Liver metastasis

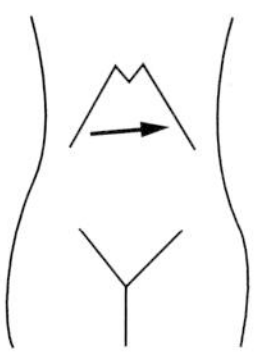

Figure 5-38. Carcinoma of the pancreas, diffuse type.
Extensive diffuse swelling of the entire pancreas with an echo-poor mass in the body region was visualized on transverse scanning. The normal contours of the pancreas were completely obliterated, and no intact parenchyma remained.

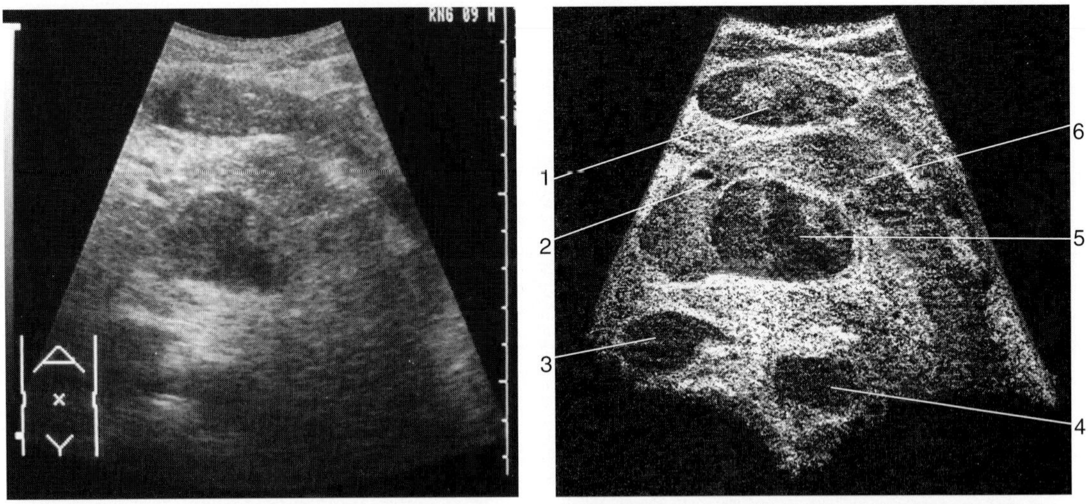

1. Stomach 2. Gastroduodenal artery 3. Inferior vena cava 4. Aorta 5. Portal vein filled with tumor thrombi 6. Pancreas

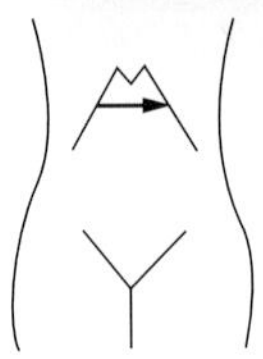

Figure 5-39. Tumor thrombi in the portal vein.
Primary hepatocellular carcinoma often produces bizarre echo patterns around the pancreas. A transverse tomogram in this patient with advanced liver cirrhosis demonstrated an echo-poor, rounded mass at the neck of the pancreas. The longitudinal scan along the portal vein trunk revealed that the mass continued superiorly to the hilum of the liver, filling the lumen of the portal vein. It was diagnosed as a tumor thrombus of the portal vein caused by hepatocellular carcinoma of the diffuse type.

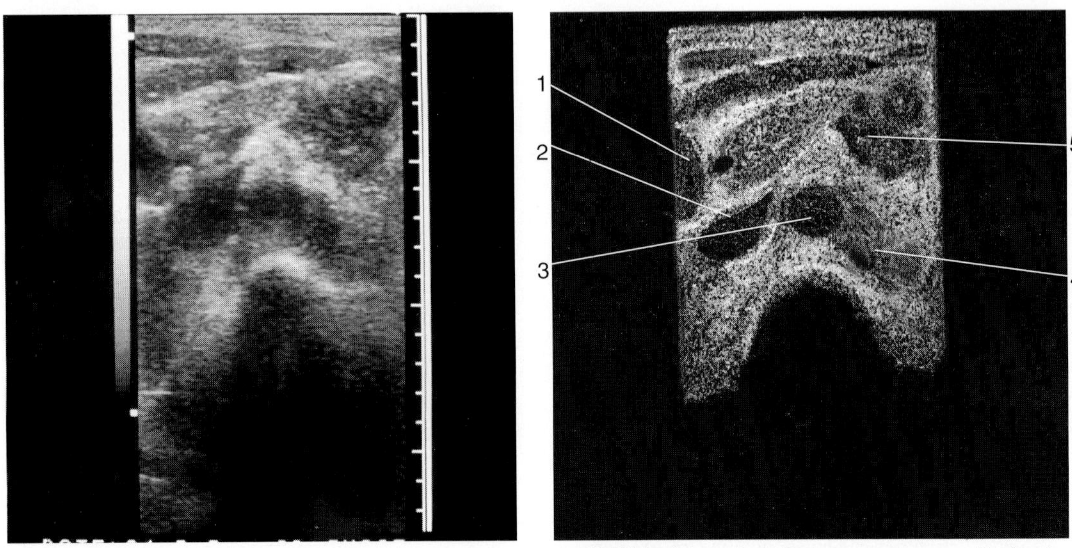

1. Gallbladder 2. Inferior vena cava 3. Aorta 4. Lymph nodes 5. Metastatic tumor at body of pancreas

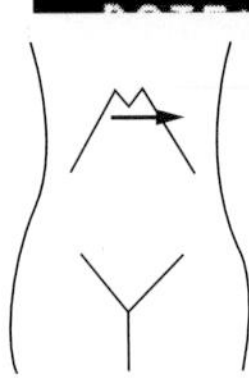

Figure 5-40. Metastatic tumor of the pancreas.
Transverse scanning of the pancreatic region revealed marked anterior displacement of the organ by extensive metastases to the retropancreatic lymph nodes. The source was a primary liver carcinoma.

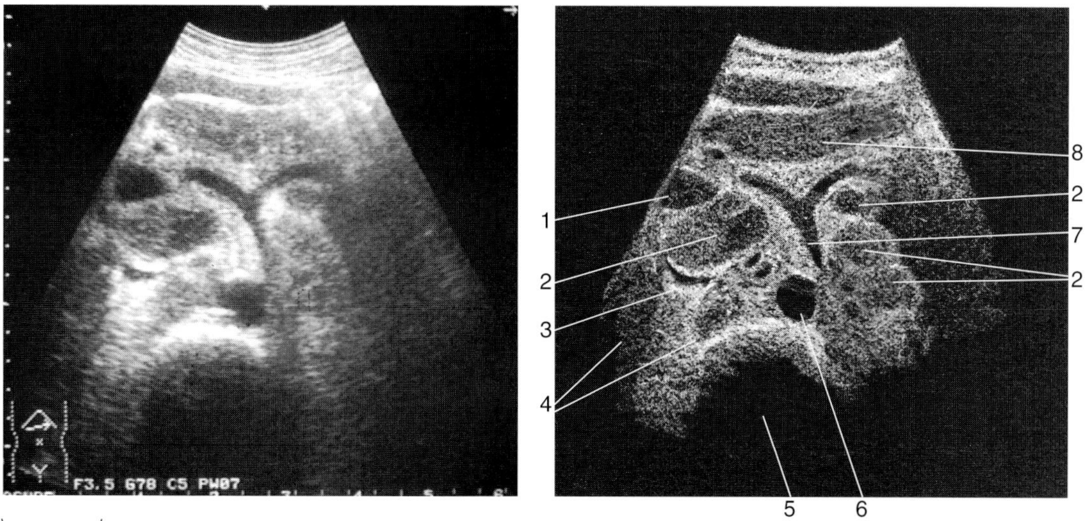

1. Portal vein 2. Lymph nodes 3. Inferior vena cava 4. Lymph nodes 5. Vertebra 6. Aorta 7. Celiac trunk 8. Body of pancreas

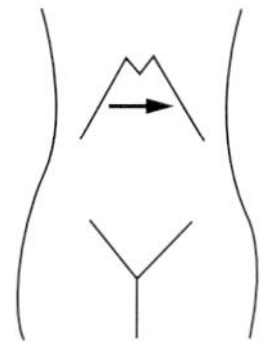

Figure 5-41. Metastatic tumor of the pancreas.
Metastatic tumor of the pancreas is relatively rare. This sonogram was obtained from a patient with gastric carcinoma operated on 1.5 years before. An ill-defined mass with low-level echogenicity was demonstrated in the body of the pancreas. At necropsy, a metastatic tumor in the pancreas was identified, along with multiple metastases to the para-aortic and retropancreatic lymph nodes.

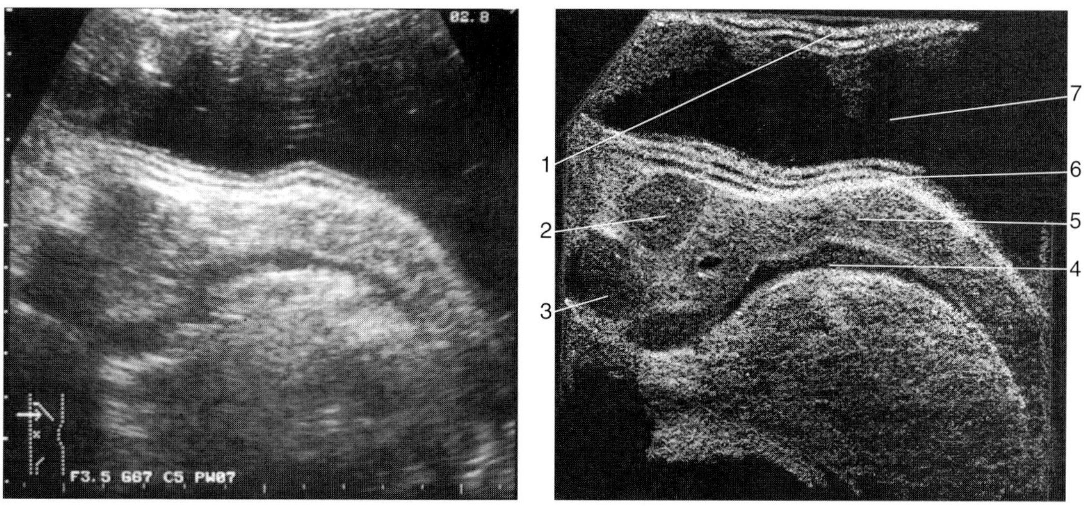

1. Anterior gastric wall 2. Metastasis 3. Metastasis
4. Splenic vein 5. Body of pancreas
6. Posterior gastric wall 7. Liquid-filled stomach

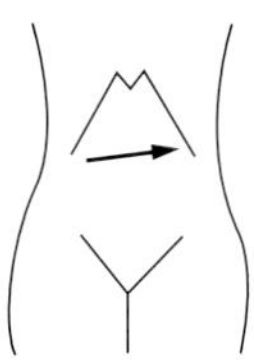

Figure 5-42. Metastatic pancreatic tumor from renal carcinoma.
In this patient being followed for carcinoma of the kidney, the head of the pancreas showed marked irregular swelling with altered echogenicity, compatible with a metastatic tumor mass originating from renal carcinoma. No dilatation of the main pancreatic duct was noted.

REFERENCES

1. Ammann R: Diagnosis and therapy of chronic alcoholic pancreatitis. A critical review of the status. Schweiz Med Wochenschr Suppl 19 : 42-51, 1985.
2. Aranha GV, Prinz RA, Esguerra AC, et al: The nature and course of cystic pancreatic lesions diagnosed by ultrasound. Arch Surg 118 : 486-488, 1983.
3. Armstrong CP, Dixon JM, Taylor TV, et al: Surgical experience of deeply jaundiced patients with bile duct obstruction. Br J Surg 71 : 234-238, 1984.
4. Baker MK, Kopecky KK, Wass JL: Perirenal pancreatic pseudocysts: Diagnostic management. AJR 140 : 729-732, 1983.
5. Berger M, Smith EH, Bartrum RJ Jr: False-positive diagnosis of pancreatic tail lesions caused by colon. JCU 5 : 343-345, 1977.
6. Blangy S, Cornyd F, Sibert A, et al: Real time echographic study of the normal Wirsung duct. Comparison with retrograde catheterization. J Radiol 65 : 35-39, 1984.
7. Bolondi L, Gaiani S, Gullo L, et al: Secretin administration induces dilatation of main pancreatic duct. Dig Dis Sci 29 : 802-808, 1984.
8. Bondestam S: Sonographic pitfalls in the diagnosis of pancreatic neoplasms. Diag Imaging 52 : 224-229, 1983.
9. Busilacchi P, Rizzatto G, Bazzocchi M, et al : Pancreatic cystadenocarcinoma: Diagnostic problem. Br J Radiol 55 : 558-561, 1982.
10. Carroll B, Sample F: Pancreatic cystadenocarcinoma: CT body scan and gray-scale ultrasound appearance. AJR 131 : 339-341, 1978.
11. Coleman BG, Arger PH, Rosenberg HK, et al: Gray-scale sonographic assessment of pancreatitis in children. Radiology 146 : 145-150, 1983.
12. Cotton PB, Lees WR, Vallon AG, et al: Gray-scale ultrasonography and endoscopic pancreatography in pancreatic disease. Radiology 134 : 453-459, 1980.
13. Crade M, Taylor KJW, Rosenfield AT: Water distension of the gut in the evaluation of the pancreas by ultrasound. AJR 131 : 348-349, 1981.
14. Dennis JW, Aranha GV, Greenlee HB, et al: Carcinoma masquerading as a pancreatic pseudocyst on ultrasound. Am J Surg 50 : 334-339, 1984.
15. DeWin JL, Rosenbusch G, Lamaers CB, et al: Radiodiagnosis of glucagonoma and vipoma, 2 rare endocrine pancreatic tumors. ROFO 140 : 537-544, 1984.
16. Donovan PJ, Sanders RC, Siegelman SS: Collection of fluid after pancreatitis: Evaluation of computed tomography and ultrasonography. Radiol Clin North Am 20 : 611-633, 1982.
17. Doust BD, Pearce JD: Gray-scale ultrasonic properties of normal and inflamed pancreas. Radiology 120 : 653-657, 1976.
18. Farman J, Dallemand S, Schneider M, et al: Pancreatic pseudocysts involving the spleen. Gastrointest Radiol 1 : 339-343, 1977.
19. Filley RA, London SS: The normal pancreas: Acoustic characteristics and frequency of imaging. JCU 7 : 121-124, 1974.
20. Foley LC, Teele RL: Ultrasound of epigastric injuries after blunt trauma. AJR 132 : 593-598, 1979.
21. Friedman AC, Lichtenstein JE, Dachman AH: Cystic neoplasms of the pancreas. Radiological-pathological correlation. Radiology 149 : 45-50, 1983.
22. Fukuda M: Ultrasonic tissue characterization of hepatic and pancreatic malignancies by mean of various pulse-echo ultrasound. International Congress Series No. 505 Ultrasound in Medicine and Biology. Amsterdam, Excerpta Medica, 1979, pp151-158.
23. Fukuda M: Assessment of diagnostic accuracy of imaging diagnosis, XCT and realtime ultrasound on pancreatic malignancy, 1988. Report of Joint Study Group Sponsored by Japanese Ministry of Health and Welfare, Tokyo, 1987, pp5-11.
24. Ghorashi B, Rector WR: Gray scale sonographic anatomy of the pancreas. JCU 5 : 25-29, 1977.
25. Gold J, Rosenfield AR, Sostman D, et al: Nonfunctioning islet cell tumors of the pancreas: Radiographic and ultrasonographic appearance of two cases. AJR 131 : 515-517, 1978.
26. Goldberg BB: The pancreas. Clin Diagn Ultrasound 23 : 165-193,1988.
27. Goldman ML, Naib ZM, Galambos JT, et al: Preoperative diagnosis of pancreatic carcinoma by percutaneous aspiration biopsy. Am J Dig Dis 22 : 1076-1082, 1977.
28. Gonzalez AC, Bradley EL, Clements JL Jr: Pseudocyst formation in acute pancreatitis: Ultrasonographic evaluation of 99 cases. AJR 127 : 315-317, 1976.

29. Gooding GAW, Laing FC: Rapid water infusion: A technique in the ultrasonic discrimination of gas-free stomach from a mass in pancreatic tail. Gastrointest Radiol 4 : 139-141, 1979.
30. Gooding GAW: Ultrasound of superior mesenteric artery aneurysm secondary to pancreatitis: A plea for real time ultrasound of sonolucent masses in pancreatitis. JCU 9 : 255-256, 1981.
31. Gosink BB, Leopold GR: The dilated pancreatic duct: Ultrasonic evaluation. Radiology 126 : 475-478, 1978.
32. Goulet RJ, Goodman J, Schaffer R, et al: Multiple pancreatic pseudocyst disease. Ann Surg 199 : 6-13, 1984.
33. Grant EG, Richardson JD, Smirniotopoulos JG, et al: Fine-needle biopsy directed by real-time sonography : Technique and accuracy. AJR 141 : 29-32, 1983.
34. Gronvall J, Gronvall S, Hegedus V: Utrasound-guided drainage of fluid-containing masses using angiographic catheterization techniques. AJR 129 : 997-1002, 1977.
35. Gunther RW, Klose KJ, Ruckert K, et al: Islet-cell tumors : Detection of small lesions with computed tomography and ultrasound. Radiology 148 : 485-488, 1983.
36. Haber K, Freimanis AK, Asher WM: Demonstration and dimensional analysis of the normal pancreas with gray-scale echography. AJR 126 : 624-628, 1976.
37. Hancke S, Pedersen JF: Percutaneous puncture of pancreatic cysts guided by ultrasound. Surg Gynecol Obstet 142 : 551-552, 1976.
38. Hashimoto BE, Laing FC, Jeffrey RB Jr, et al: Hemorrhagic pancreatic fluid collections examined by ultrasound. Radiology 150 : 803-808, 1984.
39. Hill MC: Pancreatic sonography: An update, in Sanders RC (ed), Ultrasoud Annual 1982. New York, Raven Press, 1982, pp1-42.
40. Hospitel S, Guinot B, Teyssou H, et al: Intrahepatic localization of a pancreatic pseudocyst. J Radiol 64 : 355-358, 1983.
41. Houlbert D, Roche A, Dorf G, et al: Preoperative localization of insulinoma is necessary. Ann Med Interne (Paris) 135 : 16-20, 1984.
42. Itoh K, Yamanaka T, Kasahara K, et al: Definitive diagnosis of pancreatic carcinoma with percutaneous fine needle aspiration biopsy under ultrasound guidance. Am J Gastroenterol 71 : 469-472, 1979.
43. Jacobson P, Crade M, Taylor KJW: The upright position while giving water for the evaluation of the pancreas. JCU 6 : 353-354, 1978.
44. Kaude JV, McInnis AN: Pancreatic ultrasound following blunt abdominal trauma. Gastrointest Radiol 7 : 53-56, 1982.
45. Kolmannskog G, Larsen S, Swensen T, et al: Reproducibility and observer variation at computed tomography and ultrasound of the normal pancreas. Acta Radiol [diagn] (Stockh) 24 : 21-25, 1983.
46. Kuhn FP, Gunther R, Ruckert K, et al: Ultrasonic demonstration of small pancreatic islet cell tumors. JCU 10 : 173-175, 1982.
47. Kunzman A, Bowie JD, Rochester D: Texture patterns in pancreatic sonograms. Gastrointest Radiol 4 : 353-357, 1979.
48. Lawson TL, Berland LL, Foley WD: Coronal upper abdominal anatomy: Technique and gastrointestinal applications. Gastrointest Radiol 6 : 115-128, 1981.
49. Lawson TL: Acute pancreatitis and its complications. Computed tomography and sonography. Radiol Clin North Am 21 : 495-513, 1983.
50. Lindsell DR: Ultrasound imaging of pancreas and biliary tract. Lancet 335(8686) : 390-393, 1990.
51. Lloyd TV, Antonmattei S, Freimanis AK: Gray-scale sonography of cystadenoma of pancreas: Report of two cases. JCU 7 : 149-151, 1979.
52. MacMahon H, Bowie JD, Beezhold C: Erect scanning of pancreas using a gastric window. AJR 132 : 587-591, 1979.
53. Marks WM, Filly RA, Callen PW: Ultrasonic evaluation of normal pancreatic echogenicity and its relationship to fat deposition. Radiology 137 : 475-479, 1980.
54. McGahan JP: The posterior gastric wall: A possible source of confusion in the identification of the pancreatic duct. JCU 12 : 366-368, 1984.
55. Meire HB: Ultrasound in gastroenterology. Clin Gastroenterol 13 : 183-203, 1984.
56. Neoptolemos JP, Hall AW, Finlay DF, et al: The urgent diagnosis of gallstones in acute pancreatitis : A prospective study of three methods. Br J Surg 71 : 230-233, 1984.
57. Niederau C, Sonnenberg A, Muller JE, et al: Sonographic measurements of the normal liver, spleen, pancreas and portal vein. Radiology 149 : 537-540, 1983.
58. Ohto M, Saotome N, Saisho H, et al: Real-time sonography of the pancreatic duct: Application to percutaneous pancreatic ductography. AJR 134 : 647-652, 1980.

59. Paivansalo M: Normal pancreatic echogenicity: Relation to structural unevenness and thickness in CT. Ann Clin Res 16 : 60-71, 1984.
60. Paivansalo M, Makarainen H, Siniluoto T, et al: Ultrasound compared with computed tomography and pancreatic angiography in the detection of endocrine tumours of the pancreas. Eur J Radiol 9 : 173-178, 1989.
61. Parulekar SG: Ultrasonic evaluation of the pancreatic duct. JCU 8 : 457-463, 1980.
62. Pollock D, Taylor KJW: Ultrasound scanning in patients with clinical suspicion of pancreatic cancer : A retrospective study. Cancer 47 : 1662-1665, 1981.
63. Sarti DA, King W: The ultrasonic findings in inflammatory pancreatic disease, in Raymond HW, Zweibel WJ (eds), Seminars in Ultrasound, Vol 1. New York, Grune and Stratton, 1980, pp178-191.
64. Savarino V, Mansi C, Bistolfi L, et al: Failure of new diagnostic aids in improving detection of pancreatic cancer at a resectable stage. Dig Dis Sci 28 : 1078-1082, 1983.
65. Schrever T, Gunther R, Ruckert K, et al: Microcystic pancreas adenoma. Rontgenblatter 36 : 384-387, 1983.
66. Schulz RD, Willi U: Ultrasound diagnosis following blunt abdominal injury in childhood. Ultraschall Med 4 : 154-159, 1983.
67. Schwerk WB, Durr HK, Schmitz-Moorman P: Ultrasound guided fine needle biopsies in pancreatic and hepatic neoplasms. Gastrointest Radiol 8 : 219-225, 1983.
68. Shawker TH, Doppman JL, Dunnick NR, et al: Ultrasonic investigation of pancreatic islet cell tumors. JCU 1 : 193-200, 1982.
69. Shawker TH, Linzer M, Hubbard VS: Chronic pancreatitis: The diagnostic significance of pancreatic size and echo amplitude. JCU 3 : 267-272, 1984.
70. Silverstein W, Isikoff MB, Hill MC, et al: Imaging of acute pancreatitis: Prospective study using CT and sonography. AJR 137 : 497-502, 1981.
71. Simeone JF, Dembner AF, Mueller PR: Invasion of the pancreas by gastric carcinoma: Ultrasonic appearance. JCU 8 : 501-503, 1980.
72. Smith EH, Bartrum RJ, Chang YC: Ultrasonically guided percutaneous aspiration biopsy of the pancreas. Radiology 112 : 737-738, 1974.
73. Stolte M: Chronische Pancreatitis: Morphologie-Pancreatographie-Differentialdiagnose. Erlangen, Perimed Fachbuch Verlagsgesellschaft, 1984, pp1-167.
74. Suramo I, Myllyla V, Kairaluoma MI: Ultrasonographic diagnosis of pancreatic carcinoma supplemented with CT or ERCP. Ann Clin Res 16 : 44-46, 1984.
75. Szebeni I, Tulassay Z, Papp J, et al: Ultrasonography and endoscopy in the diagnosis of obstructive icterus. Fortschr Med 101 : 901-906, 1983.
76. Tatsuta M, Yamamoto R, Yamamura H, et al: Cytologic examination and CEA measurement in aspirated pancreatic material collected by percutaneous fine-needle aspiration biopsy under ultrasonic guidance for the diagnosis of pancreatic carcinoma. Cancer 52 : 693-698, 1983.
77. Taylor KJW: Anatomy of pancreas by gray-scale ultrasonography. J Clin Gastroenterol 1 : 67-75, 1979.
78. Taylor KJW, Brant MH: Ultrasonic biopsy guidance in the management of patients with pancreatic cancer. J Clin Gastroenterol 1 : 267-272, 1979.
79. Triller J, Klauser H: Current value of sonography in pancreas diagnosis. Computertomographie 3 : 42-48, 1983.
80. Warren KW, Christophi C, Aremendariz R, et al: Current trends in the diagnosis and treatment of carcinoma of the pancreas. Am J Surg 145 : 813-818, 1983.
81. Warren PS, Garrett WJ, Kossoff G: The liquid-filled stomach: A new sonic window. JCU 6 : 315-320, 1978.
82. Weber W, Von Essen CF, Metzger U, et al: Pancreatic cancer, epidemiology, etiology, diagnosis and therapy. Schweiz Med Wochensch 113 : 417-426, 1983.
83. Weighall SL, Wolfman NT, Watson N: The fluid-filled stomach: A new sonic window. JCU 7 : 353-356, 1979.
84. Weill F, Schraub A, Eisenscher A, Bourgoin A: Ultrasonography of the normal pancreas: Success rate and criteria for normality. Radiology 123 : 417-423, 1977.
85. Weill F, Brun P, Rohmer P, et al: Migrations of fluid of pancreatic origin: Ultrasonic and CT study of 28 cases. Ultrasound Med Biol 9 : 485-496, 1983.
86. Weinstein DP, Wolfman NT, Weinstein BJ: Ultrasonic characteristics of pancreatic tumors. Gastrointest Radiol 4 : 245-251, 1979.
87. Weinstein DP, Weinstein BJ: Ultrasonic demonstration of the pancreatic duct: An analysis of 41 cases. Radiology 130 : 729-734, 1979.

88. Weinstein BJ, Weinstein DP, Brodmerkel FJ Jr: Ultrasonography of pancreatic lithiasis. Radiology 134 : 185-189, 1980.
89. Wise SR, Johnson J, Sparks J, et al: Gastrinoma: The predictive value of preoperative localization. Surgery 106 : 1087-1092, 1989.
90. Wittenberg J, Simeone J, Ferrucci J Jr, et al: Non-focal enlargement in pancreatic carcinoma. Radiology 144 : 131-135, 1982.
91. Wolson AH, Walls WJ: Ultrasonic characteristics of cystadenoma of the pancreas. Radiology 119 : 203-205, 1976.
92. Worthen NJ, Beabeau D: Normal pancreatic echogenicity: Relation to age and body fat. AJR 139 : 1095-1098, 1982.
93. Zirinsky K, Abiri M, Baer JW: Computed tomography demonstration of pancreatic microcystic adenoma. Am J Gastroenterol 79 : 139-142, 1984.

CHAPTER 6

THE SPLEEN

NORMAL ANATOMY

The spleen lies in the left upper quadrant of the abdomen immediately beneath the left hemidiaphragm. The diaphragmatic surface is smooth and convex, whereas the visceral surface is concave and faces the posterior surface of the stomach, the lateral border of the left kidney, and the tail of the pancreas (Figure 6-1).[10, 24, 44] The spleen is overlain by the 8th to 11th ribs. It is an approximately triangular organ and has a centrally located hilum on the visceral surface containing the splenic vessels, the lienogastric and lienorenal ligaments. The splenic vein runs medially along the upper border of the tail and body of the pancreas and joins the superior mesenteric vein to form the main trunk of the portal vein. The splenic artery is more tortuous and is located superior to the splenic vein. The spleen is covered with peritoneum except at its hilum. It is held and fixed in position between the left diaphragm and the stomach by the lienorenal, lienogastric, and phrenicocolic ligaments.

The spleen is the largest reticuloendothelial organ in the body. Its size changes in a variety of clinical conditions including vascular congestion, infections, storage diseases, proliferation of hematopoietic cells and when infiltrated by tumor tissues.[4, 8, 10, 35, 40]

The normal spleen weighs approximately 150-170 grams.[14] Theoretically, its volume could be calculated by summing the sequential splenic areas obtained with parallel planes separated by known distances, e.g., 1 cm or the distance between intercostal spaces,[15, 17, 27, 29, 38, 49] however, this method is cumbersome and difficult to perform with ultrasound. A more practical method is to use an index obtained by multiplying the largest values of the breadth(B), thickness(T) and length(L) of the spleen divided by 27(splenic volumetric index, SVI).[44] In normal individuals the value lies between 8 and 34, and in most clinical conditions the index is sensitive to enlargement allowing a consistent diagnosis of splenomegaly. Simpler methods are to estimate its volume (V) on the assumption that it has an ellipsoidal shape ($V\ cm^3 = 0.523 \times B \times T \times L$ - $\pi/6 = 0.523$) or to use the "Splenic index" obtained by multiplying the largest diameter×longitudinal diameter.[29]

In most cases, however, the classification of splenomegaly as mild, moderate or marked by visual estimation is sufficient (Figure 6-2), unless it is critical to use the size of the spleen as an index of response to treatment, as in chemotherapy for leukemia or lymphoma. The shape and location of the spleen are also important in the evaluation of splenomegaly.[35, 51]

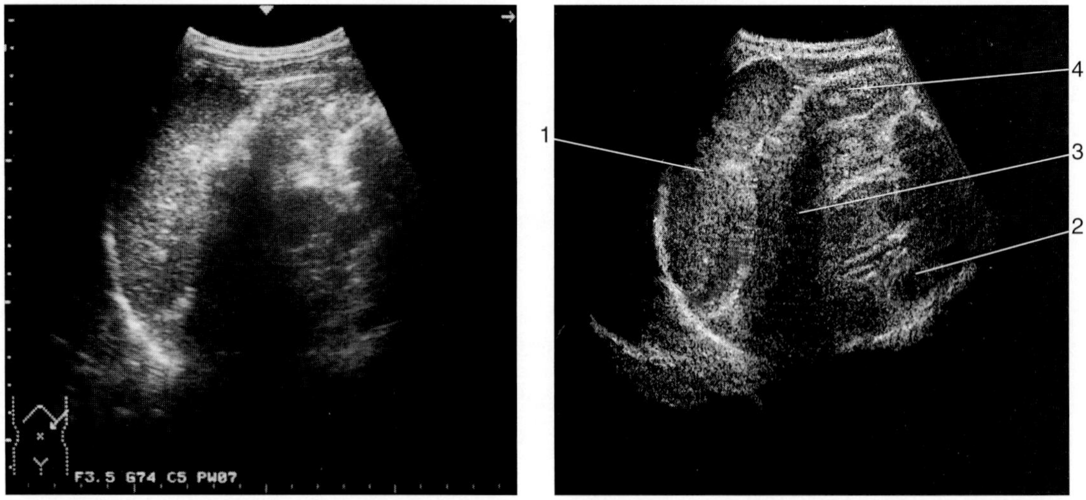

1. Spleen 2. Left kidney 3. Acoustic shadow by intestinal gas 4. Intestine

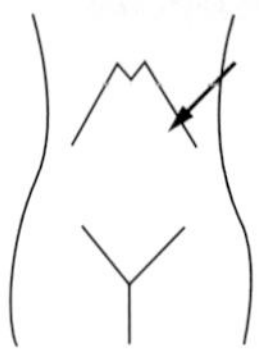

Figure 6-1. The normal spleen.
The spleen is best imaged via an intercostal space, often the 9th intercostal space is optimal. The scan head may need to be angled to optimize the image. The upper pole is generally difficult to image, even using a curvilinear or sector probe, because it is often overlaid by the lung. The size and shape of the spleen can be assessed without difficulty. The normal echo texture is a fine, uniform, speckled pattern.

a

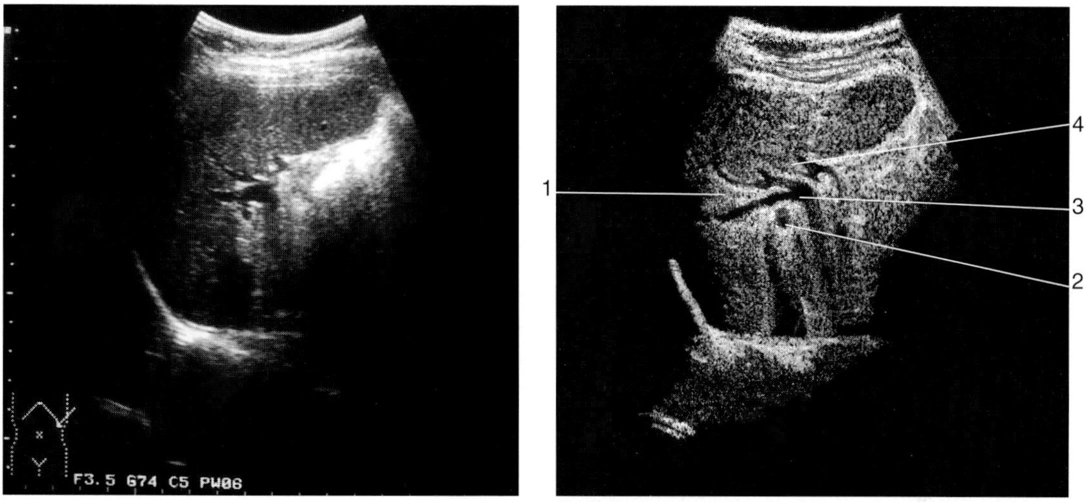

1. Spleen 2. Splenic artery 3. Splenic vein 4. Hilum of spleen

b

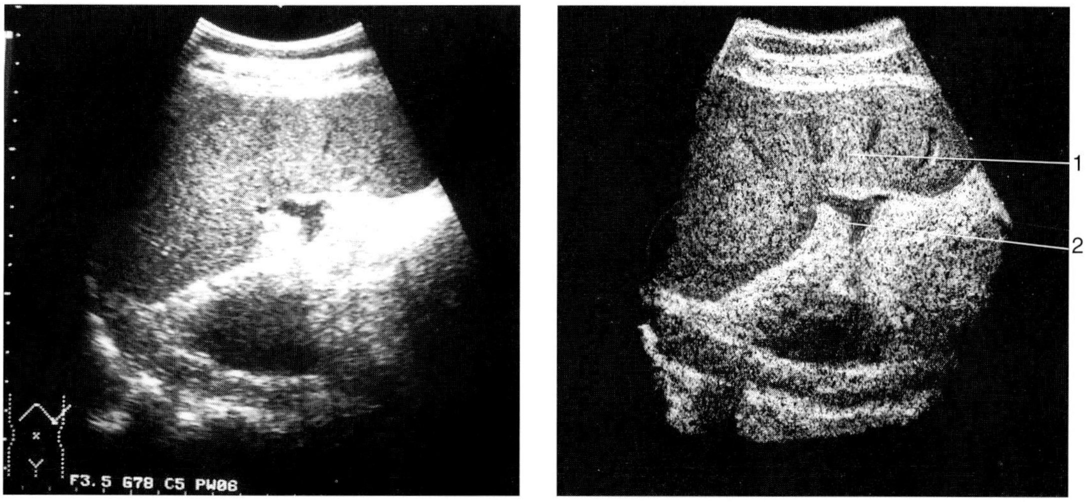

1. Spleen 2. Splenic vein

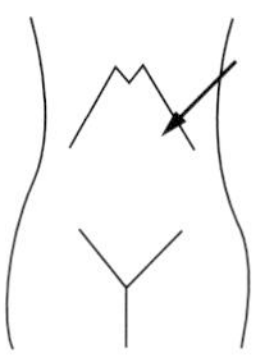

Figure 6-2. Diffuse splenomegaly, medium and marked degrees.
(a) Moderate splenomegaly in a patient with persistent chronic hepatitis. The splenic vein at the hilum showed slight dilatation. However, no specific change was observed in the splenic parenchyma. (b) Marked splenomegaly also observed in a patient with prolonged chronic active hepatitis. Liver biopsy and liver function tests indicated the presence of cirrhotic change superimposed on chronic hepatitis. The internal reflectivity is slightly increasd, but the echo texture and caliber of the splenic vein at the hilum are not significantly different from those in (a).

SCANNING TECHNIQUES

It is considerably easier to visualize the spleen with real-time scanning than with static scanning. The most complete images of the spleen are obtained with the patient in the right lateral decubitus position, scanning through the 9th or 10th intercostal space. The best landmark is the left kidney, which lies caudad to the spleen and is readily identified by its distinctive sonographic pattern (see Chapter 7). Once the left kidney has been identified, the probe may simply be moved up slightly to the intercostal space, where the triangular shaped spleen is imaged. Alternatively, scanning in the left coronal plane between the anterior and posterior axillary lines with a linear array transducer can effectively image the spleen. The upper pole of the spleen is difficult to visualize by any means because of the air in the overlying left lung, which obscures the sonogram, especially with a normal-sized spleen. Occasionally, however, it is possible to visualize the whole spleen by adjusting the tilt of the probe to match the phase of respiration.

ULTRASONIC APPEARANCES

Normally, the splenic sonogram consists of evenly distributed fine echoes; the vascular structures are not prominent within the spleen, but major vessels are seen near the hilum.[10,35] Careful manipulation of the transducer is essential for successful imaging.

The echo amplitude and distribution of the echo texture of the spleen may change slightly in various disease states, but they are so subtle that they are not diagnostically useful.

PATHOLOGICAL FINDINGS

Spleen size changes in a number of pathological states. Diffuse enlargement is common in congestion(Figure 6-2), long-standing bacterial, viral, or protozoan infections, collagen disorders, and diffuse infiltration by pathological cellular components, such as in storage diseases of congenital origin, or by diffuse infiltration of hematological cells such as malignant lymphomas,[18, 22, 30, 39] polycythemia vera or in myelofibrosis (Figures 6-3 and 6-4).[5, 23] Among these conditions, the most marked splenomegaly is encountered in patients with chronic myelogenous leukemia, hemolytic anemia and certain types of protozoan infections such as kala-azar and malaria. In patients with extreme splenomegaly, the spleen may fill the left half of the abdominal cavity, and the lower pole often crosses the midline to reach the right lower quadrant of the abdomen. Figure 6-5 shows a case of extensive splenomegaly caused by chronic hemolytic anemia of the nonspherocytic type.[52]

The echo patterns of diffuse splenomegaly generally lack specific features, except for changes in the caliber of the splenic vessels. However, in patients with a long history of hemolytic episodes, multiple scattered, echogenic, strands may be found, probably due to fibrosis in the parenchyma (Figure 6-5).

Congestion can cause enormous splenomegaly, particularly in patients with essential portal hypertension in whom marked dilatation of the portal vein and engorgement of the splenic artery are present.[53, 54, 55] Calcification of the splenic artery often coexists and is seen as plaques casting acoustic shadows. The presence of engorged collaterals in the vicinity of the splenic hilum is particularly striking; they can often be traced extending in the direction of the venous plexus around the esophagus (Figure 6-6). Figure 6-7 shows a splenic sonogram of a moderately enlarged spleen with an aneurysm of the splenic artery together with dilated splenic veins in a case of cirrhosis accompanied by a small hepatocellular carcinoma.

Less marked, diffuse splenomegaly is observed in a number of liver diseases, including chronic hepatitis and cirrhosis, as well as in symptom-free carriers of hepatitis B or hepatitis C virus. In many acute inflammatory conditions such as sepsis or bacteremia, less pronounced splenomegaly with lower echo levels is found. In cirrhosis or chronic hepatitis, splenomegaly is generally accompanied by dilatation of the splenic vein and its tributaries, including varices (Figures 6-8 and 6-9). Chronic infections also cause enlargement of the spleen and in tuberculosis echogenic foci of calcified granuloma may appear (Figure 6-10). *Echinococcus granulosus* infection also can cause calcification in the spleen.

Hematological diseases, such as non-Hodgkin's disease and Hodgkin's lymphoma (Figure 6-11), chronic lymphatic leukemia, and acute myelogenous leukemia, commonly cause splenic enlargement (Figures 6-4 and 6-12). The proliferative splenomegaly that accompanies hematological diseases produces characteristically blunt thickening of the anterior splenic border even in mild cases (Figure 6-12).

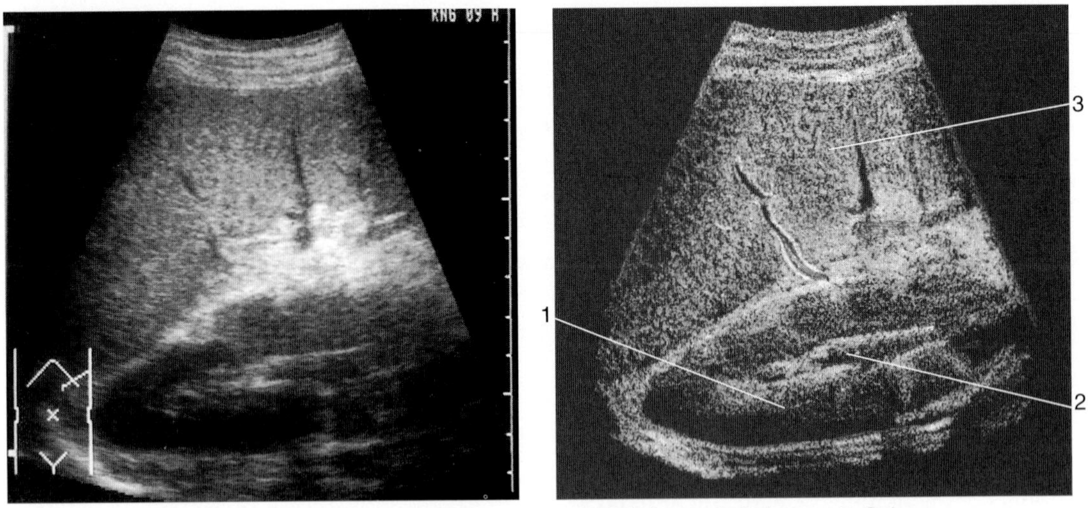

1. Left kidney 2. Calyces 3. Spleen

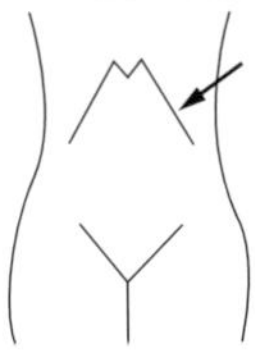

Figure 6-3. Diffuse swelling of the spleen in chronic myelofibrosis.
Unlike the marked venous dilatation accompanying splenomegaly caused by portal congestion, the splenic vein dilate only in proportion to spleen size in other types of splenomegaly. A patient with chronic myelofibrosis, with a characteristic clinical course including hematological change, showed no dilatation of the splenic vein. The ultrasonic texture of the splenic parenchyma, however, seemed somewhat coarser than normal, consistent with fibrosis.

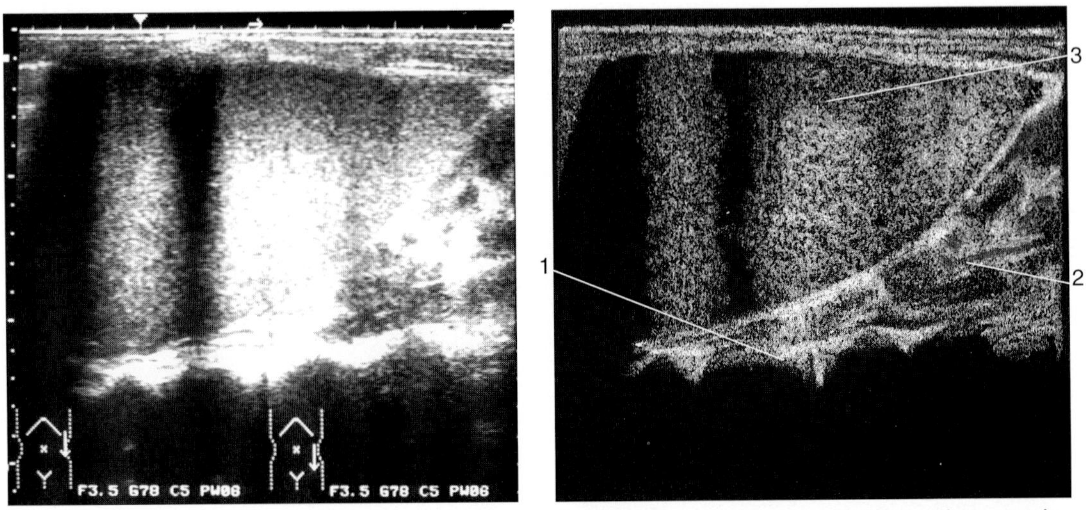

1. Vertebra 2. Left kidney 3. Huge splenomegaly

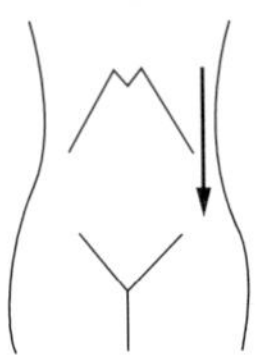

Figure 6-4. Extensive splenomegaly in hairy cell leukemia.
Chronic myelogenous or monocytic leukemia is frequently accompanied by marked splenomegaly. In this patient, a young male, with the diagnosis of hairy cell leukemia, extensive splenomegaly occupied the left side of the abdomen, extending to the right lower abdomen. In the near-coronal scan (two scans are combined in this composite image), the spleen, over 16 × 10 cm in size, is visualized. The spleen completely occupied the space between the abdominal wall and the spine and left kidney is markedly displaced.

a 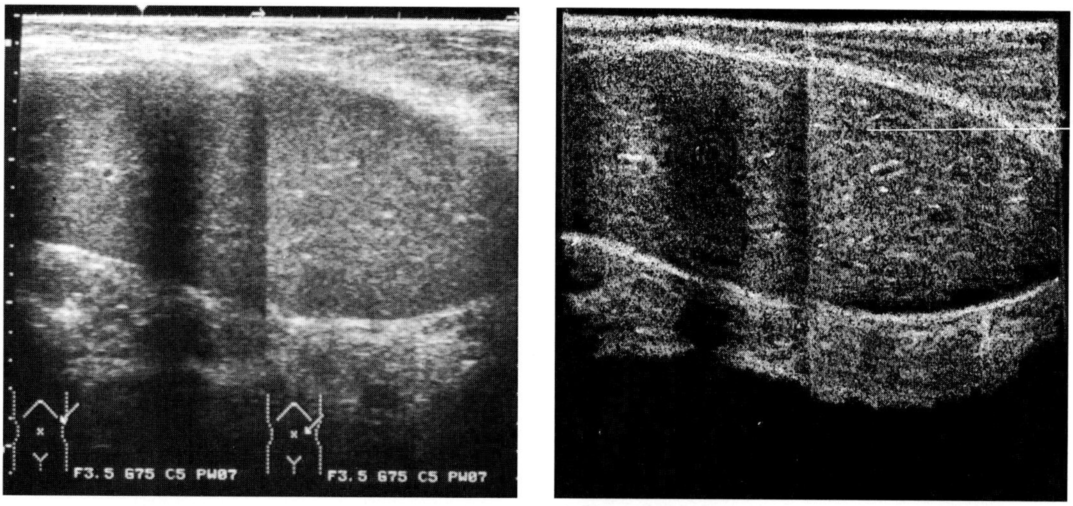

1. Enlarged spleen

b 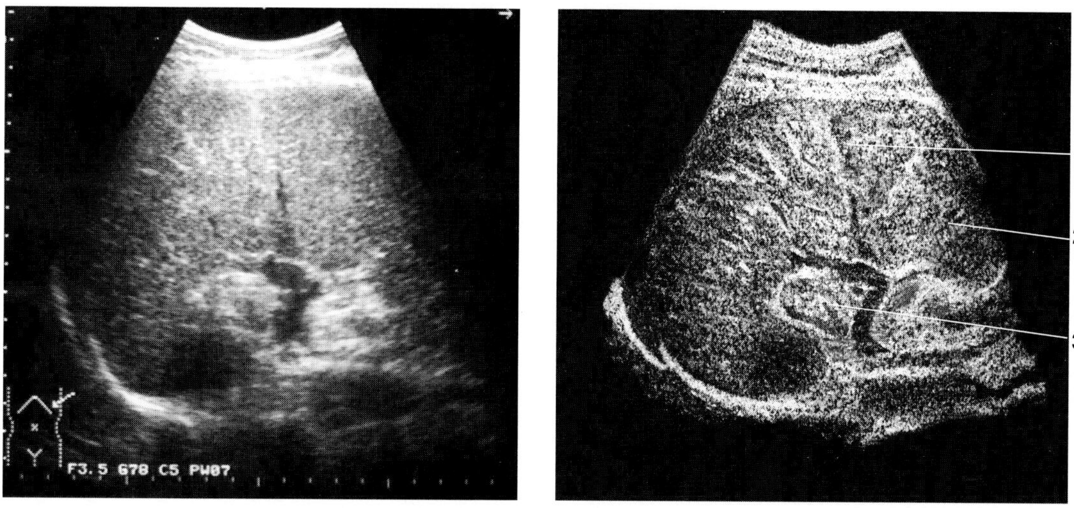

1. Fibrotic strands 2. Spleen 3. Splenic vein

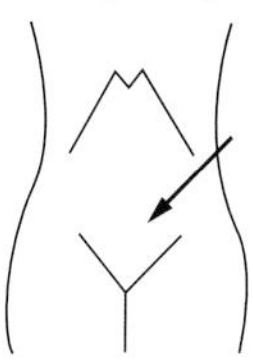

Figure 6-5. Marked splenomegaly in hemolytic anemia.
Patients with prolonged hemolytic anemia, either sickle cell or spherocytic, often develop marked splenomegaly. This sonogram shows a massive spleen extending to the iliac crest and across to the midline of the abdomen(a). The characteristic coarse network pattern of fibrosis is found throughout the splenic parenchyma, reflecting persistent episodes of hemolysis(b).

a

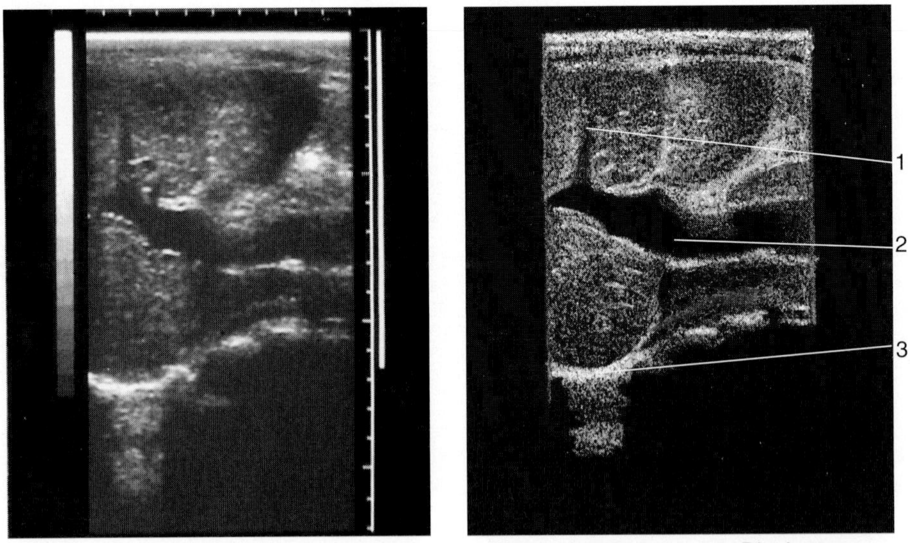

1. Liver 2. Portal vein 3. Diaphragm

b

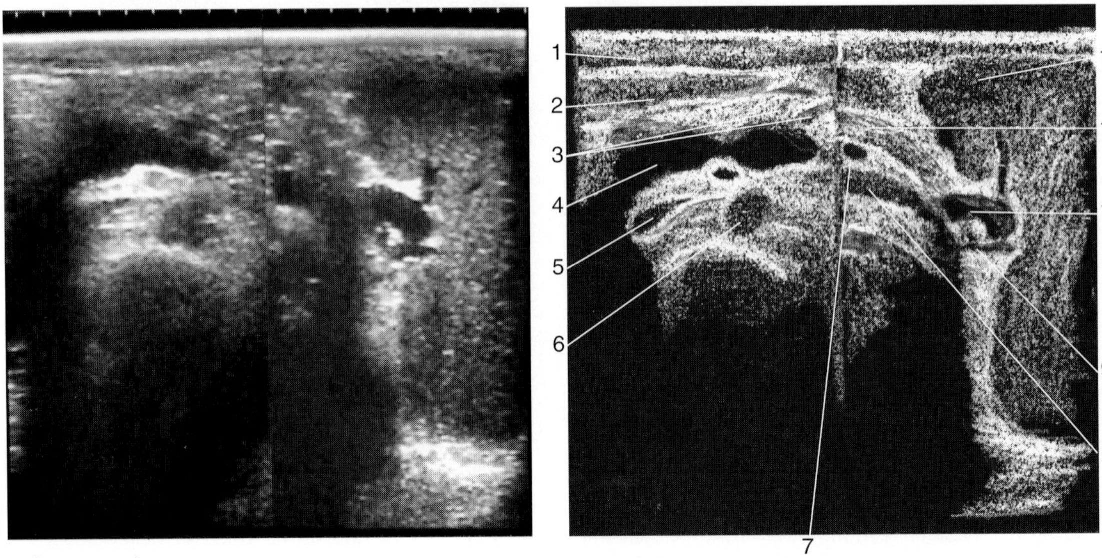

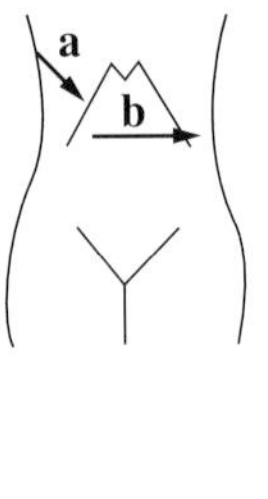

1. Rectus muscle 2.Left lobe of liver 3. Coronary veins (collateral vein) 4. Splenic vein 5. Inferior vena cava 6. Aorta 7. Superior mesenteric artery 8. Left renal vein 9. Splenic artery 10. Splenic vein 11. Pancreas 12. Spleen

Figure 6-6. Splenomegaly in advanced cirrhosis.
Advanced cirrhosis is characterized by shrinkage of the liver, with bluntening of the angle of the free edge of the liver and dilatation of the portal vein. Vascular congestion of the entire portal circulation is manifested by dilatation of the splenic vein, detected throughout its course, and by the collateral circulation that develops. Pronounced splenomegaly is a usual finding.

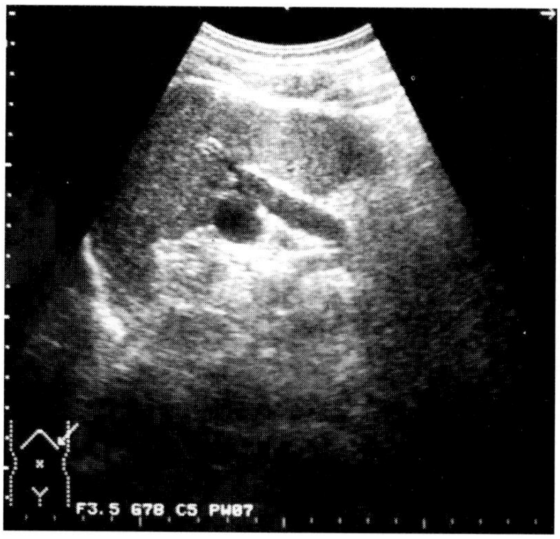

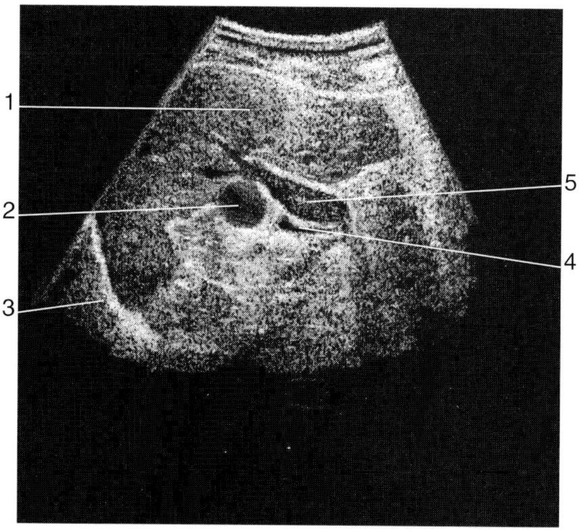

1. Spleen 2. Aneurysm 3. Diaphragm 4. Splenic artery 5. Splenic vein

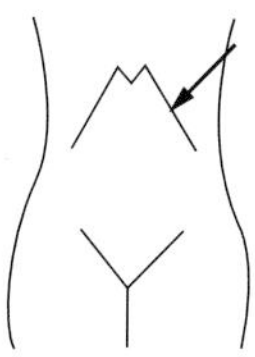

Figure 6-7. Aneurysm of the splenic artery.
Portal hypertension is often accompanied by the formation of aneurysms of the splenic artery. The sonogram demonstrated moderate splenomegaly with dilatation of the splenic vein at the splenic hilum. Deep to the dilated splenic vein is a round, echo-free mass; the Doppler signals from it were unequivocally arterial, whereas the dilated vein showed the characteristic portal pattern. Careful scanning revealed a direct connection between the cystic mass and the splenic artery, shown adjacent to the aneurysm. Angiography confirmed the sonogrpahic findings.

a

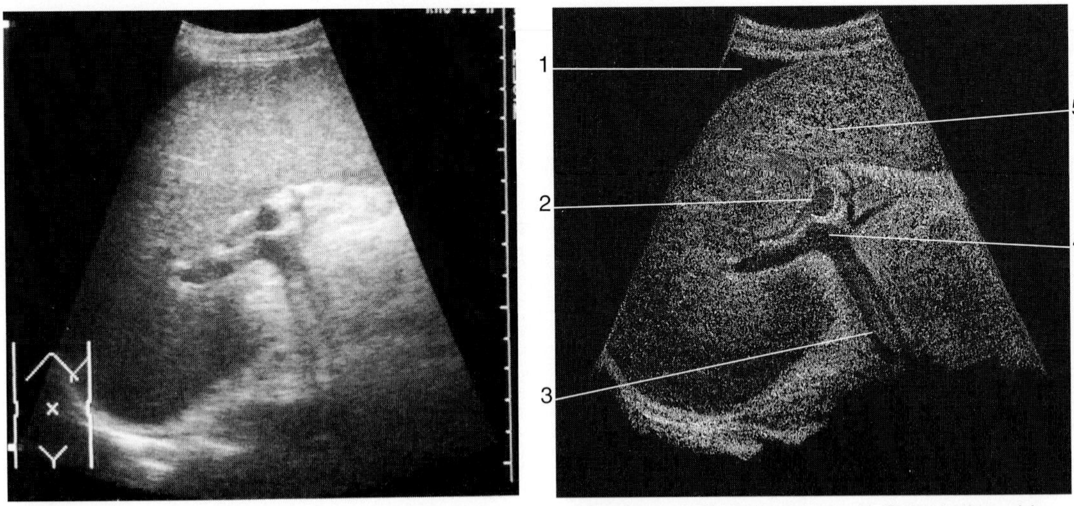

1. Ascites 2. Splenic artery 3. Splenic thrombi
4. Splenic vein 5. Spleen

b

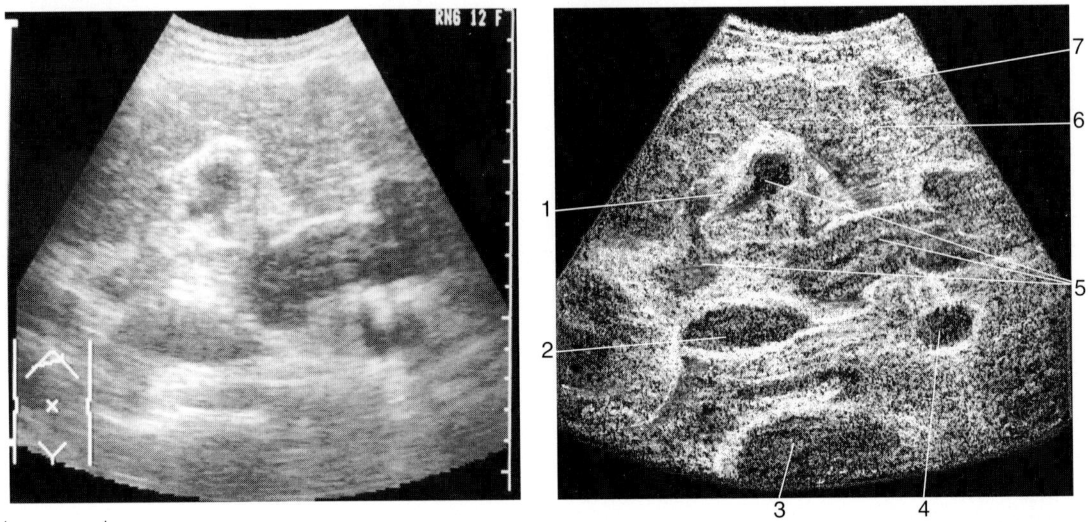

1. Periportal fatty tissue (parenchymal atrophy)
2. Inferior vena cava 3. Vertebra 4. Aorta
5. Dilated portal vein (with tumor thrombi) 6. Left lobe of liver 7. Protrusion

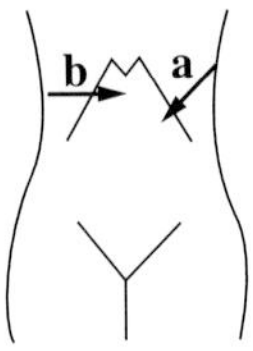

Figure 6-8. Marked splenomegaly in a case of liver carcinoma with massive tumor thrombi in the portal vein.

Hepatocellular carcinoma(HCC) has the characteristic of growth into the bloodstream, creating tumor thrombi in the portal or hepatic veins. This case is particularly informative because no discrete mass formed in the liver (diffuse type of HCC), but there was massive tumor thrombus filling the main portal vein and causing marked dilatation of the extrahepatic portal vein, which extended to the level of pancreatic neck (b). The splenic sonogram (a) shows marked splenomegaly, with dilatation of splenic vessels and perisplenic ascites.

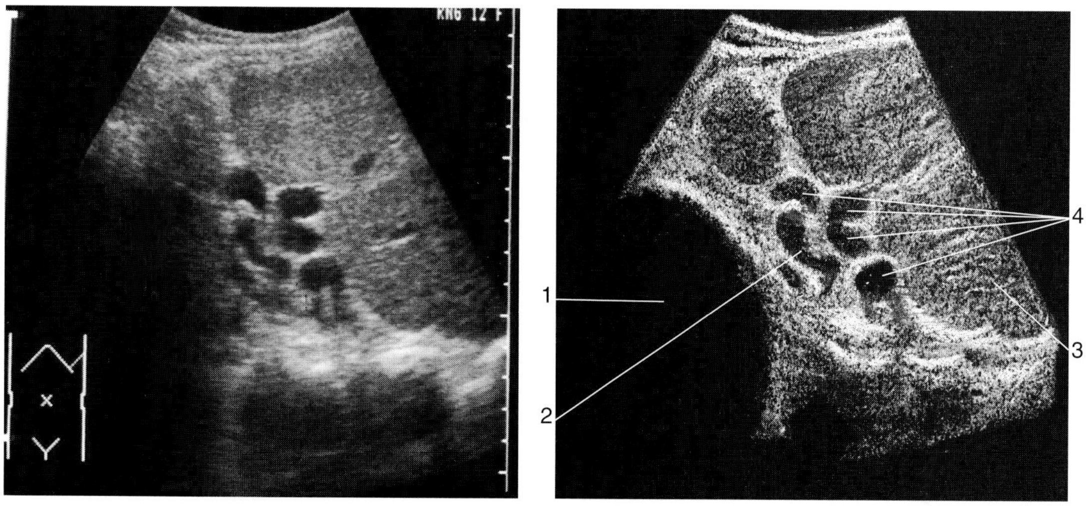

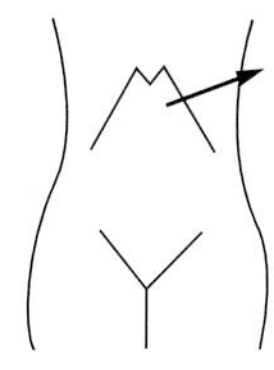

1. Vertebra 2. Splenic artery 3. Splenomegaly 4. Varices

Figure 6-9. Splenomegaly and collateral formation in cirrhosis.
Sustained portal congestion in advanced liver cirrhosis usually results in collateral circulation with marked splenomegaly. In a near-transverse scan through the splenic hilum in a patient with cirrhosis, multiple engorged collaterals are disclosed together with the dilated splenic vein. The reflectivity of the splenic parenchyma is not significantly changed.

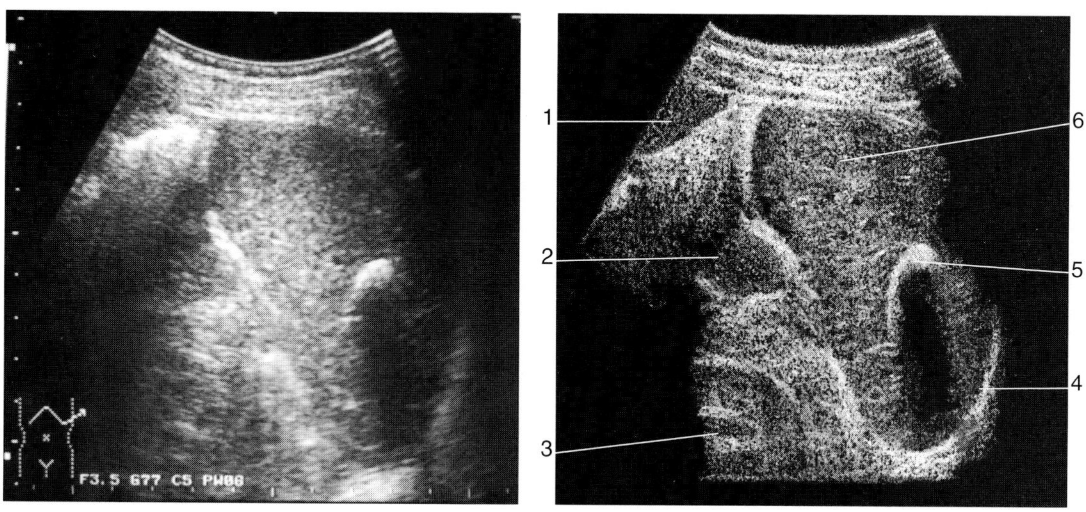

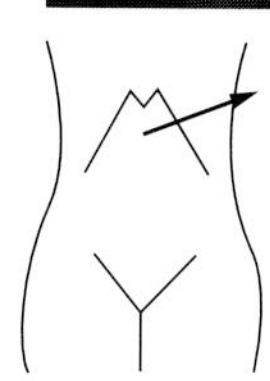

1. Left lobe of liver 2. Tail of pancreas 3. Left kidney 4. Diaphragm 5. Calcification 6. Spleen

Figure 6-10. Calcification in the spleen.
Calcification in the spleen in a case of old pulmonary tuberculosis is demonstrated on an intercostal scan. A bright echo casting an acoustic shadow behind was found in a slightly enlarged spleen; the pattern simulated a stone. Roentgenographic study also disclosed a calcified spot in the spleen, presumably caused by calcification of a caseous granuloma from tuberculosis.

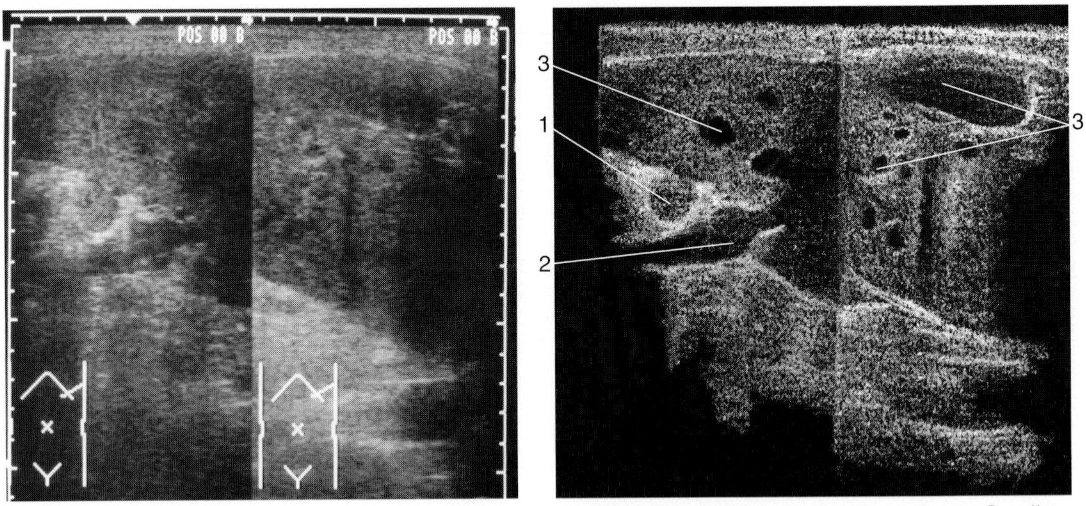

1. Accessory spleen 2. Splenic vein 3. Small to large intrasplenic masses

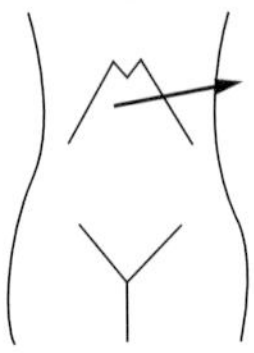

Figure 6-11. Splenomegaly in Hodgkin's lymphoma.
Hodgkin's lymphoma often causes marked enlargement of the spleen, sometimes with discrete masses in the spleen. This case showed marked splenomegaly accompanied by extensive abdominal lymphadenopathy.

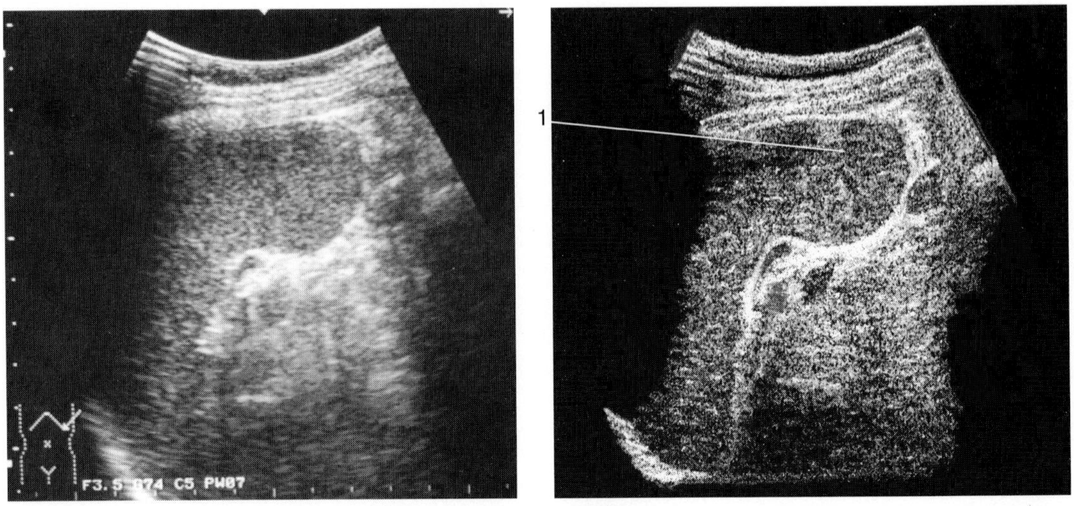

1. Spleen

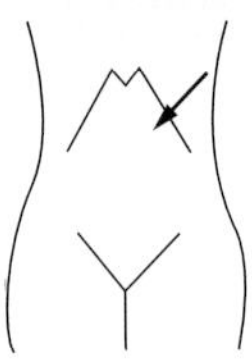

Figure 6-12. Splenomegaly in acute myelogenous leukemia.
Acute myelogenous leukemia is accompanied by splenomegaly, but it is less pronounced than in chronic myelogenous leukemia. Although the enlargement is less pronouced, a blunted anterior edge is a characteristic finding in infiltrative splenomegaly including leukemia, and the internal echo texture is much coarser than that or nonleukemic splenomegaly. Attenuation of the ultrasound signal is not apparent.

FOCAL LESIONS OF THE SPLEEN

Cysts

The most obvious benign lesion of the spleen is the cyst. There are rarely true cysts,[6, 7, 12, 35] secondary cysts (pseudocysts without epithelial lining caused mostly by trauma) being more common. The wall of a pseudocyst consists of fibrous tissue with evidence of old hemorrhage[13, 27, 37, 45, 46, 50] (Figure 6-13). Splenic pseudocysts may also result from acute pancreatitis affecting the tail of the pancreas.[41]

Cysts are characteristically seen as smoothly outlined, anechoic masses with marked posterior acoustic enhancement. They are usually encircled by clear, rounded margins with no solid lesion or thickened portions (Figure 6-14). However, rarely an isolated lymphoma nodule can mimick a cyst.[10]

Hemangioma

Cavernous hemangiomas of the spleen are often similar in appearance to hemangiomas in the liver and usually are entirely asymptomatic. Therefore, they are found accidentally during routine sonographic examinations.[31, 40a] The lesions appear as single or multiple echogenic, irregularly outlined mass(es) (Figure 6-15). They may appear at any site within the organ. As in the liver, the echogenicity and shape of the mass are not necessarily characteristic of hemangioma, therefore, a definitive diagnosis depends upon angiography. However, the diagnosis can be confirmed if there is absolutely no change in the size and character of the mass on repeated examinations.[10] In difficult cases, the use of other diagnostic modalities such as dynamic x-ray CT or MRI will give supportive evidence. When there are multiple lesions in the spleen, they do not necessarily have a uniform appearance. Some may be diffusely echogenic, while others may be echo-poor or intermediate.

In nonmalignant lesions, the sonographic findings of splenic infarctions, splenic abscesses[19, 46] and traumatic rupture of the spleen[15, 20] deserve special mention.

Acute splenic infarction which usually produces acute splenic pain, may occasionally be overlooked until calcified plaques are found accidentally on sonography[33, 59, 60] (Figure 6-16). The previous debate concerning the multiplicity of echo pattern characteristics of splenic infarction has almost been settled following a number of reports describing the echographic patterns of proven infarctions at various stages[31, 34, 62, 66] and the increased frequency of accidental splenic infarction during transarterial embolization of the hepatic artery, the mostly hypoechoic, triangular lesion having had the base toward the surface of the spleen[56, 57] (Figure 6-17).

Abscesses of the spleen are also uncommon in this era of widespread use of antibiotics. When they occur they are usually the sequelae of the septicemia in an immunocompromised host in whom antibiotics have limited value in combating infection.[24, 31, 41, 48] The mixed echo pattern is similar to those of bacterial abscesses in other parenchymatous organs, with a poorly defined, echo-poor lesion with shaggy walls often containing echogenic foci representing debris or gas. It may be difficult to distinguish splenic abscesses from a hematoma, tumor metastasis, or infarction. The presence of general symptoms such as fever, abdominal pain and local tenderness of the left upper quadrant help the differential diagnosis.

Ultrasound has been reported to have accuracy of 96% in detecting abscess and of 99% in excluding their presence.[35]

Splenic hematoma is usually caused by blunt trauma, such as by a traffic accident or a penetrating trauma as from a sharp knife[43, 58](Figure 6-18). A partially marginated, round lesion with a complex echo pattern caused by laceration of the splenic parenchyma is seen and it may be possible to demonstrate a thin echo-poor line indicating the bleeding into the parenchyma. The pattern of hematoma vary in relation to the location and the time since the trauma. A lesion with a stellate configuration may be seen and an echogenic mass with echo-poor linear bands extending to the capsule is characteristic.

Ultrasound is extremely valuable in the follow-up examination of hematomas. Thin peripheral lacerations may disappear within weeks, large intrasplenic hematomas may persist for much longer and sometimes evolve into posttraumatic splenic cysts.

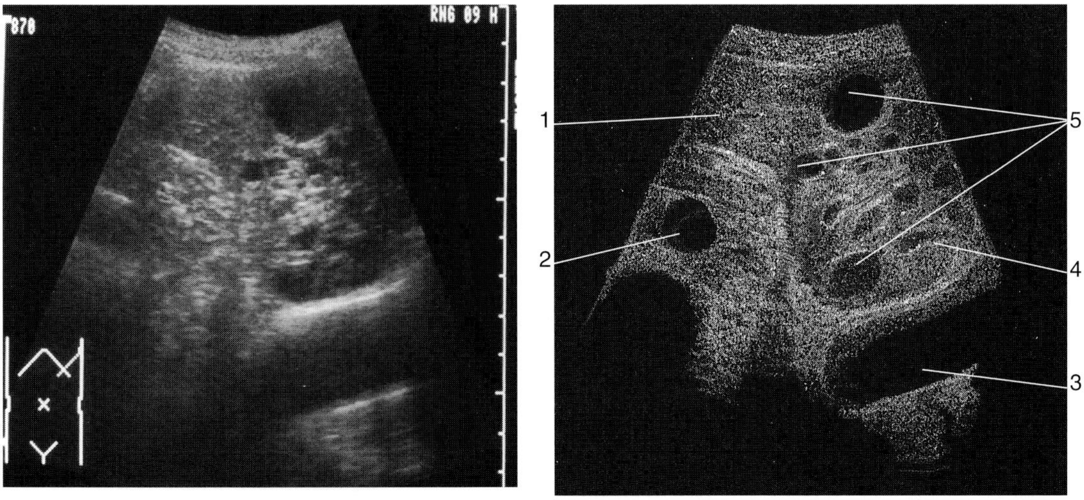

1. Spleen 2. Aorta 3. Stomach 4. Spleen 5. Cysts

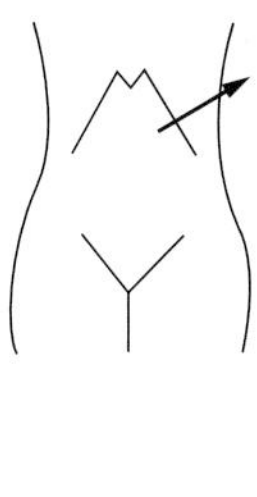

Figure 6-13. Splenic cyst.
Splenic cyst may be solitary genuine cysts but more often are pseudocysts following other lesions, such as traumatic hematoma or pancreatic pseudocyst. In this case, multiple round cysts of varying size with distal acoustic enhancement were found. There were also multiple cysts in the liver. The splenic cysts did not show any contrast enhancement with dynamic CT, which supported the diagnosis of benign splenic polycystic disease.

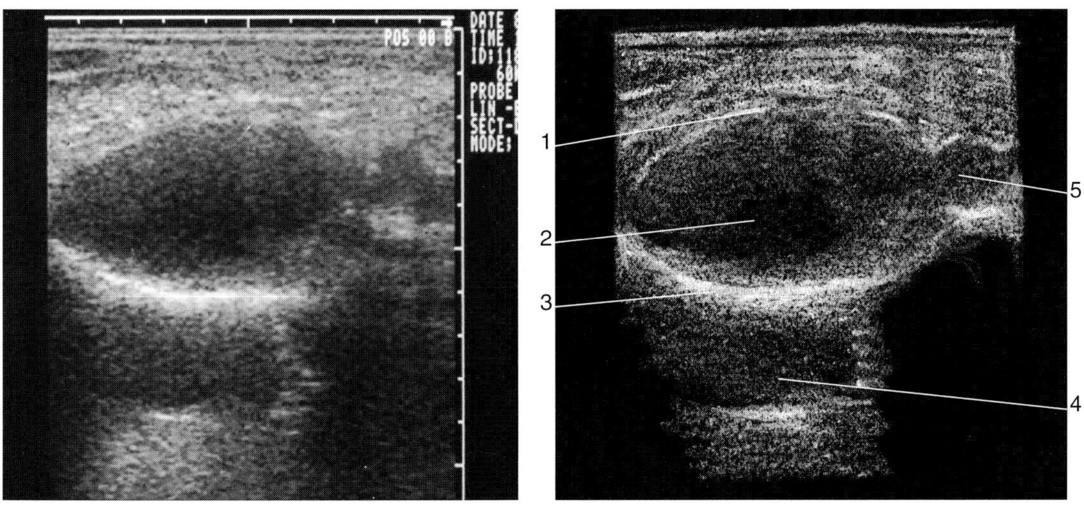

1. Anterior wall of cyst 2. Splenic cyst 3. Calcified posterior wall of cyst 4. Gastric lumen 5. Spleen

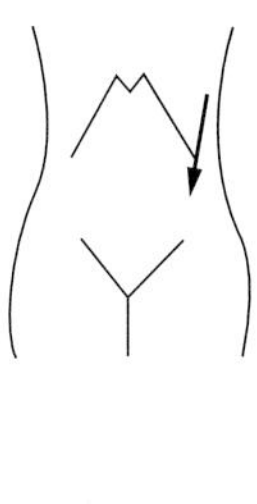

Figure 6-14. A calcified splenic cyst.
A large splenic cyst was first detected by endoscopy when moderate extragastric compression was demonstrated. Endoscopic ultrasound failed to penetrate the lesion because of marked sound attenuation by the wall of the mass. On transabdominal ultrasound with a convex probe of 3.5 MHz, a solitary cyst was found adjacent to the stomach; it was strongly echogenic, with marked acoustic shadowing. Surgery revealed a single large splenic cyst with a calcified wall, possibly secondary to previous intrasplenic bleeding.

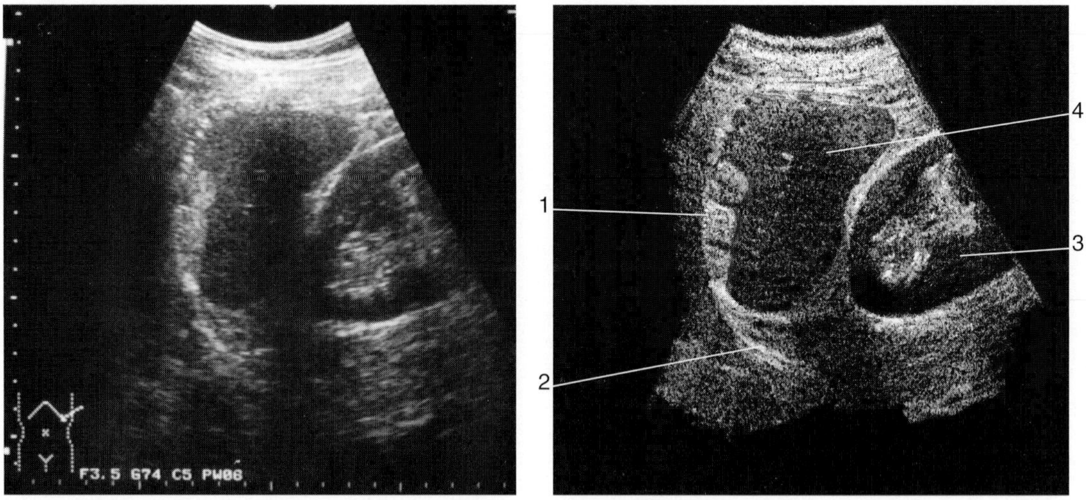

a

1. Hemangiomas (three) 2. Diaphragm 3. Left kidney 4. Spleen

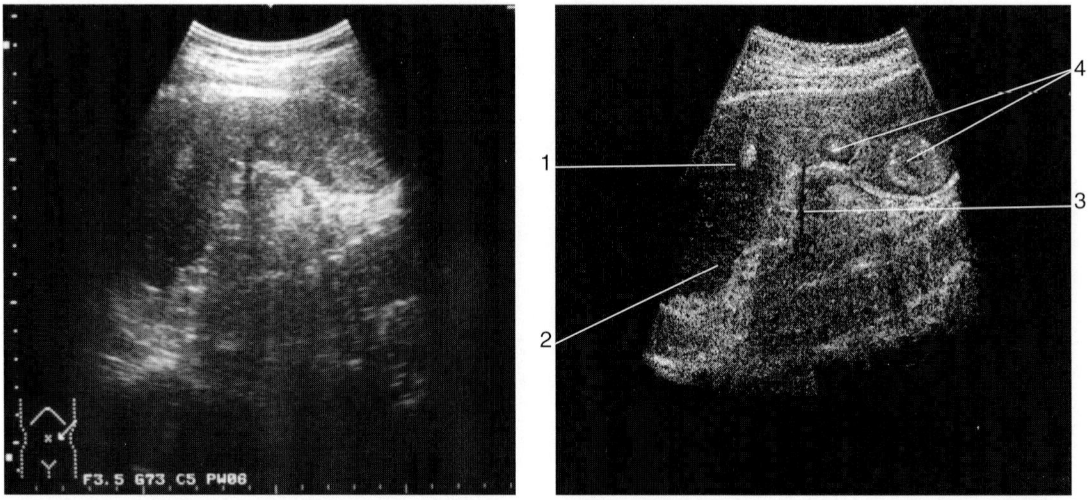

b

1. Hemangioma 2. Spleen 3. Splenic hilum 4. Hemangiomas

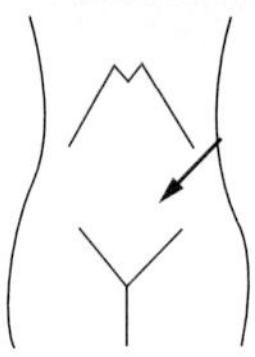

Figure 6-15. Multiple hemangiomas of the spleen.
Hemangiomas in the spleen produce the same echo patterns observed in the liver. In (a), three small, echogenic masses lying inferior to the left dome of the diaphragm. In (b), three hemangiomas with different echogenicity are demonstrated. Plain and dynamic CT scanning disclosed characteristic findings confirming the diagnosis. A follow-up study over 1 year later showed no change in the lesions confirming their benign nature.

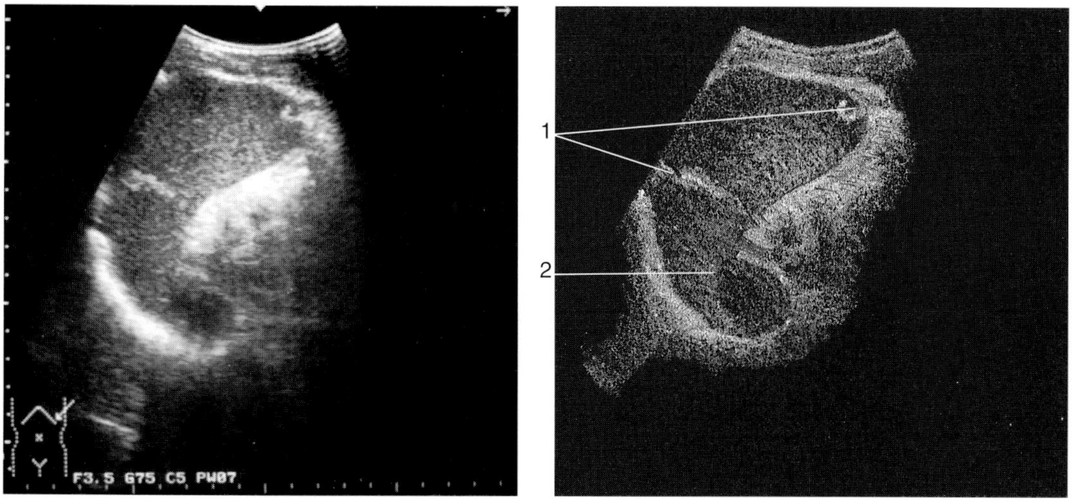

1. Calcified infarction 2. Spleen

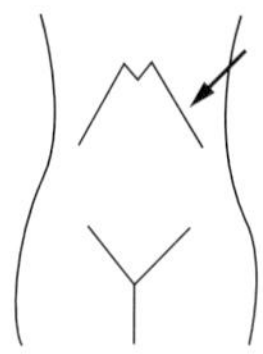

Figure 6-16. Splenic infarction.
This sonogram, obtained from a patient with cardiac failure due to valvular disease, shows a highly echogenic, strand-like structure extending from near the splenic hilum to the surface of the spleen. At the lower pole, a small area of similar change was noted. The cause was thought to be spontaneous arterial emboli from chronic mural thrombi in the left atrium.

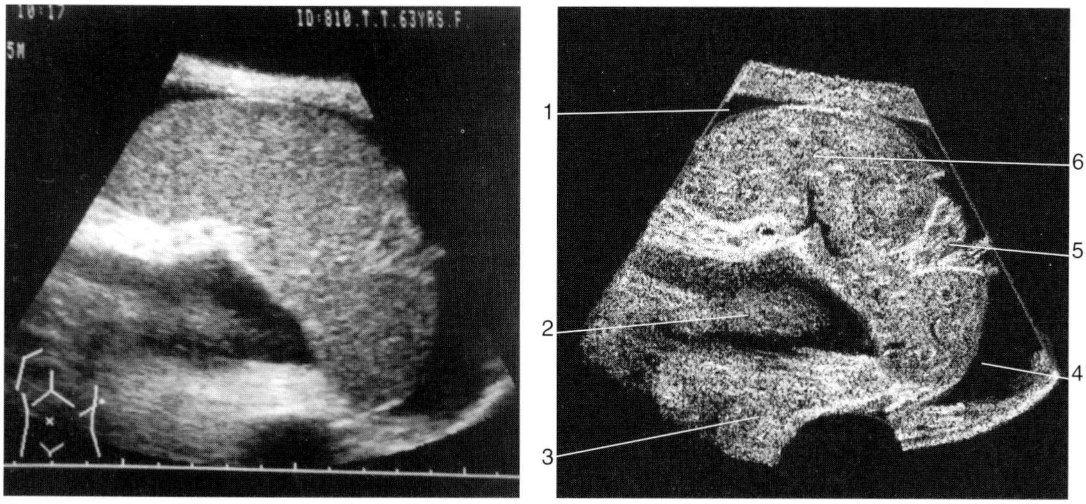

1. Ascites 2. Lesser omentum 3. Left kidney
4. Ascites 5. Infarction 6. Spleen

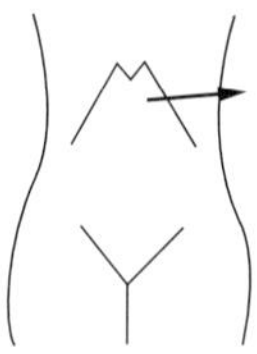

Figure 6-17. Splenic infarction.
Various sonographic characteristics of splenic infarction have been reported, mostly in cases of portal congestion. The incidence of secondary splenic infarction is also increasing rapidly following the introduction of transarterial embolization, for example, in inoperable hepatocellular carcinoma. The sonogram shows a relatively fresh splenic infarction in such a case. On the lateral border of the enlarged spleen, a triangular infarction is imaged via a left intercostal scan. Accumulation of ascitic fluid is demonstrated.

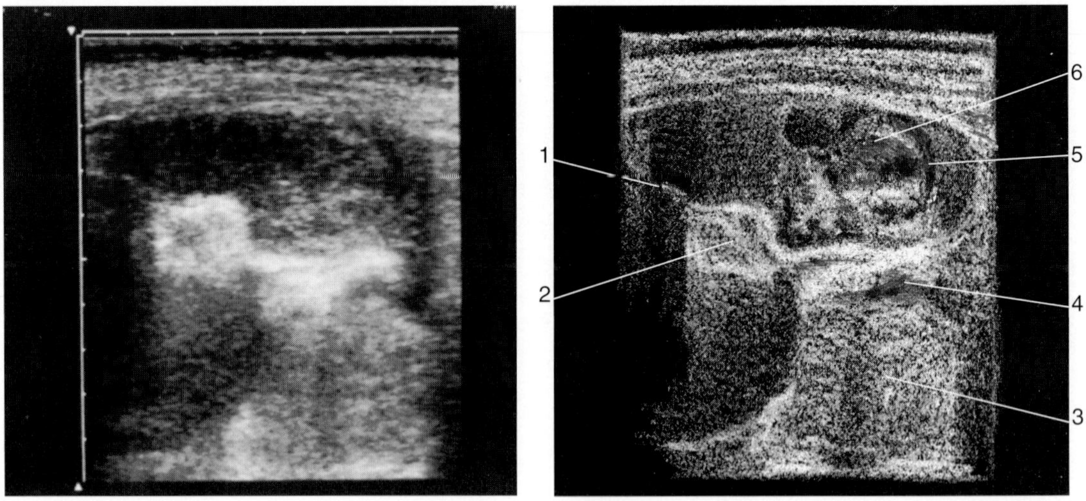

1. Spleen 2. Splenic hilum 3. Posterior echo enhancement 4. Intestine 5. Anechoic rim (subcapsular bleeding) 6. Hematoma (ruptured)

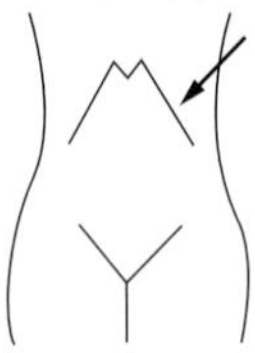

Figure 6-18. Hematoma of the spleen.
This figure shows a fresh splenic hematoma recorded by real-time ultrasound scanning of a patient 3 hr following an autombile accident, with blunt trauma of the left hypochondrium. A partially marginatcd, round, cxpanding lcsion with a complex stellate echo pattern is found at the midportion of the spleen, accompanied by a thin, hypoechoic slit suggesting bleeding into the splenic parenchyma. The round hematoma is also accompanied by marked distal echo enhancement, indicating decreased attenuation by the hematoma.

MALIGNANT TUMORS

Primary malignant tumors of the spleen are extremely rare. Generally they are sarcomas such as malignant hemangioendothelioma. Metastatic tumors in the spleen are also uncommon, and in most instances occur along with generalized metastatic involvement of other organs.[32, 36, 51] Examples of tumors that metastasize to the spleen are malignant melanoma [36, 42, 56] (Figure 6-19), and occasionally lung or breast cancers[32, 50, 51] (Figures 6-20 and 6-21).

Contiguous spread of carcinoma from neighboring organs is also infrequent; however, continuous spread from the stomach or pancreas can occur. Intraperitoneal dissemination in ovarian cancer is well recognized (Figure 6-22).

Nonepithelial splenic malignancies of hematological origin can create discrete tumor mass(es) in the parenchyma of the spleen.[1, 3, 5, 11] As shown in Figure 6-11, Hodgkin's disease, non-Hodgkin's lymphoma and lymphatic leukemia can cause single or multiple tumor masses of low echogenicity in the splenic parenchyma [52, 60, 63] (Figure 6-23). Regression can be demonstrated following successful antileukemic treatment, however, complete eradication of the mass rarely occurs.[28]

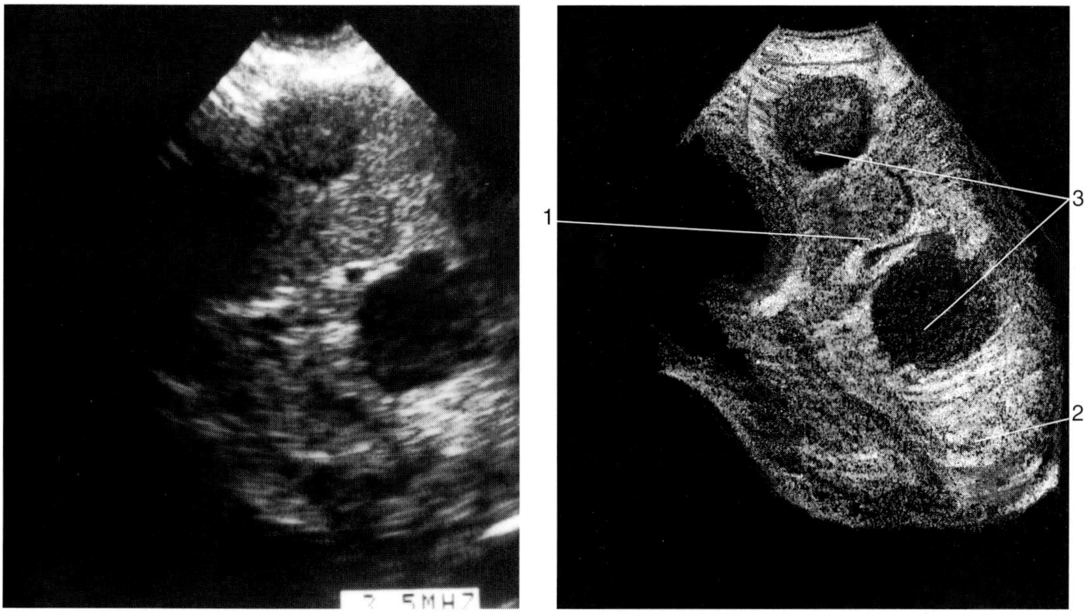

1. Spleen 2. Posterior echo enhancement
3. Melanoma metastasis

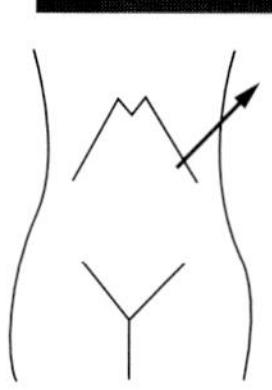

Figure 6-19. Malignant melanoma of the spleen.
Metastatic spread to the spleen is rare compared to spread to the liver; metastasis from disseminated melanoma is most frequently observed. Two echo-poor masses with irregular contours were found in the splenic parenchyma. Echo enhancement is noted distal to one nodule indicating lower attenuation by the tumor tissue (Courtesy of Dr. Schmillevitch, São Paulo, Brazil).

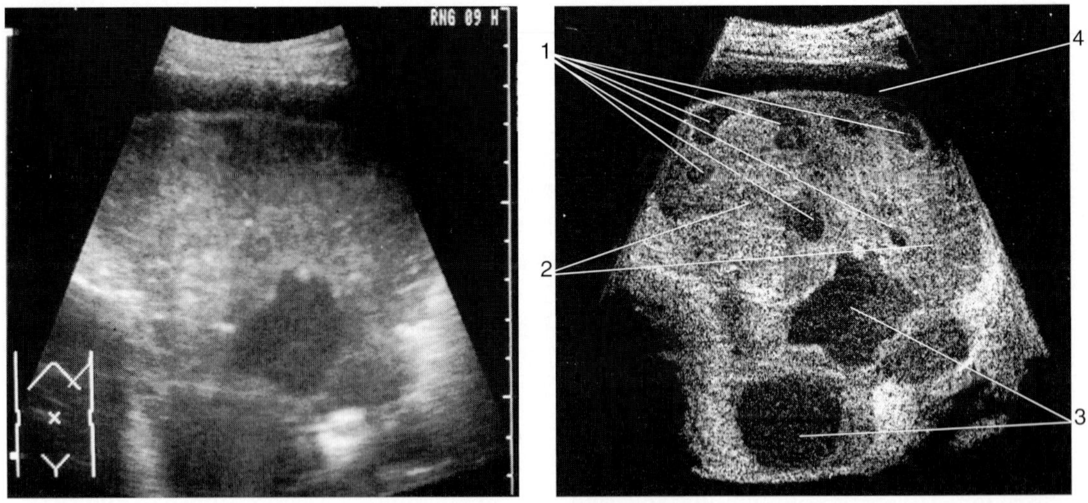

1. Metastatic tumors 2. Spleen 3. Metastatic tumors (hypoechoic) 4. Ascites

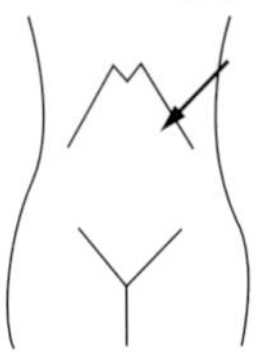

Figure 6-20. Metastatic splenic tumor in lung carcinoma.
Splenic sonograms obtained from a patient suffering from anaplastic bronchial carcinoma disclosed tumor masses with irregular contour and generally decreased echo levels together with ascites.

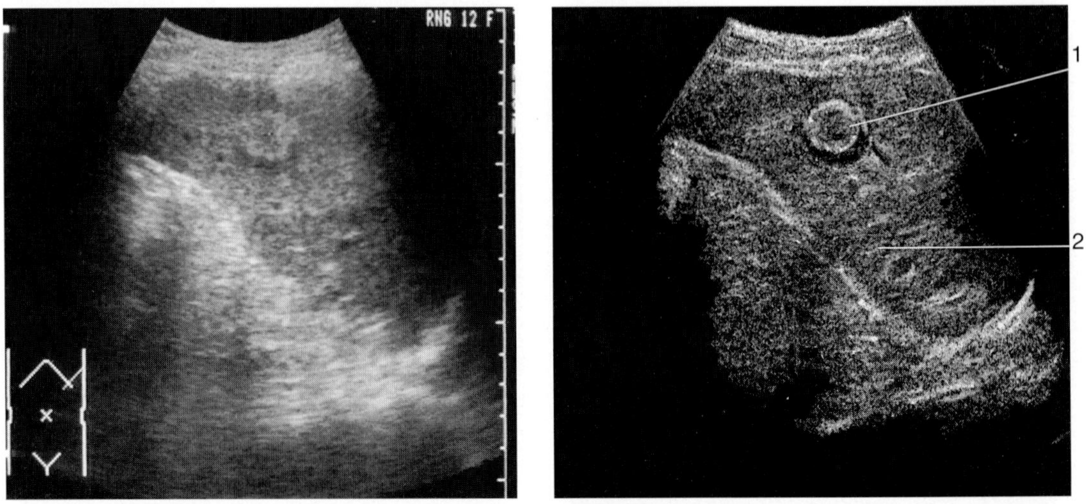

1. Echogenic mass with hypoechoic rim 2. Spleen

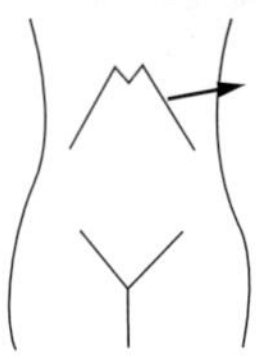

Figure 6-21. Metastatic tumor of the spleen of breast carcinoma.
Less frequently, splenic metastasis occurs from breast carcinoma. An ill-defined, slightly echogenic tumor mass surrounded by a hypoechoic rim was demonstrated in this minimally enlarged spleen. Neither acoustic enhancement nor attenuation was found.

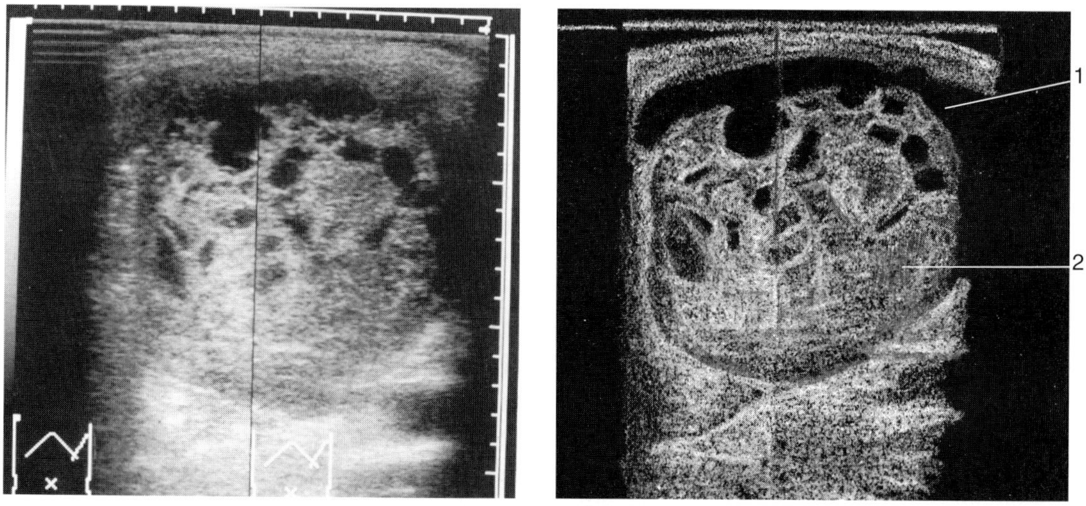

1. Spleen 2. Mixed type tumor (ovarian cancer origin)

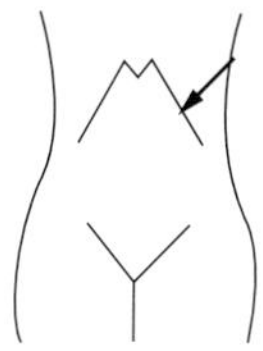

Figure 6-22. Metastatic tumor of the spleen from ovarian carcinoma.
A round tumor mass with a complex echo pattern was visualized in a follow-up study of a female patient with a previous history of ovarian carcinoma. The diagnosis was suggested by the similarity of the echo pattern to the appearance of the primary tumor and also by the presence of identical metastasis in the liver.

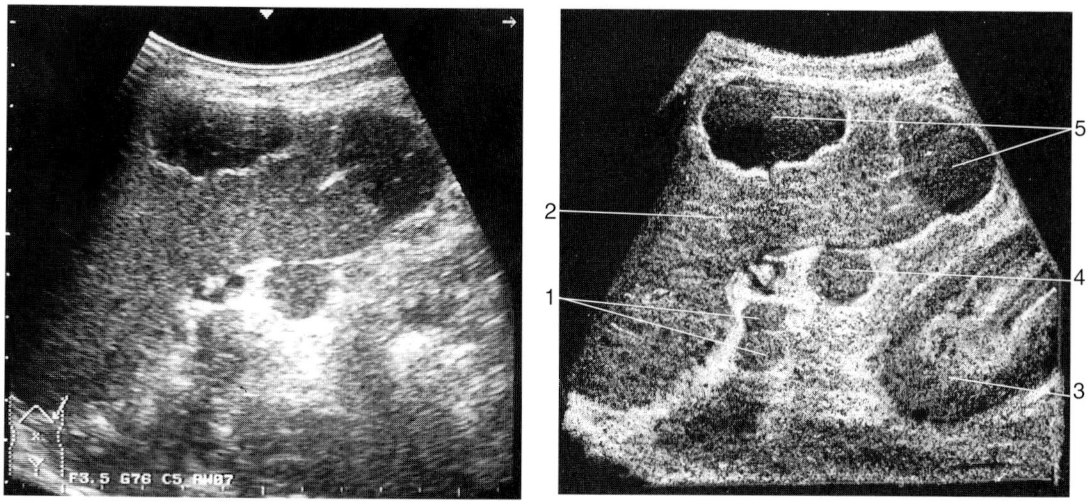

1. Lymph nodes 2. Spleen 3. Left kidney 4. Accessory spleen 5. Hypoechoic masses

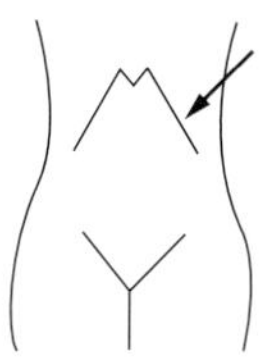

Figure 6-23. Hypoechoic splenic masses in B-cell leukemia.
In leukemia, splenic sonograms generally show diffuse enlargement reflecting infiltration of leukemia cells into the splenic parenchyma. However, it is not so uncommon to see localized lesions in the spleen as well. Two localized lesions with irregular contours and decreased echo levels were found in the spleen of this patient with B-cell lymphatic leukemia. Following combined chemotherapy, the lymphadenopathy and intrasplenic masses decreased slightly in size, indicating partial remission. An accessory spleen is also found at the splenic hilum.

CONDITIONS INVOLVING THE PERISPLENIC REGION

The spleen is also involved in a number of disease states not due to splenic pathology per se but rather to pathological processes around the spleen. Pancreatic pseudocysts, renal cysts, or adrenal masses may all simulate splenic lesions. Identification of the normal splenic parenchyma is helpful; this may be difficult, however, in the presence of perisplenic collections[2, 24, 25, 64] (Figure 6-24).

The differentiation of ascites from hematoma requires diagnostic tap, though a history of blunt trauma to the splenic region should raise a suspicion. The bleeding may also follow splenic portography or other penetrating wounds; the splenic hematomas produced can rupture subsequently, producing hemoperitoneum.

Hypertrophy of the left lobe of the liver can also simulate splenic enlargement, the differentiation depending upon the demonstration of normal spleen, as shown in Figure 6-25. This patient underwent successful partial hepatectomy for hepatic echinococcosis; however, the remaining lobe hypertrophied markedly, enlarging to cover the normal-sized spleen and simulating extensive splenomegaly. Careful scrutiny of the parenchymal echo pattern is necessary to avoid erroneous interpretation.

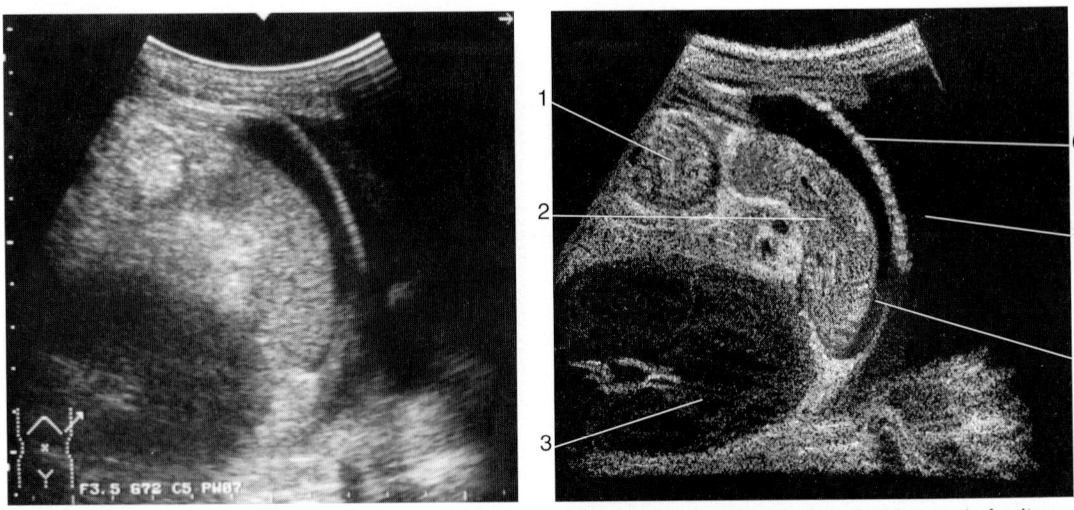

1. Intestine 2. Spleen 3. Left kidney 4. Ascites
5 Pleural fluid 6. Diaphragm

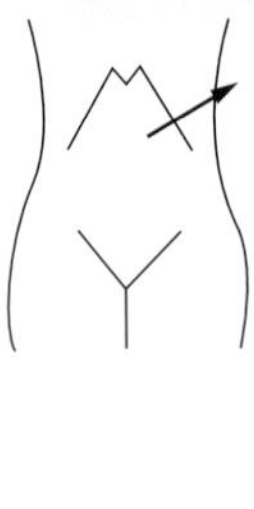

Figure 6-24. Delineation of the spleen by ascitic fluid accumulation.
Accumulation of ascitic fluid often delineate the spleen floating in the fluid. This case showed an entirely normal spleen in the ascites, renal insufficiency was the cause. Part of a swollen, hypoechoic kidney was visualized in the lower left portion of the image. There was also a pleural effusion.

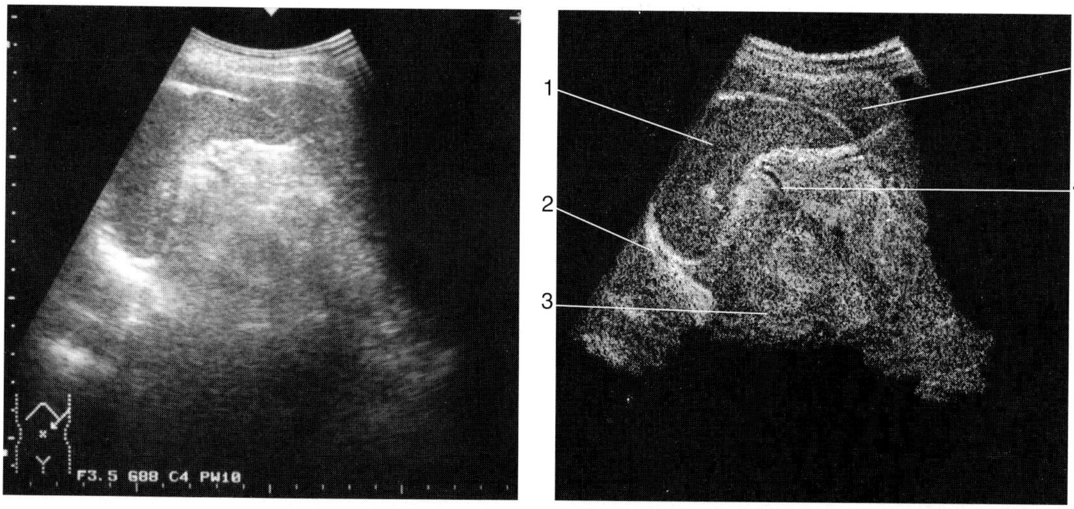

a

1. Spleen 2. Diaphragm 3. Small intestine 4. Splenic vessel 5. Enlarged left lobe of liver

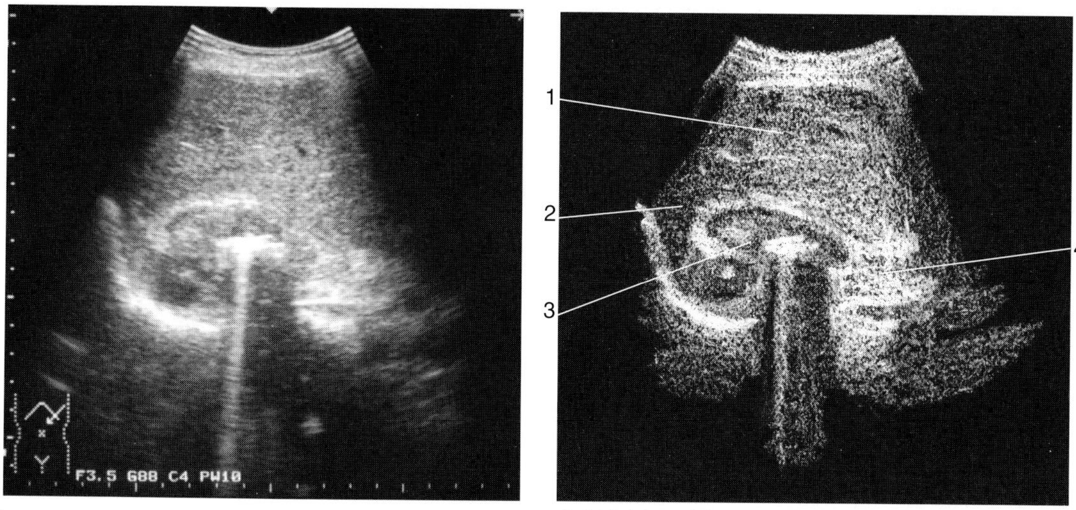

b

1. Left lobe of liver 2. Spleen 3. Stomach 4. Left kidney

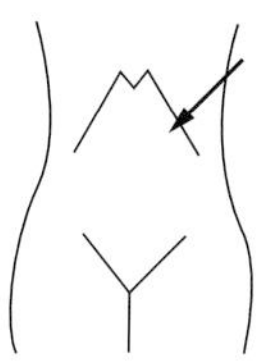

Figure 6-25. A normal spleen simulating splenomegaly.
In patients with massive enlargement of the liver, a normal sized spleen may seem to be enlarged, being imaged together with the enlarged left lobe of the liver. This patient made a complete recovery after extensive hepatectomy for involvement of the right lobe by Echinococcus granulosus. However, hypertrophy of the remaining left lobe of the liver lying between the rib cage and the spleen displaced the normal spleen inferiorly, simulating splenomegaly. The liver boundary was defined in intercostal sonograms at the 8th intercostal space; this demarcated the spleen, with its entirely normal echo texture, from the hypertrophied left lobe of the liver. The similarity in echogenicity of the liver and spleen on modern equipment further complicated the interpretation.

ANOMALIES

Congenital variations of the spleen include asplenia, splenic separation, accessory spleen, and polysplenia with multiple small spleens.[9, 12, 14, 19, 26, 47, 49, 58] Wandering spleen, alternatively known as the floating spleen or splenic ptosis, is rare.[18]

Accessory spleen, on the other hand, commonly occur at the hilar region (Figure 6-26). The result of failure of fusion of one small splenic mass during fetal development, it is reported to have an incidence of more than 10 % at necropsy. It is completely asymptomatic. Splenculi are seen as round or oval masses with internal echoes identical to those of the spleen, though they are easily confused with lesions such as lymphadenopathy, pancreatic or adrenal tumors.

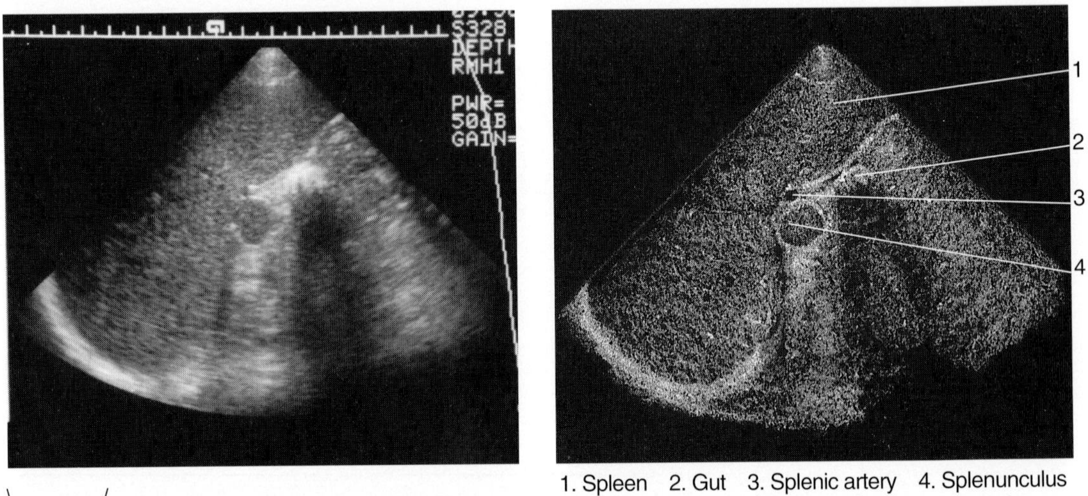

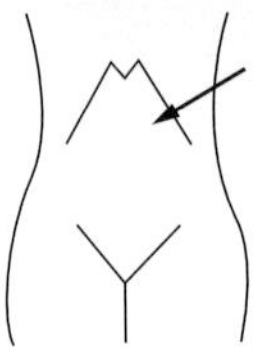

Figure 6-26. Accessory spleen.
Accessory spleen is found in 10 % of patients at careful autopsy. Though usually too small to be demonstrated on ultrasound, larger splenunculi are visualized as rounded nodules with the same pattern as the spleen, often located close to its hilum. Distinction from an enlarged node may be difficult. The texture and typical position is helpful features, but a careful search must be made for additional masses if lymphadenopathy is suspected.

REFERENCES

1. Ahmann DL, Kiely JM, Harrison EG, et al: Malignant lymphoma of the spleen. Cancer 19 : 461-469, 1966.
2. Asher WM, Parvin S, Virgillo RW, et al: Echographic evaluation of splenic injury after blunt trauma. Radiology 118 : 411-415, 1976.
3. Barloon TJ, Lu C: Lymphoma presenting as an abdominal mass involving an ectopic spleen. Am J Gastroenterol 79 : 684-686, 1984.
4. Berge T: Splenic metastases : Frequencies and patterns. Acta Path Microbiol Scand 82 : 499-501, 1974.
5. Brauner M, Buffard MD, Jeantils V, et al: Sonography and computed tomography of macroscopic tuberculosis of the liver. JCU 17 : 563-568, 1989.
6. Breiman RS, Castellino RA, Harell GS, et al: CT-pathologic correlations in Hodgkin's disease and non-Hodgkin's lymphoma. Radiology 126 : 159-166, 1978.
7. Brinkley AA, Lee JKT: Cystic hamartoma of the spleen : CT and sonographic findings. JCU 9 : 136-138, 1981.
8. Chulay JD, Landerani MR: Splenic abscess: Report of ten cases and review of the literature. Am J Med 61 : 513-522, 1976.
9. Clark RE, Korobkin M, Palubinskas AJ: Angiography of accessory spleens. Radiology 102 : 41-44, 1972.
10. Cooperberg P: Ultrasonography of the spleen, in Sarti DA, Sample WF (eds), Diagnostic Ultrasound: Text and Cases. Boston, GK Hall, 1980, pp244-245.
11. Cunningham JJ: Ultrasonic findings in isolated lymphoma of the spleen simulating splenic abscess. JCU 6 : 412-414, 1978.
12. D'Altorio RA, Cano JY: Upside-down spleen as cause of suprarenal mass. Urology 11 : 442-444, 1978.
13. Daneman A, Martin DJ: Congenital epithelial splenic cysts in children. Emphasis on sonographic appearances and some unusual features. Pediatr Radiol 12 : 119-125, 1982.
14. DeMaeyer P, Wilms G, Baert AL: Polysplenia. J Comput Assist Tomogr 5 : 104-105, 1981.
15. Dittrich M, Milde S, Dinkel E, et al: Sonographic biometry of liver and spleen size in children. Pediatr Radiol 13 : 206-211, 1983.
16. Ein SH, Shandling B, Simpson JS, et al: Nonoperative management of traumatic spleen in children: How and why. J Pediatr Surg 113 : 117-119, 1978.
17. Frank K, Linhart P, Bettendorf U, Christl HL: Sonographic determination of spleen size and spleen weight. Ultraschall Med 5 : 104-107, 1984.
18. Glees JP, Taylor KJW, Gazet JC, et al: Accuracy of gray scale ultrasonography of liver and spleen in Hodgkin's disease and other lymphomas compared with isotope scans. Clin Radiol 28 : 233-238, 1977.
19. Gordon DH, Burrell MI, Levin DC, et al: Wandering spleen: The radiological and clinical spectrum. Radiology 125 : 39-46, 1977.
20. Heartzanu Y, Mendelsohn DB, Goudie E, et al: Splenic abscess: A review with the value of ultrasound. Clin Radiol 34 : 661-667, 1983.
21. Hertzanu Y, Mendelsohn DB: Delayed splenic rupture: A true entity. Clin Radiol 35 : 393-396, 1984.
22. Honegger HP, Otto R, Maurer R, et al: What does computer tomography and abdominal ultrasound studies accomplish in the staging of Hodgkin's disease? Schweiz Med Wschr 114 : 475-481, 1984.
23. Hunter TB, Haber K: Unusual sonographic appearance of the spleen in a case of myelofibrosis. AJR 128 : 138-139, 1977.
24. Johnson MA, Cooperberg PL, Boisvert J, et al: Spontaneous splenic rupture in infectious mononucleosis : Sonographic diagnosis and follow-up. AJR 136 : 111-114, 1981.
25. Kathrein H, Judmaier G: Sonographic study of the spleen and retroperitoneal space-occupying masses. Wien Med Wochenschr 133 : 489-494, 1983.
26. Katz JF, Kane RA: Sonographic appearance of accessory spleen. JCU 12 : 163-165,1984.
27. Kim EE: Focal splenic defect. Semin Nucl Med 9 : 320-321, 1979.
28. King DJ, Dawson AA, Bayliss AP: The value of ultrasonic scanning of the spleen in lymphoma. Clin Radiol 36 : 473-474, 1985.
29. Koga, T: Correlation between sectional area of the spleen by ultrasonic tomography and actual volume of the removed spleen. JCU 7 : 119-120, 1979.
30. Kuntz DJ, Leonard-Kitschke RM, et al: An evaluation of diagnostic techniques utilized in the initial workup of pediatric patients with acute lymphocytic leukemia. Clin Nucl Med 9 : 405-408, 1984.
31. Lupien C, Sauerbrei EE : Healing in the traumatized spleen: Sonographic investigation. Radiology 151 : 181-185, 1984.
32. Manor A, Starinsky R, Garfinkel D, et al: Ultrasound features of asymptomatic splenic hemangioma. JCU

12 : 95-97, 1984.

33. Maresca G, Mirk P, De Gaetano M, et al: Sonographic patterns in splenic infarct. JCU 14 : 23-28, 1986.
34. Marymount JH, Gross S: Patterns of metastatic cancer in the spleen. Am J Clin Path 40 : 58-66, 1963.
35. Mittelstaedt CA, McCartney WH, Mauro MA, et al: Spleen, in Simeone J (ed), Clinics in Diagnostic Ultrasound: Coordinated Diagnostic Imaging. New York, Churchill Livingstone, 1984, pp235-273.
36. Mittelstaedt CA, Partain CL: Ultrasonic-pathologic classification of splenic abnormalities: Gray-scale patterns. Radiology 134 : 697-705, 1980.
37. Moran C, Geisse G: Epidermoid cysts of the spleen. J Can Assoc Radiol 28 : 150-152, 1977.
38. Murphy JF, Bernardino ME: The sonographic findings of splenic metastases. JCU 7 : 195-197, 1979.
39. Myers MJ: Spleen imaging. Clin Haematol 12 : 395-420, 1983.
40. Niederau C, Sonnenberg A, Muller JE, et al: Sonographic measurements of the normal liver, spleen, pancreas and portal vein. Radiology 149 : 537-540, 1983.

40a. Niizawa M, Ishida H, Morikawa P, et al: Color Doppler sonography in a case of splenic hemangioma: Value of compressing the tumor. AJR 157 : 965-966, 1991.

41. Okuda K, Taguchi T, Ishinara K, et al: Intrasplenic pseudocyst of the pancreas. J Clin Gstroenterol 3 : 37-41, 1981.
42. Paling MR, Shawker TH, Love I: The sonographic appearance of metastatic malignant melanoma. J Ultrasound Med 1 : 75-78, 1982.
43. Piekarski J, Federle MP, Moss AA, et al: Computed tomograpy of the spleen. Radiology 135 : 683-689, 1980.
44. Pietri H, Boscaini M: Determination of a splenic volumetric index by ultrasonic scanning. J Ultrasound Med 3 : 19-23, 1984.
45. Propper RA, Weinstein BJ, Skolnick ML, et al: Ultrasonography of hemorrhagic splenic cysts. JCU 7 : 18-20, 1979.
46. Rao BK, AuBuchon J, Lieberman LM: Cystic lymphangiomatosis of the spleen: A radiologic-pathologic correlation. Radiology 141 : 781-782, 1981.
47. Rosenkranz W, Klamhi B, Horowits M: Retroperitoneal accessory spleen simulating a suprarenal mass. Br J Radiol 42 : 939-942, 1969.
48. Rudick MG, Wood BP, Lerner RM: Splenic abscess diagnosed by ultrasound in the pediatric patient : Report of three cases. Pediatr Radiol 13 : 269-271, 1983.
49. Setiawan H, Harrell RS, Perret RS: Ectopic spleen. A sonographic diagnosis. Pediatr Radiol 12 : 152-153, 1982.
50. Shanser JD, Moss AA, Clark RE, et al: Angiographic evaluation of cystic lesions of the spleen. AJR 119 : 166-174, 1973.
51. Shirkhoda A, McCartoney WH, Staab EV, et al: Imaging of the spleen: A proposed algorithm. AJR 135 : 195-198, 1980.
52. Siler J, Hunter TB, Weiss J, et al: Increased echogenicity of the spleen in benign and malignant disease. AJR 134 : 1011-1014, 1980.
53. Solbiati L, Bossi MC, Bellotti E, et al: Focal lesions in the spleen: Sonographic patterns and guided biopsy. AJR 140 : 59-65, 1983.
54. Sommer FG, Hoppe RT, Fellingham L, et al: Spleen structure in Hodgkin disease: Ultrasonic characterization. Work in progress. Radiology 153 : 219-222, 1984.
55. Steinmaurer HJ, Jirak P, Walchshofer J, et al: Accuracy of sonography in the diagnosis of diffuse liver parenchymal diseases: Comparison of sonography and liver histology. Ultraschall Med 5 : 98-103, 1984.
56. Stutte H, Muller PH, d'Hoedt B, et al: Ultrasonographic diagnosis of melanoma metastasis in liver, gallbladder and spleen. J Ultrasound Med 8 : 541-547, 1989.
57. Subramanyam BR, Balthazar EJ, Raghavendra BN, et al: Sonographic evaluation of patients with portal hypertension. Am J Gastroenterol 78 : 369-373, 1983.
58. Subramanyam BR, Balthazar EJ, Horii SC: Sonography of the accessory spleen. AJR 143 : 47-49, 1984.
59. Taniguchi N, Itoh K, Mori H, et al: Echographic study of focal lesions in the spleen. Jap J Med Ultrason 16 : 438-447,1989.
60. Takayasu K, Moriyama N, Muramatsu K, et al: Splenic infarction, a complication of transcatheter hepatic arterial embolization. AJR 151 : 371-375, 1984.
61. Vansonnenberg E, Simeone JF, Mueller PR, et al: Sonographic appearance of hematoma in liver, spleen and kidney: A clinical, pathologic, and animal study. Radiology 147 : 507-510, 1983.
62. Verheyden CN, Van Heerden JA, Carney JA: Symptomatic metastatic melanoma of the spleen. Minn Med 57 : 693-696, 1974.
63. Vicary FR, Souhami RL: Ultrasound and Hodgkin's disease of the spleen. Br J Radiol 50 : 521-522, 1977.

64. Vick CW, Simeone JF, Ferrucci JT, et al: Pancreatitis associated fluid collections involving the spleen: Sonographic and computed tomographic appearance. Gastrointest Radiol 6 : 247-250, 1981.
65. Weill F, Didier D, Coche G: Ultrasound of the traumatized spleen: Left butterfly sign in lesions masked by echogenic blood clot. Gastrointest Radiol 13 : 169-172, 1988.
66. Weingarten MJ, Fakhry J, McCarthy J, et al: Sonography after splenic embolization: The wedge-shaped acute infarct. AJR 141 : 957-959, 1983.

CHAPTER 7

THE KIDNEYS AND RETROPERITONEUM

NORMAL ANATOMY

The Retroperitoneum

The central ridge formed by the spine determines the shape of the retroperitoneum and thus the disposition of the soft tissue organs within it[22,49] (Figures 7-1 and 7-2). Midline structures lie anteriorly, often to a surprising extent, so that, for example, the neck of the pancreas may be only a few centimeters below the surface in a thin subject. Structures that run transversely are more anteriorly placed at the midline. The duodenum is an example where the second part lies posteriorly to the right, with the third and fourth parts sweeping anteriorly across the midline. The long left renal vein passes anteriorly from the hilum of the left kidney, crossing over the aorta to reach the inferior vena cava.

The forward curve of the lumbar lordosis also brings inferior structures relatively anteriorly. Thus the aortic bifurcation may lie only a few centimeters deep to the skin. The psoas muscle, arising from the bodies of lower thoracic and lumbar vertebrae, sweeps anteriorly as it passes down over the iliac bone to fuse with the iliacus muscle, both inserting on the femur. The kidney lies on the quadratus lumborum muscle, with the psoas posteromedially. The lower poles of the kidneys are tilted anteriorly as well as laterally by the increasing bulk of the psoas as it thickens inferiorly.

The retroperitoneal space contains the great vessels, the kidneys, the adrenals, and the pancreas together with their blood vessels and lymphatics. Fatty tissue fills the spaces between the organs. It is divided into two compartments by a fascial sheet of variable integrity known as the renal or Gerota's fascia; it surrounds the kidneys and adrenals and separates the perirenal from the pararenal spaces. The perirenal space is continuous across the midline and encloses the great vessels. Gerota's fascia is open inferiorly, so that here the two spaces merge. When well formed, it acts to confine inflammatory and malignant processes.

A foramen of the diaphragm at T-12 marks the level of entry of the aorta in the abdomen[38] (Figure 7-3). It is formed by the two diaphragmatic crura, which cross over the anterior wall of the aorta and then pass inferiorly along the vertebrae, attaching to them as far down as L-4. The uppermost portion of the aorta seen on ultrasound is actually intrathoracic and lies in the retrocrural space. From here the aorta passes inferiorly, closely applied to the spine, to its bifurcation into the common iliac arteries at approximately the umbilical level (L-4/L-5). It tapers steadily from a maximum luminal diameter of 2.5 cm superiorly to 1.5 cm at the bifurcation.[42] The midline celiac axis (or trunk) and superior mesenteric artery are usually well visualized on ultrasound, whereas the inferior mesenteric artery is generally obscured by gassy bowel. Of the paired branches, the renal arteries are often visualized but the smaller vessels (intercostals, lumbars) are rarely delineated.

The inferior vena cava, lying to the right of the aorta and originating from the common iliac veins at umbilical level, has a somewhat different course (Figure 7-4). It passes to the right superiorly and curves anteriorly to an indentation on the posterior surface of the liver, where it is embedded just below the diaphragm. The hepatic veins enter the cava here and lie very close to the diaphragm (see Chapter 3). Immediately above the diaphragm, the inferior vena cava discharges directly into the right atrium. The renal veins join the inferior vena cava in the epigastrium, that from the right kidney being very short and running anteromedially since the inferior vena cava often overlies the medial portion of the kidney. The left renal vein is longer, passing anteromedially from the renal hilum between the aorta and the superior mesenteric artery before discharging into the cava. It often appears to be compromised as it crosses the aorta, with a wider upstream portion.[52] There are no other large tributaries to the inferior vena cava, all of the flow from the splanchnic bed passing via the portal venous system.

Imaging of the superior parts of the aorta and inferior vena cava is usually straightforward, using the liver as a window. Below this level, intestinal gas tends to interfere and may preclude adequate viewing. Using a sector scanner, it is often possible to find a window through which exposure can be maximized. With persistent, gentle probe pressure it is often possible to move enough gas out of the way to obtain good images. An alternative view through the flank in the coronal plane often allows the great vessels to be imaged in their entirety(Figure 7-3b). If the patient is turned into the decubitus position, the intestines drop forward, improving visualization.[27]

The aorta is seen as an echo-free space with echogenic walls. The walls taper smoothly except where atheroma produces irregularity. Pulsation in the aorta consists of simple expansion in systole. The inferior vena cava, on the other hand, undergoes a more complex opening and closing movement in sympathy with the right atrial pressure changes. It has thinner walls, and its lumen varies from round to slit-like, presumably with hydration and cardiovascular status, since it acts as a blood pool (so-called capacitance vessel). Moving particles of low reflectivity are often visible in the inferior vena cava. They are due to red cell aggregates and provide useful confirmation of caval patency. Doppler (pulsed or color flow) is a more precise method of demonstrating essentially the same phenomenon.

The Kidneys

The paired kidneys usually lie in the upper abdomen in the paraspinal gutters. They rest on the muscles of the posterior abdominal wall (quadratus lumborum and trapezius) and the lowest ribs (12, 11, and sometimes 10 as well). Anteriorly, the kidneys are covered by peritoneum with the hepatorenal recess (Morison's pouch) separating the right kidney from the liver. Often the gallbaldder overlies the kidney here, with the duodenum anteromedially. On the left, the spleen lies superiorly and the stomach anteromedially, both separated by peritoneum. The tail of the pancreas crosses the upper pole of the left kidney as it passes toward the splenic hilum. On both sides, the lower portions of the kidneys are covered by colon. Since these portions of the gut are usually gas-filled, they limit access to the kidneys from in front. Access posteriorly is usually possible, though the sound beam has to traverse the paraspinal muscles and their fascial layers, which distort the beam and degrade the images. Views from the flanks in the coronal plane are ideal and have the added advantage of displaying the kidney sectioned along its anatomical axis.

Renal position is very variable. Since the kidneys are not firmly anchored in the retroperitoneum, they drop inferiorly on standing, move with breathing, and are easily displaced by nearby space-occupying lesions. Congenital variations include ectopia (e.g., crossed, pelvic) and duplication, as well as atresia. In the horseshoe kidney, the lower poles are fused across the midline (usually at umbilical level) and the renal sinuses face anteriorly.

Each bean-shaped kidney consists of a set of about 12 lobes arranged around the hilum, which faces anteromedially and through which the blood vessels and ureters pass[1, 12] (Figure 7-5). Each lobe is bilayered, with a peripheral zone, the cortex (containing the glomeruli and convoluted tubules) encasing the central medullary region on three sides. The medulla, which contains tubules and collecting ducts only, is pyramid-shaped, with its apex, the papilla, facing the hilum. Each papilla protrudes into a calyx, into which its tubules discharge urine. The calyces join to form the renal pelvis which empties into the upper ureter. This lobar architecture of the kidney is sometimes apparent as grooves on the renal surface and, since the lobes vary somewhat in size, the thickness of the cortical layers may vary, especially where the layers are contiguous between two pyramids, the septa of Bertin.[41] When prominent ("hypertrophic"), they may simulate a space-occupying lesion radiologically.[34] When the embryological lobes fuse into two groups instead of one, a duplex kidney is formed. A continuum of variations occurs, from totally separated moieties (rare) to minor variations in which the calyces form discrete upper and lower groups. When there are two ureters, it is common for the upper one to have a compromised junction with the bladder, producing hydronephrosis of the upper moiety.

On ultrasound the kidney appears as an oval with a pole-to-pole length of 9 to 12 cm[4] (Figures 7-6 to 7-8). The central portion, the renal sinus, is strongly echogenic due to the abundant interfaces produced by the blood vessels and drainage system and to the intervening fatty tissue. Short portions of the blood vessels may be discerned under good imaging conditions[9] (Figures 7-9, 7-14, and 7-15), and there may be slight separation of the pelvicalyceal walls in patients undergoing diuresis[11] (Figure 7-10). This physiological distention can be increased by a full bladder, a condition that often obtains when pelvic scanning is carried out, and the maximum separation can amount to 5 mm. The sinus is usually about the same thickness as one parenchymal layer, so that a "sandwich" of three equal layers is seen. However, excess fat deposition in the sinus makes it thicker (so-called sinus lipomatosis), a change that is of no pathological significance (Figure 7-11).

The portions of renal parenchyma are usually well defined, especially if high-frequency transducers are used, with the triangular, centrally situated, medullary pyramids having lower reflectivity than the surrounding cortical layer. The cortex is slightly less echogenic than the liver, with about the same reflectivity as the spleen. Arcuate vessels, lying at the corticomedullary junctions, can often be discerned as small, echogenic foci. The renal outline is usually smooth, but lobation may be detected (Figure 7-12). The fat spaces surrounding the kidney can also sometimes be made out (Figure 7-13), and portions of the renal vessles are usually seen (Figures 7-14 and 7-15).

In the neonate, the kidney has a somewhat different appearance; because of immaturity of the cortex, this layer is thinner than in the adult and more echogenic so the pyramids are more striking.[19, 25] They must not be mistaken for dilated calyces. Lobation is often marked.

The Adrenals

The adrenals lie superior to the kidneys, and both are in contact with the respective crus of the diaphragm medially.[22, 39] On the right, the adrenal lies posterior to the upper part of the inferior vena cava and superior to the upper pole of the kidney. It is most easily imaged in the transverse plane, taking small sector views through an intercostal space laterally and using the right lobe of the liver as a window[46] (Figure 7-16). Working superiorly from the upper pole of the kidney, the echo-poor line of the crus of the diaphragm is located up against the spine posteriorly and separating the inferior vena cava from the aorta anteriorly. The adrenal is often (but not always) imaged as a second echo-poor, linear structure posterior to the cava and close to the crus. It may also be imaged in longitudinal section lying posterior to the upper inferior vena cava.

The left adrenal lies medial to the upper pole of the kidney with the aorta lying medial to it. Working in the coronal plane in the triangle between the upper pole and the spleen, the crus of the diaphragm must be located running parallel to the aorta (Figure 7-17). The adrenal appears as a linear, echo-free structure lateral to the crus.

In the neonate the adrenals are much larger; with atrophy they acquire adult proportions within the first year. They are seen as layered V- or Y-shaped bands applied to the upper pole of the kidney and must not be mistaken for pathology here.

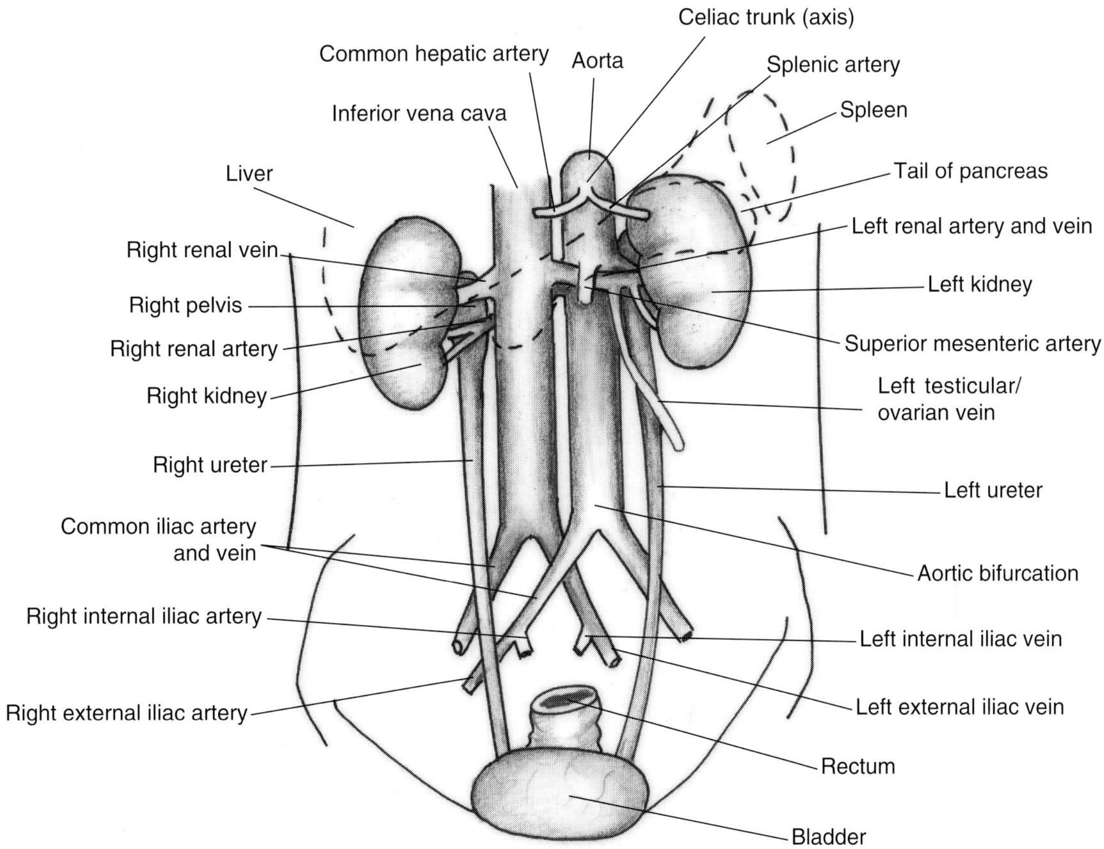

Figure 7-1. Position and relations of the kidneys.
The paired kidneys are shown from in front together with their vessels and ureters. The peritoneum has been removed. The liver, spleen, and pancreas are indicated by broken lines.

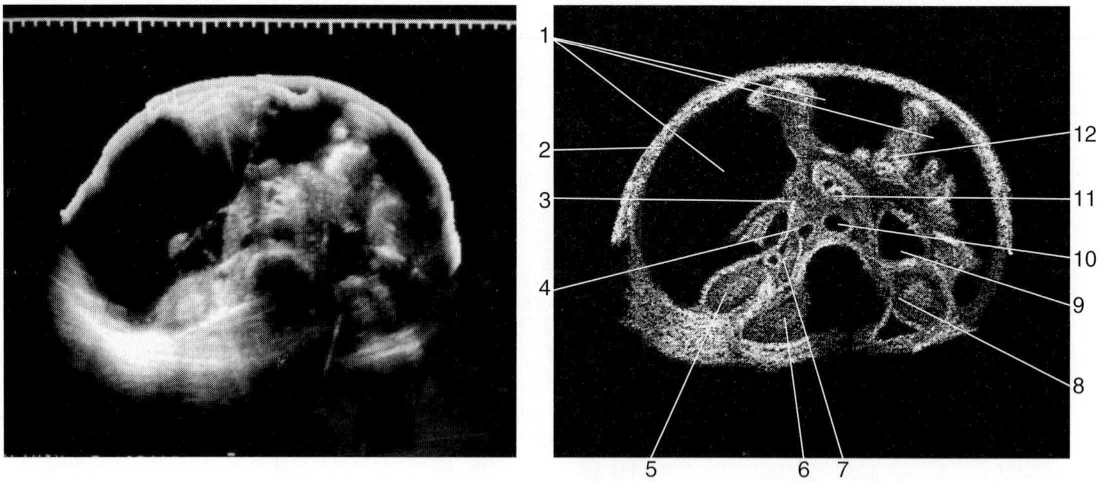

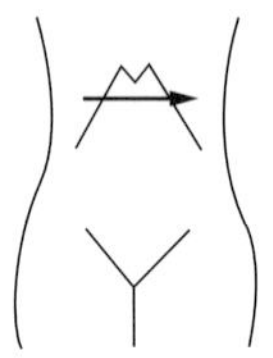

1. Greater sac 2. Parietal peritoneum 3. Visceral peritoneum 4. Inferior vena cava 5. Right kidney 6. Sacrospinalis muscle 7. Psoas muscle 8. Left kidney 9. Lateral recess of lesser sac 10. Aorta 11. Superior mesenteric artery 12. Superior mesenteric vein

Figure 7-2. The retroperitoneum, transverse section of the epigastrium.
The soft tissues of the retroperitoneum (shaded) are draped across the pronounced convexity of the spine so that the lateral structures lie relatively posteriorly. Thus the kidneys lie in a plane posterior to the great vessels, and the medial portion of the right kidney is found immediately posterior to the inferior vena cava. The renal vessels pass anteriorly from the kidneys. The pancreas also follows this anteroposterior curve, so that its neck and body lie anterior to the head on the right and even more markedly to the tail on the left.

a

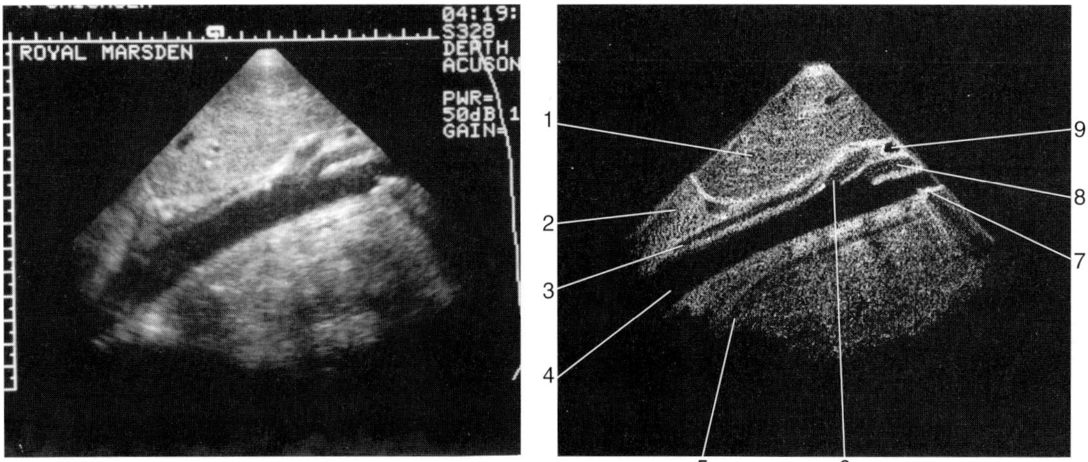

1. Left lobe of liver 2. Esophagus 3. Crus of diaphragm 4. Aorta 5. Spine 6. Celiac trunk 7. Calcific alteration with shadow 8. Superior mesenteric artery 9. Hepatic artery

b

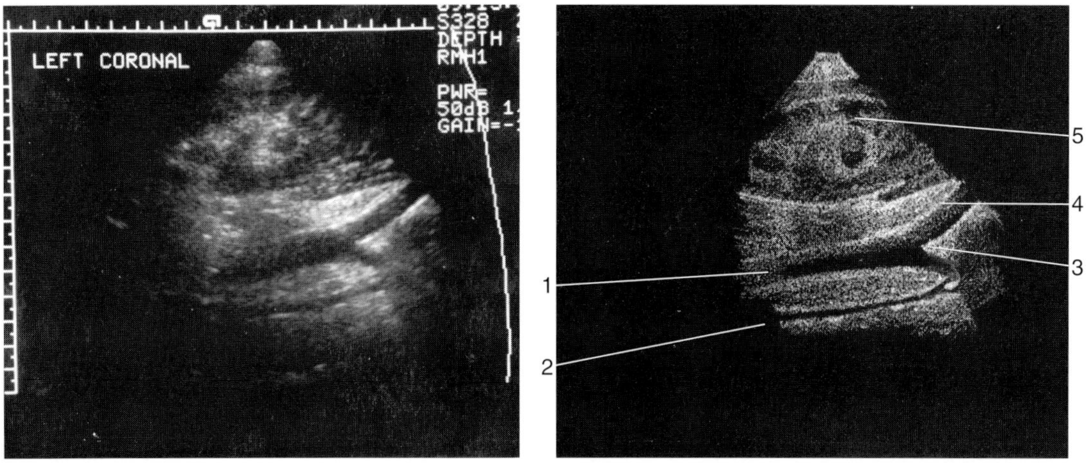

1. Aorta 2. Inferior vena cava 3. Aortic bifurcation 4. Left common iliac artery 5. Gut loops (descending colon)

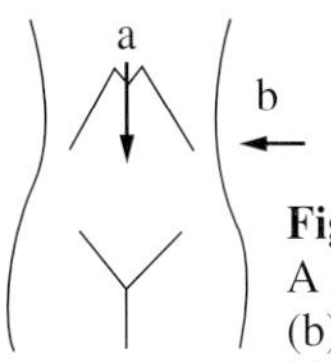

Figure 7-3. The aorta.
A midline sagittal section (a) demonstrates the aorta lying in front of the spine. In the coronal view (b) just anterior to the spine, the inferior part of the aorta can usually be demonstrated, with its bifurcation into the two common iliac arteries at the umbilical level (= L-5). The inferior vena cava lies to its right.

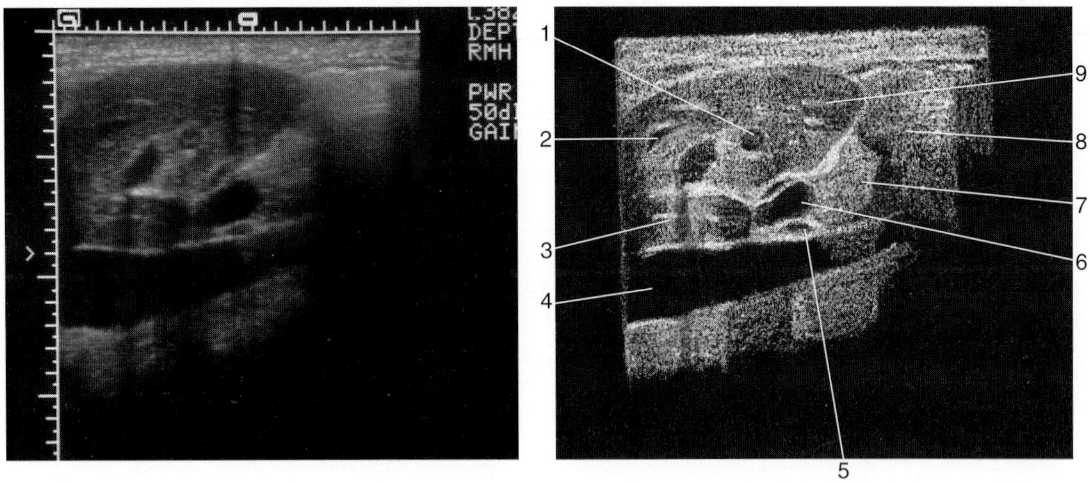

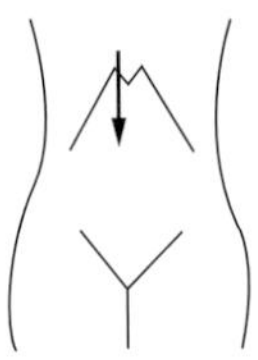

1. Left portal vein 2. Left hepatic vein 3. Caudate lobe of liver 4. Inferior vena cava 5. Hepatic artery (anomalous position) 6. Splenic vein 7. Pancreas 8. Stomach 9. Left lobe of liver

Figure 7-4. The inferior vena cava.
The origin of the inferior vena cava from the common iliac veins (at the umbilical level) is usually obscured by intestinal gas, but in the epigastrium its anterior curve can be demonstrated as it passes through the liver and diaphragm to empty into the right atrium. With a high-frequency probe, flowing particles due to red cell aggregates can often be demonstrated within it. Note the marked increase in caliber at the level where the renal veins empty into the cava.

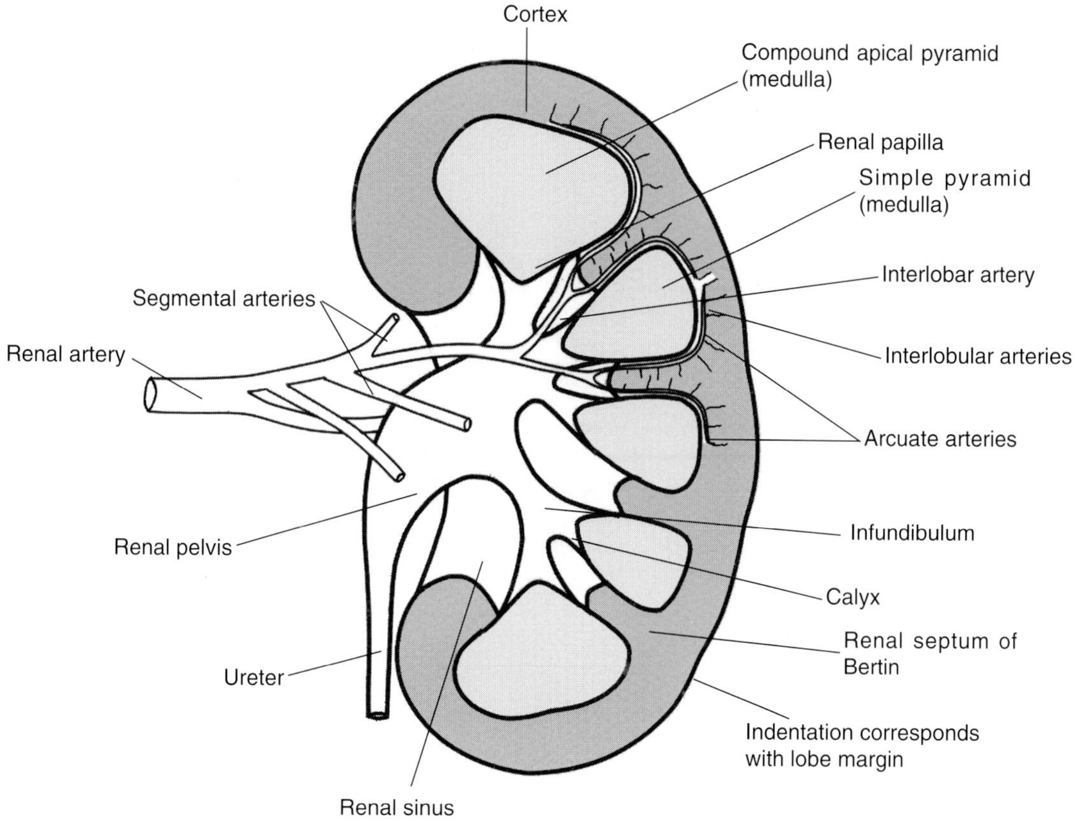

Figure 7-5. Anatomy of the kidney.
The kidney is diagrammed as though bivalved in its long axis to display the hilum. The drainage system is shown under minimal distention. Parts of the arterial system are illustrated.

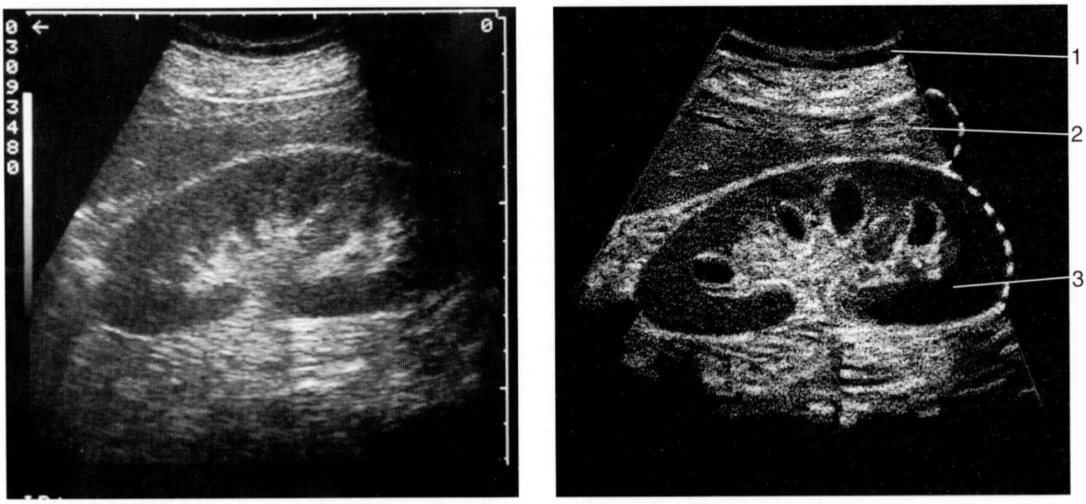

1. Skin line 2. Liver 3. Kidney

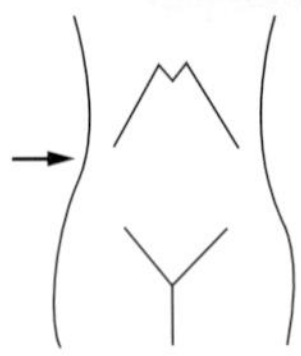

Figure 7-6. Normal kidney, coronal view.
In this section, the kidney is bivalved in its anatomical long axis through the hilum. The parenchyma is seen enveloping the sinus, which has strong echoes due to the vessels and pelvicalyceal system together with the fat occupying the intervening spaces. The lobar structure of the human kidney is well shown. Each lobe consists of a central medulla (the pyramid); its collecting ducts empty into the associated calyx, into which it protrudes. Each pyramid is surrounded by glomerular-bearing cortex, which is more echogenic.

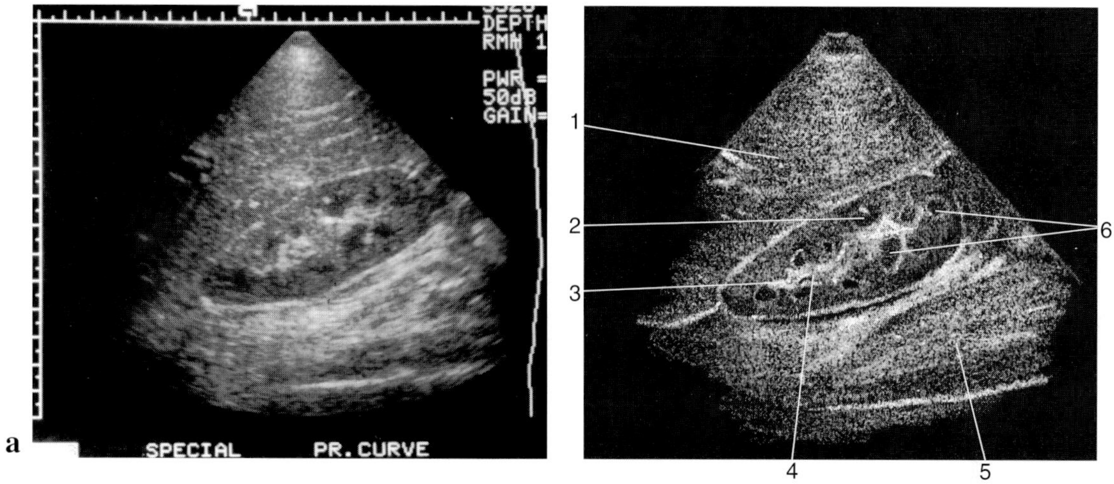

1. Liver 2. Arcuate vessel 3. Renal sinus 4. Interlobar vessels 5. Psoas muscle 6. Medullary pyramids

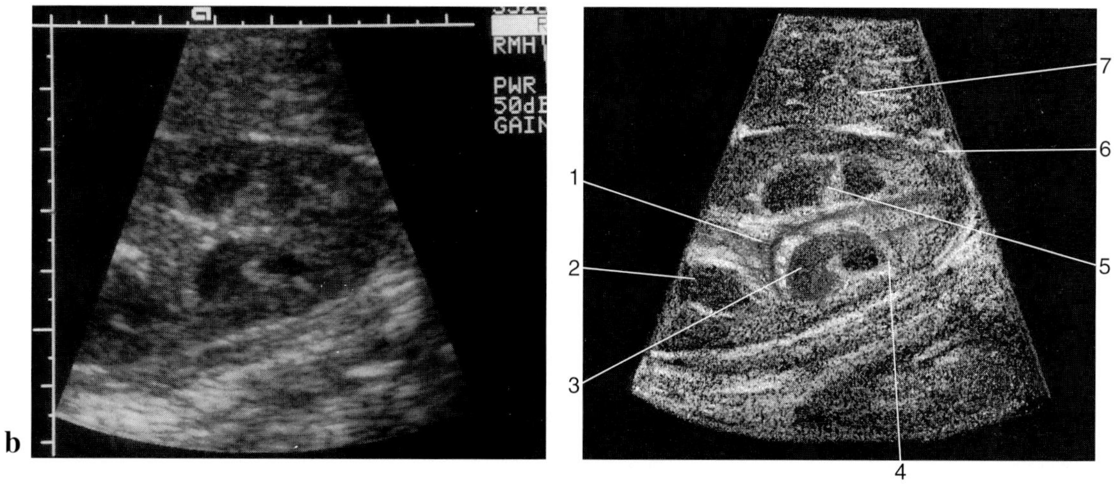

1. Renal sinus 2. Simple pyramid 3. Compound pyramid 4. Peripheral part of cortex 5. Septal part of cortex (Septum of Bertin) 6. Renal capsule 7. Liver

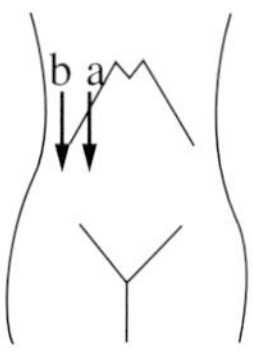

Figure 7-7. Normal kidney.
In longitudinal section the parenchyma is seen as a layer surrounding the more echogenic sinus, with its fat and blood vesssels. The parenchyma comprises the relatively echo-poor medullary pyramids, which lie centrally, surrounded by the cortical layer. Under good imaging conditions, the varying shapes of simple and compound pyramids and the position of the arcuate vessels may be discerned.

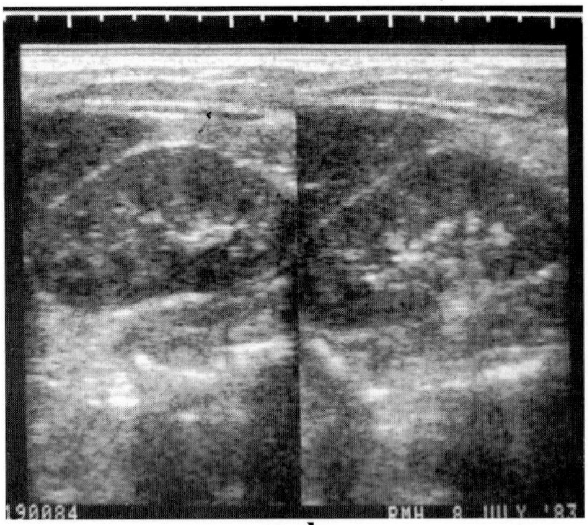

a b

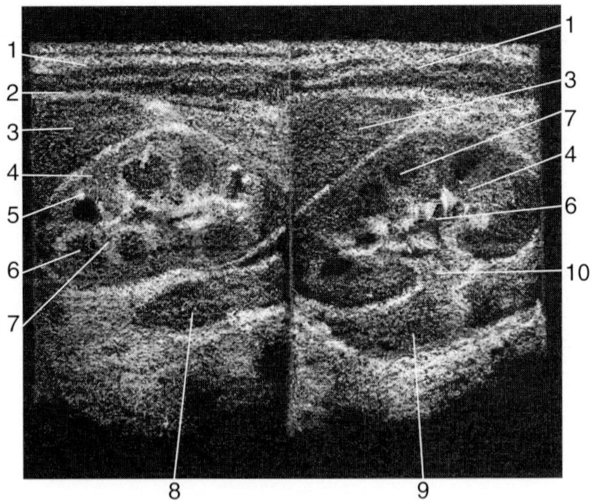

1. Abdominal wall 2. Peritoneum 3. Liver 4. Cortex 5. Arcuate vessel 6. Pyramid 7. Sinus 8. Quadratus lumborum muscle 9. Psoas muscle 10.Hilum

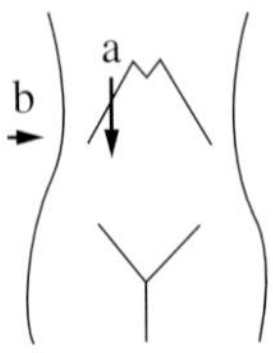

Figure 7-8. Normal kidney, linear-array scans.
The different appearances of the same kidney in sagittal (a) and coronal (b) tomograms can be appreciated in these scans. The arcuate vessels can be discerned marking the corticomedullary junction.

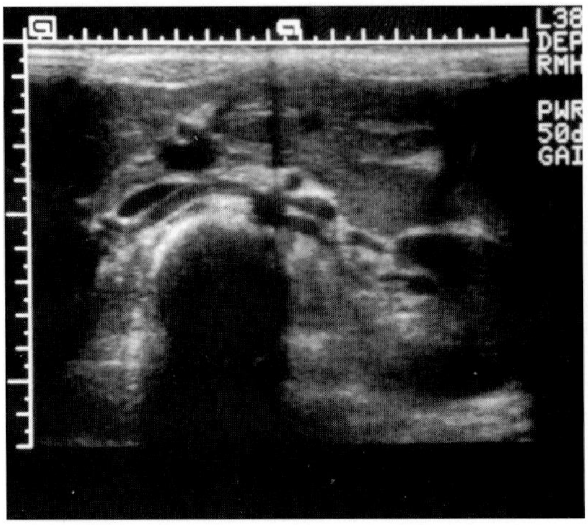

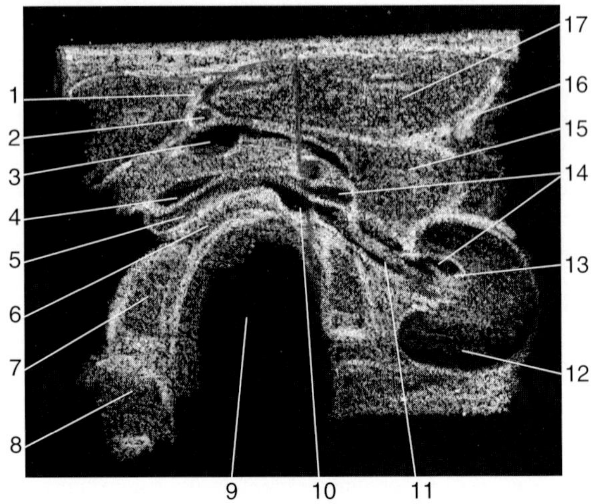

1. Ligamentum teres 2. Hepatic artery 3. Portal vein 4. Inferior vena cava 5. Right renal artery 6. Right crus 7. Psoas muscle 8. Sacrospinalis muscle 9. Spine 10. Aorta 11. Left renal artery 12. Left kidney 13. Renal hilum 14. Left renal vein 15. Tail of pancreas 16. Stomach 17. Left lobe of liver

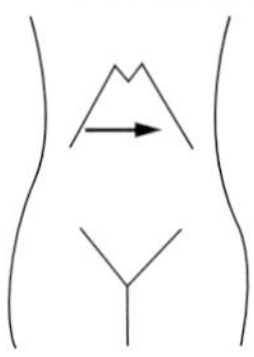

Figure 7-9. The renal hilum.
In transverse section the anteromedial lie of the sinus is shown. Portions of the renal vessels are imaged; the veins lie anterior, as is the rule in the upper part of the abdomen.

a

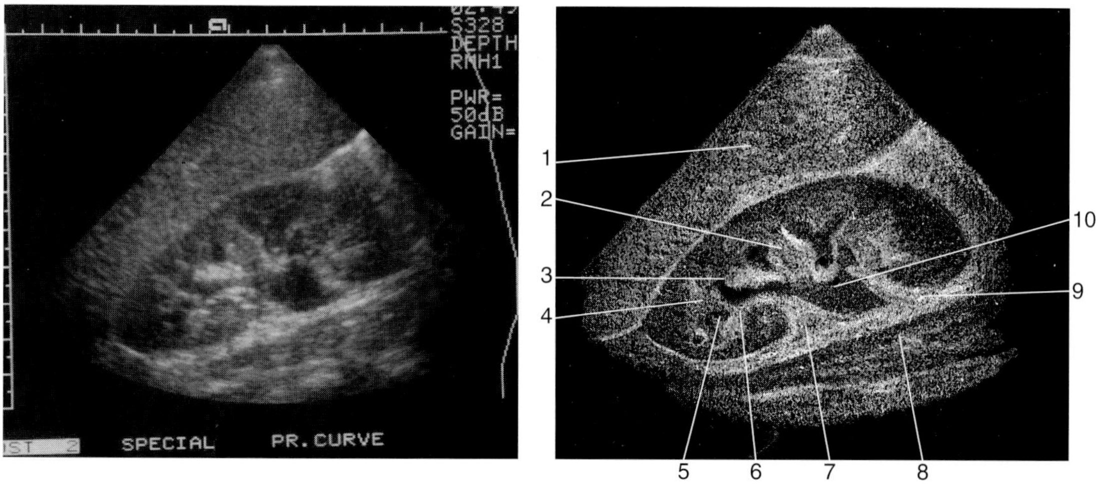

1. Liver 2. Septum of Bertin 3. Infundibulum 4. Arcuate vessel 5. Pyramid 6. Interlobar vessel 7. Renal hilum 8. Psoas muscle 9. Ureter 10. Pelvis

b

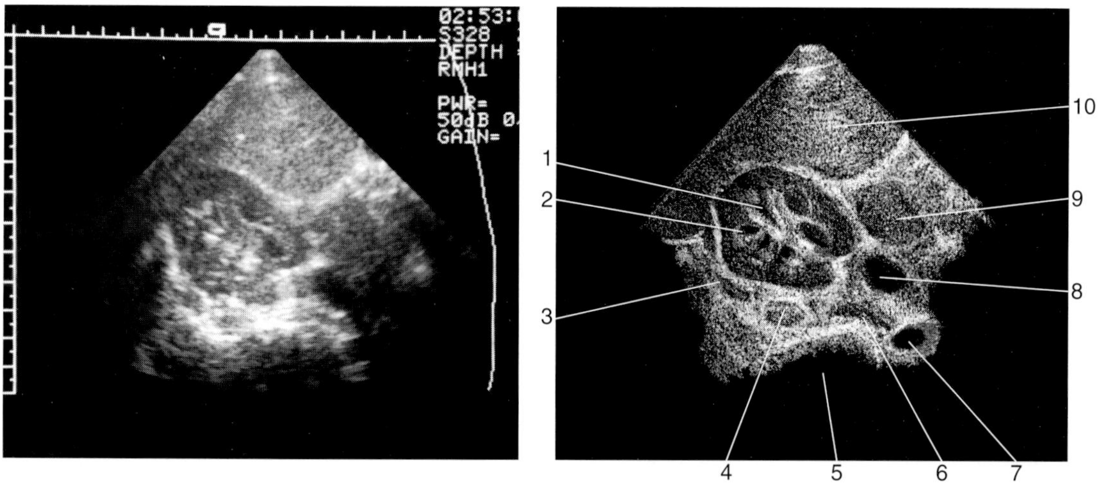

1. Interlobar vessel 2. Pyramid 3.Quadratus lumborum muscle 4. Psoas muscle 5. Spine 6. Crus of diaphragm 7.Aorta 8. Inferior vena cava 9. Duodenum 10. Liver

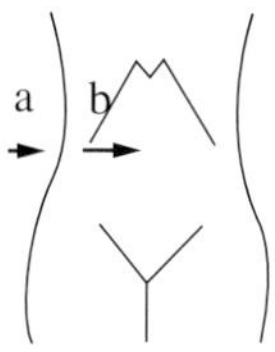

Figure 7-10. Normal kidney, physiological pelvic filling.
During a diuresis the normal collecting systems may fill and so may be visualized on ultrasound as an echo-free space in the sinus. In this subject the infundibulum was demonstrated leading to the renal pelvis (a). Pyramids and intrarenal blood vessels can also be discerned (b).

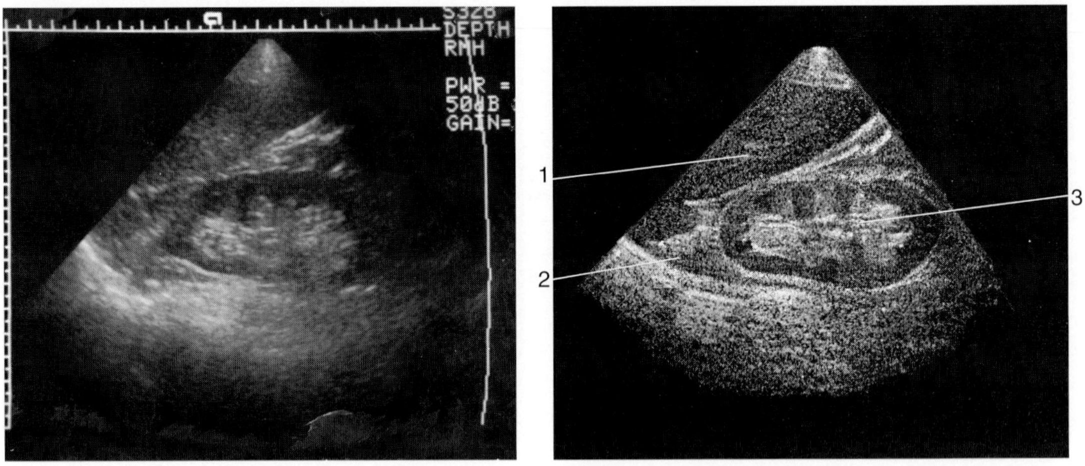

1. Spleen 2. Crus of diaphragm 3. Fatty sinus

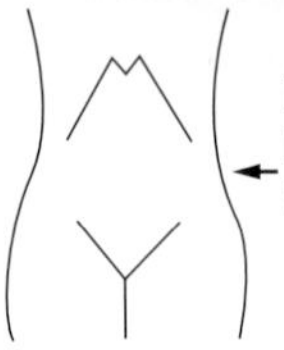

Figure 7-11. Sinus lipomatosis.
Excess fat in the renal sinus produces an expansion of the echogenic central region of the kidney. It is of no clinical significance.

a

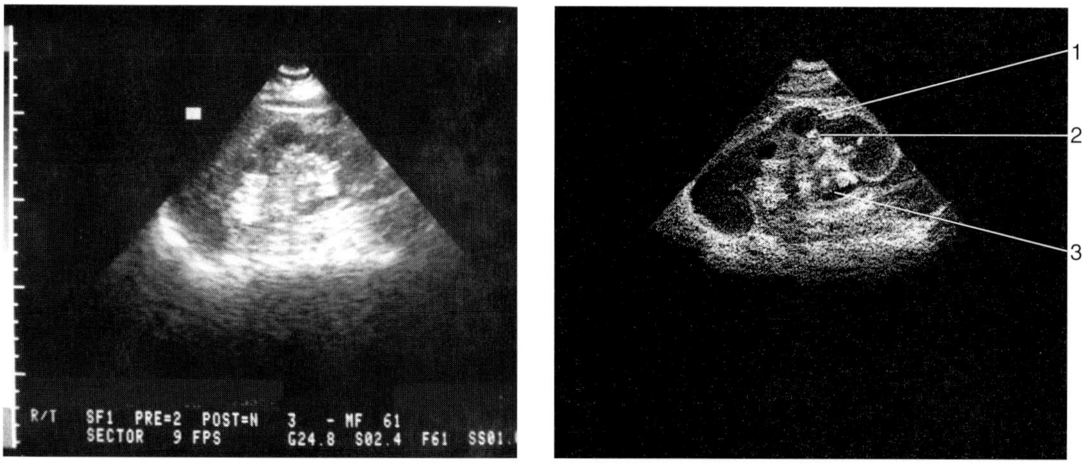

1. Hump 2. Pyramid 3. Sinus

b

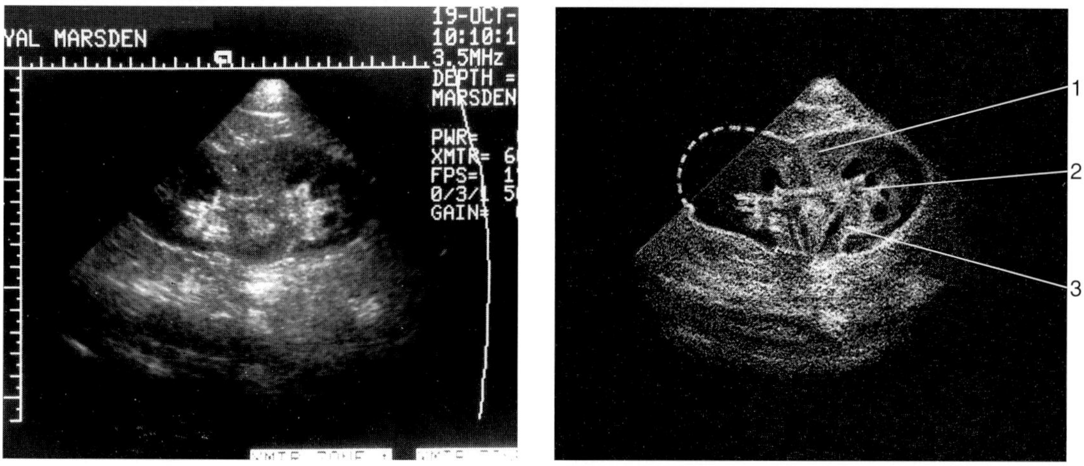

1. Septum of Bertin 2. Pyramid 3. Sinus

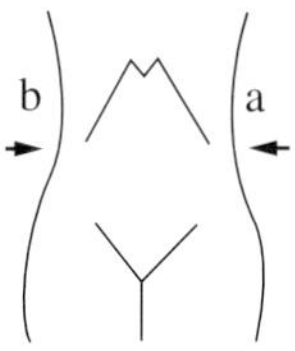

Figure 7-12. Fetal lobation and septum of Bertin.
The outline of the kidney is usually smooth, but traces of the fetal lobar pattern may persist into adult life as nodularity of the renal outline (a). Where the layers of cortex from adjacent lobes are prominent, a band of echogenic cortical tissue extending in toward the sinus results (b). It may separate the calyces and may simulate a mass on the intravenous urogram (IVU).

a

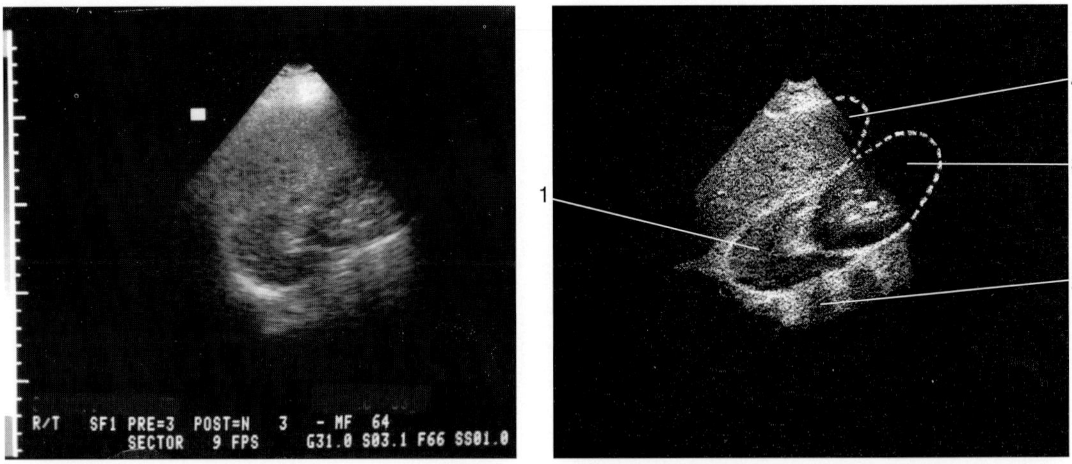

1. Fat space 2. Rib 3. Kidney 4. Liver

b

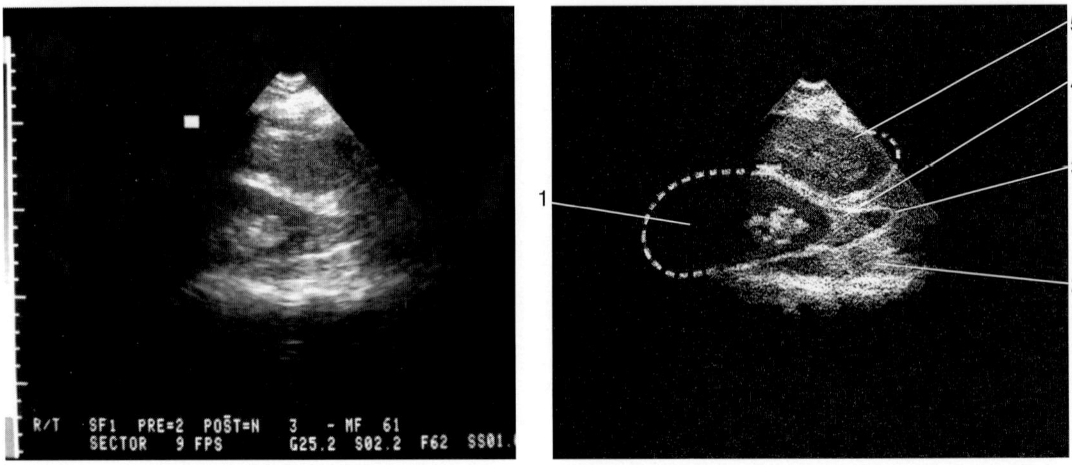

1. Kidney 2. Pararenal fat 3. Gerota's fascia
4. Perirenal fat 5. Liver

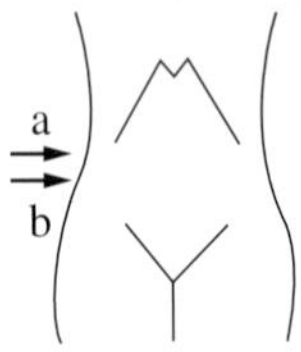

Figure 7-13. Fat around the kidney.
The kidney is embedded in fat, which is especially thick at its two poles. A fascial sheet (Gerota's fascia) separates it into two layers, the peri- and pararenal compartments, which can sometimes be distinguished on ultrasound.

a

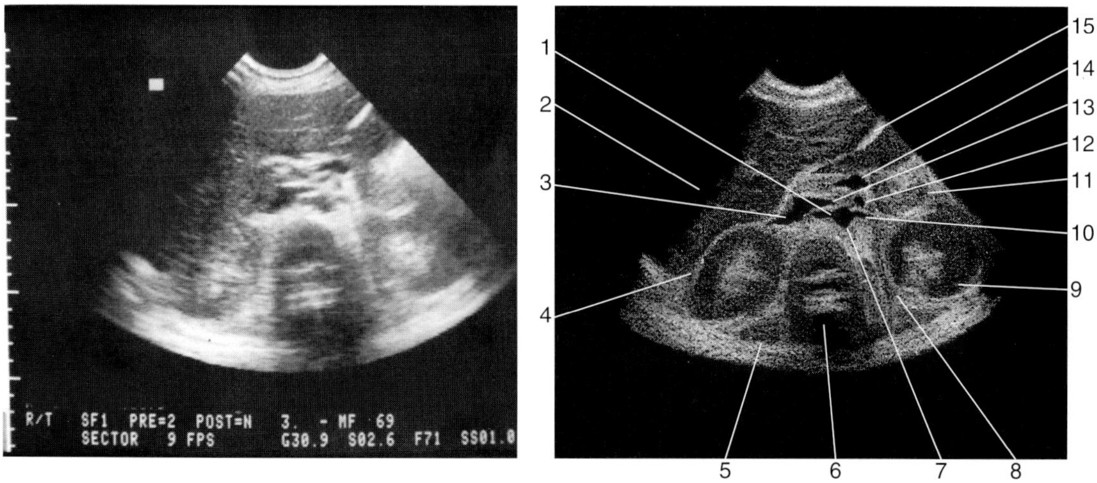

1. Right renal artery 2. Liver 3. Inferior vena cava 4. Right kidney 5. Quadratus lumborum muscle 6. Spinal canal 7. Aorta 8. Psoas muscle 9. Left kidney 10. Left renal artery 11. Pancreas 12. Superior mesenteric artery 13. Left renal vein 14. Splenic vein 15. Stomach gas bubble

b

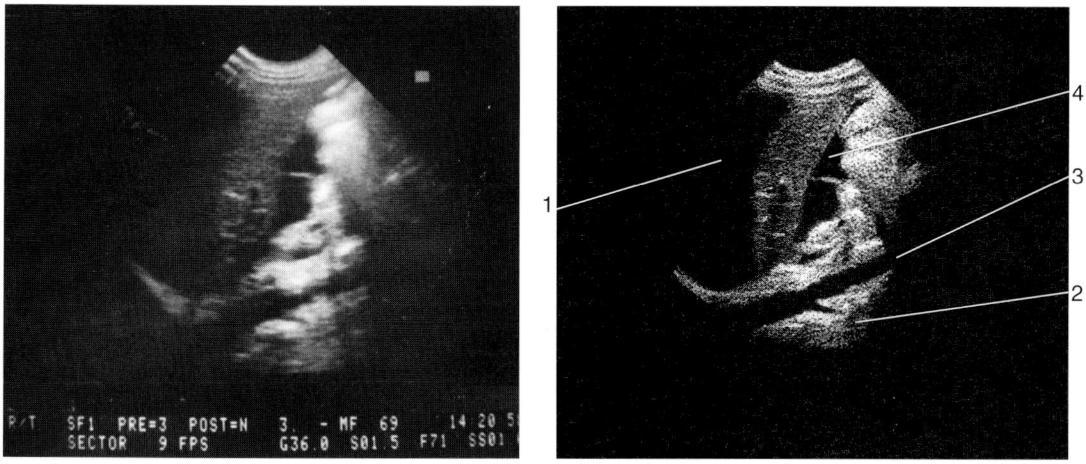

1. Liver 2. Left renal artery 3. Aorta 4. Ascites

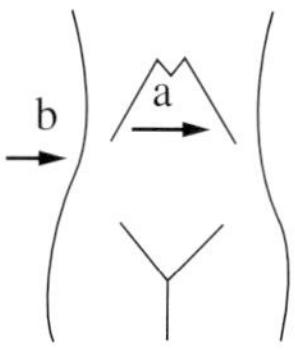

Figure 7-14. Renal vessels.
The origins of the renal arteries can be discerned, as well as the terminal portion of the left renal vein as it empties into the cava (a). The renal arteries commonly arise at the same level as the superior mesenteric artery, as in this case. In the coronal projection, the renal artery origin may be discerned as a projection from the aorta; the shape has been likened to that of a rose thorn (b).

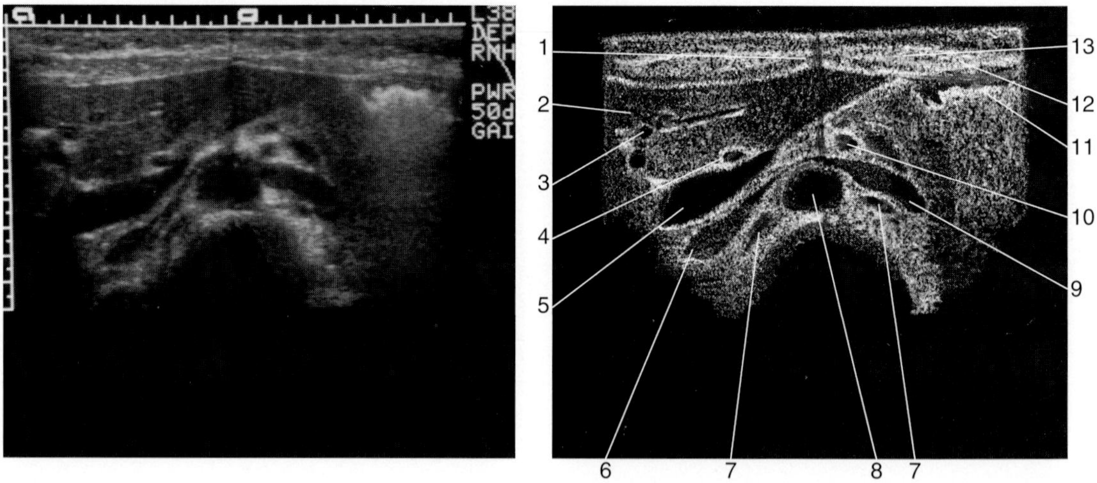

1. Linea alba 2. Liver 3. Left portal vein 4. Hepatic artery 5. Main portal vein 6. Inferior vena cava 7. Crura of diaphragm 8. Aorta 9. Left renal vein 10. Superior mesenteric artery 11. Stomach 12. Peritoneal layer 13. Rectus abdominis muscle

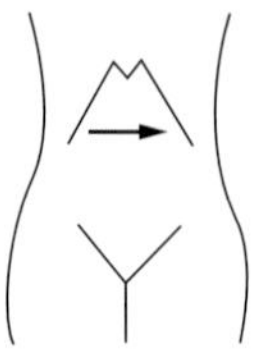

Figure 7-15. The left renal vein.
The left renal vein has a long course, passing anteriorly over the aorta; here it is overlain by the superior mesenteric artery, and it may be narrowed so that the upstream segment (to the left of the aorta) is dilated. This is a normal finding that should not be misinterpreted as an aneurysm or a para-aortic mass.

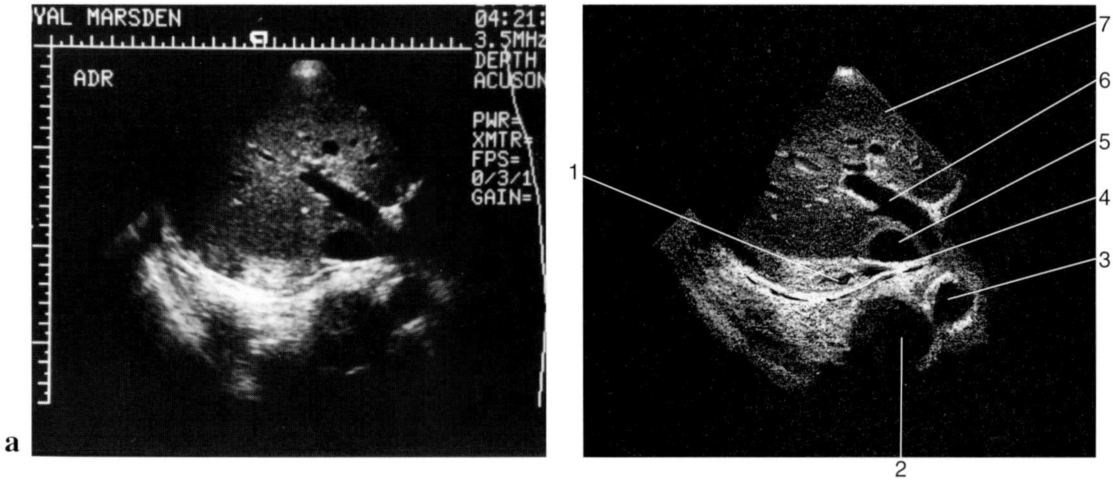

1. Right adrenal 2. Spine 3. Aorta 4. Crus of diaphragm 5. Inferior vena cava 6. Portal vein 7. Right lobe of liver

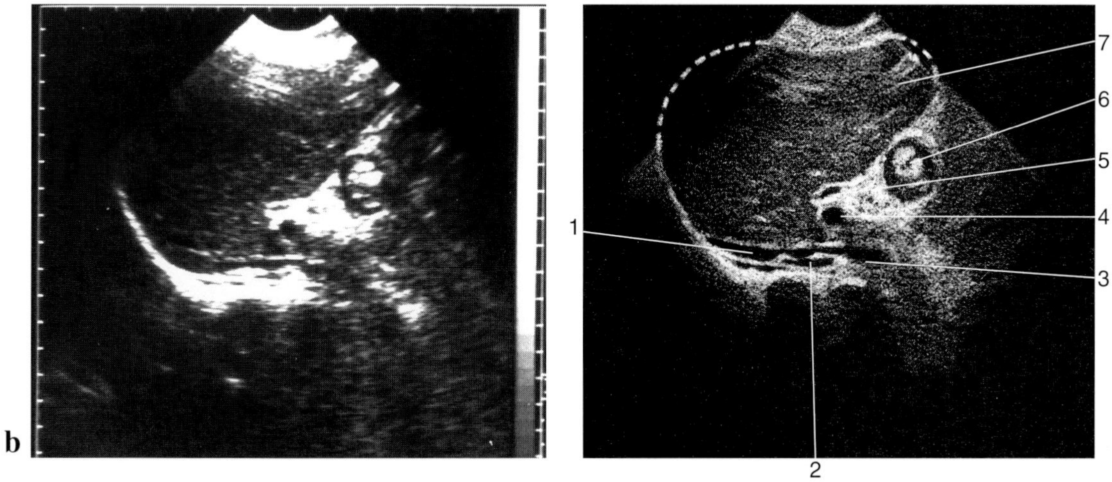

1. Crus of diaphragm 2. Right adrenal 3. Inferior vena cava 4. Portal vein 5. Common bile duct 6. Duodenum 7. Liver

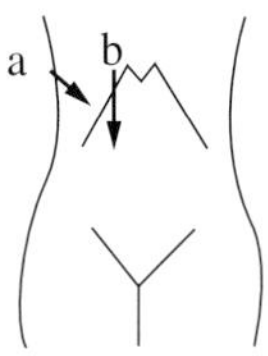

Figure 7-16. The right adrenal.
The right adrenal gland lies in a retrocaval position alongside the cava. Useful projections for its display are an angled transverse view through one of the right intercostal spaces (a) to display the crus of the right diaphragm. The adrenal may be imaged lying immediately posterior to the cava as an echo-poor linear or Y-shaped structure. The same anatomy may be discerned in the longitudinal projection (b) through the liver to show the crus posteromedial to the cava. The adrenal appears as an echo-poor, linear structure separating these two structures.

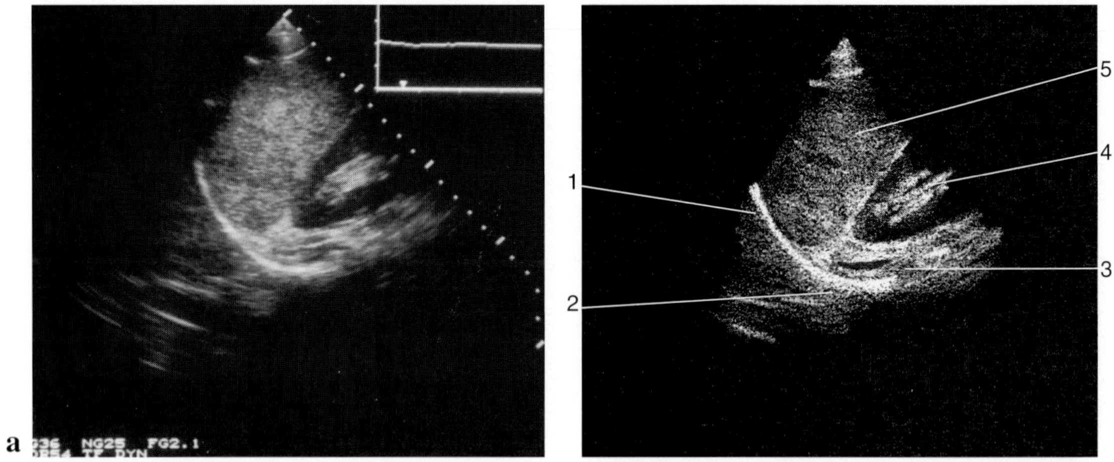

1. Diaphragm 2. Crus 3. Left adrenal 4. Left kidney 5. Spleen

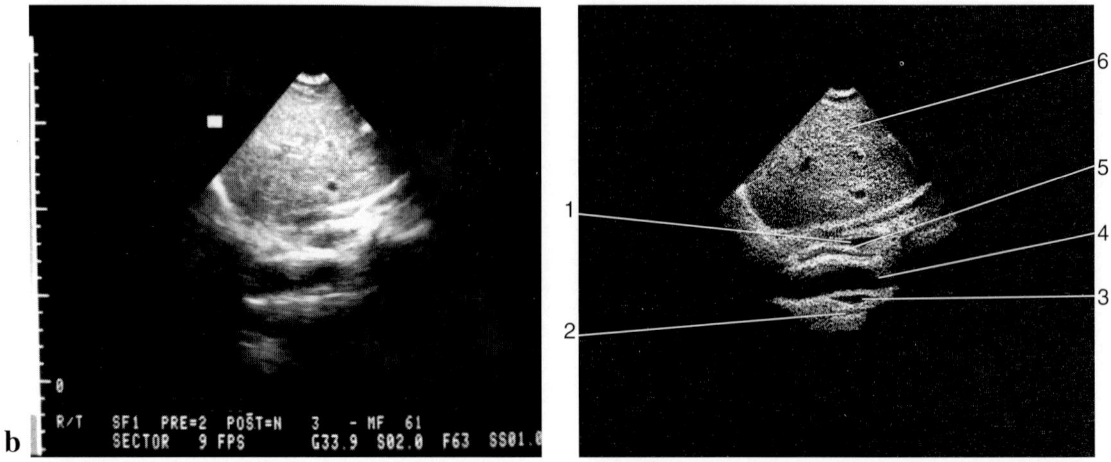

1. Inferior vena cava 2. Left adrenal 3. Left crus of diaphragm 4. Aorta 5. Right crus of diaphragm 6. Liver

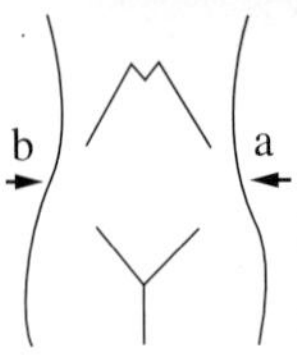

Figure 7-17. The left adrenal.
The left adrenal gland also lies against the crus of the diaphragm, but on this side the thoracic aorta is the related vessel and it lies medial to the crus. Coronal views through the spleen show the crus medial to the upper pole of the right kidney. The adrenal gland is an echo-poor, linear structure lying against the crus (a). An alternative view that may be very useful is a right coronal approach, lining up the cava and the aorta, with the two crura spanning the aorta. The left adrenal is visualized alongside the left crus. The right adrenal is often also demonstrated in this projection (b).

ABNORMALITIES OF THE KIDNEYS

Developmental Anomalies

Developmental anomalies of the renal tract are common, many being the consequence of its complex embryology.[38] Complete duplication of the kidney is rare; it can be recognized on ultrasound by the detection of two separate kidneys in the renal bed. In most cases the renal parenchyma is fused, but the collecting systems are duplicated. A difficulty arises when one of the duplex ureters is obstructed, giving rise to hydronephrosis with parenchymal atrophy. This usually affects the upper moiety, when the sonogram simulates a simple cyst at the upper pole of an otherwise normal kidney. Careful scanning in the coronal plane may reveal the cone-shaped pelviureteric junction. Since the normal ureter is rarely imaged, ureteric duplication is undetectable on ultrasound but may be inferred by the demonstration of division of the sinus by a central portion of the renal parenchyma (Figure 7-19). A variant of this arrangement, when the two joined moieties are slightly offset relative to each other, may produce the "dromedary hump" of normal renal tissue on the lateral margin of the kidney. Similarly, where two pyramids and their associated calyces are separated by an unusual thickness of cortex, the so-called hypertrophic septum of Bertin results; confusing at urography, this is readily distinguished from a mass on ultrasound since it has the same echo pattern as normal renal tissue.[33, 35]

In the horseshoe kidney, fusion of the lower poles of the two kidneys occurs. The bridge may contain functioning renal parenchyma or may merely be a fibrous strand. The natural migration of the developing kidneys is interrupted, so that the ascent is arrested when the bridge reaches the inferior mesenteric vessels. The horseshoe kidney therefore lies low in the abdomen, with the lower poles drawn medially. The fusion also interferes with the normal rotation of the hila and they face anteriorly, often with minor compromise of drainage resulting in hydronephrosis (Figure 7-20).

Disorders of the Renal Sinus

Hydronephrosis is easily detectable as abnormal separation of the layers of the sinus by fluid (Figures 7-21 and 7-22). There is usually no urine in the pelvis or calyces, though during a diuresis, a small amount of collects, separating the walls by a fluid space a few millimeters thick. Separation greater than 5 mm is abnormal and suggests dilatation.[11] With greater degrees of hydronephrosis the calyces also become dilated, and are seen as sacular spaces around the sinus and communicating with the bag-like pelvis (Figure 7-23). A coronal section gives an optimal display, since the connection between the calyces and pelvis can be lined up to give the so-called "Mickey Mouse" or "inflated-glove" pattern. When dilated, the upper part of the ureter can often be traced as it emerges medially from the pelvis to give a funnel shape (Figure 7-24).

The pattern on ultrasound is easy to recognize. Multiple renal cysts occasionally seem similar, but cysts do not intercommunicate, usually arise in the periphery, and are of varying sizes, in contrast to the central, equal-sized spaces of hydrocalycosis[17, 30, 32] (Figure 7-25). Renal papillary necrosis produces enlargement of the fluid space in the calyces.[21] The pattern may simulate hydronephrosis, but the lack of dilatation of the pelvis points to the diagnosis. In pyonephrosis the fluid contains echogenic material, which often layers out with gravity[8, 55] (Figure 7-26). A solitary cyst arising deep in the parenchyma (parapelvic cyst) can be confusingly similar to a hydropelvis (Figure 7-27). Though the classic Mickey Mouse pattern is absent, an intravenous urogram (IVU) may be needed for definitive diagnosis. The common normal variant of a baggy extrarenal pelvis can be distinguished from hydronephrosis by the intrarenal position of the latter (Figure 7-28). A transverse section, perhaps through the flank, may enable this distinction to be made.

In gross hydronephrosis the renal substance may atrophy, leaving simply a bag of fluid without other recognizable features, the calyces having been taken up into the pelvis. A large, simple cyst displacing the kidney, which then becomes difficult to locate, may cause confusion.

While ureteric reflux can be the cause, hydronephrosis is usually due to ongoing obstruction, though it must be borne in mind that a previous obstructive episode may leave the pelvicalyceal system permanently dilated. Like other imaging techniques, ultrasound displays only anatomy; unfortunately, the pressure of the fluid in a hydronephrosis cannot be deduced from the degree of dilatation. Duration is a more important determinant of the severity of hydronephrosis than the completeness of the obstruction. Indeed, in some cases with sudden, complete obstruction, urine output ceases, so there may be no hydronephrosis at all.

Other conditions of the sinus are less important in sonography. Sinus lipomatosis should be mentioned; not truly pathological, this is simply the accumulation of fatty tissue around the blood vessels and the pelvicalyceal system. The sinus appears abnormally widened, forming more than the normal one-third of the kidney's thickness (see Figure 7-11). The sinus remains echogenic.

Renal stones produce strong echoes, regardless of their chemical composition. However, they are often difficult to detect against the background of the echogenic renal sinus unless they are large enough (25 mm in diameter) to obstruct the ultrasound beam and thus produce the telltale shadowing[37] (Figure 7-29). Tumors in the sinus are imaged only when large; pyelography is much more sensitive.[2]

Focal Renal Pathology

Cystic disease

Simple renal cysts are common incidental findings, increasing in frequency with age, so that they are seen in 50% of patients over 50. They are usually very easy both to detect and to differentiate from other conditions. Classically, a renal cyst is an echo-free, rounded, smooth-walled mass with distal echo enhancement (Figures 7-30 to 7-32). Typically, they lie superficially in the renal parenchyma or protruding from the renal surface, but deeply buried cysts are not uncommon, the so-called parapelvic cyst. Multiple cysts may also occur, especially in the elderly. Though a cyst should be echo-free, artifactual reverberant echoes are often seen in the superficial parts of the cyst. It is usually obvious that these are reverberations, but for lesions smaller than 1 or 2 cm in diameter, it may be impossible to decide whether the internal echoes represent true structures or artifacts. Distal enhancement may be inapparent for smaller cysts because the short fluid path produces only a small amount of enhancement. It may also be difficult to demonstrate with cysts that lie against the renal sinus because the strong echoes from the sinus saturate the display, so that no further intensification is possible.

A cyst with classic features (smooth walls, echo-free contents, and enhancement) is, for practical purposes, always benign and no further investigation is needed. Any deviation from these strict criteria indicates a significant risk that the lesion is a tumor with a cystic element, and further investigation is mandatory (usually by ultrasound-guided aspiration). However, most such atypical cysts prove to be benign complications. Hemorrhage into a cyst is common and produces internal echoes. Superinfection likewise gives echoes within the lesion.

In adult polycystic disease, the lesions have a spectrum of sizes[15, 30, 32] (Figure 7-33). Close packing distorts their rounded shape, so that they become polygonal. Hemorrhage into one or several of the cysts is common, so that a confusingly heterogeneous appearance may result. The gross anatomical distortion may make it exceedingly difficult to discern additional pathology such as hydronephrosis, abscess or tumor formation. Hepatic, pancreatic, and splenic cysts may coexist.

Cystic disease may also be encountered in the neonate. The most common form, the dysplastic kidney, results from ureteric stenosis; the fetal response to back pressure is different from that of the adult. Often the kidney atrophies, and characteristically contains a bizarre mixture of cell types, ciliated epithelium, muscle, and cartilage being found.[43, 53] Sometimes large cysts develop and present as an abdominal mass. On ultrasound, these are seen as multiple cysts of varying sizes with echogenic intervening septa. The lack of intercommunication distinguishes dysplasia from hydronephrosis. Ultrasound can be useful to confirm that the other kidney is normal, important because of the higher incidence of contralateral anomalies such as pelviureteric junction obstruction. The prognosis is good.

Polycystic disease may also occur in the neonate as an infantile form.[3] This is a rare disease causing severe renal failure that is usually rapidly fatal. Unlike the adult version, the cysts are minute, too small to be resolved on ultrasound. Instead, the multiple small interfaces give the kidneys an overall increased reflectivity, with obliteration of the corticomedullary distinction.

Cysts are also a feature of medullary sponge kidney, but here they are restricted to the medullary tubules.[15] They may be large enough to be detected on ultrasound but, in other cases, the small cysts and associated calculi produce a reversed ultrasound pattern with stronger echoes from the pyramids (Figure 7-34).

Trauma

The kidneys are vulnerable to injury in blunt and penetrating abdominal trauma. Renal biopsy is a frequent cause. Hematoma confined by the renal capsule is most common, but extension into the retroperitoneum occurs if the kidney is ruptured. A hematoma is seen on ultrasound as a focal mass of mixed but predominantly low reflectivity, with an ill-defined margin[6, 28, 29] (Figure 7-35). Perirenal or retroperitoneal extravasation produces an echo-free space around the kidney. The identical appearances of abscesses must be borne in mind. Intraperitoneal blood has the same appearance as ascites; the clinical context suggests its true nature, which should be confirmed by an abdominal tap.

Infection

The pathological changes of acute inflammation, particularly the increased tissue water, reduce echo levels. Focal acute inflammation in the kidney is usually due to ureteric reflux. The refluxed bacteria produce regions of acute "nephronia" involving a single renal lobe. The upper pole is more commonly affected, due partly to its position in the direct line of refluxed urine and partly to the compound pyramids that occur at the poles. The lower pole is the next most often involved. A region of reduced echoes is seen on ultrasound [13, 45] (Figure 7-36). The functional defect is best seen on a ^{99m}Tc-DMSA scan. In adults the condition usually resolves completely, whereas in the developing child, kidney scarring is often produced. On ultrasound these depressed scars appear as bands of strong echoes associated with an indentation of the renal surface, often with dilatation of the underlying calyx as well.

Focal nephronia may evolve into a frank abscess; septicemia and sepsis around a renal stone are other causes. The ultrasound findings are the same as for abscesses elsewhere, with an irregular walled cavity filled with variably echogenic contents[14, 20] (Figure 7-37). The fibrosis of chronic inflammation give high level echoes especially in tuberculosis where the associated calcification accentuates the echogenicity. The renal architecture is usually very distorted.

Tumors

Adenomas are common incidental findings at autopsy, especially in the elderly, but are usually too small to be detected by ultrasound. Larger adenomas appear as rounded, uniformly echogenic, parenchymal masses, but non-invasive verification of the true nature of such lesions is difficult.[56]

Angiomyolipoma is a curious hamartomatous tumor with a very strongly echogenic appearance on ultrasound which is often distinctive enough to suggest the diagnosis. The strong echoes are due to the abundant fat and blood vessels they contain.[18] The fat gives a characteristically low attenuation on CT scanning. The combination of high ultrasound reflectivity and low CT attenuation is pathognomonic. Hemorrhage is common. If this is confined to the tumor, irregular, echo-poor regions result but, if it extends, fluid is seen in the perinephric or peritoneal spaces. Biopsy should be avoided.

Nephroblastomas (Wilms' tumor) are often large at presentation and produce a mass with gross distortion of the retroperitoneal anatomy (Figure 7-38). Hemorrhage is common. Thus, the ultrasound texture is often very heterogenous, sometimes with frank fluid spaces.[36] Ultrasound is useful in confirming the diagnosis by ruling out other causes of a palpable mass in a child, and also to some extent in assessing operability, though CT scanning is more valuable in this respect. Ultrasound is also used in follow-up to check the remaining kidney, since a significant proportion of nephroblastomas are bilateral. The renal bed can also be evaluated. Careful observation with real-time scanning is required to distinguish tumor recurrence from the gut loops that fall back into the nephrectomy site, a task that is facilitated by color Doppler.

Adenocarcinomas (Grawitz tumor, hypernephroma) often present with hematuria. Commonly they produce a focal renal mass that is obviously solid on ultrasound, usually consisting of predominantly low-level echoes together with some echogenic regions due to necrosis or hemorrhage [7] (Figure 7-39). Sometimes the echogenic portions dominate the appearance, giving a very heterogeneous pattern while small (< 2 cm) tumor may be very echogenic. Rarely, the lesion is predominantly cystic, though there is always some irregularity of the "cyst" wall, and the fluid contains some echoes due to hemorrhage or debris. Any atypical renal cyst must be aspirated for pathological examination. Another difficult but uncommon pattern occurs when the tumor infiltrates the whole kidney. A large, echo-poor kidney with distortion or simply loss of anatomical detail results. The changes may be subtle and easily missed. Local invasion of the renal bed is difficult to detect, but nodal and liver metastases can be assessed, as can the common invasion of the renal vein and inferior vena cava.[38] Renal carcinomas are usually vascular, as can be demonstrated on Doppler.[12]

Metastatic tumor in the kidney is not uncommon, especially in lymphoma, where the focal type produces echo-poor masses which are usually multiple. Diffuse infiltration produces renal enlargement with nonspecific appearances (see discussion under "Diffuse Renal Diseases"). Carcinoma metastatic to the kidney variable, echo-poor or echogenic lesions (Figure 7-40).

Diffuse Renal Diseases

Because the kidney's response to a wide variety of injuries is limited, the ultrasound changes observed are usually nonspecific.[54] In addition, as the pathology progresses, the changes evolve through a sequence, so that the point in the course of a disease when an examination is performed may be critical to interpretation. Enlargement of the kidney, for example, occurs in the early stages of most inflammatory and congestive disorders, but later, with progressive scarring and tubular atrophy, the kidney shrinks.

The most common ultrasound change in diffuse diseases is a general increase in reflectivity of the renal parenchyma.[23,46] Normally, the renal cortex is more reflective than the medulla but somewhat less reflective than the adjacent liver. A mild increase in reflectivity makes the cortex equal to the liver (grade 1) and this is within normal limits; with a moderate increase, it is more echogenic than the liver (Figure 7-41a). With a severe increase (grade 3), the cortex is as reflective as the renal sinus (Figures 7-41b and 7-42). A wide range of inflammatory and infiltrative disorders produce this pattern; they are often associated with a cellular infiltrate (interstitial nephritis). There is a rough correspondence between the severity of infiltration and the echogenicity.

Low reflectivity is produced by conditions with increased water without infiltration. Renal vein thrombosis is the most important. The affected kidney is enlarged and echo-poor, and the internal anatomy is effected.[5,44] Diffuse lymphoma and leukemic involvement also produce this pattern, though usually it is bilateral.

Calcification in the medulla (nephrocalcinosis) reverses the normal pattern, so that the pyramids become more reflective than the cortex[16] (Figure 7-43).

The Transplanted Kidney

Because of its superficial position, high-frequency transducers can be used to give detailed images of the transplanted kidney[26, 36, 48] (Figure 7-44).

Surgically produced fluid collections are easily imaged by ultrasound.[11, 51] Appearance, size, and timing often allow an accurate diagnosis. Hematoma around the transplant creates an irregular, echo-poor space often lying close to the hilum. Such spaces may be found immediately postoperatively or may appear over the first 2 weeks after surgery. They usually contain a few scattered echoes but on occasion they are truly echo-free. Lymphoceles enlarge slowly over a period of weeks. They form close to the kidney and are usually echo-free initially but later develop septations. Urinomas develop early and are also echo-free but lie close to the bladder since they arise from a leak at the uretero-vesical implant site. If they rupture into the peritoneum, their appearance is identical to that of ascites or persistent peritoneal dialysate. Abscesses associated with the transplant have the typical shaggy-walled appearance seen elsewhere. Hydronephrosis is easily detected (Figure 7-45), but it is important to note that a minor degree of pelvicalyceal dilatation is normal in transplanted kidneys.

Acute tubular necrosis is the invariable accompaniment of the warm ischemia associated with cadaver transplants; it occurs in live donor transplants as well, but here is less severe. The renal enlargement it produces in the first few days can be documented on ultrasound; it reverses in 1 or 2 weeks. There are no specific structural changes in the parenchyma, though sometimes the distinction between cortex and pyramids is increased.[40, 50]

Rejection also produces renal enlargement, but this commences after 10 day or so. It is progressive until suppressed by anti-immune drugs. Within the kidney the changes are variable. Often nothing abnormal is detectable but, in some cases, striking accentuation of the appearance of the pyramids is noted. Frequently the sinus echoes appear compressed and thin, as though distorted by the intense renal parenchyma.[24] In severe cases there may be infarction of the parenchyma, seen as irregular, echo-poor patches in the renal substance (Figure 7-46). Because in many cases rejection produces a vasculitis with obliteration of the smaller vessels, Doppler is more sensitive than imaging in its detection. An increased resistance to flow occurs first as a drop in diastolic perfusion. In severe cases, this progresses to complete absence of diastolic flow.

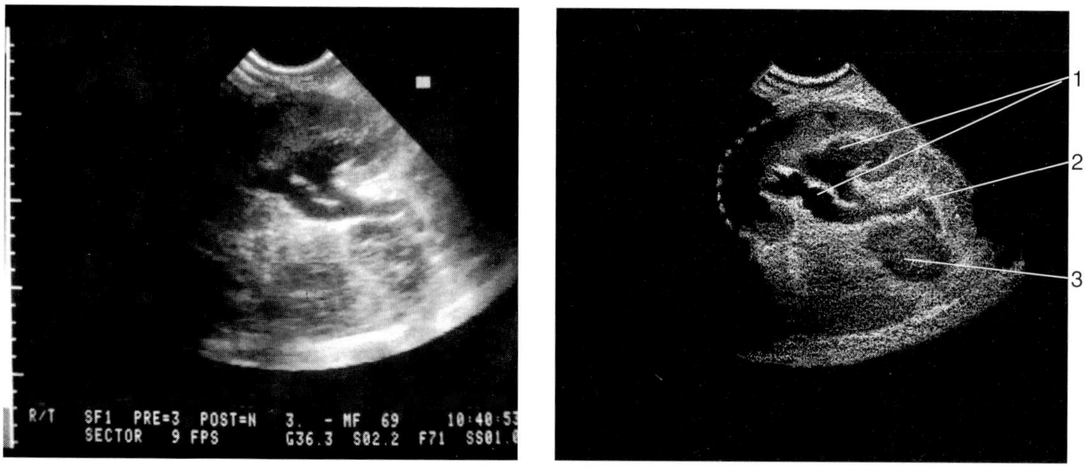

1. Duplex pelvicalyceal system 2. Ureter 3. Psoas muscle

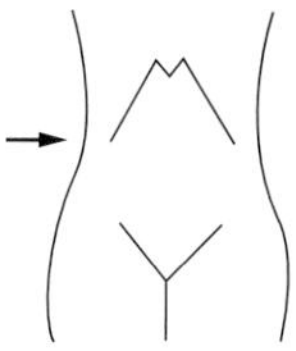

Figure 7-18. Duplex pelvicalyceal system.
The duplex upper drainage system in this patient with a pelvic tumor is clearly revealed by the hydronephrosis. The oblique-coronal cut taken to align the drainage system presents the psoas muscle in an unusual projection.

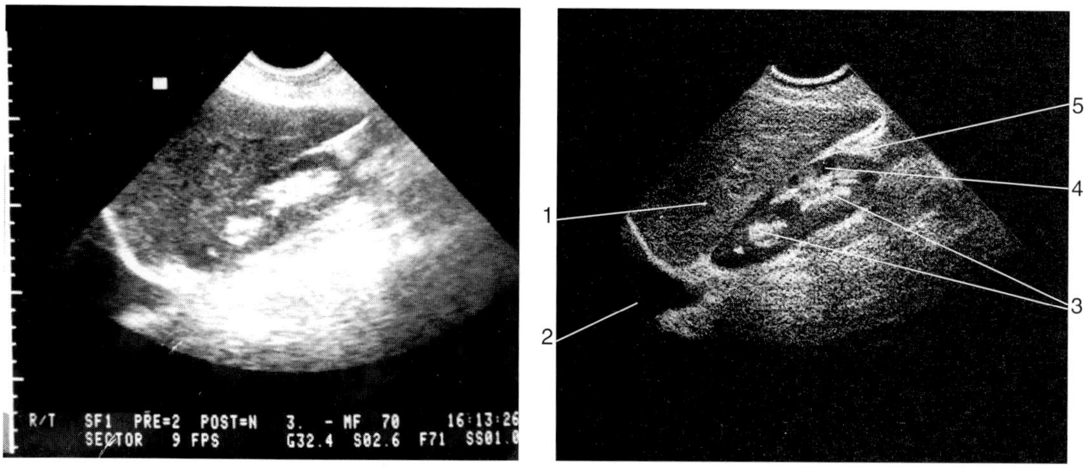

1. Liver 2. Effusion 3. Duplex calyceal pattern 4. Pyramid 5. Colon

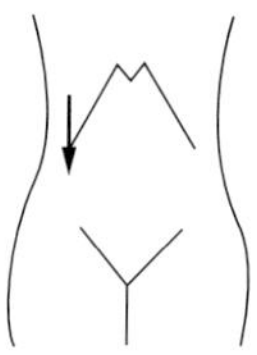

Figure 7-19. Duplex calyceal pattern.
An early division of the major calyces appears as though the kidney contains a bridge of parenchyma dividing the sinus. This is a common normal variant and was an incidental finding in this patient being investigated for a pleural effusion.

a

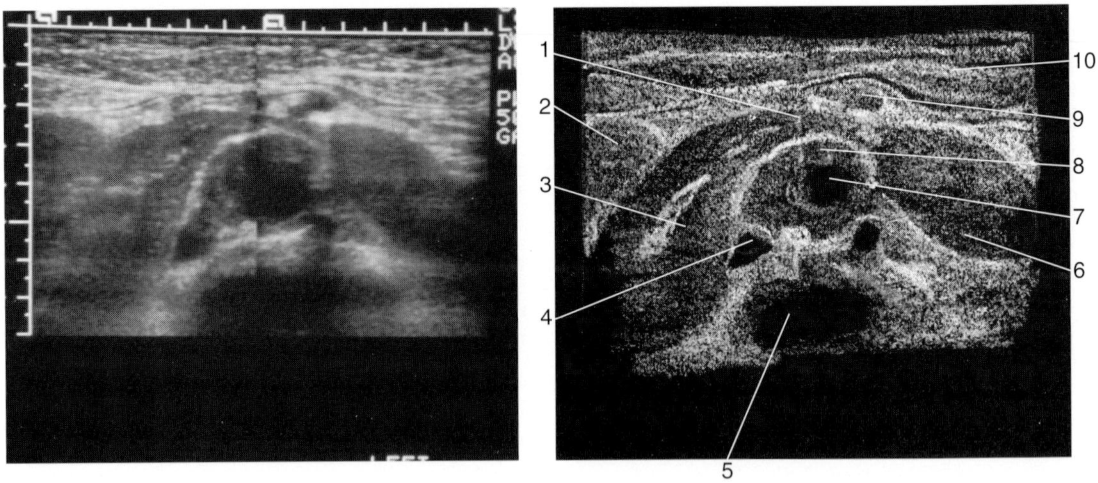

1. Bridge of horseshoe kidney 2. Liver 3. Right renal mass 4. Inferior vena cava 5. Spine 6. Left renal mass 7. Lumen of aneurysmal aorta 8. Thrombus of aneurysmal aorta 9. Mesenteric artery 10. Rectus abdominis muscle

b

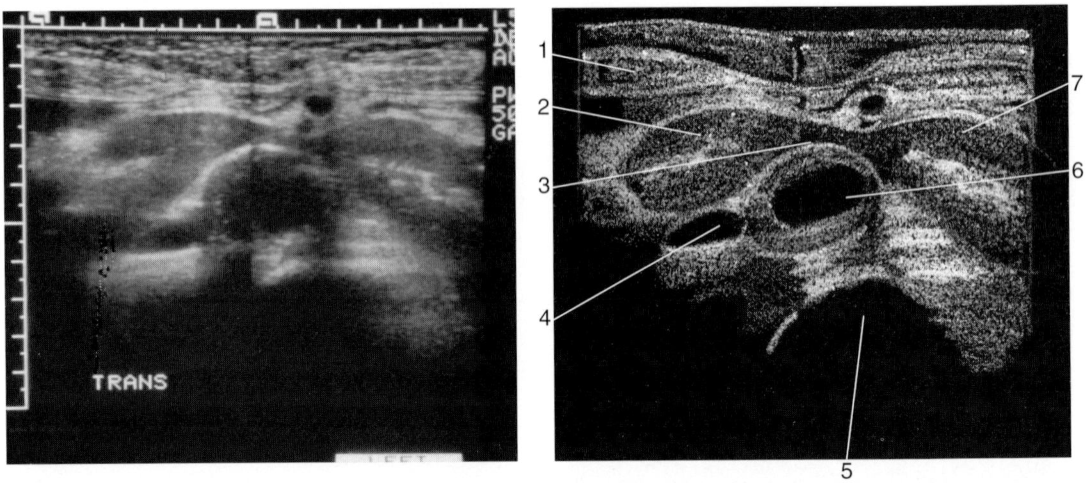

1. Rectus abdominis muscle 2. Right part of horseshoe kidney 3. Bridge of horseshoe kidney 4. Inferior vena cava 5. Spine 6. Aorta 7. Left part of horseshoe kidney

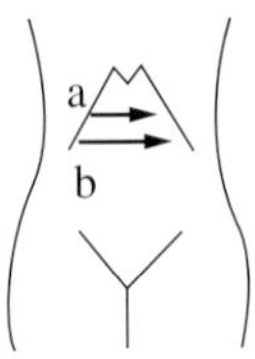

Figure 7-20. Horseshoe kidney and aortic aneurysm.
The components of a typical horseshoe kidney are demonstrated in these transverse sections. The two main renal moieties are low and medially positioned, with an attenuated bridge connecting their lower poles. Typically, this bridge lies immediately inferior mesenteric artery. The aorta is dilated, with an eccentrically thickened wall due to thrombus deposition there. Aneurysms are commonly found in patients with a horseshoe kidney.

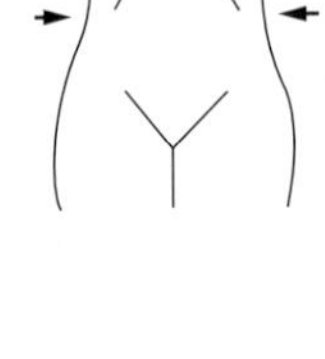

Figure 7-21. Hydronephrosis, dilated renal pelvis.
The coronal view lines up the renal sinus with the pelvis and displays the dilated renal pelvis to best advantage. The pattern of calyces emptying into a dilated pelvis forms the Mickey Mouse pattern. The shape is like that of a surgical glove inflated with water; the fingers are the calyces, and the hand is the pelvis. a: minimal dilatation ; b: moderate dilatation ; c: gross dilatation with parenchymal atrophy.

►

a

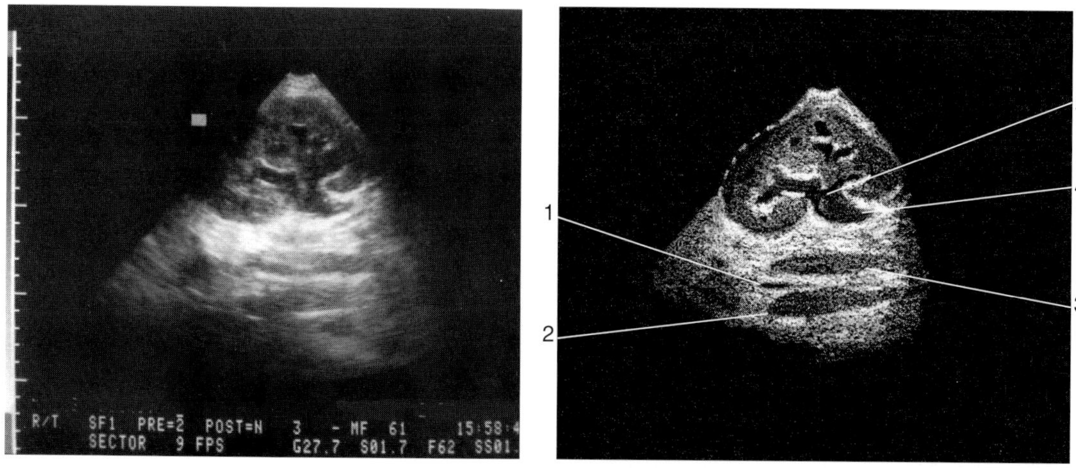

1. Crus of diaphragm 2. Aorta 3. Inferior vena cava 4. Ureter 5 . Pelvis

b

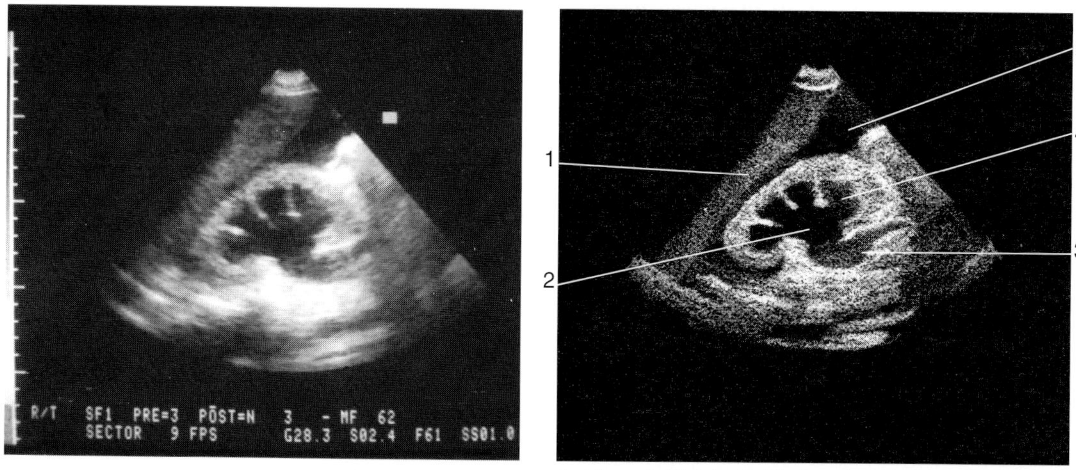

1. Liver 2. Pelvis 3. Ureter 4. Calyces 5. Ascites

c

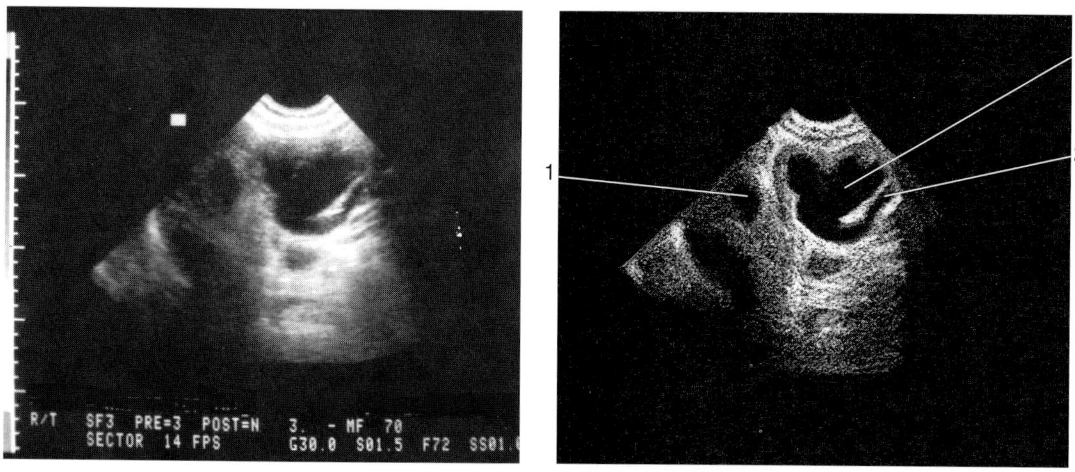

1. Spleen 2. Ureter 3. Pelvis

Figure 7-21. (See legend on opposite page)

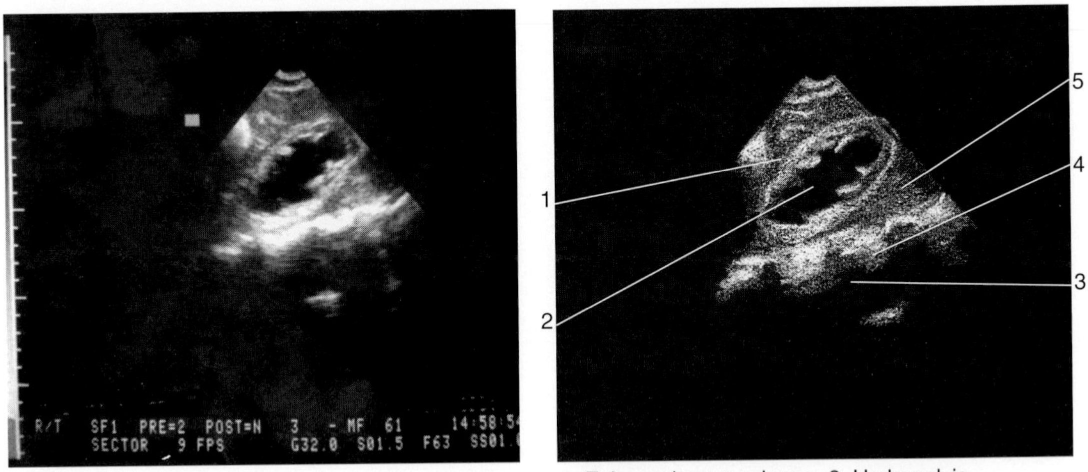

1. Echogenic parenchyma 2. Hydropelvis
3. Vertebral body 4. Disc 5. Psoas muscle

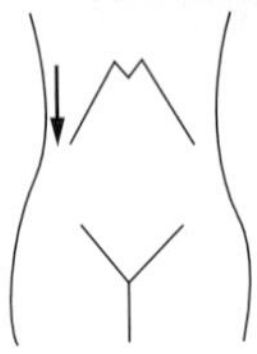

Figure 7-22. The renal parenchyma in hydronephrosis.
The compressed renal parenchyma in severe hydronephrosis may show an increase in echo intensity, as in this case(cf. also Fig.7-21b). Such a change is not necessarily due to coexistent diffuse disease, and the degree to which renal function can be recovered cannot be predicted on the basis of the structure revealed by ultrasound.

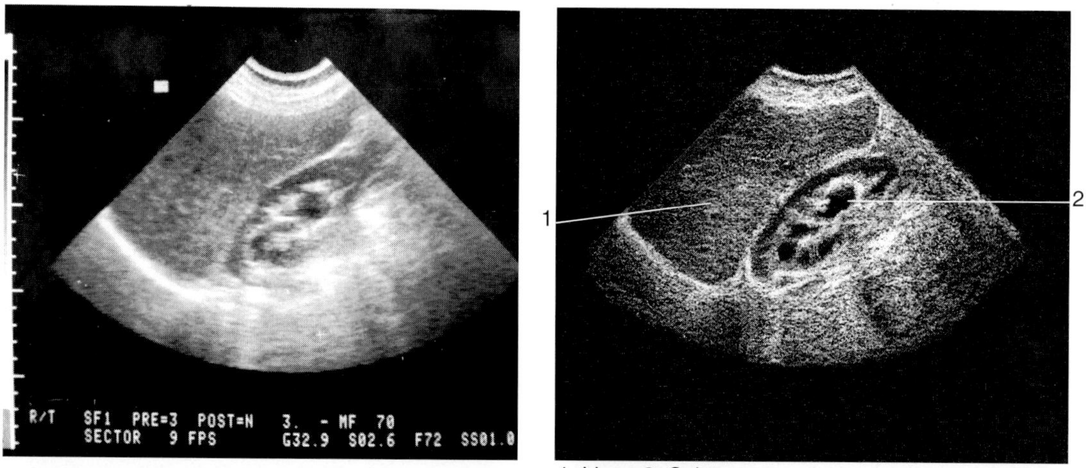

a

1. Liver 2. Calyx

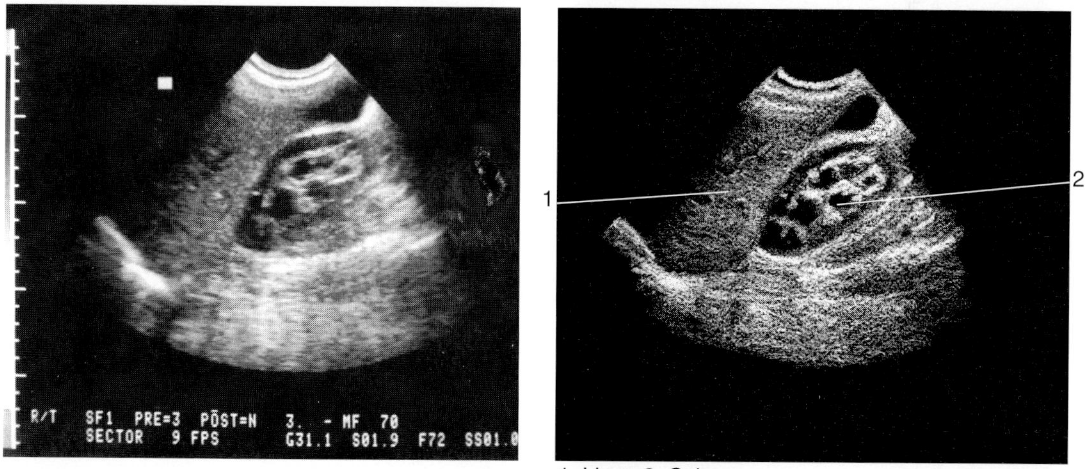

b

1. Liver 2. Calyx

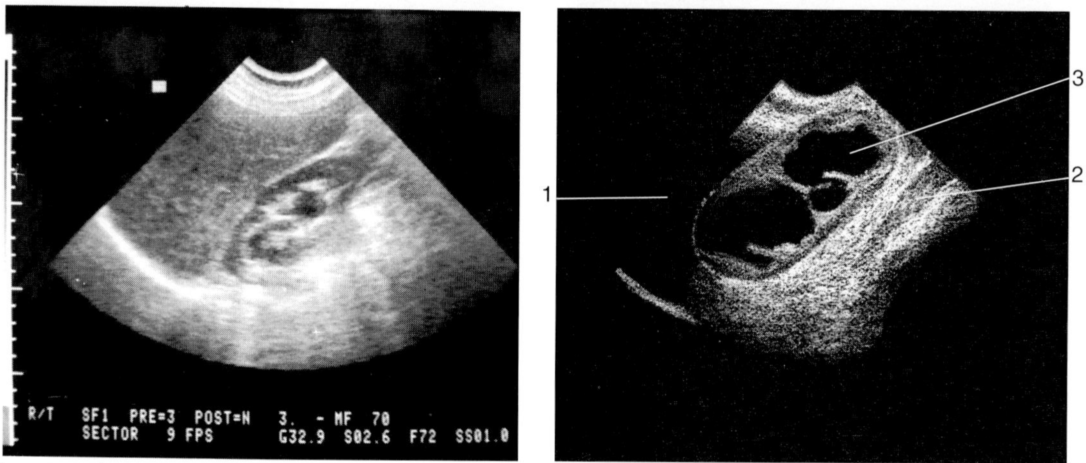

c

1. Liver 2. Psoas muscle 3. Calyx

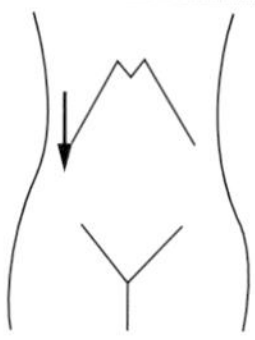

Figure 7-23. Hydronephrosis—calyctasis.
Progressive dilatation of the calyces is shown in this series of cases. The calyces lie within the renal sinus and so are enclosed in reflective tissue, unlike renal pyramids with which minor degrees of dilatation might be confused. In (c) little of the renal parenchyma can be identified. Nevertheless, the amount of recoverable renal function may be surprising; ultrasound is a poor index of function.

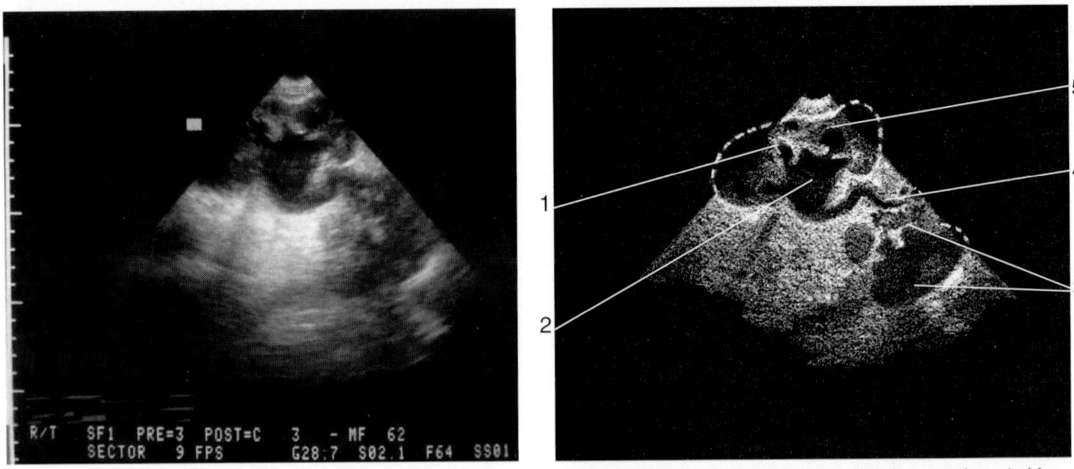

1. Pyramid 2. Pelvis 3. Lymphadenopathy 4. Ureter 5. Calyx

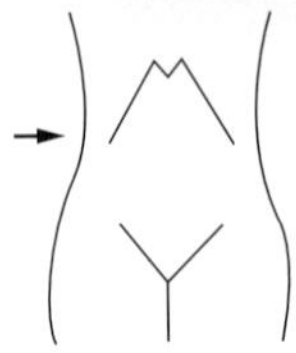

Figure. 7-24 The upper ureter.
The ureter is often very tortous, making the task of tracing its course difficult. The tortuosity may be accentuated by the lengthening that accompanies dilatation. In this case, the enlarged retroperitoneal lymph nodes causing the obstruction are well seen, with the tortuous ureter running into them.

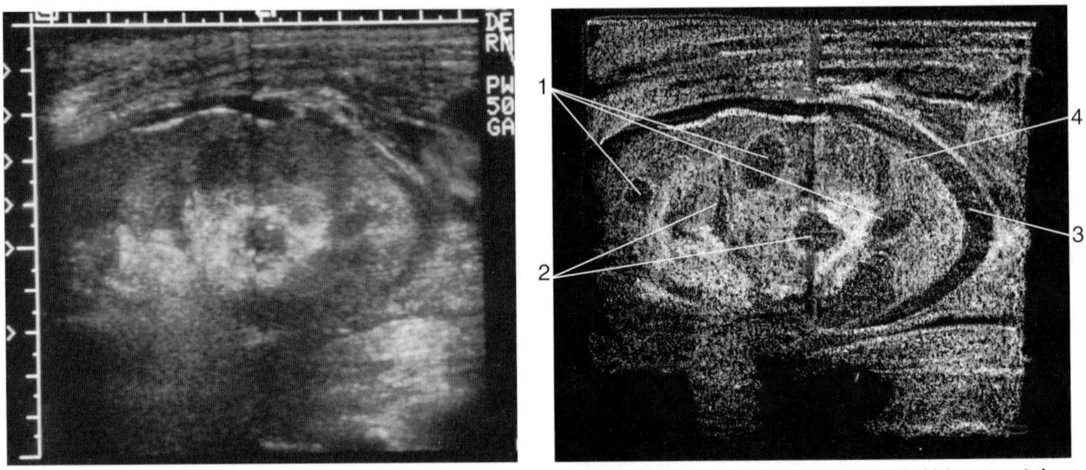

1. Pyramids 2. Collecting system 3. Urinoma 4. Arcuate vessels

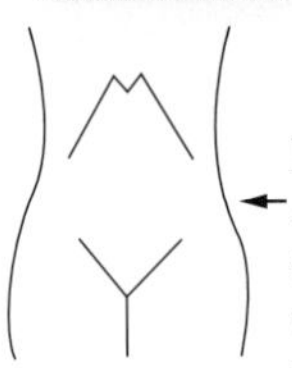

Figure 7-25. Urine extravasation.
A crescentic fluid space covers the lower pole and lateral aspect of the kidney in this patient with acute ureteric obstruction. The pattern suggests extravasated urine. This was confirmed on subsequent percutaneous nephrostomy, at which blood-stained urine was aspirated before the kidney was punctured. Note the slight dilatation of the pelvicalyceal system. This is typical of acute obstruction and poses diagnostic problems in view of the capacity of the normal collecting system under diuresis.

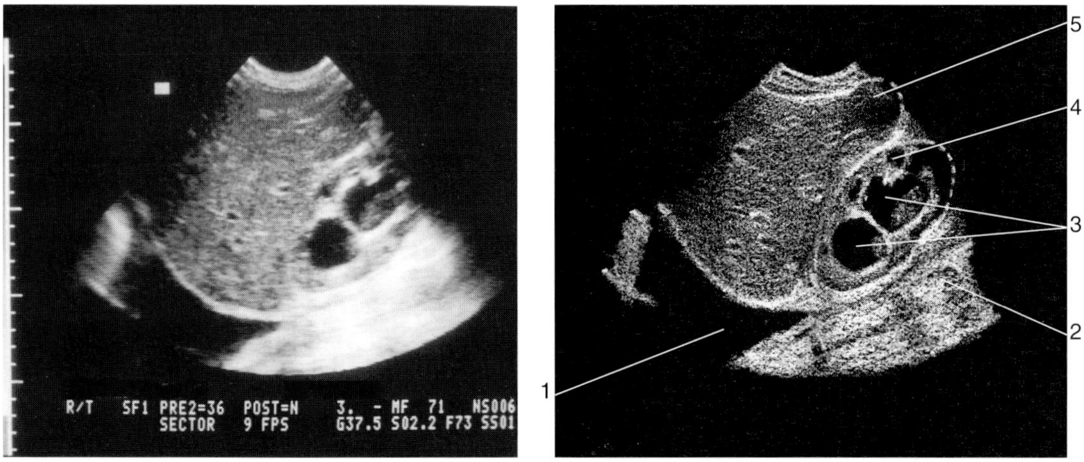

a

1. Pleural effusion 2. Rib 3. Pus 4. Renal pyramid 5. Liver

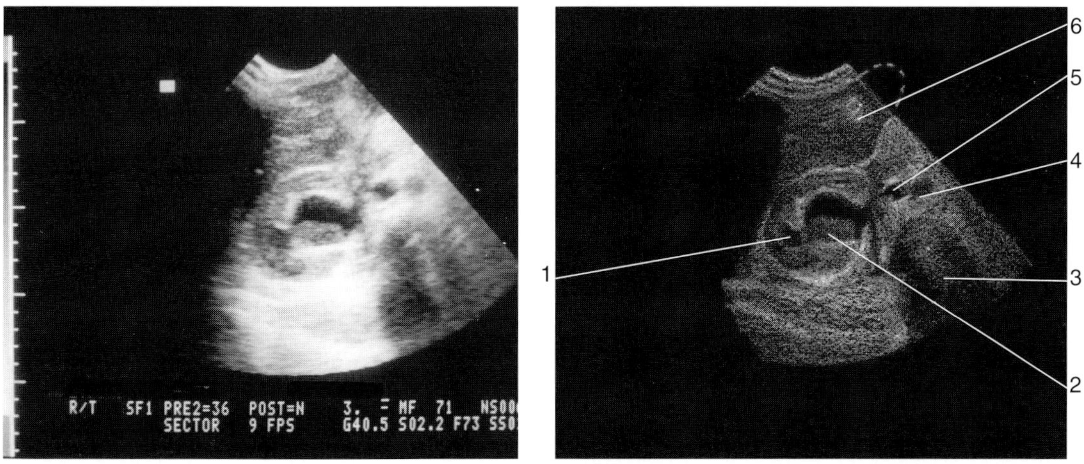

b

1. Renal pyramid 2. Pus 3. Spine 4. Aorta 5. Inferior vena cava 6. Ligamentum teres

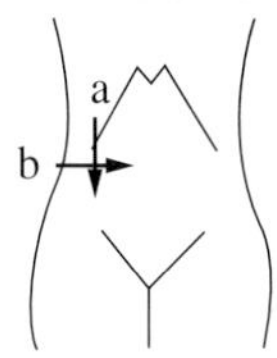

Figure 7-26. Pyonephrosis.
Superinfection of a hydronephrosis produces echoes in the fluid filling the renal pelvis. The entire pelvis may be filled with purulent material or it may form layers, as in this example. (Note the incidental pleural effusion.)

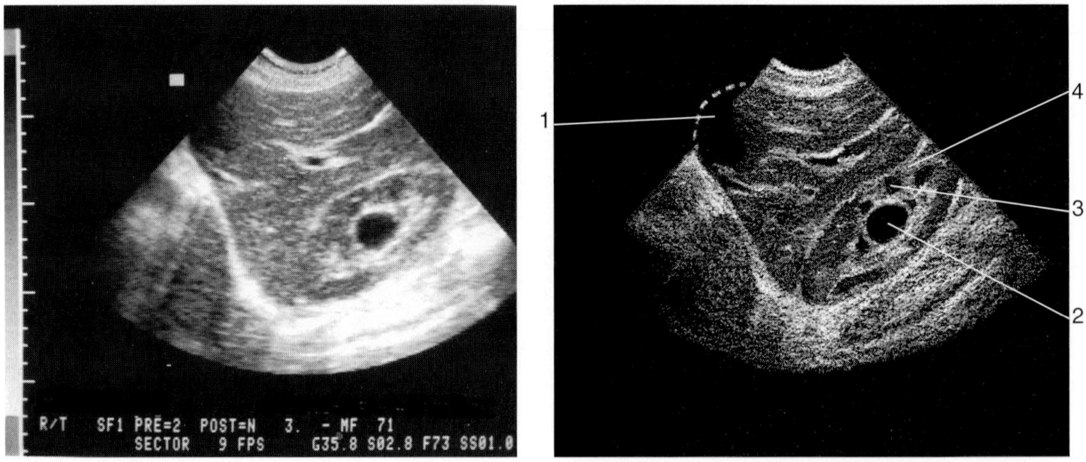

1. Liver 2. Cyst 3. Pyramid 4. Cortex

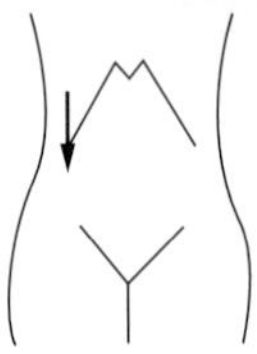

Figure 7-27. Parapelvic cyst.
This rounded, smooth-walled cyst has the typical features of a simple cyst lying within the renal sinus. Calyectasis has a more complex, "fingers-of-a-glove" pattern (cf. Figure 7-21). However, the distinction between a solitary dilated calyx, as might occur in tuberculous scarring, and a parapelvic cyst requires a urogram.

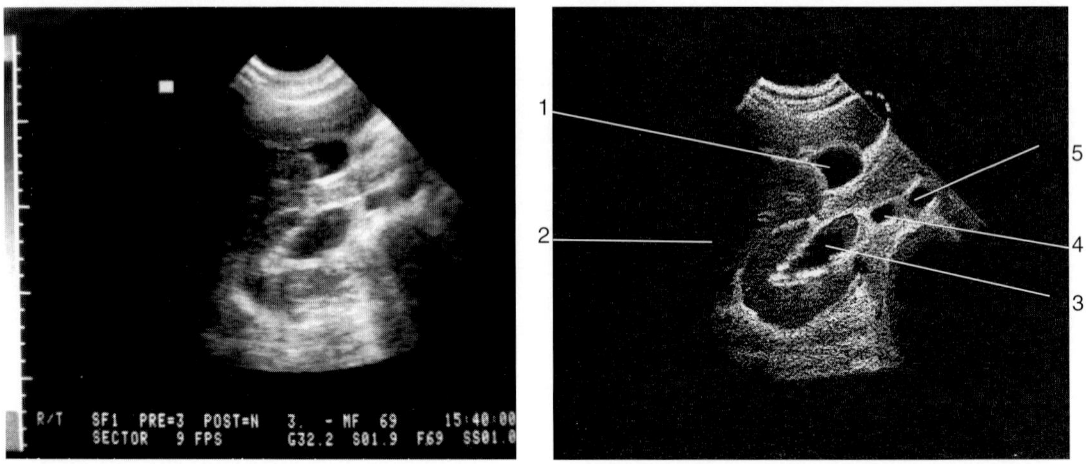

1. Gallbladder 2. Liver 3. Extrarenal pelvis
4. Inferior vena cava 5. Aorta

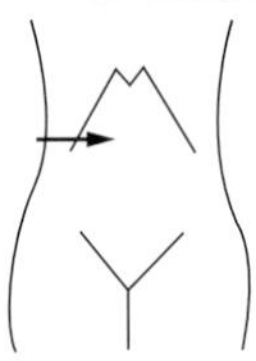

Figure 28. Extrarenal pelvis.
The extrarenal pelvis is commonly baggy, as in this case. This normal variant should not be mistaken for hydronephrosis.

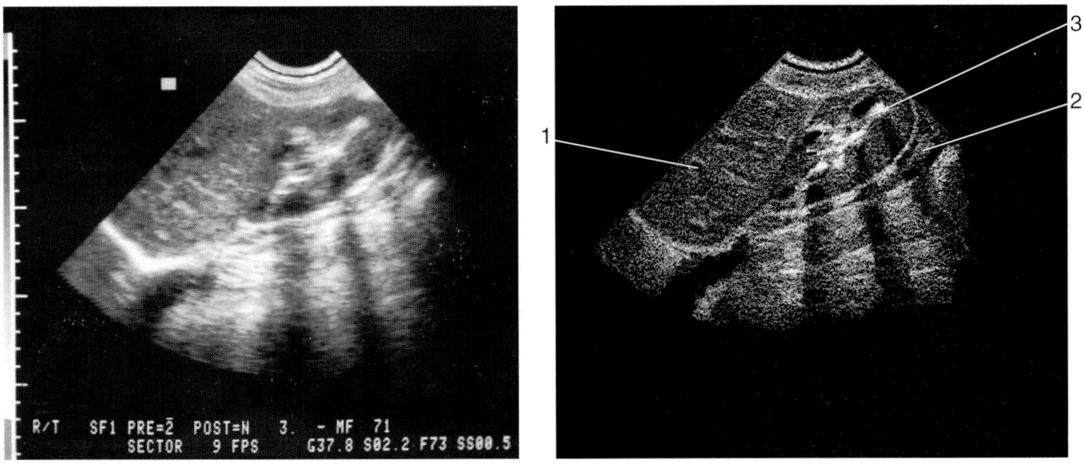

1. Liver 2. Shadow 3. Renal stone

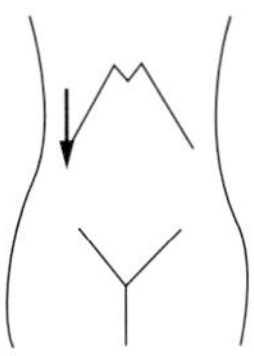

Figure 7-29. Renal stones.
The echogenic foci produced by a large staghorn calculus in this renal pelvis are masked by the strong sinus echoes. The stone is mainly revealed by the distal shadowing, which occurs only with large stones. X-ray studies are more sensitive than ultrasound in this problem.

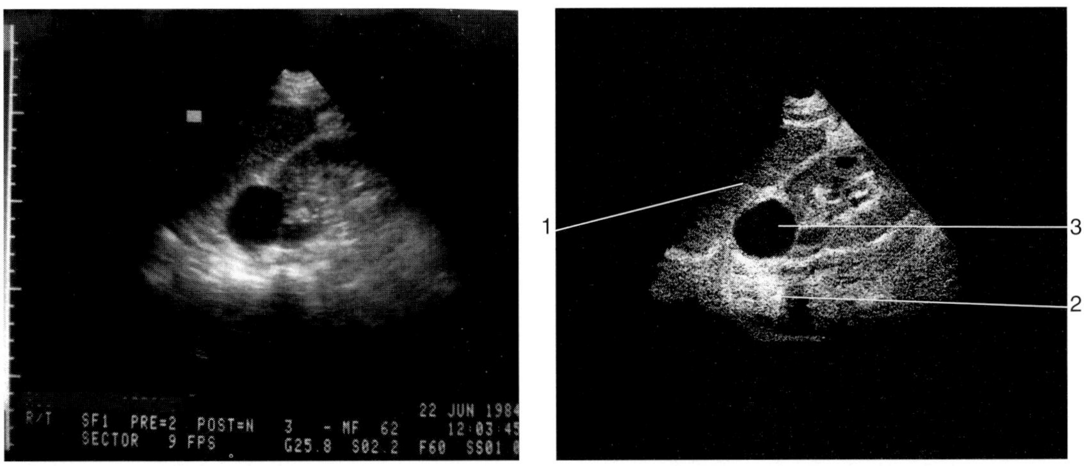

1. Liver 2. Enhancement 3. Renal cyst

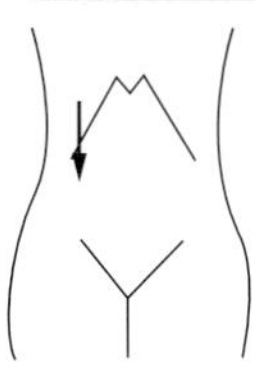

Figure 7-30. Renal cysts.
The typical features of a benign renal cyst are shown. The cyst is echo-free, with smooth walls, and exhibits distal enhancement. (Scanning through the back showed more pronounced enhancement because the enhancement fell across the liver, which is less echogenic than the normally reflective perirenal fat.)

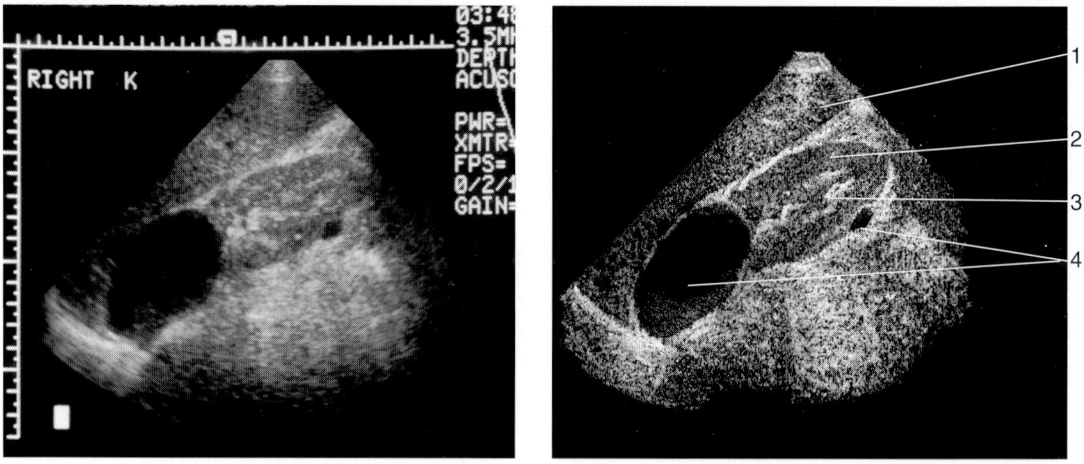

1. Liver 2 .Margin of renal hilum 3. Renal sinus
4. Simple cysts

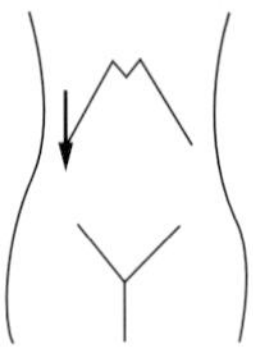

Figure 7-31. Renal cysts.
A small cyst and a larger cyst are seen projecting from the surface of this right kidney. They have well defined, smooth walls. The smaller cyst is echo-free but shows no distal enhancement because it is so small. Enhancement is apparent posterior to the larger cyst; it contains low-level echoes that on real-time scanning were interpreted as noise. The classical features of renal cysts may not always be present.

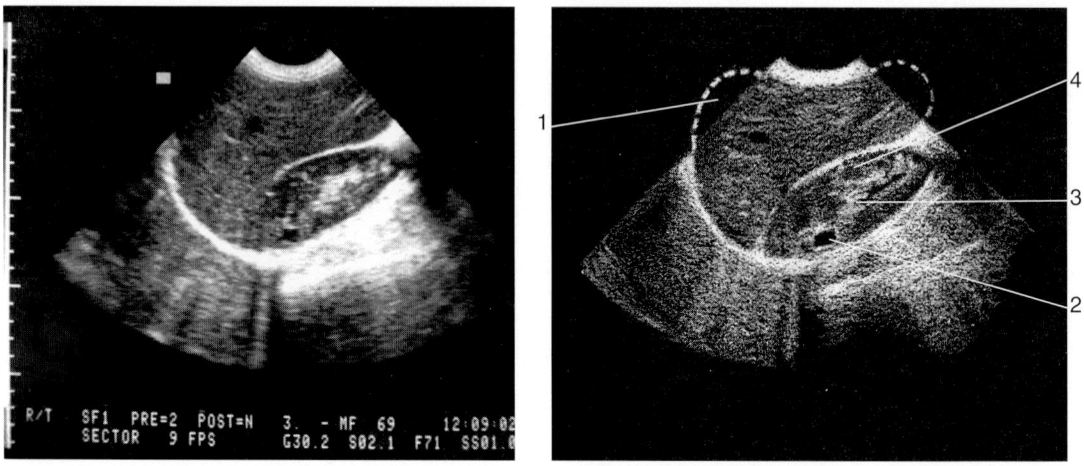

1. Liver 2. Renal cyst 3. Sinus 4. Pyramid

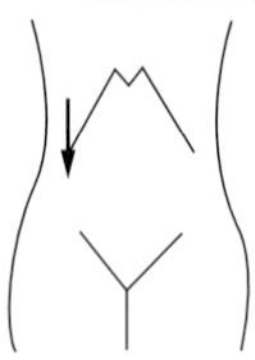

Figure 7-32. Small renal cyst.
This minute lesion has smooth walls and is echo-free, but there is no enhancement because the amount of fluid is too small to produce this effect. Such small lesions often contain echoes that may be artifactual (due to beam-width effects). A lesion that does not display the classical features of a simple cyst must be treated with suspicion.

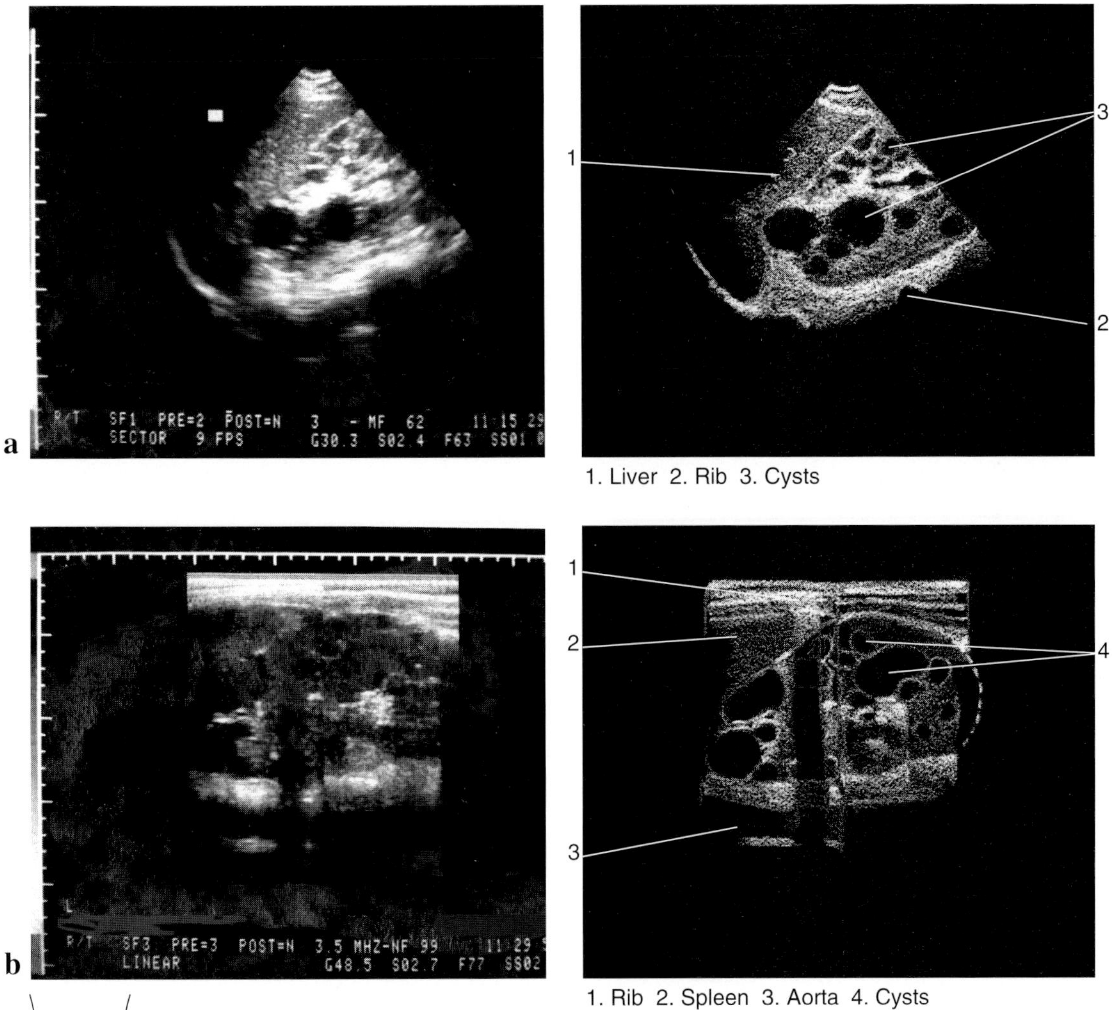

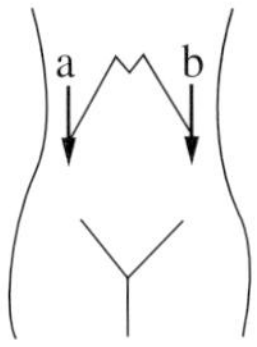

Figure 7-33. Polycystic disease.
Numerous cysts pack the renal parenchyma; such enlarged kidneys are usually palpable. Typically, the cysts are of varying sizes, and their close packing partially flattens them. Hemorrhage into some of the cysts is common; this leads to low-level echoes in the otherwise echo-free spaces.

a

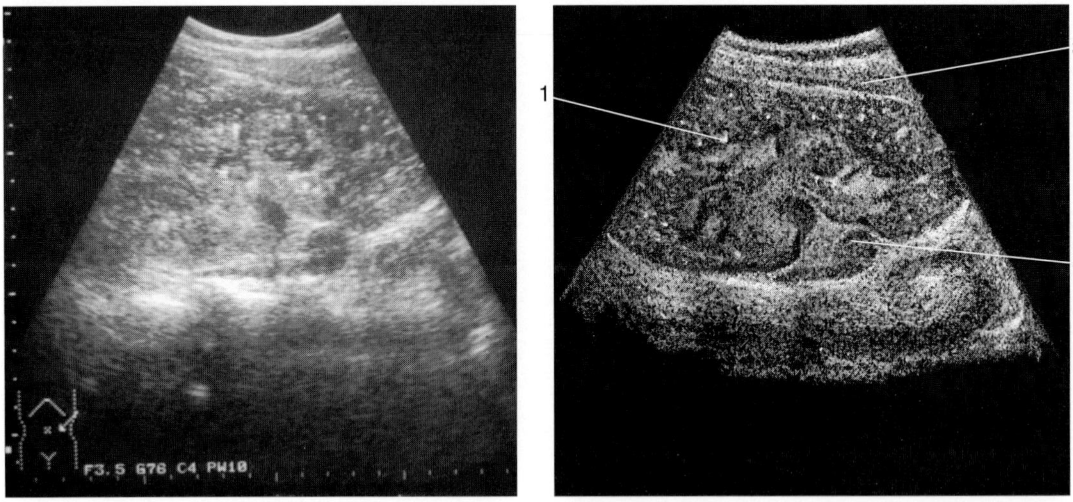

1. Swollen echogenic renal parenchyma 2. Very indistinct renal vessels 3. Multiple small stones

b

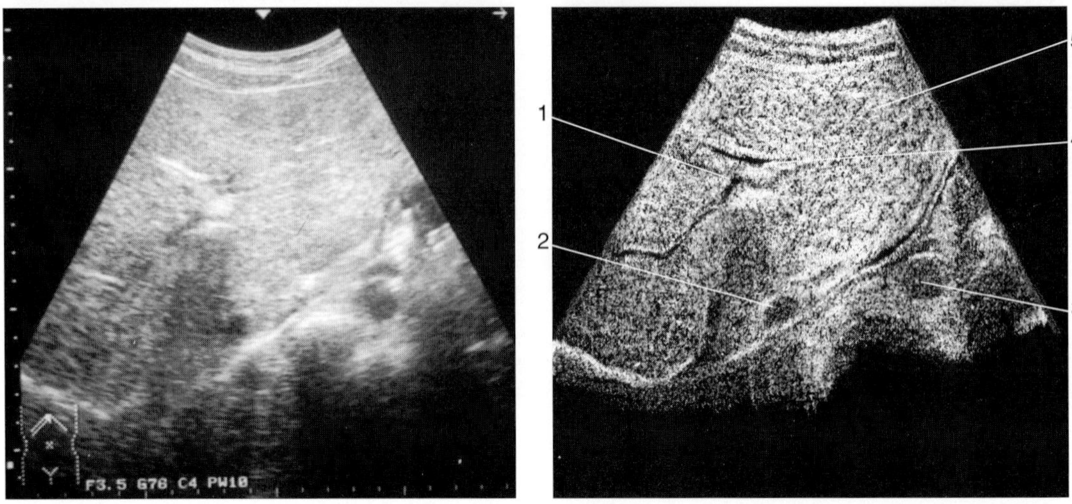

1. Left portal vein (umbilical portion) 2. Inferior vena cava 3. Aorta 4. Branches of hepatic artery 5. Left lobe of liver, diffusely echogenic

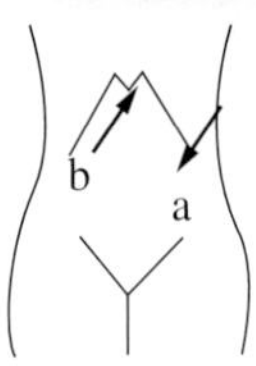

Figure 7-34. Juvenile nephronophthisis.
A 12-year-old girl suffered from severe renal and hepatic dysfunction. The kidneys showed an echogenic parenchyma with multiple small stones throughout. Examination of the upper abdomen revealed extensive hepatic fibrosis accompanied by marked portal hypertension and a splenorenal shunt.

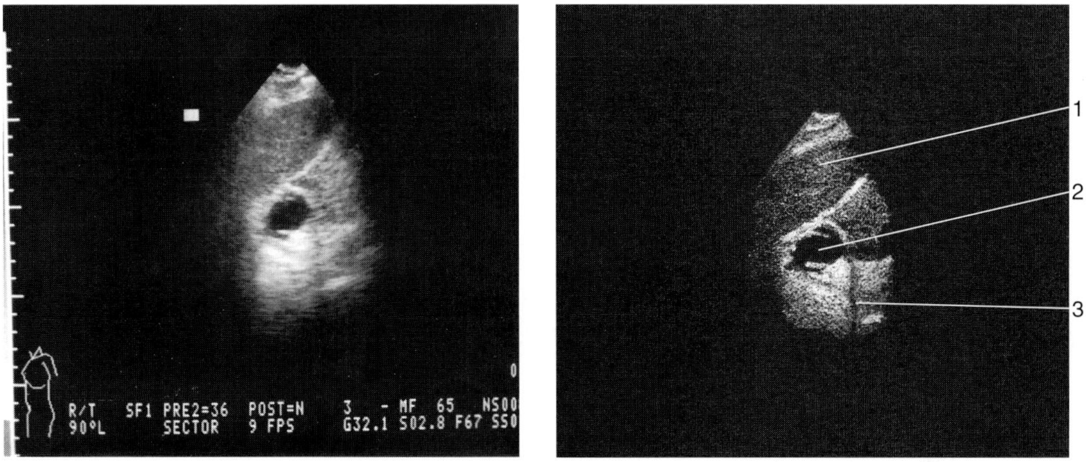

1. Spleen 2. Hematoma 3. Edge shadow

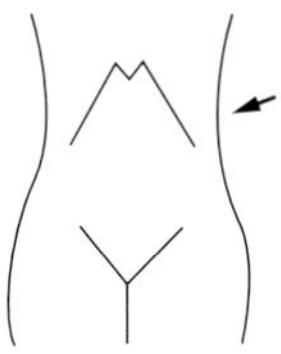

Figure 7-35. Hematoma.
Scanning after a partial nephrectomy revealed this fluid space with irregular walls and some internal echoes. Abscesses and hematomas have identical appearances on ultrasound. On clinical grounds the latter seemed likely in this patient but, when there is suspicion of sepsis, aspiration of the fluid for culture is required. Note the edge shadow from the inferior margin of the hematoma; it should not be interpreted as indicating gas or calcification.

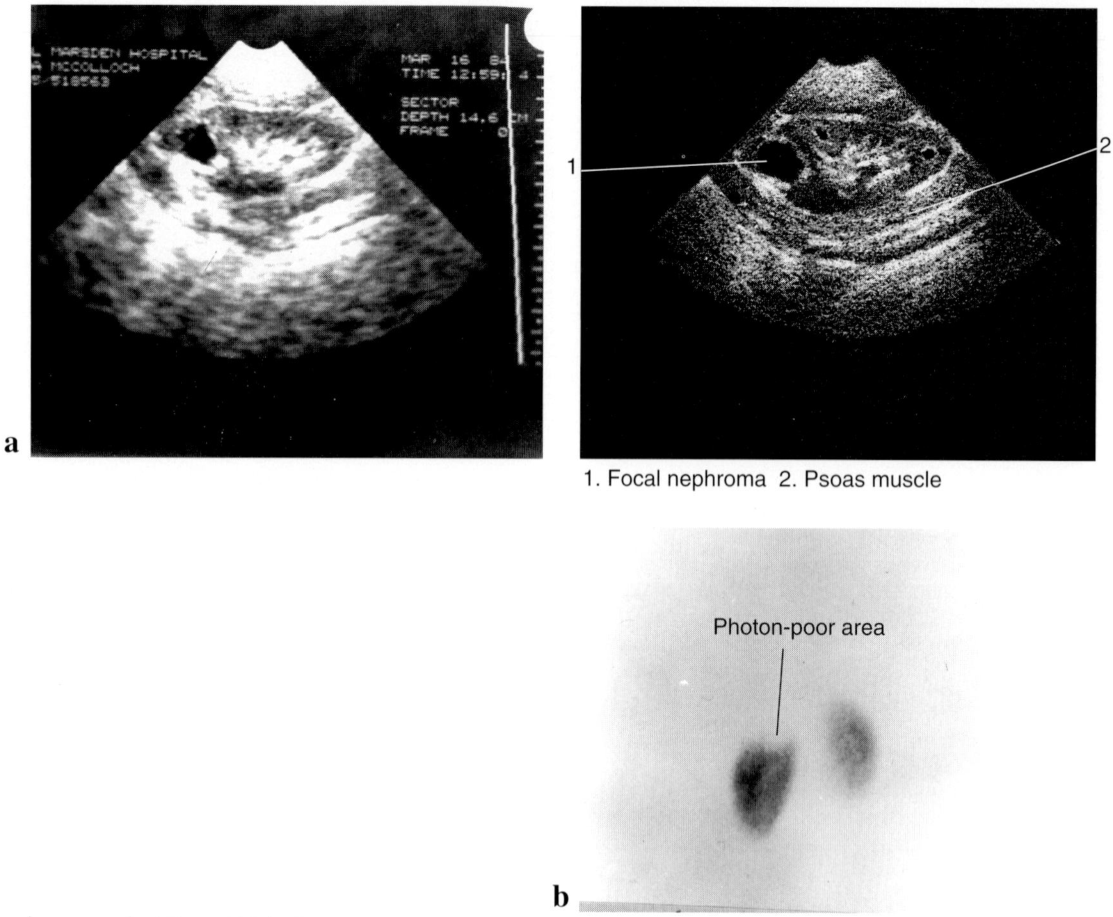

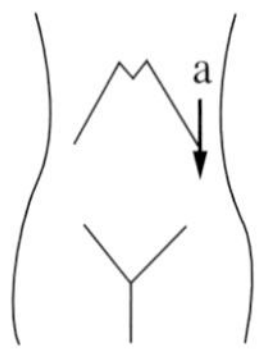

Figure 7-36. Fecal nephronia.
The reduced echoes of acute inflammation are well shown in this case of focal nephronia. Often the ultrasound features are less obvious, and the scintigram (^{99m}Tc-DMSA, L.P.O.) is more sensitive. (Figure courtesy of Dr. S. Meller.)

a
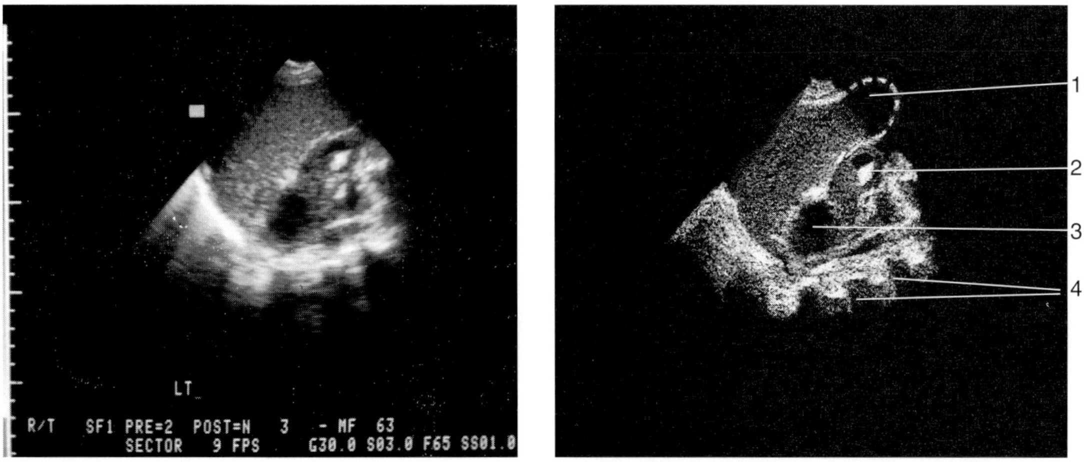

1. Spleen 2. Renal stone 3. Abscess 4. Ribs

b
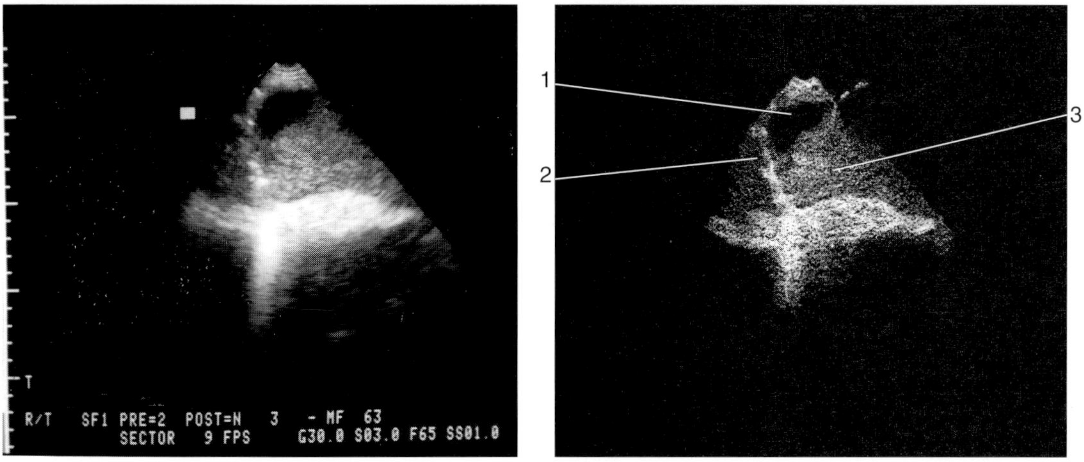

1. Subphrenic abscess 2. Left hemi-diaphragm
3. Spleen

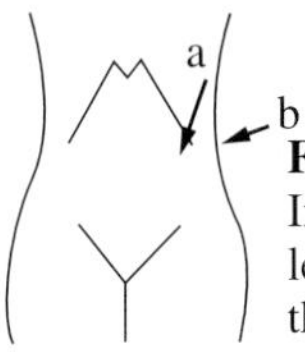

Figure 7-37. Renal abscess.
Investigation of fever in this patient with staghorn calculi revealed this irregular fluid space at the left upper pole (a). It is not echo-free and is therefore not a simple cyst. A hematoma could produce the same appearance (cf. Figure 7-35), but the aspirate grew *Pseudomonas*. An important and unexpected additional finding was a subphrenic collection (b).

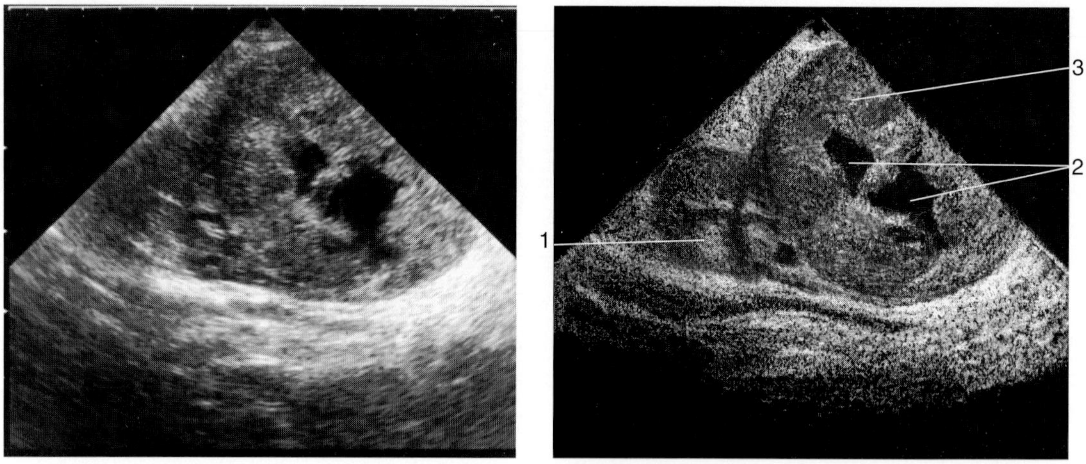

1. Left kidney 2. Central liquefaction 3. Tumor

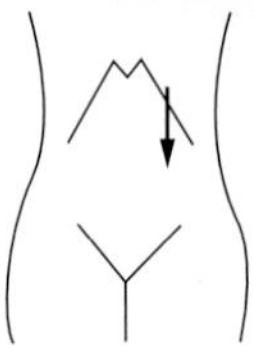

Figure 7-38. Wilms' tumor.

A 7-month-old boy with a large mass of the left abdomen. A huge tumor was visualized arising from the left kidney. The tumor measured 8 cm in the largest diameter, with mostly echogenic parenchyma and irregularly shaped, anechoic parts due to central liquefaction. Histological examination showed nephroblastoma.

a

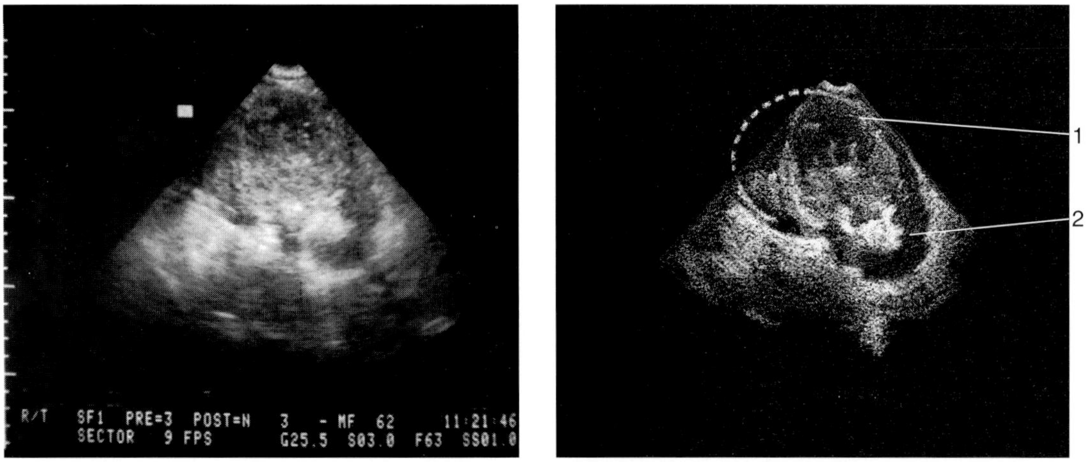

1. Tumor 2. Lower pole of kidney

b

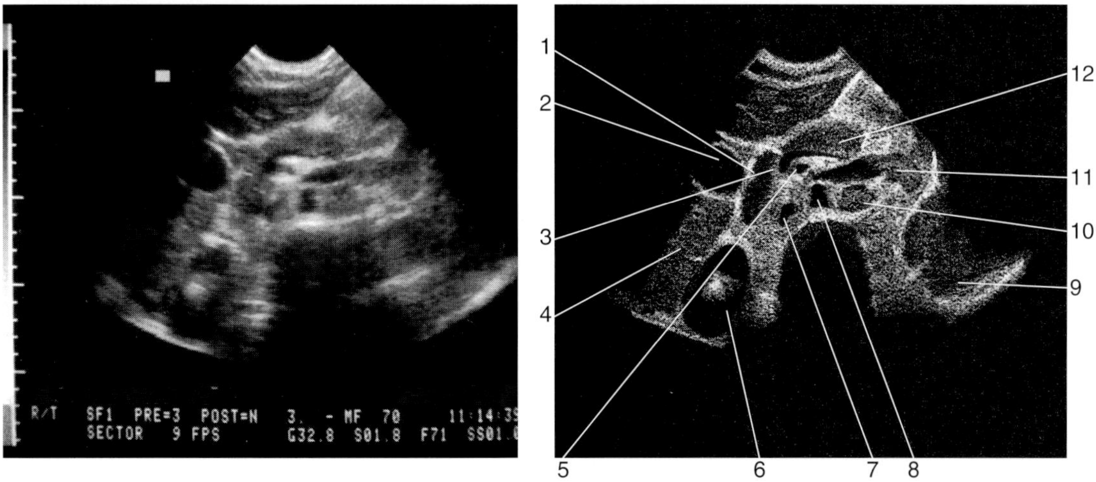

1. Duodenum 2. Gallbladder 3. Origin of portal vein 4. Liver 5. Superior mesenteric artery 6. Right kidney 7. Inferior vena cava 8. Aorta 9. Part of renal carcinoma 10. Involved renal lymph node 11. Pancreas 12. Tumor thrombus in left renal vein

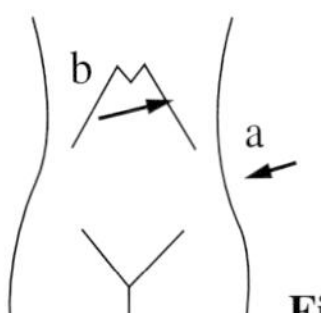

Figure 7-39. Renal carcinoma.

The upper pole of this left kidney is replaced by a solid mass with mixed, irregular echoes (a). These are typical features of carcinoma of the kidney. Spread to regional lymph nodes is common (b), as is direct invasion of the renal vein, often with extension into the cava and even the right atrium.

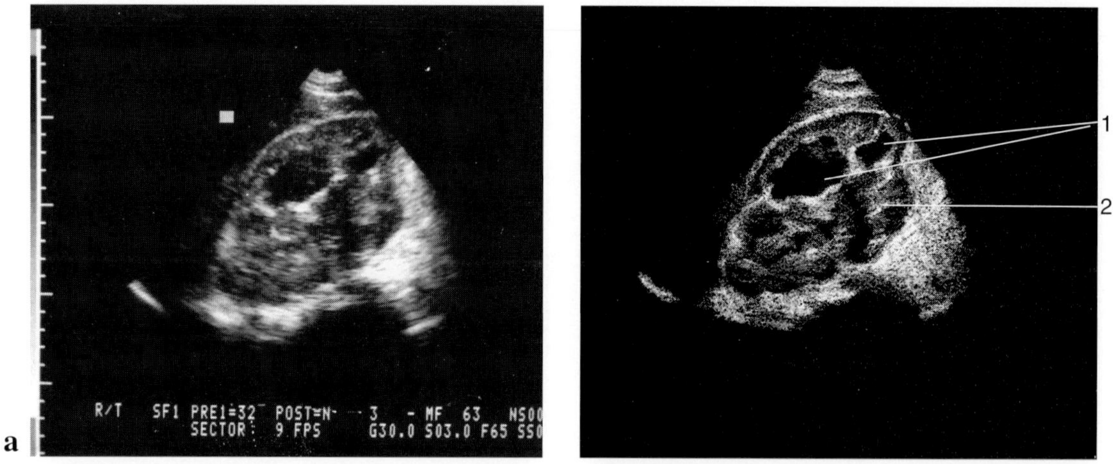

1. Dilated calyces 2. Tumor

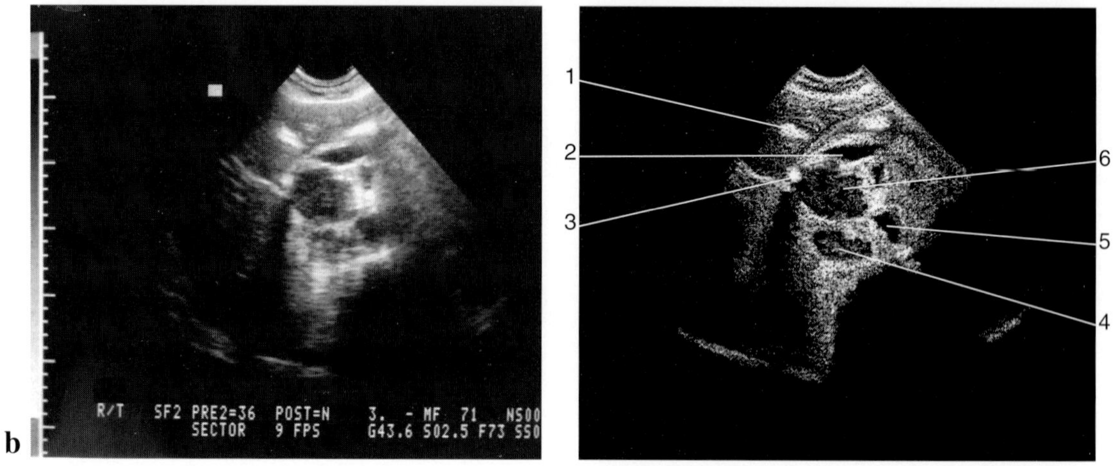

1. Ligamentum teres 2. Pancreas 3. Duodenum 4. Retroperitoneal tumor 5. Aorta 6. Tumor thrombus in inferior vena cava

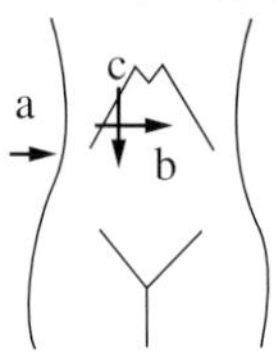

Figure 7-40. Retroperitoneal tumor.
A retroperitoneal sarcoma has invaded the right kidney, causing hydrocalycosis (a). Part of the tumor itself is shown in (b) and (c), as well as tumor thrombus in the inferior vena cava.

c

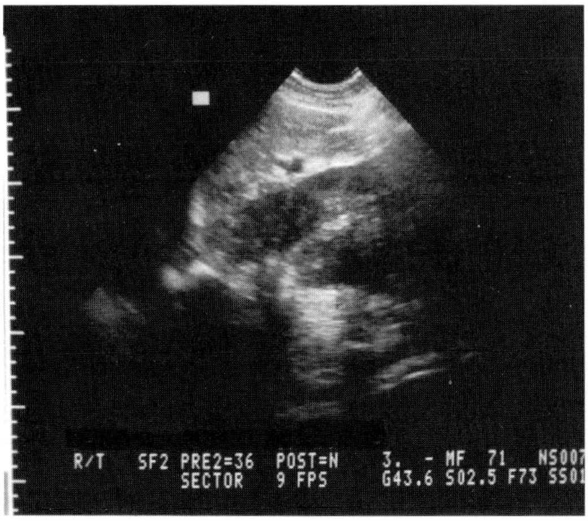

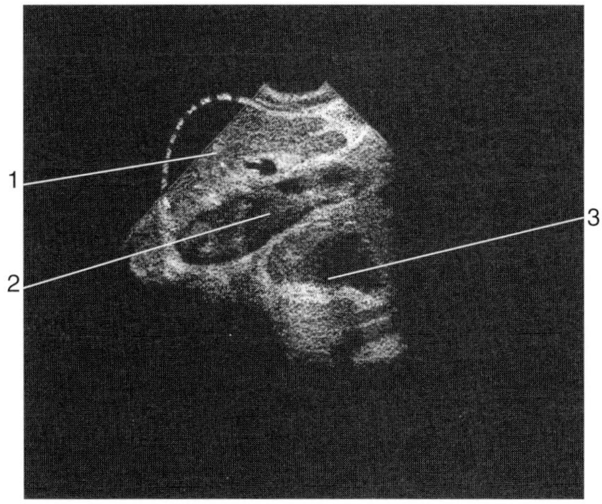

1. Liver 2. Tumor thrombus in inferior vena cava
3. Retroperitoneal tumor

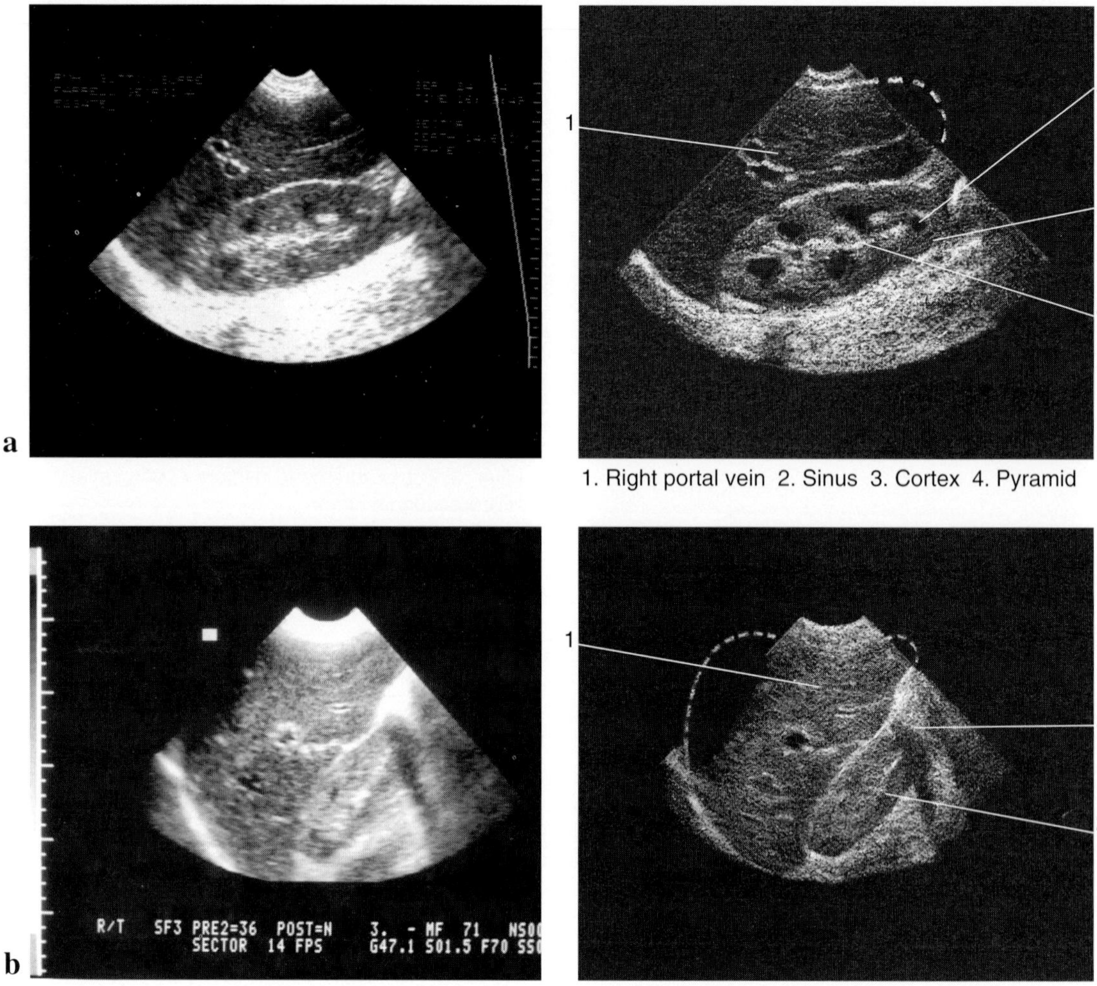

1. Right portal vein 2. Sinus 3. Cortex 4. Pyramid

1. Liver 2. Sinus 3. Hepatic flexure of colon

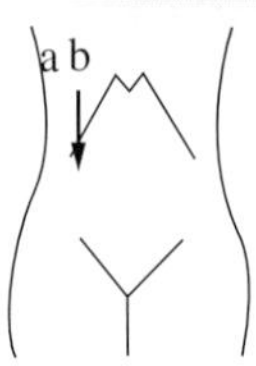

Figure 7-41. Echogenic kidney.
A common result of chronic parenchymal renal disease is a generalized increase in reflectivity, particularly affecting the cortex. Moderate degrees of increase may be recognized. The kidney is more reflective than the liver at the same depth (assuming that the liver is normal). In severe cases, the parenchyma has the same reflectivity as the renal sinus. The kidney is usually shrunken.

a

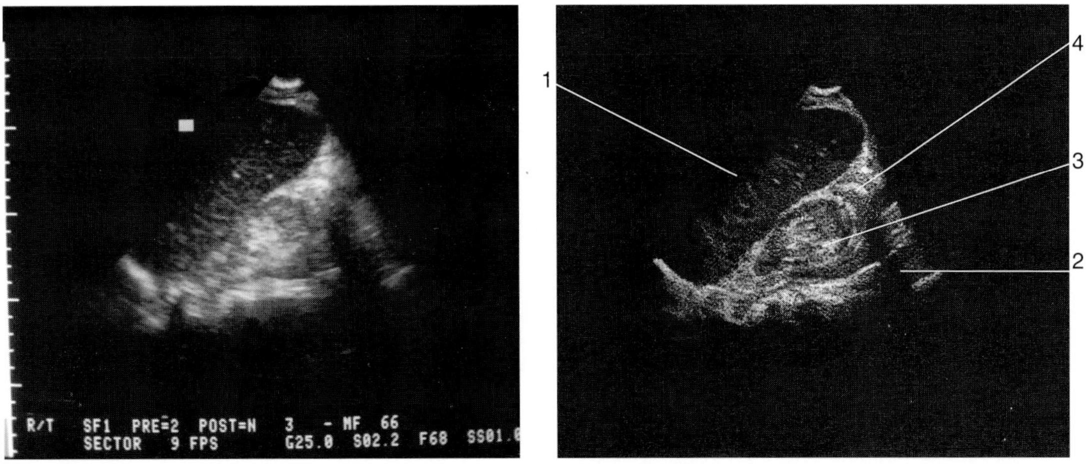

1. Liver 2. Psoas muscle 3. Kidney 4. Hepatic flexure of colon

b

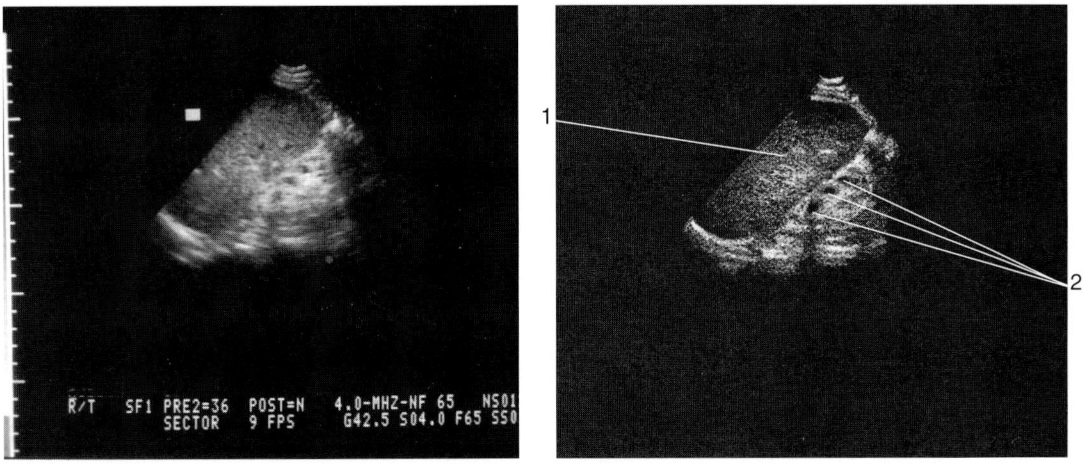

1. Spleen 2. Cysts in featureless kidney

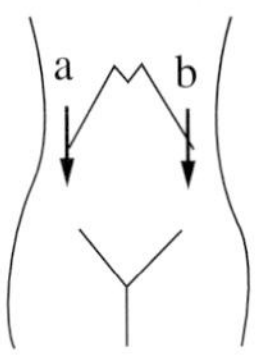

Figure 7-42. End-stage renal disease.
A shrunken, featureless kidney seen in end-stage renal failure due to any diffuse nephropathy (a). The echo levels are higher than those from the liver. In (b) an end-stage kidney shows the cysts that are common when the patient has been maintained on dialysis or with a transplant.

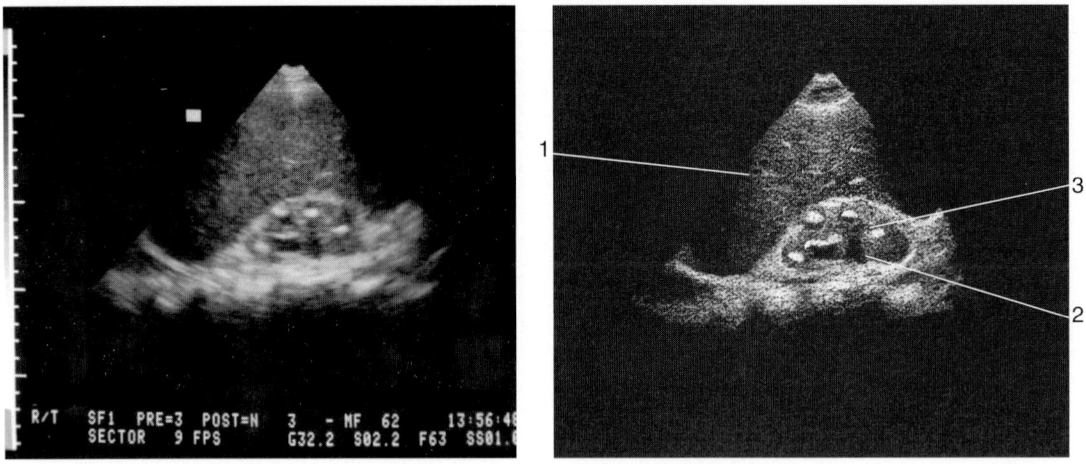

1. Liver 2. Cortx 3. Pyramid

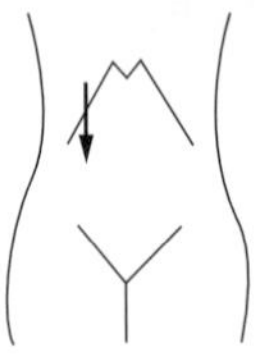

Figure 7-43. Nephrocalcinosis.
Calcification in the renal pyramids produces this characteristic reversed pattern, in which the medullary pyramids are more strongly reflective than the cortex. Ultrasound is more sensitive than conventional radiography here.

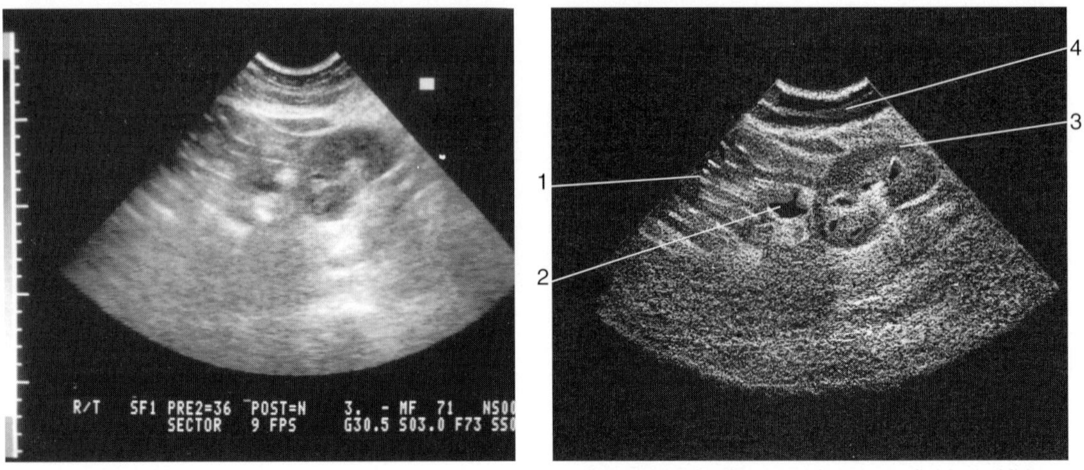

1. Gut loops 2. Pocket of dialysis fluid 3. Kidney
4. Subcutaneous fat

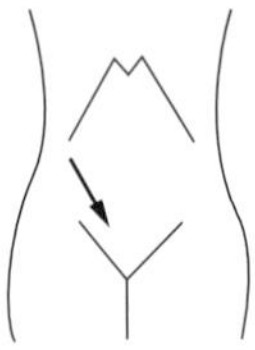

Figure 7-44. Renal transplant.
A normal appearance is seen in this allograft from a child donor. The free fluid in this patient is the residue from recent peritoneal dialysis. Without this clinical background, this appearance would raise the suspicion of intraperitoneal bleeding.

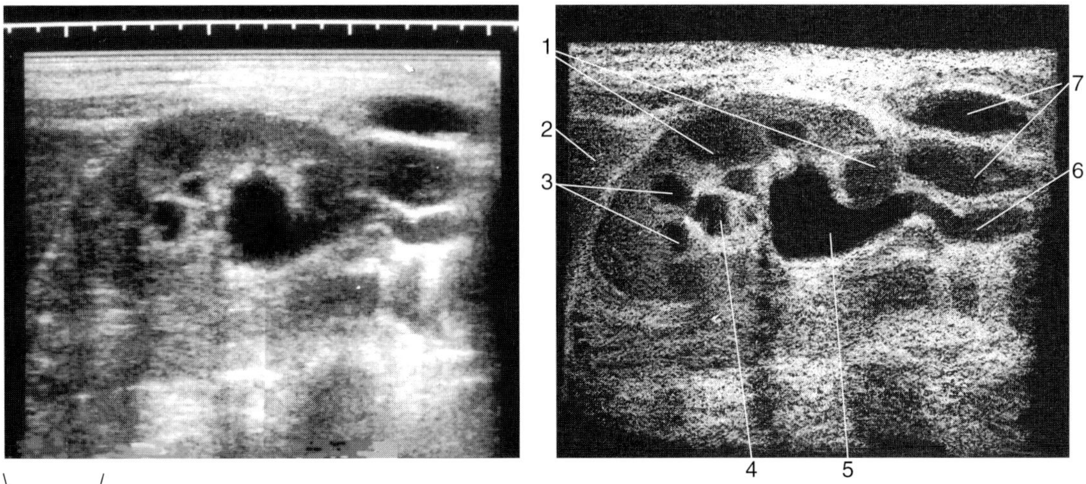

1. Echo-poor zones 2. Liver 3. Pyramids
4. Hydrocalyx 5. Hydropelvis 6. Hydroureter
7. Collection

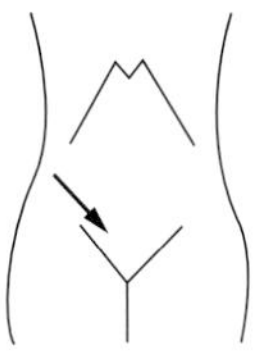

Figure 7-45. Complicated transplant.
An echo-poor, bilocular mass is seen at the lower pole of this transplanted kidney; its appearance a few days postoperatively suggested a hematoma. There is hydronephrosis with ureteric dilatation and irregular patchiness of the parenchymal echoes indicating rejection.

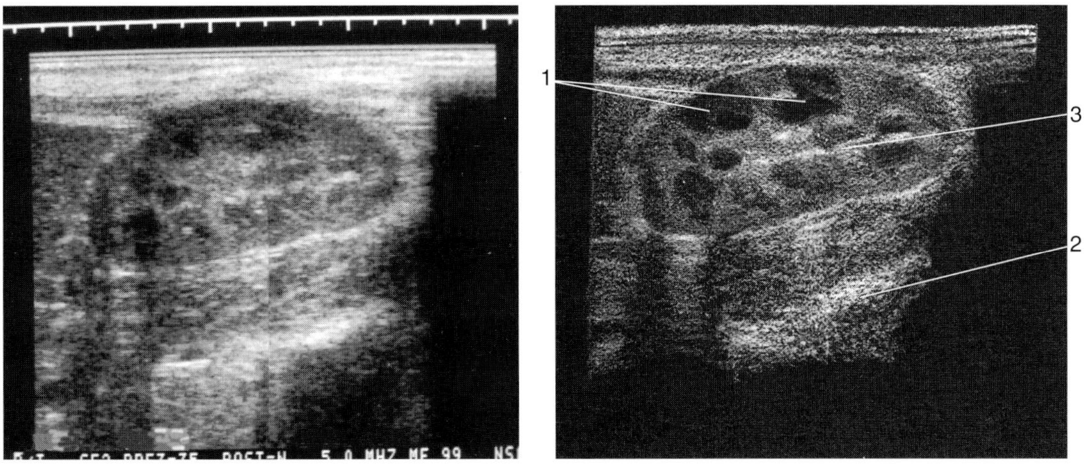

1. Necrotic regions 2. Iliac bone 3. Compressed sinus

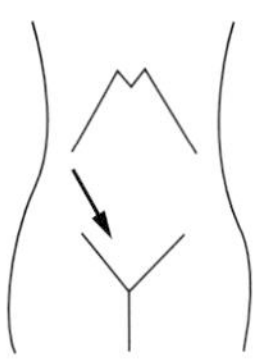

Figure 7-46. Transplant rejection.
Features of rejection (a compressed sinus and echo-poor patches in the parenchyma due to hemorrhage or necrosis) are demonstrated in this transplanted kidney, whose urine output had decreased.

ABNORMALITIES OF THE ADRENALS

The role of ultrasound in the adrenals is confined to the detection and characterization of masses. Since the normal adrenal is not always visualized, atrophy cannot be excluded; for such conditions, CT scanning is the preferred technique.

Adrenal hypertrophy causes convexity of the normally flat or concave margins of the gland. This feature may be demonstrable before measurable enlargement occurs. Cushing's syndrome can be confirmed in this way, though ultrasound is often disappointing since these patients are usually obese; CT scanning is therefore more suitable.

Tumors of the adrenal produce a localized enlargement, though often the remaining part of the adrenal is so distorted so as to be unrecognizable[56] (Figure7-47). Ultrasound then shows a mass related to the upper pole of the kidney. Its origin can be inferred by demonstrating a plane of separation from the kidney; when this is impossible, doubt will remain as to whether the mass is renal or adrenal. It is usually posssible to determine whether such a mass lies within the liver or spleen, as opposed to a retroperitoneal site, by observing that the intraperitoneal organs move across the retroperitonel lesion with respiration. This useful feature fails if the liver or spleen has been invaded or where diaphragmatic movement is poor.

Adrenal adenomas are rarely demonstrated on ultrasound (Figure 7-48). Malignant lesions, primary or metastatic, usually show heterogeneous echoes. Their margins may be well defined or indeterminate, depending on their degree of invasiveness.

In the neonate, the adrenal is much larger than in the adult. It is seen as a layered V- or Y-shaped band applied to the upper pole of the kidney. In adrenal hemorrhage this is replaced by an irregular, predominantly echo-poor mass. Ultrasound is useful in following the resolution of this self-limiting condition. Neonatal adrenal tumors have the same appearance as in the adult.

Adrenal infection usually cannot be detected with ultrasound, but cysts are easily defined and characterized as echo-free, rounded structures with distal enhancement lying in the adrenal bed. They are not clinically important. Calcification produces strongly echogenic bands or foci with distal shadowing.

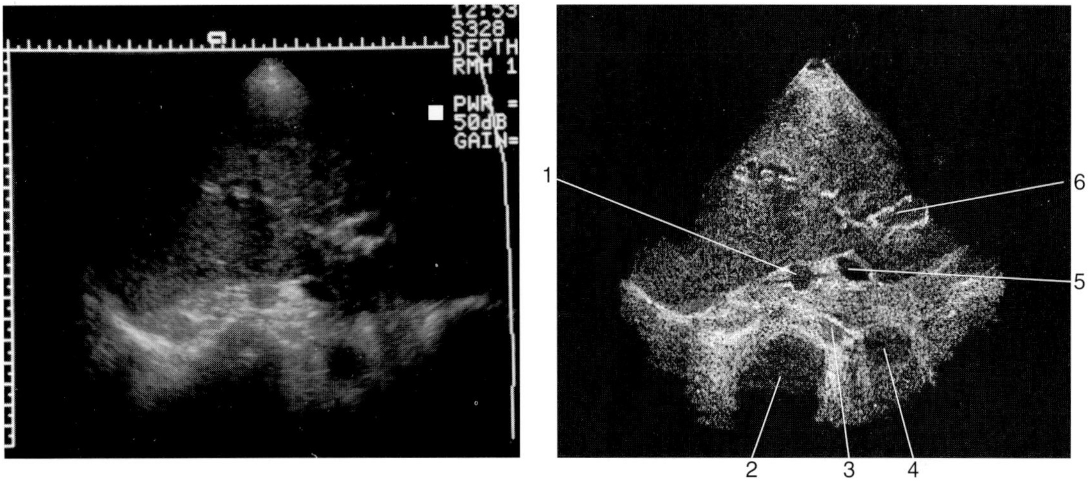

1. Mass in right adrenal 2. Spine 3. Crus of diaphragm 4. Aorta 5. Inferior vena cava 6. Portal vein branch

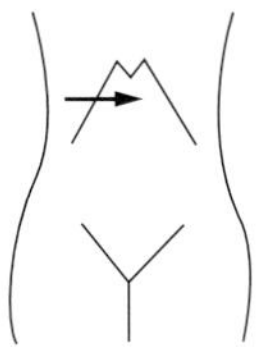

Figure 7-47. Adrenal mass.
A small nodule is seen lying within the right adrenal in this patient with carcinoma of the breast. A metastasis or an adrenal adenoma could both have this appearance. Follow-up scans would be required to distinguish between them.

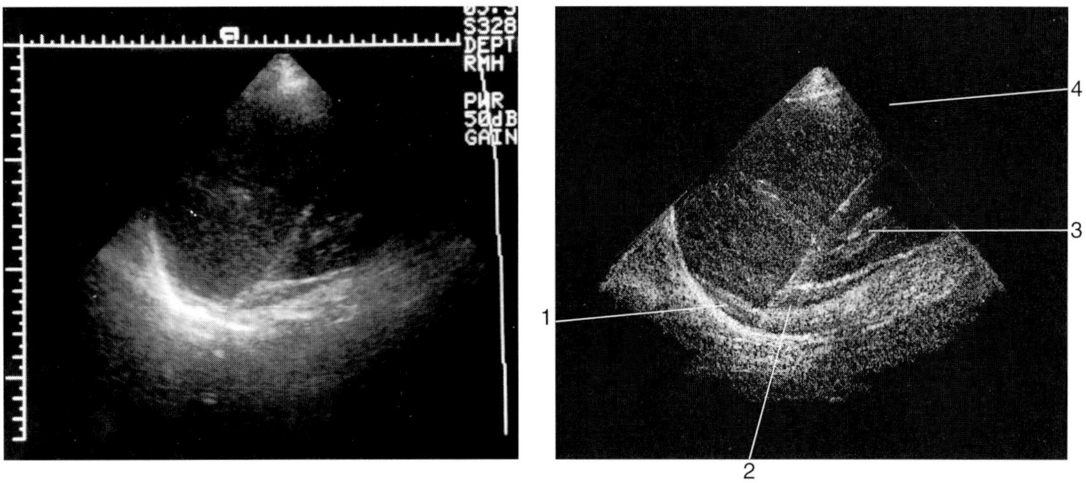

1. Crus of diaphragm 2. Enlarged left adrenal 3. Kidney 4. Spleen

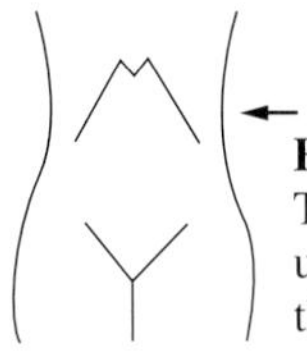

Figure 7-48. Adrenal hyperplasia.
The left adrenal also lies against the crus of the diaphragm, but it is more difficult to image with ultrasound because the window provided by the spleen is more restricted than that of the liver. In this case, the gland is diffusely enlarged in a patient with a bronchial carcinoma that was secreting ectopic adrenocorticotropic hormone (ACTH).

ABNORMALITIES OF THE RETROPERITONEUM

Dilatation of the aorta is easy to demonstrate as a loss of the normal tapering shape seen in a longitudinal section.[42] Mild degrees of this type of ectasia, due to atheroma, are common in older subjects and are not associated with dysfunction. The aortic wall is usually irregular due to ulcerated plaque. Echogenic foci represent calcification and, when extensive, produce shadowing. Aneurysmal dilatation appears as a tubular or saccular enlargement and mainly affects the lower aorta just above the bifurcation (Figure 7-49). Thrombus produces a rim or an eccentric, ring-shaped band of low-level echoes applied to the aortic wall. It is an advantage of ultrasound that both the overall and luminal diameters can be measured. Serial studies are easily carried out, and ultrasound is the best method of following patients with small aneurysms (<4 cm) when surgery is not considered urgent. Limitations to the use of ultrasound are the difficulty of demonstrating extension into the common iliac arteries and demonstrating the position of the renal arteries. Since the latter is important in planning aortic grafting, CT or aortography is required. Leakage may be demonstrated as an echo-poor space extending from the aneurysm; hematoperitoneum simulates ascites. Aortic dissection may be demonstrated on ultrasound as a fine flap in the lumen, but since this is thin, it is easily missed. Color Doppler, by showing the differing flows in the true and false lumens, makes this diagnosis much simpler.

Aortic grafts are strongly echogenic, and ultrasound is a useful way to demonstrate their integrity. Hematomas or pseudoaneurysms may be detected as an echo-poor mass, usually at one end of the graft. On color Doppler, the to-and-fro flow of blood into or out of the pseudoaneurysm is striking. Infection in a graft or hematoma does not give a specific ultrasound pattern unless gas is formed. Here the distinction from nearby gut is possible only when exceptionally good images are obtained. CT scanning is the preferred technique.

Thrombus of the inferior vena cava gives rise to echoes within the cava; blood thrombus tends to have low-level echoes, while tumor thrombus is often strongly echogenic and may show arterial Doppler signals from the neovascularization. Occlusion of the inferior vena cava results in loss of the normal cardiorespiratory pulsation and absence of the Valsalva response. Blood flow is best assessed using Doppler. It is surprising how massive a thrombus can become without causing frank obstruction to flow. The position of intracaval umbrellas can usually be defined as they are intensely echogenic.

Normal para-aortic nodes are not detectable on ultrasound but, when enlarged, they appear as rounded masses which have a lobulated contour when they coalesce[47] (Figure 7-50). They are almost always echo-poor; exceptions are the echogenic nodes due to calcification in chronic sepsis, especially tuberculosis. In general, nodes lie along the major blood vessels. In the upper abdomen, most are retroperitoneal and are associated with the aorta, the inferior vena cava, and the celiac, splenic, renal, and superior mesenteric arteries. There are also major groups in the porta hepatis and lying along the mesenteric border of the gut. Porta nodes often simulate intrahepatic metastases because they indent the soft liver. Because of intestinal gas, only larger mesenteric nodes are detectable on ultrasound. Their anterior position and the mesenteric blood vessels running through the nodal masses are characteristic features. In addition, careful observation often shows moderate respiratory movement, in contrast to the fixity of retroperitoneal nodes. Para-aortic nodes often lie posterior to the aorta and inferior vena cava, which are lifted anteriorly when they enlarge. This displacement especially affects the cava, which is easily deformed. Similarly, precaval and preaortic nodes may lift the pancreas and its vessels anteriorly. Carefull observation of these subtle features is important in arriving at the correct diagnosis. Inflammatory and malignant nodes are indistinguishable on ultrasound.

Other retroperitoneal pathologies are uncommon apart from pancreatic pseudocysts; developmental cysts and retroperitoneal abscesses may be encountered. Retroperitoneal fibrosis gives rise to sheets of echo-poor tissue over the aorta which often extend below the bifurcation. Hydronephrosis is usually present.

a

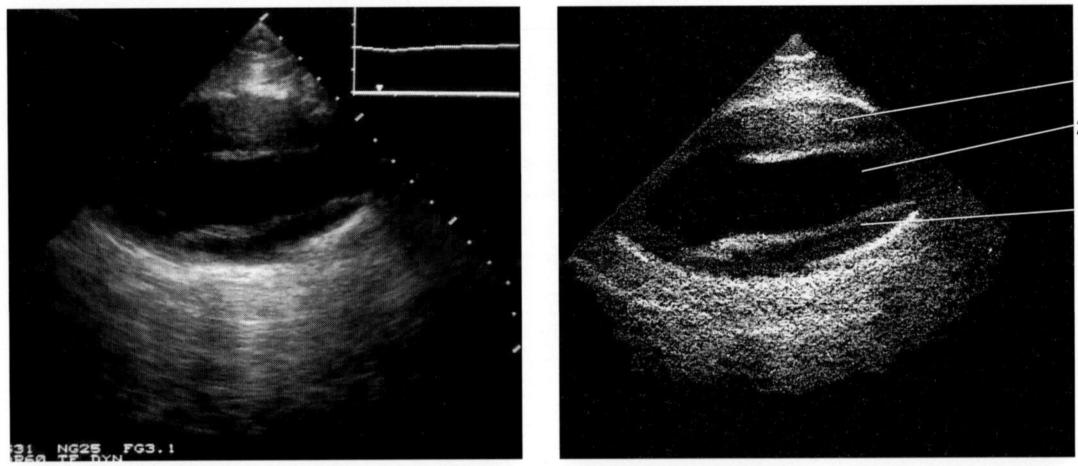

1. Thrombus 2. Lumen

b

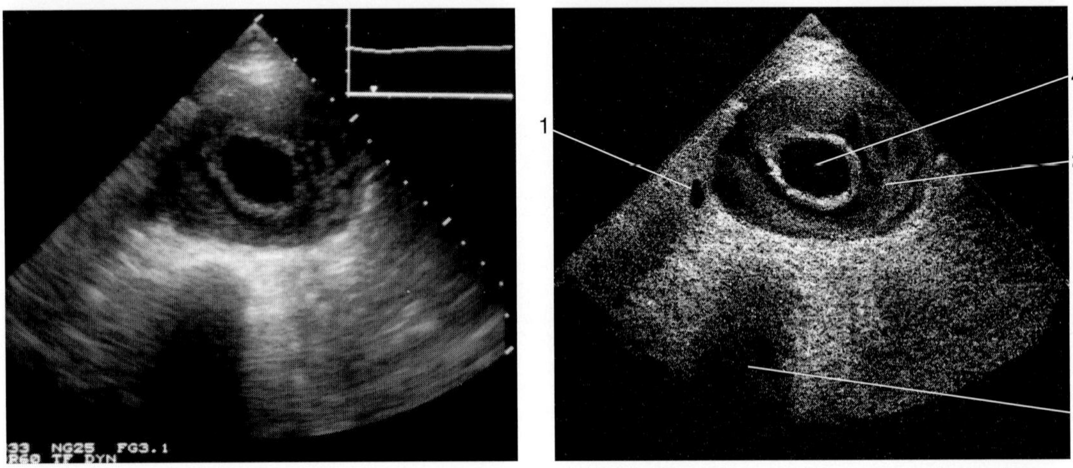

1. Inferior vena cava 2. Spine 3. Laminated thrombus 4. Lumen

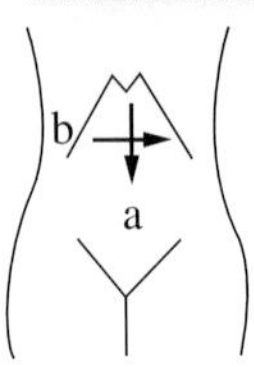

Figure 7-49. Aortic aneurysm.
This fusiform aneurysm shows the layer of thrombus encircling the lumen.

a

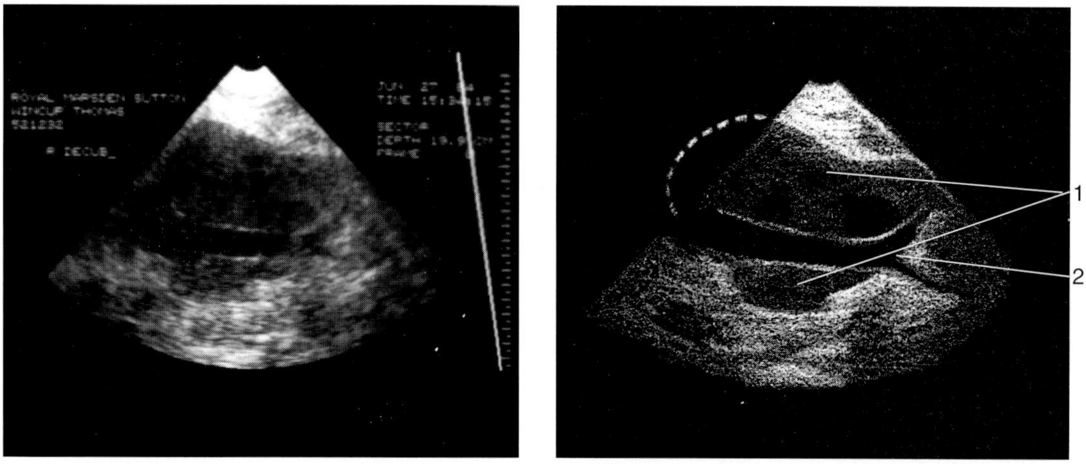

1. Para-aortic mass 2. Bifurcation of aorta

b

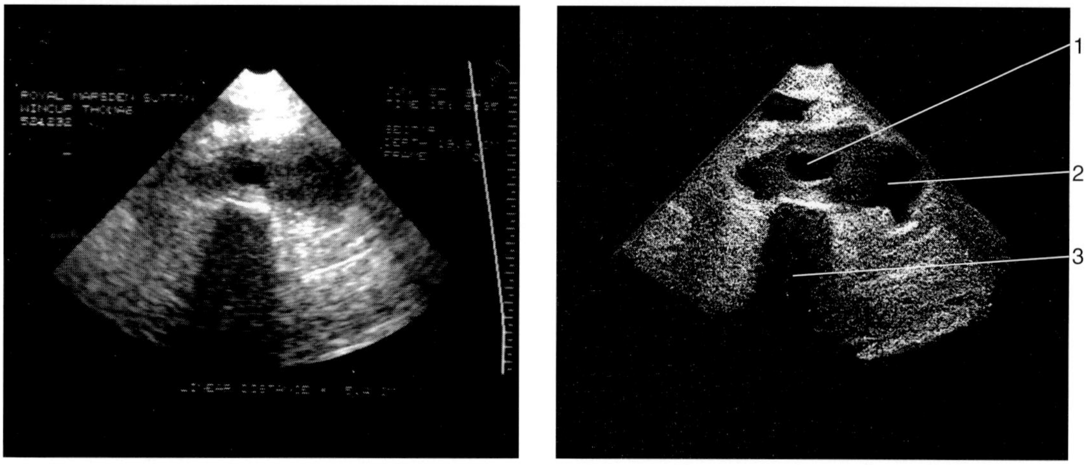

1. Aorta 2. Peri-aortic node mass 3. Spine

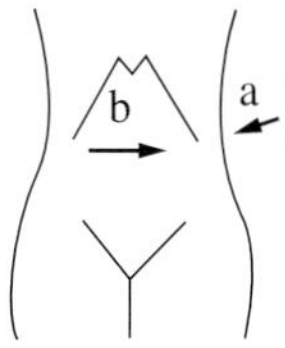

Figure 7-50. Para-aortic nodes.
The echo-poor mass surrounding the aorta at its bifurcation is a mass of nodes involved with tumor (testicular teratoma). The coronal view (a) is particularly helpful in demonstrating the lower aorta.

REFERENCES

1. Asher AW, Moffat DB, Sanders E: Nephrology Illustrated. London, Pergamon Medical, 1982.
2. Blei CL, Hartman DS, Friedman AC, et al: Papillary renal cell carcinoma: Ultrasonic/pathologic correlation (abstract). Radiology 148 : 604, 1983.
3. Boal DKB, Teele RL: Sonography of infantile polycystic kidney disease. Radiology 135 : 575-577, 1980.
4. Brandt TB, Neiman HL, Dragovsky MJ, et al: Ultrasound assessment of normal renal dimensions. J Ultrasound Med 1 : 49-56, 1982.
5. Braun B, Weilmann LS, Weigand W: Ultrasonographic demonstration of renal vein thrombosis. Radiology 138 : 157-160, 1981.
6. Buchberger W, Penz T, Wicke K, et al: Diagnosis and staging of blunt kidney trauma. A comparison of urinalysis, i.v. urography, sonography and computed tomography. Rofo Fortschr Geb Rontgenstr Neuen Bildgeb Verfahr 158 : 507-512, 1993.
7. Coleman BG, Arger PH, Mulhern CB, et al: Gray-scale sonographic spectrum of hypernephromas. Radiology 137 : 757-780, 1980.
8. Coleman BG, Arger PH, Mulhern CB, et al: Pyonephrosis: Sonography in the diagnosis and management. Am J Radiol 137 : 939-943, 1981.
9. Cook JH, Rosenfield AT, Taylor KJW: Ultrasonic demonstration of intrarenal anatomy. Am J Roentgenol 129 : 831-835, 1977.
10. Coyne SS, Walsh JW, Tisnado J, et al: Surgically correctable renal transplant complications. Am J Radiol 136 : 1113-1121, 1981.
11. Curry NS, Gobien RP, Schabel SI: Minimal dilatation, obstructive nephropathy. Radiology 143 : 531-534, 1982.
12. Dalla Palma L, Bazzocchi M, Cressa C, et al: Radiological anatomy of the kidney revisited. Br J Radiol 63 : 680-690, 1990.
13. Edell SL, Bonavita JA: Sonographic appearance of acute pyelonephritis. Radiology 132 : 683-691, 1979.
14. Fieglar W: Ultrasound in acute renal inflammatory lesions. Eur J Radiol 3 : 354-357, 1983.
15. Garel LA, Habib R, Pariente D, et al: Juvenile nephronophthisis: Sonographic appearance in children with severe uraemia. Radiology 151 : 93-95, 1984.
16. Glazer GN, Callan PW, Filly RA: Medullary nephrocalcinosis: Sonographic evaluation. Am J Radiol 138 : 55-58, 1982.
17. Grossman H, Rosenberg ER, Bowie JD: Sonographic diagnosis of renal cystic diseases. Am J Radiol 140 : 81-88, 1983.
18. Hartman DS, Goldman SM, Friedman AC, et al: Angiomyolipoma: Ultrasonic-pathologic correlation. Radiology 139 : 451-458, 1981.
19. Haller JO, Berdon WE, Friedman AP: Increased renal cortical echogenicity: A normal finding in neonates and infants. Radiology 142 : 173-179, 1982.
20. Hoddick W, Jeffrey RB, Goldberg HI, et al: CT and sonography of severe renal and perirenal infections. Am J Radiol 140 : 517-525, 1983.
21. Hoffman JC, Schnur MJ, Koenigsberg M: Demonstration of renal papillary necrosis by sonography. Radiology 145 : 785-793, 1982.
22. Hollinshead WH: Anatomy for Surgeons, Vol 2; The Thorax, Abdomen and Pelvis, ed 3. New York, Harper & Row, 1983, pp270-313.
23. Hricak H, Cruz C, Romanski RN, et al: Renal parenchymal disease: Sonographic-histologic correlation. Radiology 144 : 141-152, 1982.
24. Hricak H, Romanski RN, Eyler WR: Renal sinus during allograft rejection: Sonographic and histopathologic findings. Radiology 142 : 693-701, 1982.
25. Hricak H, Slovis TL, Callen CW, et al: Neonatal kidneys: Sonographic-anatomic correlation. Radiology 147 : 699-712, 1983.
26. Hricak H, Toledo-Pereyra LH, Eyler WR, et al: Role of ultrasound in the diagnosis of kidney allograft rejection. Radiology 132 : 667-680, 1979.
27. Isikoff MB, Hill MC: Sonography of the renal arteries: Left lateral decubitus position. Am J Roentgenol 134 : 1177-1179, 1980.
28. Jeffrey RB, Federle MP: CT and ultrasonography of acute renal abnormalities. Radiol Clin North Am 21 : 515-525, 1983.
29. Kay CJ, Rosenfield AT, Armm M: Gray-scale ultrasonography in evaluation of renal trauma. Radiology 134 : 461-474, 1980.
30. Kelsey JA, Bowie JD: Gray-scale ultrasonography in the demonstration of polycystic kidney disease.

Radiology 122 : 791-795, 1977.
31. Kier R, Taylor KJ, Feyock AL, et al: Renal masses: Characterization with Doppler US. Radiology 176 : 703-707, 1990.
32. Lawson TL, McClennan BL, Shirkhoda A: Adult polycystic kidney disease: Ultrasonographic and computed appearance. Radiology 131 : 286-298, 1979.
33. Leekham RN, Matzinger MA, Brunelle M, et al: The sonography of renal columnar hypertrophy. JCU 11 : 491-494, 1983.
34. Levine E, Maklad NF, Rosenthal SJ, et al: Comparison of computed tomography and ultrasound in staging of renal cancer (abstract). Radiology 138 : 765, 1981.
35. Mahony BS, Jeffrey RB, Laing FC: Septa of Bertin: A sonographic pseudotumor. JCU 11 : 317-319, 1983.
36. Maklad NF : Ultrasonic evaluation of renal transplants. Semin Ultrasound 2 : 88-96, 1981.
37. Marshall FF, Smith NA, Murphy JB, et al: Comparison of ultrasonography and radiography in the localization of renal calculi. Radiology 144 : 726-734, 1982.
38. Mascatello VJ, Smith EH, Carrera GF, et al: Ultrasonic evaluation of the duplex kidney. Am J Roentgenol 129 : 113-120, 1977.
39. Netter FH: Ciba Collection of Medical Illustrations, Vol 6, Kidneys, Ureters and Urinary Bladder. Summit, NJ, Ciba Pharmaceutical Co, 1973.
40. Nomura G, Kinoshita E, Yamagata Y, et al: Usefulness of renal ultrasonography for assessment of severity and course of acute tubular necrosis. JCU 12 : 135-139, 1984.
41. Patriquin H, Lefaivre JF, Lafortune M, et al: Fetal lobation. An anatomo-ultrasonographic correlation. J Ultrasound Med 9 : 191-197, 1990.
42. Raskin MM: Ultrasonography of the abdominal aorta, in Sarti DA, Sample WF (eds), Diagnostic Ultrasound. Boston, GK Hall, 1980, pp226-243.
43. Rego JD, Laing FC, Jeffrey RB: Ultrasonographic diagnosis of medullary cystic disease. J Ultrasound Med 2 : 433-436, 1983.
44. Rosenberg ER, Trought WS, Kirks DR, et al: Ultrasonic diagnosis of renal vein thrombosis in neonates. Radiology 134 : 35-39, 1980.
45. Rosenfield AT, Glickman MG, Taylor KJ, et al: Acute focal bacterial nephritis (acute lobar nephronia). Radiology 132 : 553-557, 1979.
46. Rosenfield AT, Siegel NJ: Renal parenchymal disease: Histopathologic-sonographic correlation. Am J Radiol 137 : 793-808, 1981.
47. Sample WF: Adrenal ultrasonography. Radiology 127 : 461-463, 1978.
48. Scanlon MH, Karasick SR: Acquired renal cystic disease and neoplasia: Complications of chronic hemodialysis. Radiology 147 : 837-841, 1983.
49. Schneck CD: Tha abdominal basis of abdomino-pelvic sectional imaging, in Joseph AE, Cosgrove DO (eds), Ultrasound in Inflammatory Diseases. New York, Churchill Livingstone, 1983, pp12-41.
50. Sefczek RJ, Beckman I, Lupetin AR, et al: Sonography of acute renal cortical necrosis. Am J Radiol 142 : 553-554, 1984.
51. Silver TM, Campbell D, Wicks JD, et al: Peritransplant fluid collections: Ultrasound evaluation and clinical significance. Radiology 138 : 145-155, 1981.
52. Spira R, Kwan E, Gerzof SG, et al: Left renal vein varix simulating a pancreatic pseudocyst by sonography. Am J Radiol 138 : 149-159, 1982.
53. Stuck KJ, Koff SA, Silver TM: Ultrasonic features of multicystic dysplastic kidneys. Radiology 143 : 217-234, 1982.
54. Wardle EN: Guidelines in Medicine, Vol 2, Renal Medicine. Lancaster, UK, MTP Press, 1979.
55. Yoder IC, Pfister RC, Lindfors KK, et al: Pyonephrosis: Imaging and intervention. Am J Radiol 141 : 735-742, 1983.
56. Zeman RK, Taylor KJW, Rosenfield AT: Sonographic features of kidney, adrenal and bladder tumors, in Kossoff G, Fukuda M (eds), Ultrasonic Differential Diagnosis of Tumors. New York, Igaku-Shoin, 1983, pp212-230.

CHAPTER 8

THE GASTROINTESTINAL TRACT

Ultrasound examination of the gastrointestinal tract has long been ignored as of limited value because imaging gastrointestinal organs is prevented by intestinal gas and because bowel contents may imitate tumor masses.[6, 19, 35, 46]

A number of reports have focused, however, on the value of static contact scanning in the visualization masses arising from the gastrointestinal tract. The pseudokidney sign, which is most commonly caused by a malignant tumor arising either from the stomach or the colon, is characterized by a mass having a central irregular echo cluster with an echo-poor surrounding region.[7, 26, 32, 37] The name clearly describes the characteristic echo pattern by analogy to that appearance of the kidney.

Beside masses of the gastrointestinal tract, ileus, colonic inflammatory diseases such as Crohn's disease and ulcerative colitis, as well as ascitic fluid accumulation can be identified on ultrasound.[3, 26, 52] It soon became apparent, however, that the static scanner has limited resolution and cannot visualize minute lesions such as early gastric or colonic cancers, which are diagnosed easily and precisely by routine endoscopy. The introduction of real-time scanners with improved resolution has changed the perspective views on imaging of these hollow viscera. It is now considered routine to survey the gastrointestinal tract during a sonographic examination.

ULTRASONIC APPEARANCES OF THE NORMAL GASTROINTESTINAL TRACT

Of the various parts of the gastrointestinal tract, the esophagus, because of its intrathoracic localization, is rarely accessible to ultrasonic scanning, except for the uppermost part immediately posterior to the left lobe of the thyroid and the lowermost part connecting to the cardiac portion of the stomach. High-resolution real-time scanning clearly identifies the esophagogastric junction by virtue of its characteristic sonographic pattern with an echogenic central region surrounded by a hypoechoic zone (Figure 8-1).

The stomach, on the other hand, can be imaged ultrasonographically, either when empty or when filled by fluid. A high-resolution sector or convex array probe applied to the midepigastrium or at the lower left costal margin clearly demonstrates the stomach (Figures 8-2 and 8-3). In the midline sagittal sonogram, the antral portion of the stomach can be imaged routinely as an elliptical shape representing the cross-section of the stomach, with an echogenic inner layer surrounded by thin echo-poor zone that corresponds to the muscularis propria. This layer tends to be thicker toward the pylorus. The thickness of the muscular layer varies considerably according to the amount of the gastric content, being thinner when the stomach is distended. When high-resolution equipment is used, the five-layered structure of the gastric wall can frequently be made out.[22] From the internal surface of the stomach, layers of alternating reflectivities are seen. The mucosal layer is echogenic with a surrounding hypoechoic layer, the submucosal layer is echogenic, the muscularis propria is hypoechoic, and the relatively thin serosal layer, together with its attached fat, is again echogenic (Figure 8-4). Peristaltic movement of the stomach is well appreciated after it is filled with water. Changes in the wall of the stomach can be detected ultrasonographically, except at the cardiac portion of the stomach, which is rather difficult to scan with a linear-array probe, but much easier with a sector or convex-array scan head.

Another important capability of real-time ultrasound is dynamic observation. The wall motility of the digestive tract and the transit time of the gastric contents to the intestine can be assessed accurately and continuously with real time ultrasound without the use of x-rays.

The duodenum, because of its particular localization, can easily be identified by the movement of its contents, though visualization of the wall is not complete because it is thin and because of the rapid peristalsis, which carries intensely echogenic content due to admixed air bubbles. Once the duodenal loop has been filled with anechoic fluid such as degassed water, the location and movement of the duodenal wall can be identified more easily. On the other hand, the duodenojejunal junction, if filled with echogenic material, often simulates a mass in the body of the pancreas (Figure 8-5). It is imperative, therefore, to take care caution not to misinterpret these pseudotumors in the body region of the pancreas by using the fluid-filled stomach method, which, in turn, helps identify the junction by filling it with moving particles. These structures are much better visualized by endoscopic US (see Chapter 9).

Similarly, the lower colon can be examined without difficulty with a real-time scanner if an adequate acoustic window is generated by means of a water enema(see Chapter 9). Using newer high-resolution equipment in conjunction with a carefully performed water enema, it has been claimed recently that visualization of the layered structure in the wall of the normal colon is possible, and that the loss of these normal structures allows elucidation of colonic pathologies such as ulcerative colitis or Crohn's disease.[12, 25]

An important application of real-time ultrasound in clinical practice is the investigation of the acute abdomen. This will be described later in this chapter.

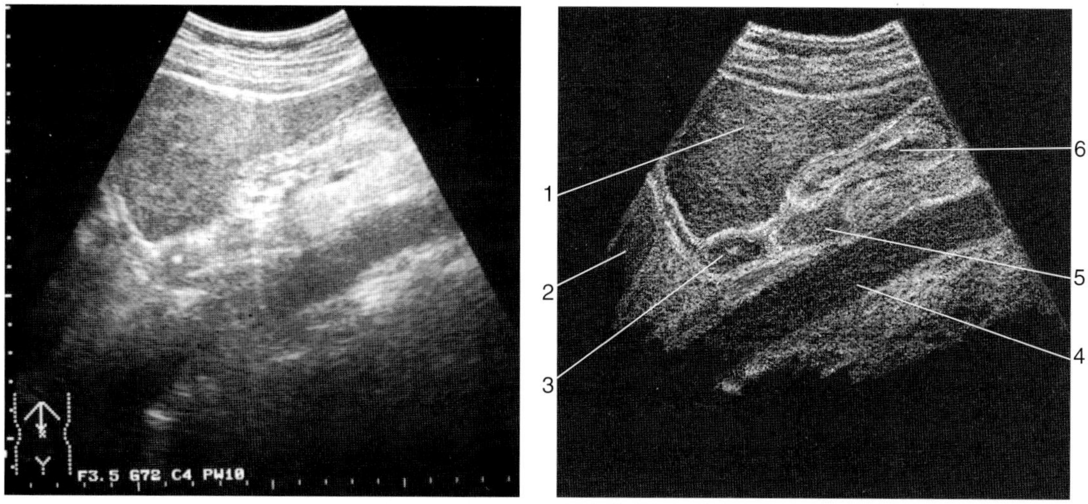

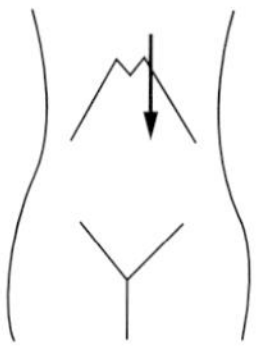

1. Left lobe of liver 2. Left ventricle 3. Esophagogastric junction 4. Aorta 5. Pancreas 6. Stomach

Figure 8-1. The esophagogastric junction, sagittal scan.
A parasagittal scan slightly left of the midline shows a cross section of the esophagogastric junction behind the left lobe of the liver. An elliptical region surrounded by a thin layer of echo-poor muscularis propria with a central echogenic cluster corresponding to the lumen is visualized. The junction can be identified by real-time observation of fluid movement through the site following a drink of water.

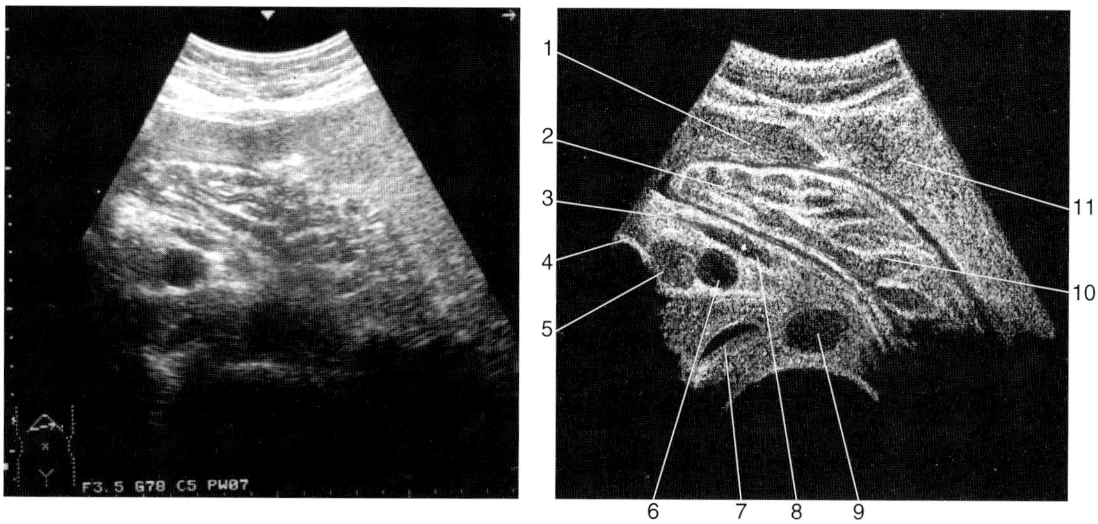

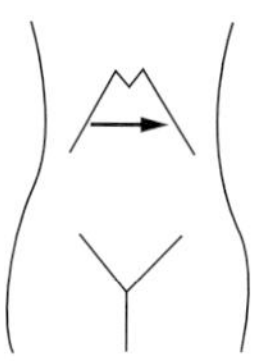

1. Liver 2. Antrum of stomach 3. Adipose tissue 4. Descending duodenum 5. Uncinate part of pancreas 6. Splenic vein 7. Inferior vena cava 8. Third portion of duodenum 9. Aorta 10. Normal stomach 11. Spleen (splenomegaly)

Figure 8-2. The normal stomach, transverse scan.
The increased resolution of newer real-time scanners has revealed clearer images of the stomach wall. A transverse scan of the normal gastric antrum tangential to the stomach wall demonstrates the complex mucosal pattern of the stomach. Part of the pancreas is also imaged together with the larger vessels : the aorta, inferior vena cava, and superior mesenteric and splenic veins.

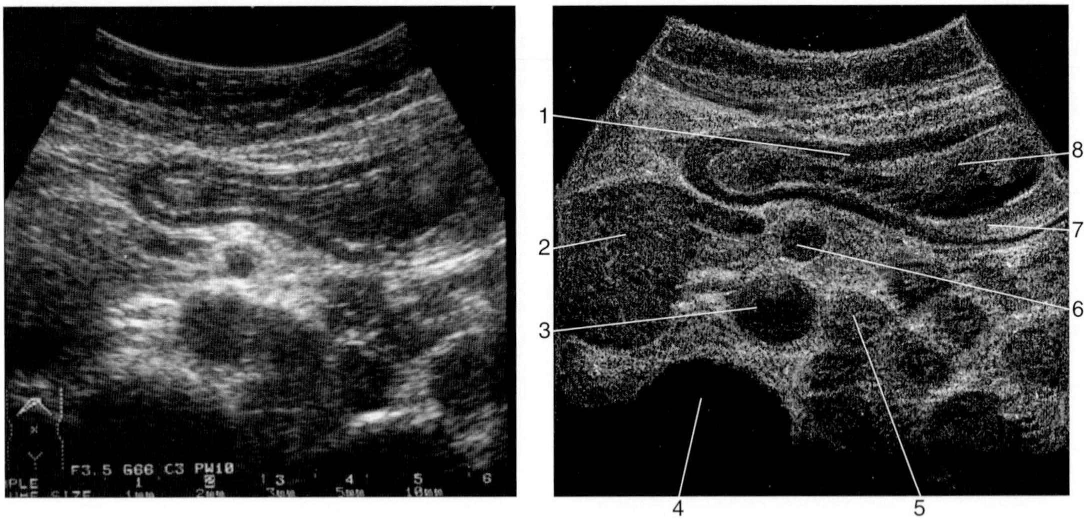

1. Anterior wall of stomach 2. Head of pancreas 3. Aorta 4. Vertebra 5. Intestinal loop 6. Superior mesenteric artery 7. Posterior wall of stomach 8. Gastric cavity

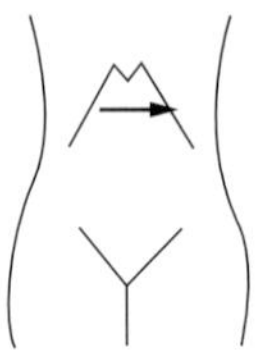

Figure 8-3. The normal stomach, transverse scan.
This image of the normal stomach, scanned longitudinally through the body of the stomach, demonstrates the echo-poor zone corresponding to the muscularis propria together with an irregular echogenic portion indicating intraluminal structures. The thickness of the muscle layer varies considerably with gastric contraction or filling of the stomach. Anterior to the stomach is the left lobe of the liver.

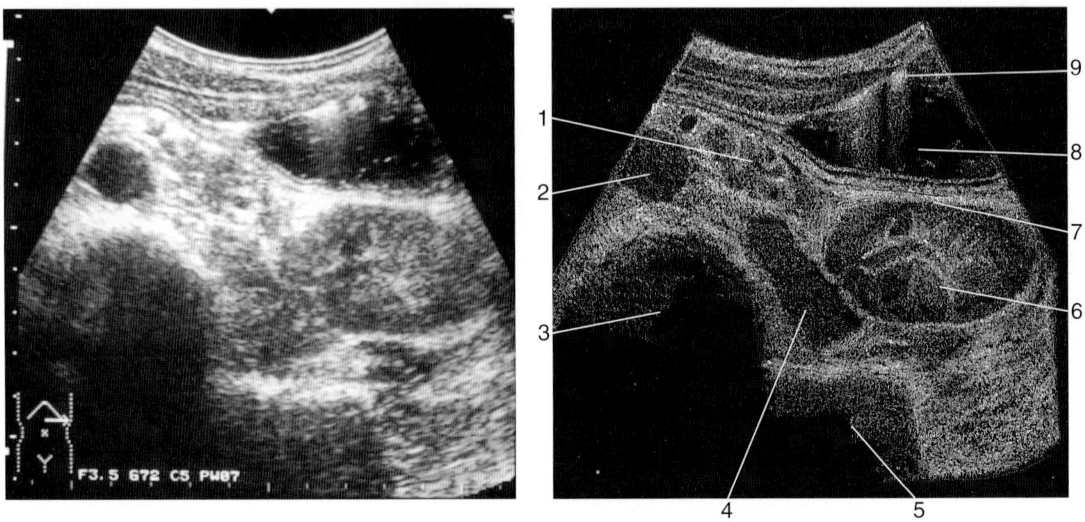

1. Duodenojejunal junction 2. Aorta 3. Vertebra 4. Psoas muscle 5. Transverse process 6. Left kidney 7. Posterior wall of stomach 8. Gastric lumen 9. Anterior wall of stomach

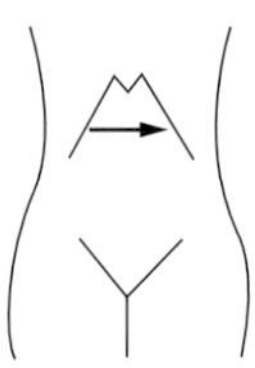

Figure 8-4. An accumulation of gastric juice in a patient with gastric ulcer.
Peptic ulceration of the stomach regularly produces accumulation of gastric juice in the stomach. Although the ulcer crater is not shown due to its location, hypersecretion suggests the abnormality by analogy with fluoroscopic findings. The layering structure of the gastric wall is well visualized through accumulated gastric juice.

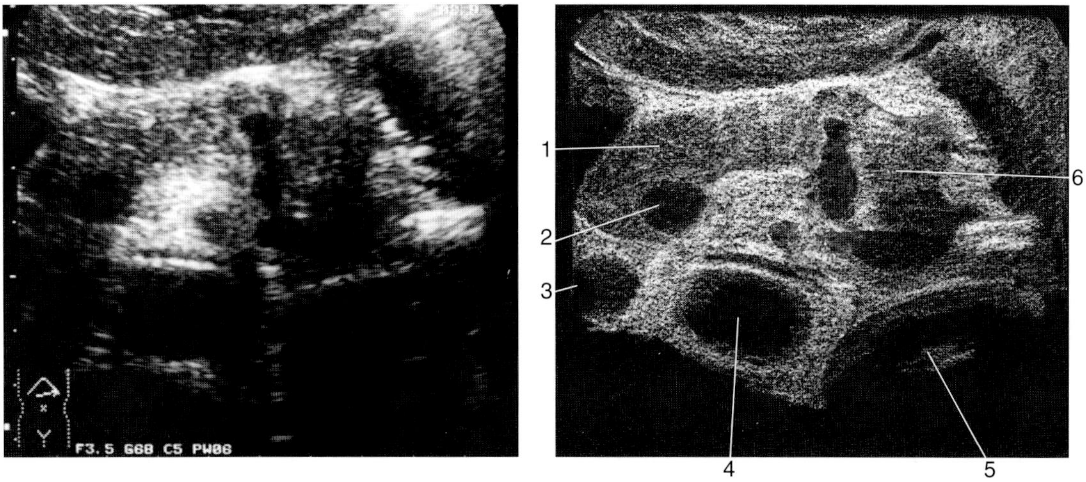

1. Head of pancreas 2. Portal vein 3. Inferior vena cava 4. Aorta 5. Left kidney 6. Pseudotumor (duodenojejunal flexure)

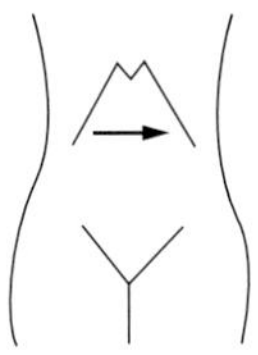

Figure 8-5. A transverse image of the duodenojejunal flexure.
The transition of the duodenum to the intestine, the duodenojejunal flexure, normally lies immediately to the pancreatic body. It usually visualized when filled; however, it often mimics the appearance of a pancreatic mass, as shown in this example. This patient underwent exploratory laparotomy, which revealed an abnormally high position of the flexure lying behind the pancreatic body. The increased level of a tumor marker, CA 19-9, also supported the erroneous diagnosis. Parenchymal biopsy revealed chronic pancreatitis, which probably caused the elevation of the tumor marker test.

DISEASES OF THE STOMACH

Tumor masses, either malignant or benign, can be depicted as a localized or diffuse thickening of the gastric wall by real-time ultrasound. Except for very large tumors, the use of a fluid-filled method is necessary. The pseudokidney sign, as described above, is indicative of advanced malignant tumor in the wall of the stomach.[32] A careful search for enlarged regional lymph nodes by an experienced examiner may allow earlier detection of tumor spread than is possible with other imaging methods, especially in the retropancreatic and para-aortic regions and sometimes also in the region of the cardia.

It is often difficult, however, to determine the precise nature of a mass, whether benign or malignant, based on the sonographic findings alone. Additional x-ray and/or endoscopic studies combined with biopsy of the mucosa are usually needed to establish the diagnosis.

Acute gastric mucosal lesions, which cause massive thickening of the gastric wall, complicating mucosal ulceration, may transiently mimic a malignant tumor of the stomach (Figure 8-6). Severe pain and thickening of the gastric wall are the cardinal signs that suggest the condition. It generally runs a fairly acute course, and therefore, is not very difficult to differentiate from neoplastic conditions.

Malignant Tumors of the Stomach

Gastric Carcinoma

In many areas of the world particularly the Far East, the most frequent gut malignancy is gastric carcinoma.[1,3,7] The onset of symptoms is generally insidious, and most patients are asymptomatic until late in the course of disease. The lesions may be fungating, ulcerated, diffuse, polypoid, or superficially infiltrating. The value of early detection of gastric carcinoma by routine gastrointestinal series and endoscopy is well documented; despite this, the late presentation of many cases leads to a tragic outcome.

Gastric carcinoma in its earlier stages invariably shows localized thickening of the gastric wall with reduction in echo levels, often accompanied by a shallow ulceration in the center, which can only be visualized with the fluid-filled stomach method (Figure 8-7).

Advanced carcinoma produces a target lesion or the pseudo-kidney pattern with altered echogenicity.[7] It is often difficult to detect lesions in the cardiac portion of the stomach because of restricted access, and those that can be detected are difficult to differentiate from carcinomas arising at the lower end of the esophagus (Figure 8-8). Sonographic identification of gastric carcinoma is relatively straightforward if the tumor is in the gastric antrum or angulus and has reached a considerable size (Figures 8-9, 8-10, and 8-11).

The fluid-filled stomach method allows a clear demonstration of a tumor mass in the stomach. Thickening of the wall with loss of peristaltic motion is indicative of a malignant neoplasm. Scirrhous carcinomas often invade the entire gastric wall (Figure 8-12).

Metastatic spread to regional lymph nodes, the liver or the peritoneal cavity can be elucidated relatively easily, provided that the echogenicity of lesions differs significantly from that of the surroundings (Figure 8-13). Gastric carcinoma may also cause partial or complete obstruction of the pylorus, producing pyloric stenosis, which again can be depicted easily by the specific echo patterns produced (Figure 8-14).

Regrettably, however, the limited resolution and difficulty in assessing various parts of the stomach, including the cardia and the lateral portions of the stomach, limit the use of transabdominal ultrasound to screening for advanced cancers and their metastases. Endoscopic ultrasound, as described in Chapter 9, is clearly the method of choice in diagnosing and staging gastric malignancy at much earlier stages.

Gastric Lymphoma

Gastrointestinal lymphoma is much less common than gastric carcinoma. It affects the stomach, the ileum, and, less frequently, the colon and rectum.[5,8] The clinical signs and symptoms and the sonographic appearance of these tumors are usually indistinguishable from those of gastric carcinoma. Advanced diffuse gastric lymphomas are demonstrated as large tumor masses with relatively echo-poor appearances or with diffuse thickening of the gastric wall (Figure 8-15). Enlargement of perigastric lymph nodes with the characteristic sandwich sign is often observed (Figure 8-16). A spokewheel pattern has also been described.[7]

Gastric Submucosal Tumors

In a small number of gastric tumors, a submucosal lesion, leiomyoma (Figure 8-17) or leiomyosarcoma (Figure 8-18), is found.[45] The fluid-filled stomach method facilitates identification of submucosal tumors and clarifies their involvement in or relationship to the respective layer(s) of the stomach wall.

Submucosal tumors often reach a considerable size without causing symptoms. Typically, they are round or elliptical in shape and have low-level internal echo intensities. They may show marked inhomogeneity in internal texture, mostly caused by the central liquefaction that is a characteristic feature of leiomyoma. The size of the mass frequently reflects the malignant nature of the lesion.[29] However, accurate differential diagnosis is possible only after direct biopsy, though this is generally difficult using ordinary endoscopic techniques.

Diagnostic pitfalls, however, may be encountered, for example, direct invasion of the stomach from adjacent malignancies may simulate a primary gastric carcinoma (Figure 8-19).

Peptic Ulcer

The diagnosis of gastric or duodenal ulcer is not an ideal indication for ultrasound. Acute ulceration can be diagnosed accurately by routine endoscopy. However, when chronic ulceration mimics gastric carcinoma, ultrasound may be useful, though the differential diagnosis remains difficult.[27,32] Another indication for ultrasonic survey of peptic ulcer is impending perforation of an ulcer crater, with or without concomitant focal peritonitis. Indicative sonographic findings, such as an echogenic, gas-containing ulcer crater in the center of the ulceration together with a thickened gastric wall, may be elicited.[27]

Extrinsic Compression of the Stomach

The differential diagnosis of extrinsic compression is also an important indication for ultrasound. A double-contrast study of the stomach by x-ray is a sensitive method for delineating subtle changes in the mucosa caused by early gastric cancer or small polyps, but it does not contribute useful information concerning an extrinsic mass that has not involved the mucosa. Here ultrasound is reliable because of its sensitivity and the specific findings it provides concerning the mass causing compression such as compression by the left lobe of the liver (Figure 8-20), a left polycystic kidney, pancreatic tumors, or a splenic cyst. All of these changes can be evaluated quickly and reliably.

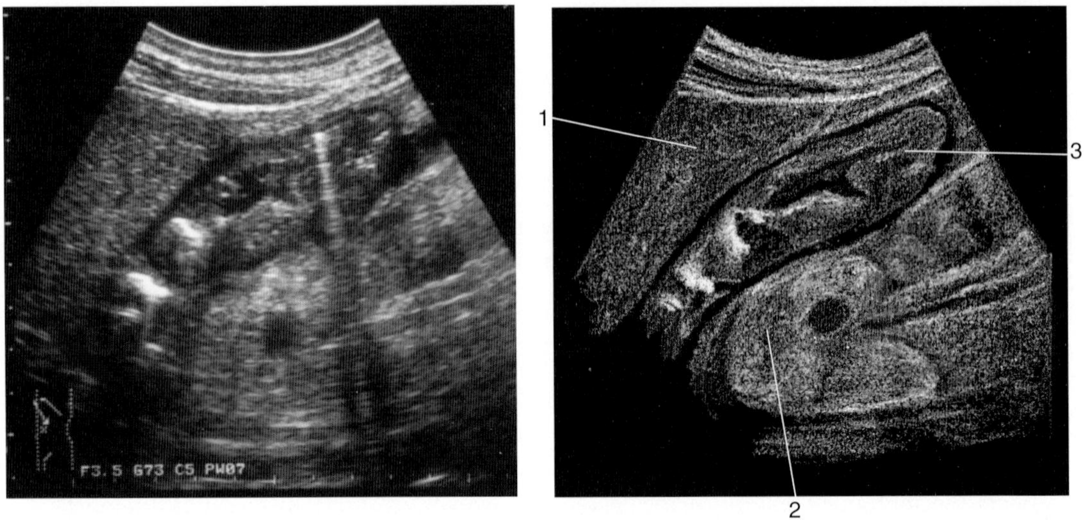

1. Liver 2. Pancreas 3. Inflamed gastric wall

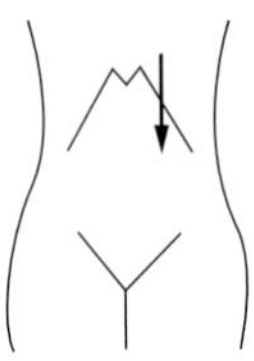

Figure 8-6. Acute gastric mucosal lesion.
Acute gastric mucosal lesions can occur in a variety of conditions, all usually accompanied by severe symptoms such as epigastric pain and vomiting. Although the endoscopic findings are very characteristic, with edematous thickening of the mucosa with massive exudation, erosions, and mucosal bleeding, ultrasonographically the thickened mucosa is similar to that of an infiltrating scirrhous carcinoma. However, after the acute phase has passed, the sonographic findings rapidly return to normal.

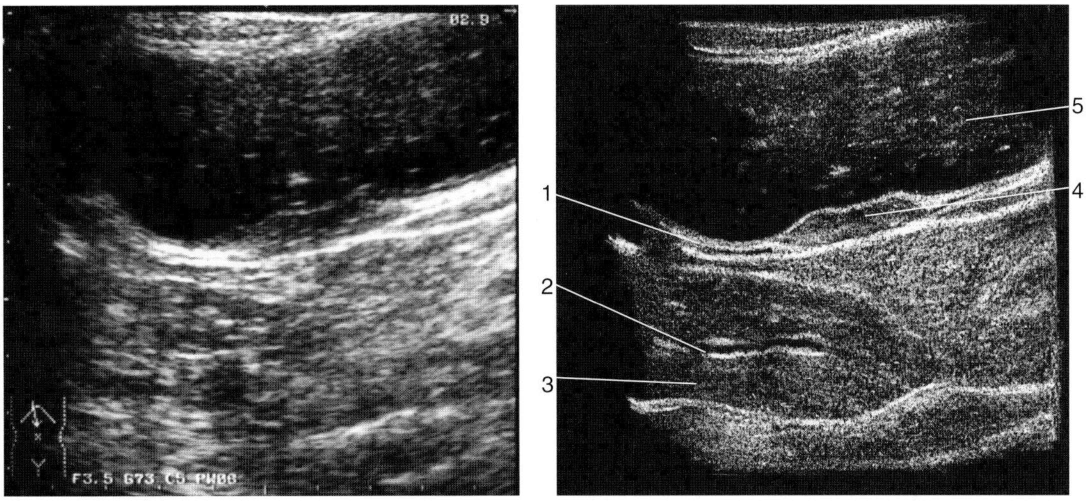

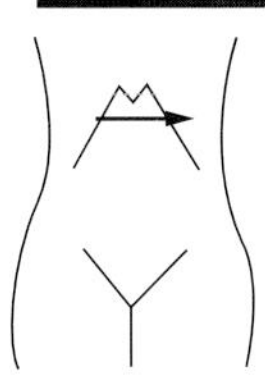

1. Posterior wall of stomach 2. Pancreatic duct
3. Pancreas 4. Ulcer crater of early gastric cancer
5. Gastric lumen

Figure 8-7 a. An early gastric carcinoma visualized via the fluid-filled stomach method. In early gastric carcinoma, the lesion itself is seldom visualized by routine ultrasound in the upper abdomen. An image obtained by scanning after filling the gastric lumen with degassed water, using high resolution equipment, is shown. A slight elevation of the hypoechoic mass on the echogenic submucosal layer suggested that the lesion is early gastric mucosal carcinoma.

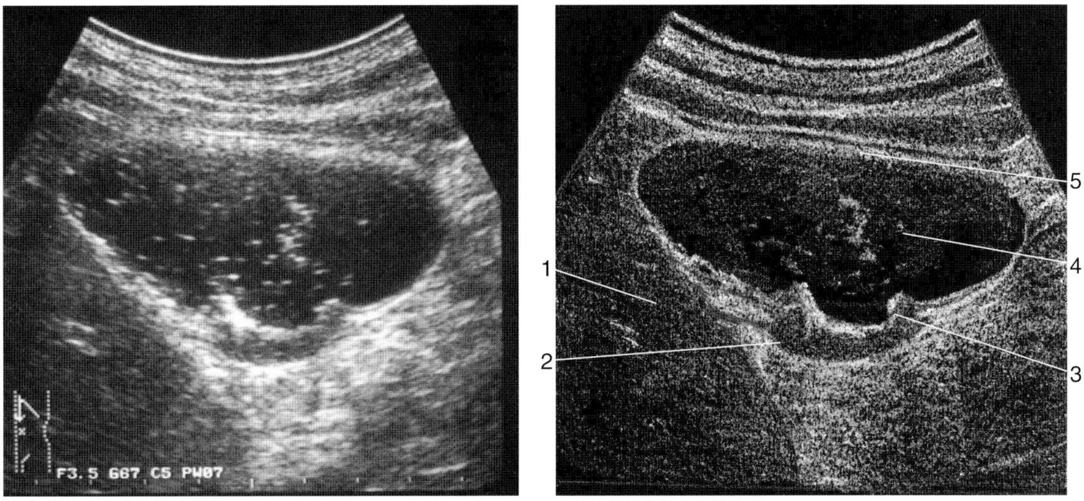

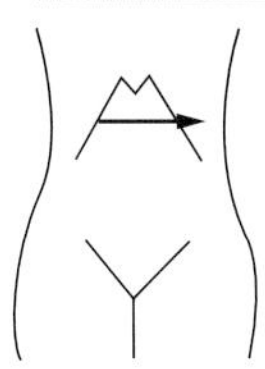

1. Liver 2. Ulcerating gastric cancer (pm cancer)
3. Disruption of submucosal (sm) layer 4. Gastric lumen 5. Gastric wall

Figure 8-7b. A small gastric cancer invading the muscularis propria layer, sagittal scan. A hypoechoic mass with a centrally located ulcer crater is shown on the posterior wall of the gastric antrum, with disruption of the echogenic submucosal layer (the stomach has been filled with water). The posterior border of the tumor is strongly reflective, indicating low attenuation by the malignant tissue. No lymph node enlargement was demonstrated.

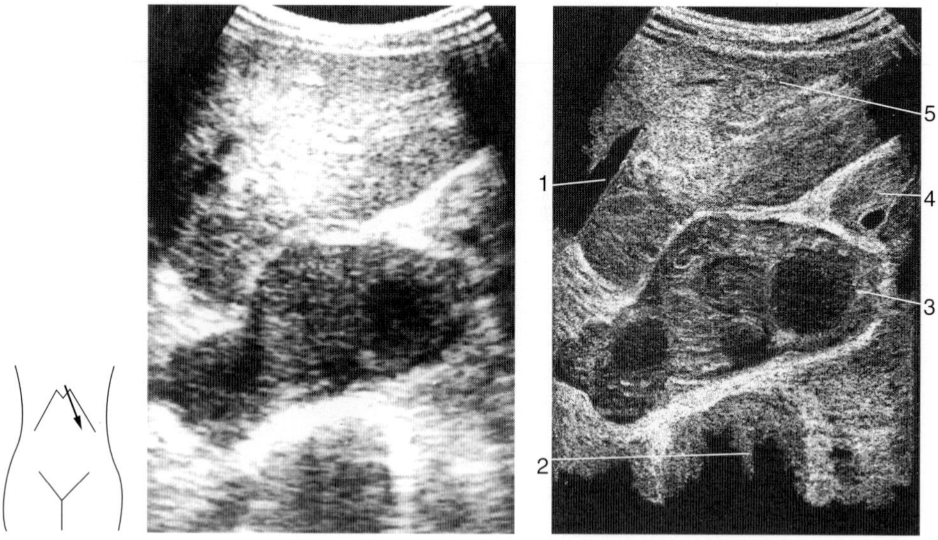

1. Left hepatic vein 2. Vertebra 3. Cancer of esophagus (abdominal portion) 4. Body of pancreas 5. Left lobe of liver

Figure 8-8. Large tumor mass at the lower end of the esophagus.
A large, irregularly shaped tumor mass in a patient with esophageal carcinoma is visualized directly posterior to the left lobe of the liver. Its position corresponds to the esophagogastric junction but the tumor has also infiltrated to the cardia of the stomach, and there is compression of the posterior surface of the liver. An irregularly shaped liver metastasis can be seen in the posterior segment of the left lobe of the liver.

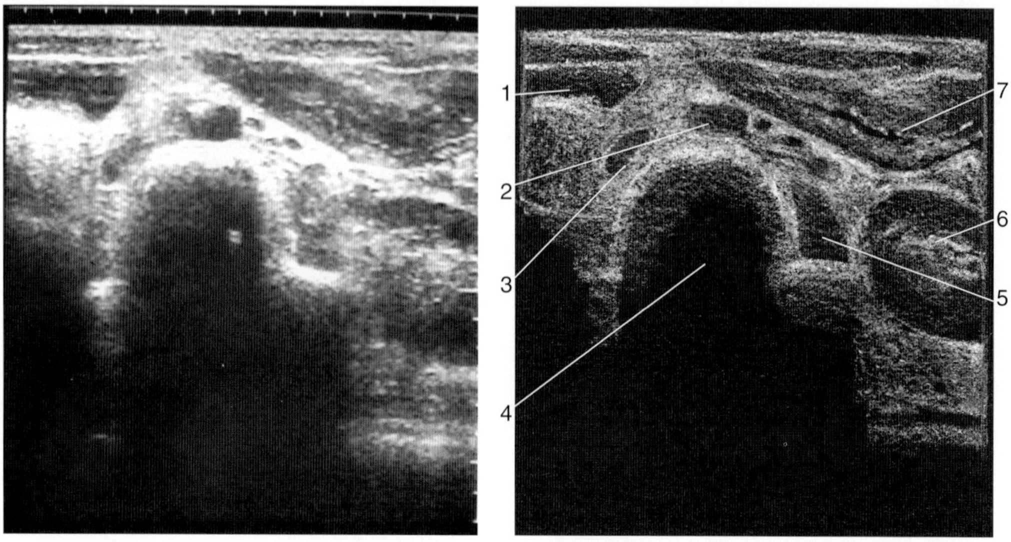

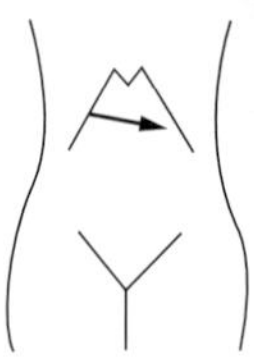

1. Gallbladder 2. Aorta 3. Inferior vena cava 4. Vertebra 5. Psoas muscle 6. Left kidney 7. Gastric cancer

Figure 8-9. A gastric tumor in the lower portion of the body of the stomach.
A triangular mass is visualized in the lower portion of the body of the stomach. It is more echogenic than the stomach wall. The mass also showed considerable respiratory excursion, indicating that the extragastric spread has not occurred.

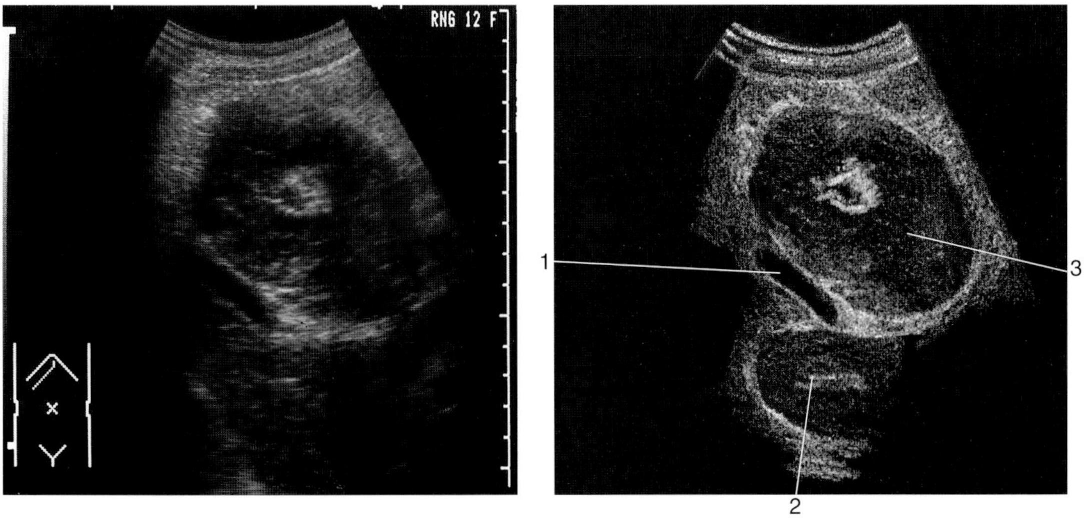

1. Gallbladder 2. Right kidney 3. Gastric cancer

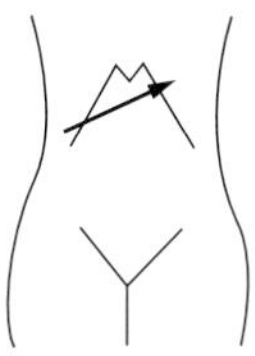

Figure 8-10. A large gastric carcinoma at the pylorus.
A large, ovoid hypoechoic mass in the pylorus is shown in this right subcostal scan. The residual central lumen is demonstrated. The patient suffered from long-standing dysphagia caused by mechanical obstruction (pyloric stenosis).

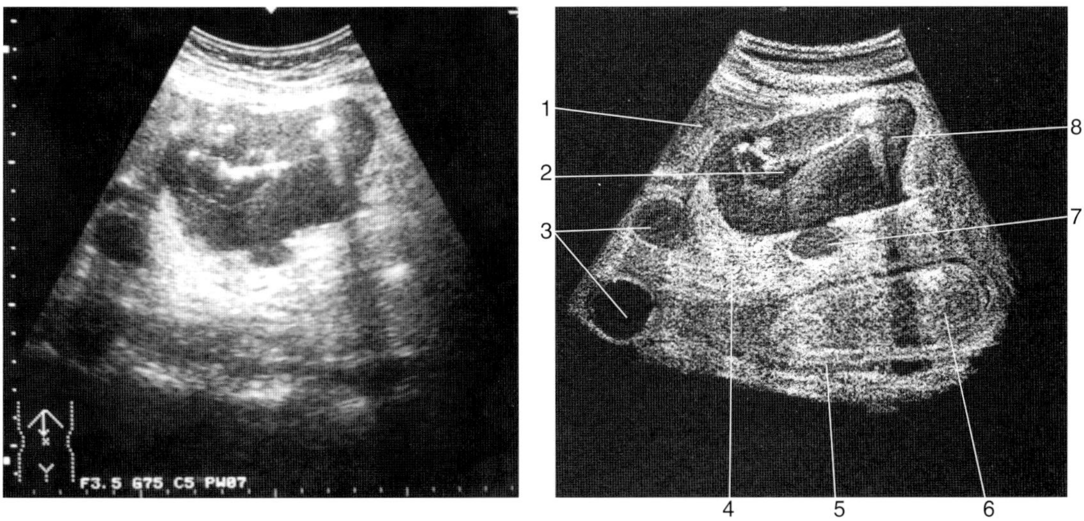

1. Liver 2. Gastric lumen 3. Lymph node metastases 4. Acoustic enhancement 5. Inferior vena cava 6. Head of pancreas 7. Lymph node metastases 8. Gastric cancer

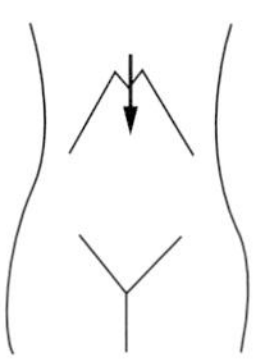

Figure 8-11. A solid tumor mass of the stomach.
A large, hypoechoic mass with irregular contours is visualized in the antrum of the stomach. A comet tail artifact producing acoustic shadowing and strong central echoes arising from the center of the mass is characteristic of a gastrointestinal tumor; the artifact is caused by air in the lumen. The echo-poor mass on the posterior surface of the tumor mass is an enlarged lymph node. The posterior part of the mass shows acoustic enhancement due to the low attenuation of the tumor.

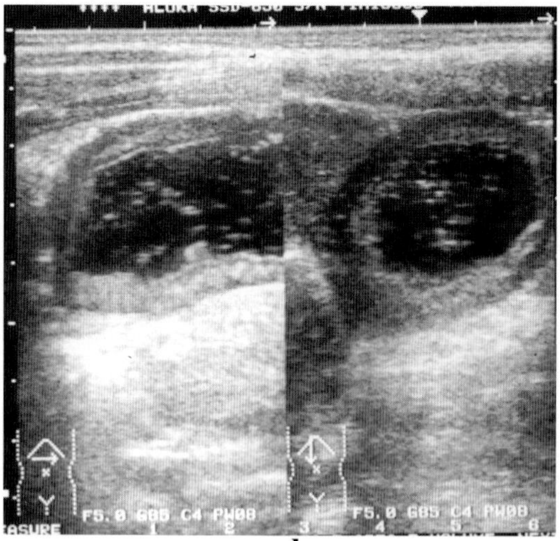

a **b**

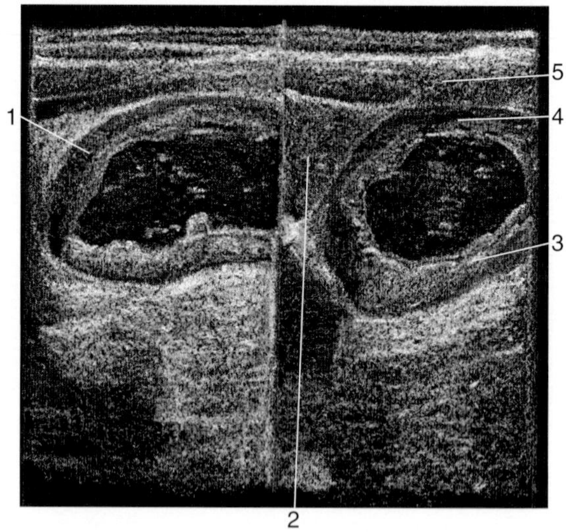

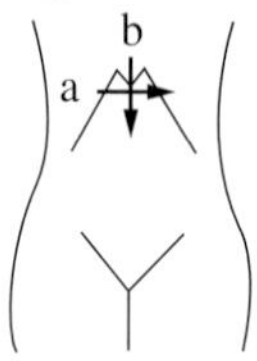

1. Gastric cancer 2. Liver 3. Gastric cancer (scirrhous cancer) 4. Anterior wall of stomach 5. Ascites

Figure 8-12. Gastric carcinoma: scirrhous carcinoma diffusely infiltrating the stomach. Diffusely infiltrating gastric carcinomas are often overlooked because of the paucity of symptoms and signs. In these two sonograms traversing the antral portion of the stomach, uniform thickening of the gastric wall with low-level echoes characteristic of gastric carcinoma are visualized. Scanning in at least two different planes, preferably orthogonal (both longitudinal and transverse), is necessary to delineate the full extent of the mass. In addition, the technique of the fluid-filled stomach is extremely useful to demonstrate the location of the tumor mass as well as loss of distensibility of the gastric wall, a characteristic feature of scirrhous carcinomas.

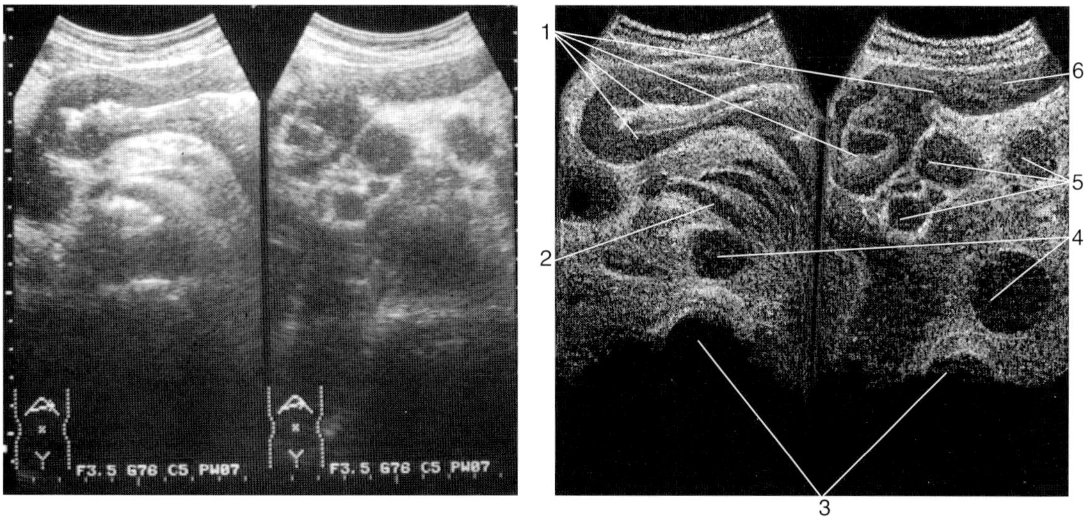

a

1. Gastric cancer at the antrum 2. Left renal vein 3. Vertebra 4. Aorta 5. Lymph nodes 6. Left lobe of liver Gastric cancer at the antrum

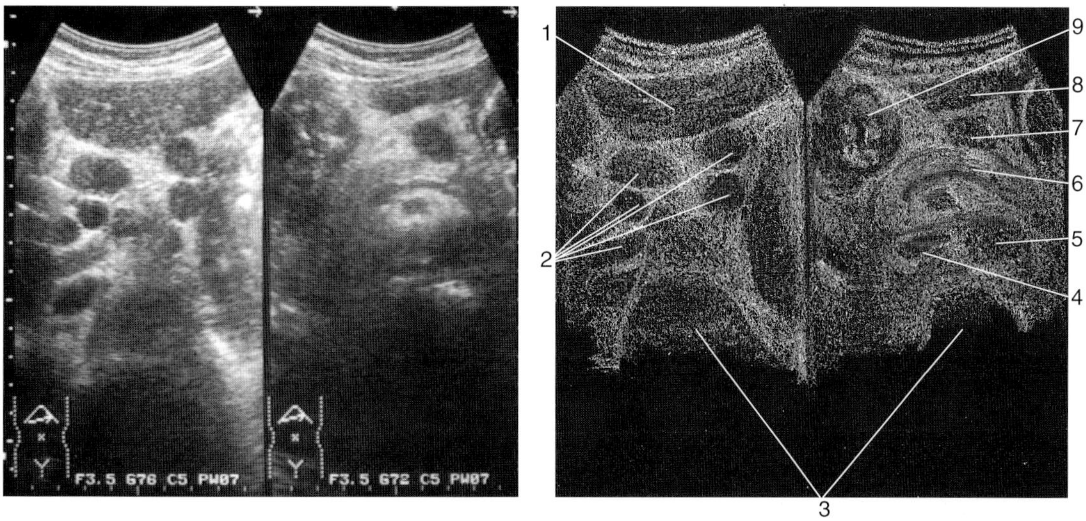

b

1. Liver 2. Lymph nodes 3. Vertebra 4. Inferior vena cava 5. Aorta 6. Pancreas 7. Lymph node 8. Liver 9. Cancer of stomach

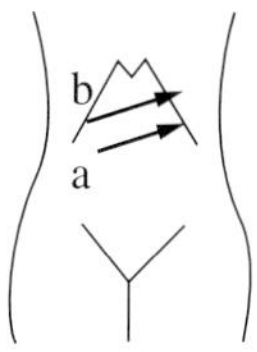

Figure 8-13. Lymph node enlargement due to metastatic dissemination of gastric carcinoma of the antrum.

These four serial images recorded in the transverse plane in the epigastrium demonstrate a tumor at the antrum together with metastatic spread to the regional lymph nodes. Multiple enlarged lymph nodes were demonstrated as round or oval-shaped, hypoechoic masses, not only in the vicinity of the original tumor but also to remote nodes. No ascitic fluid was demonstrated.

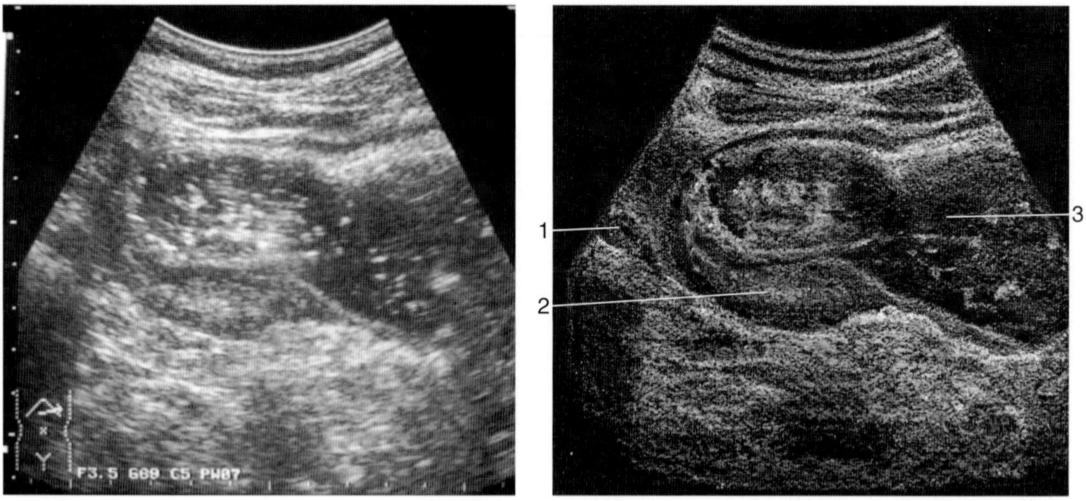

1. Lymph node 2. Gastric cancer 3. Dilated gastric lumen

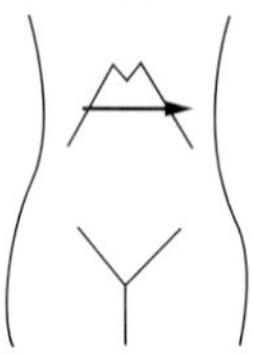

Figure 8-14. Pyloric stenosis caused by gastric cancer of the pylorus.
A transverse tomogram of the pyloric region shows a large, echo-poor mass obstructing the pyloric canal, causing stenosis and accumulation of gastric contents. Considerable gastric dilatation is evident.

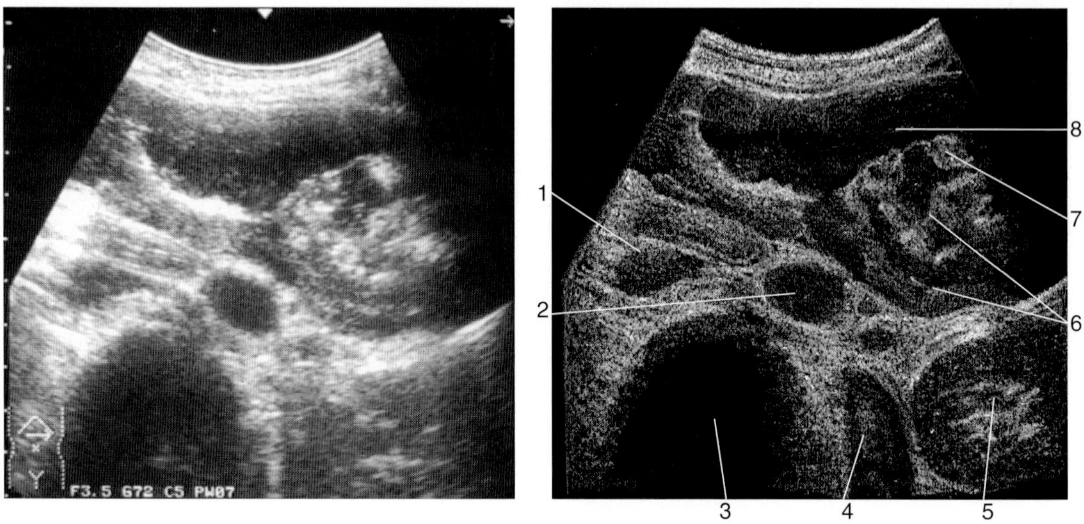

1. Inferior vena cava 2. Aorta 3. Vertebra 4. Psoas muscle 5. Left kidney 6. Gastric lymphoma 7. Ulceration 8. Gastric lumen

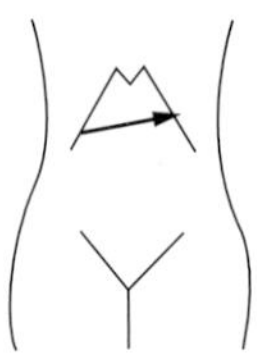

Figure 8-15. Lymphoma of the stomach.
Lymphomatous invasion of the stomach wall may occur as a primary lesion as well as the secondary to the generalized infiltration by lymphoma. A transverse tomogram of the stomach demonstrates echo-poor thickening of the entire gastric wall, the pattern closely resembles that of scirrhous carcinoma of the stomach.

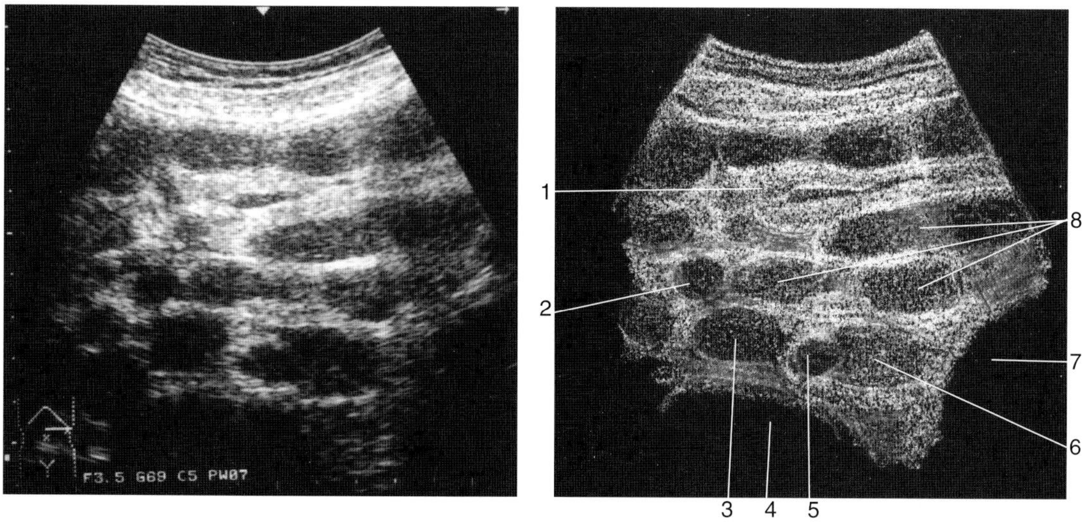

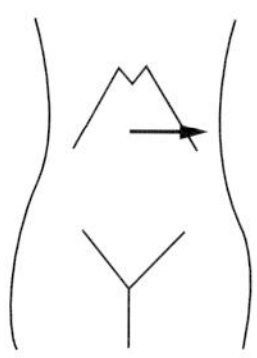

1. Body of pancreas 2. Superior mesenteric vein 3. Inferior vena cava 4. Vertebra 5. Aorta 6. Para-aortic lymph node 7. Left kidney 8. Lymph nodes

Figure 8-16. Malignant lymphoma showing the characteristic sandwich sign.
The characteristic conglomeration of enlarged lymphomatosis resembles the cut surface of a sandwich, with the layers shown.

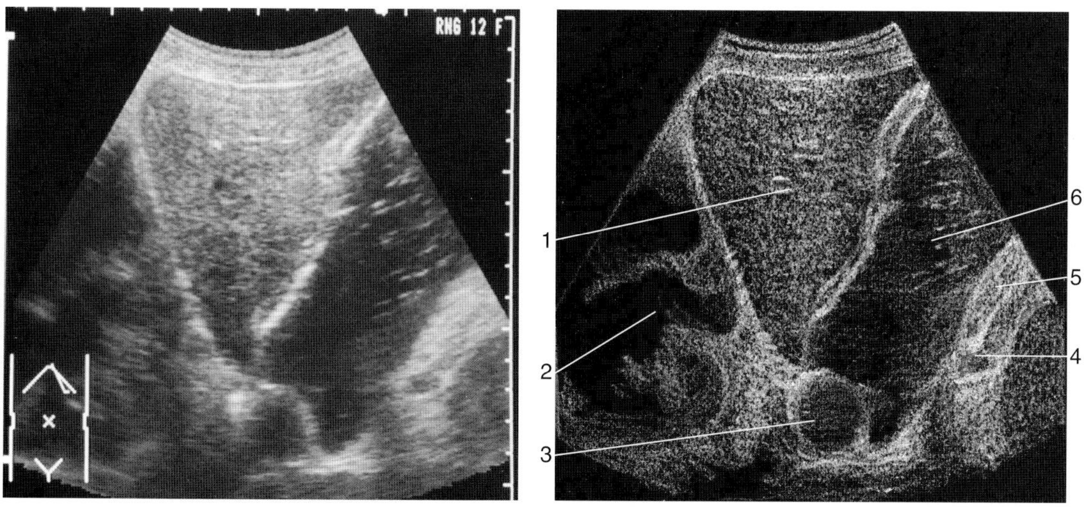

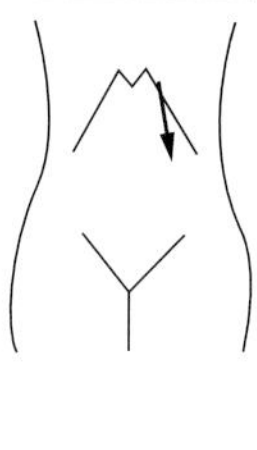

1. Left lobe of liver 2. Left ventricle of heart 3. Small leiomyoma (submucosal tumor) 4. Splenic vein 5. Tail of pancreas 6. Stomach

Figure 8-17. Submucosal tumor of the cardia of the stomach.
A small, round, echo-poor mass was visualized in the fluid-filled stomach. Gastric submucosal tumors seldom produce symptoms; this case was found during gastric screening after a barium meal. The tumor is surrounded by a thin layer of gastric mucosa. The fluid-filled stomach method was also helpful in delineating the mass.

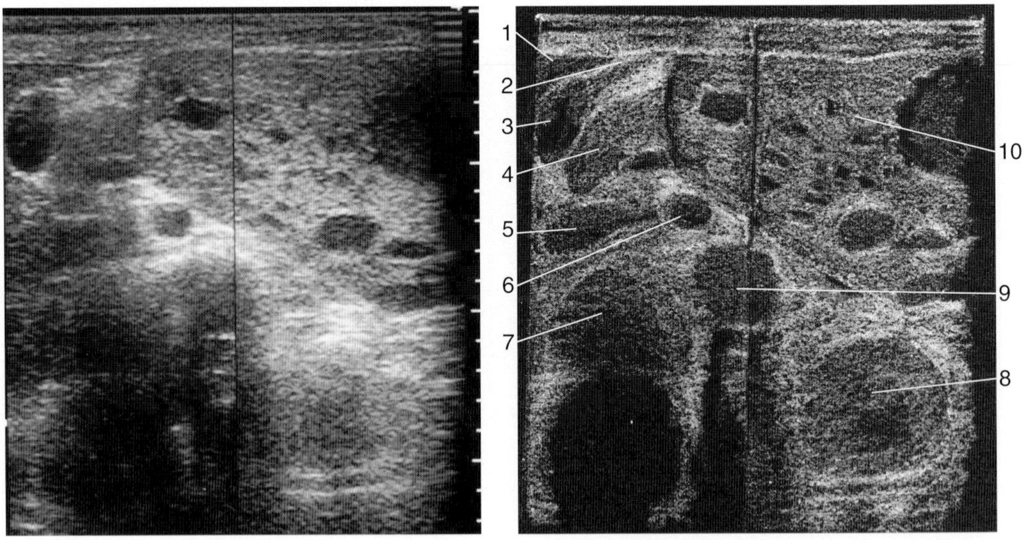

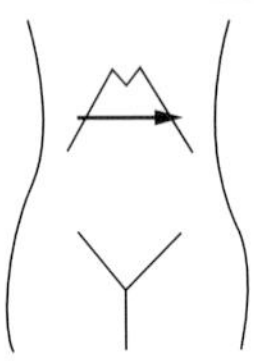

1. Liver 2. Antrum of stomach 3. Gallbladder 4. Head of pancreas 5. Inferior vena cava 6. Superior mesenteric artery 7. Vertebra 8. Left kidney 9. Aorta 10. Submucosal tumor (leiomyosarcoma)

Figure 8-18. Large gastric leiomyosarcoma.
A huge gastric tumor is visualized in this transverse scan in the epigastrium. In spite of its large size, the patient had minimum discomfort and no weight loss. However, the tumor size and the echo pattern i.e., echo-poor round mass with a markedly heterogeneous texture including partial liquefaction, supported the diagnosis of leiomyosarcoma, which was proven at operation. The contour of the mass was generally smooth, and there were no signs of metastatic spread to the surrounding lymph nodes.

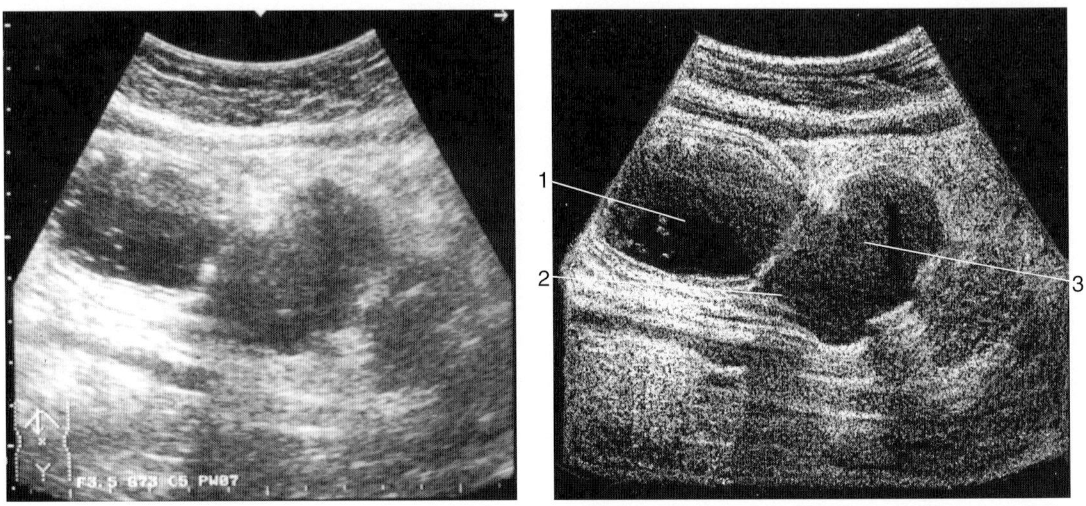

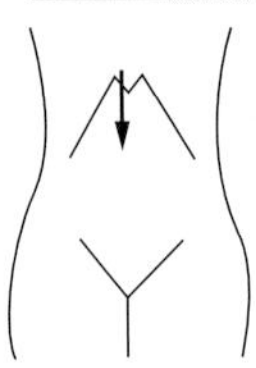

1. Gastric lumen 2. Infiltration to the muscularis propria 3. Colonic carcinoma with irregular contour

Figure 8-19. Colonic mass simulating an extragastric tumor.
A large, irregular, echo-poor mass was found in the epigastric region. The mass was connected to the muscularis propria of the stomach; however, it was later found to be a carcinoma of the transverse colon, with the typical apple core sign on barium enema. Direct infiltration of the mass into the submucosal and muscularis propria layers were identified at the time of surgical excision.

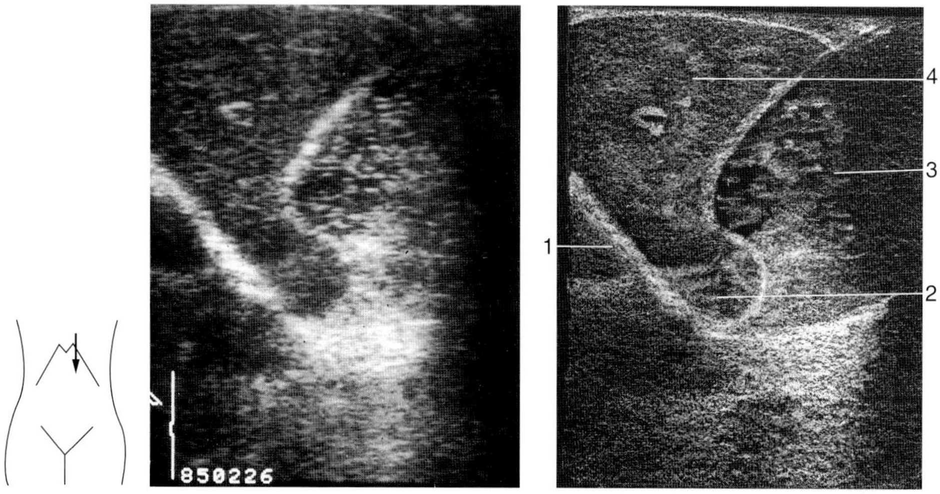

1. Diaphragm 2. Hemangioma of liver 3. Gastric lumen 4. Left lobe of liver

Figure 8-20. Extragastric compression of the cardia by hepatic hemangioma.
A small protrusion of the left lobe of the liver was demonstrated by scanning the cardia of the stomach through the water-filled stomach. This was first found during screening for gastric malignancy after a barium meal and confirmed by subsequent endoscopy. Although the lesion seemed to be isoechoic, the endoscopic ultrasound scan disclosed similar lesion with slightly increased echogenicity. Angiography demonstrated a circumscribed hemangioma of the liver, which was confirmed at laparotomy.

DISEASES OF THE INTESTINES

Intestinal Obstruction

The fluid within the dilated intestinal lumen shows to-and-fro movements, a characteristic sign of acute intestinal obstruction; it is known as the keyboard sign [12, 14, 17, 28, 34, 43, 49, 51] (Figure 8-21). The symptoms vary, most commonly presenting as an acute abdomen with severe pain and vomiting. If the obstruction is caused by a tumor at the lower end of the dilated intestine, the diagnosis is usually straightforward on real-time ultrasound, even though the clinical signs are still vague and not severe enough to suggest full-blown ileus.[21, 30, 31] It is often difficult, however, to assess the site of obstruction, especially in more severe cases caused by strangulation in which there is no mass.

Obstruction of the upper gastrointestinal tract in an infant is commonly caused by pyloric stenosis; sudden onset of propulsive vomiting is the typical feature.[2, 16, 18, 40, 47] Sonography may confirm the presence of a hypertrophic pyloric canal representing the target lesion on a transverse scan and an elongated, thick pyloric canal on a longitudinal scan (Figure 8-22).

Intestinal obstruction can also be caused by intussusception; in small children this occurs most frequently at the ileocecal region while in adults a mass in the terminal ileum is often responsible[4, 21, 30] (Figures 8-23 and 8-24). Occasionally, a foreign body can precipitate intestinal ileus, producing indistinguishable sonographic signs of obstruction. A careful search for the obstructing lesion and other gastroenterological investigations are necessary to establish the diagnosis.

Inflammatory Disorders

Acute appendicitis progresses to life-threatening complications such as local or general peritonitis due to perforation of the inflamed appendix,[8, 30] unless surgery is performed early. Real-time ultrasound has become the method of choice in the diagnosis and staging of acute appendicitis. It is possible to make the diagnosis at all stages of appendicitis, from acute catarrhal to full-blown appendiceal abscess and to diagnose perforation. In acute catarrhal stage, a thickened appendix with slightly lower wall echoes can be demonstrated (Figure 8-25). In cases with advanced inflammation, the appendix usually enlarges, and is surrounded often by local exudate. It may be accompanied by a fecolith causing local ileus (Figure 8-26). If the appendicitis is further aggravated, then inflammation may proceed rapidly to wall necrosis and localized abscess formation, the stage of gangrenous appendicitis[15] (Figure 8-27). The accuracy of sonography approaches 85% based on these findings, though expertise and meticulous technique are necessary.

Ultrasound is also useful in differentiating appendicitis from terminal ileitis, which has almost identical symptoms without the positive sonographic signs characteristic of acute appendicits. A slight but diffuse thickening of the terminal ileum with a minimal exudate are the principal findings of the lesion. However, these are not constant and the disease essentially runs a benign course of short duration.

Acute inflammation of the intestine, pseudomembranous enterocolitis or acute hemorrhagic enterocolitis, is caused by the prolonged use of antibiotics, especially oral penicillin, for infection. *Clostridium difficile* is the most commonly reported organism in severe colitis; the ultrasound findings are diffuse swelling of the colonic wall, similar to AGML of the stomach (Figure 8-28).

As shown above, real-time ultrasound is the method of choice in primary care medicine, especially in a number of acute abdominal conditions, because of the speed with which it elucidates the diagnosis and guides treatment schedules (e.g., biliary colic, perforation of the stomach or intestine, intestinal obstruction, renal stones, and even torsion of an ovarian cyst).

Crohn's disease is a chronic intestinal granulomatous inflammation causing persistent diarrhea, fever, emaciation, and a mass, often with internal and external fistulas frequently complicated by intraperitoneal abscess or intestinal obstruction.[25, 52] Diffuse thickening of the wall of the affected intestinal segment, mimicing a malignancy, requires careful clinical survey, including a barium enema, colonoscopy, and biopsy for its exclusion(Figure 8-29).

Ulcerative colitis, another inflammatory bowel disease, mostly affecting the colon, seldom causes masses despite the frequent development of pseudopolyps affecting the entire length of the colon.

Tuberculous chronic inflammation of the intestine and peritoneum has become less common since the development of effective antituberculous chemotherapy. However, sporadic cases are encountered in developed and it remains common in poorer communities, so it is important to recognize the sonographic characteristics of the lesion. Unlike the anechoic fluid of serous ascites found in decompensated liver cirrhosis and malignant peritonitis (Figure 8-30), tuberculous ascites contains low level echoes caused by cholesterol crystals (Figure 8-31) and the intestinal loops are all clearly demonstrated.

Tumors

Malignant tumors of the colon

Calcinoma of the colon has rather higher incidence in Western populations.[23] The cause is unknown, though suspicion has focused on the low-residue diet of Western countries. Over 80% of colonic carcinomas develop in the rectosigmoid region; other sites of the colon are uniformly affected.[20, 22, 41, 48]

In an advanced stage the lesion typically produces the target or pseudokidney sign, with chronic obstruction of the bowel [37, 41, 44] (Figures 8-32 and 8-33). If it presents as positive or overt occult bleeding, endoscopic examination by fiberoptic or electronic colonoscopy leads to early detection and effective therapy, with a good cure rate. Unfortunately, as with gastric malignancy, many patients present late; detection of a mass by ultrasound is usually associated with a grave outcome.

Colonic or rectosigmoid carcinoma can be staged by ultrasound, with little discomfort to the patient.[11,37] A water enema may be necessary to remove interfering colonic gas; if it is performed carefully with lukewarm water without applying excessive pressure, visualization of the mass may be simple. A careful search for the thickness of the wall, and assessment of the presence or absence of regional lymph node enlargement, are essential in confirming the extent of infiltration of the carcinoma to the surrounding tissues (Figures 8-34 and 8-35). A more detailed sonographic investigation can be performed by endosonography, either in combination with endoscopy as endoscopic ultrasound or simply by endosonography of the rectal region as described in Chapter 9.

Pararectal abscess simulating rectal malignancy is said to be identifiable by careful scanning though experience with this disorder is limited; endosonography is more likely to be definitive than routine ultrasound.

In scanning for colonic malignancies, a careful search of the liver and the retroperitoneum for possible metastatic involvement is mandatory.

Miscellaneous tumors of the colon

Lymphoma of the colon is rare and is part of generalized gastrointestinal involvement [27,37](Figure 8-36). Metastatic tumor of the colon is also relatively rare(Figure 8-37).

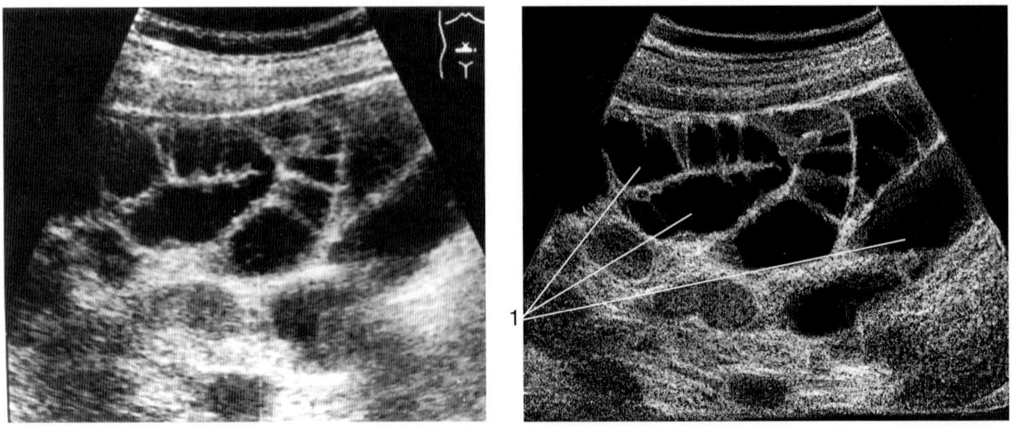

1. Dilated intestinal loops with keyboard-sign appearance

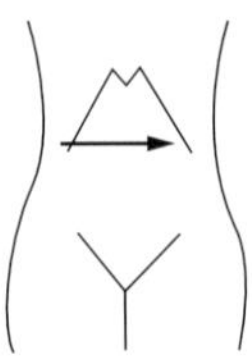

Figure 8-21. Dilated intestinal loops in a patient with intestinal obstruction.
Intestinal obstruction, either acute or chronic, is seen as dilated intestinal loops filled with liquid contents. In acute obstruction of the small intestine in particular, dilatation of the intestinal loops appears before the development of well-known fluid levels with gas on a plain abdominal film. A careful search along the dilated lumen often discloses the site of obstruction. The movement of minute echogenic particles is due to the rapid, active antiperistalsis characteristic of mechanical obstruction.

a

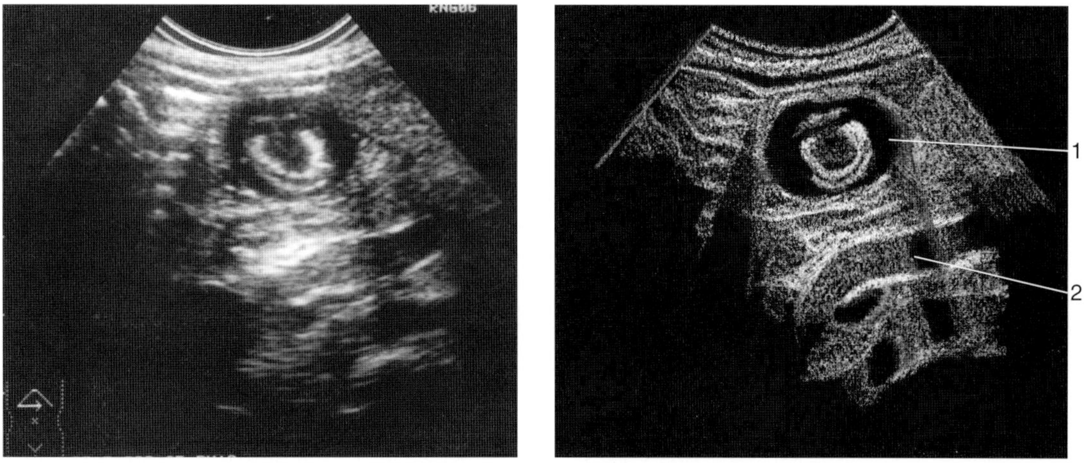

1. Thick pyloric wall 2. Pancreas

b

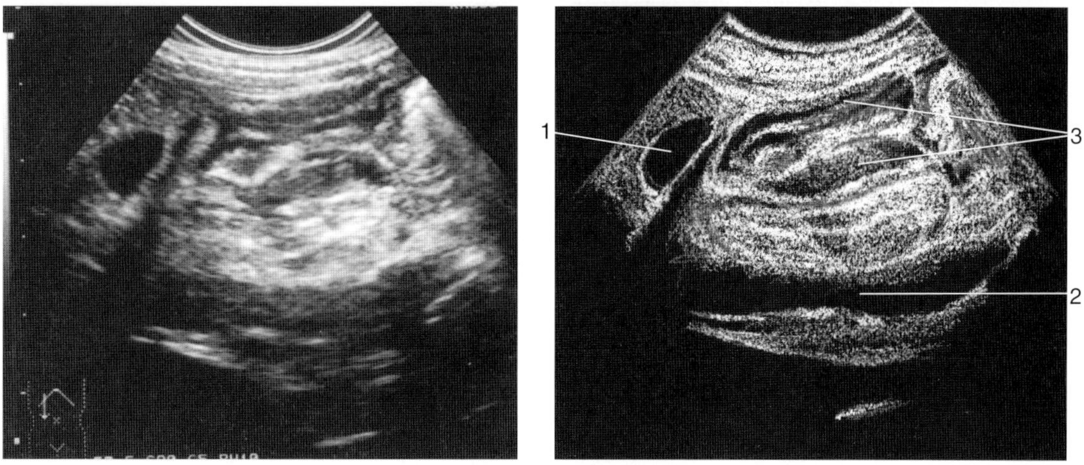

1. Gallbladder 2. Inferior vena cava 3. Thickened pyloric ring

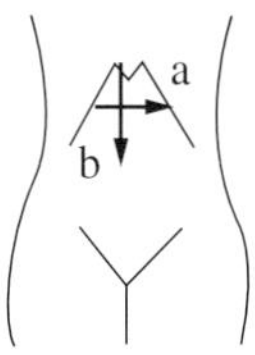

Figure 8-22. Pyloric stenosis in a 2-month-old baby.
Pyloric stenosis in infants is a relatively common disease manifested by abrupt vomiting caused by benign hypertrophy of the pyloric canal as shown here. In a transverse section (a), the pylorus appears as a round, echo-poor ring. However, the longitudinal scan(b) clearly demonstrates an elongated, thickened pyloric canal, mostly composed of echo-poor thickened muscularis propria.

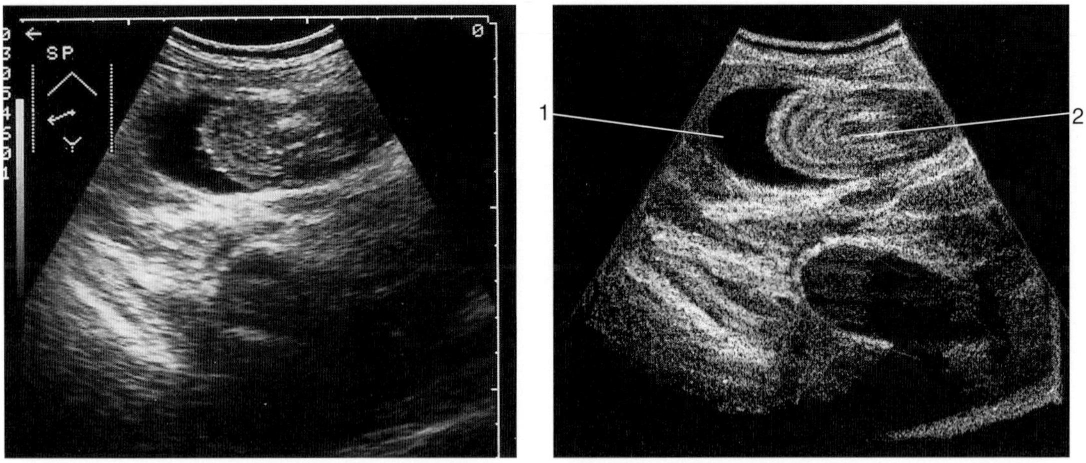

1. Cecum 2. Terminal ileum

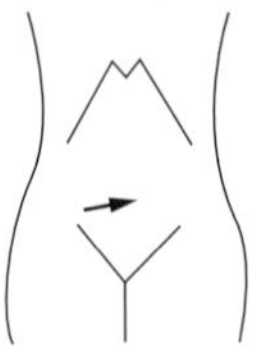

Figure 8-23. Colonic intussusception.
Colonic intussusception occurs fairly frequently in young children. This figure demonstrates intussusception of the terminal portion of the ileum into the colon in a 4-month-old boy. It shows the typical layered pattern of the intestine. (Courtesy of Drs. Lo and Wang, Shenyan Medical School Hospital, China)

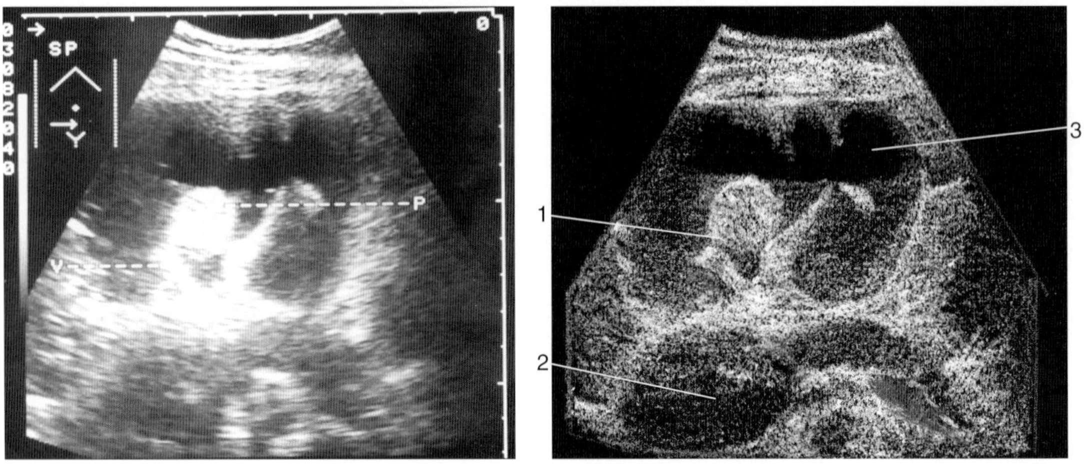

1. Polyp 2. Iliopsoas muscle 3. Dilated intestinal loop with fluid

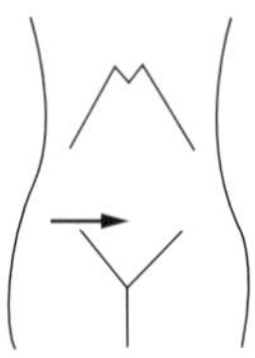

Figure 8-24. Polyp of the colon.
Colonic polyps may be single or multiple. This 30-year-old male developed a relatively large polyp in the colon with signs of chronic ileus and typhlitis. At operation a round polyp of 2.1 × 1.9 cm diameter was found. Histological examination showed a benign adenoma. (Courtesy of Drs. Lo and Wang, Shenyan Medical School Hospital, China)

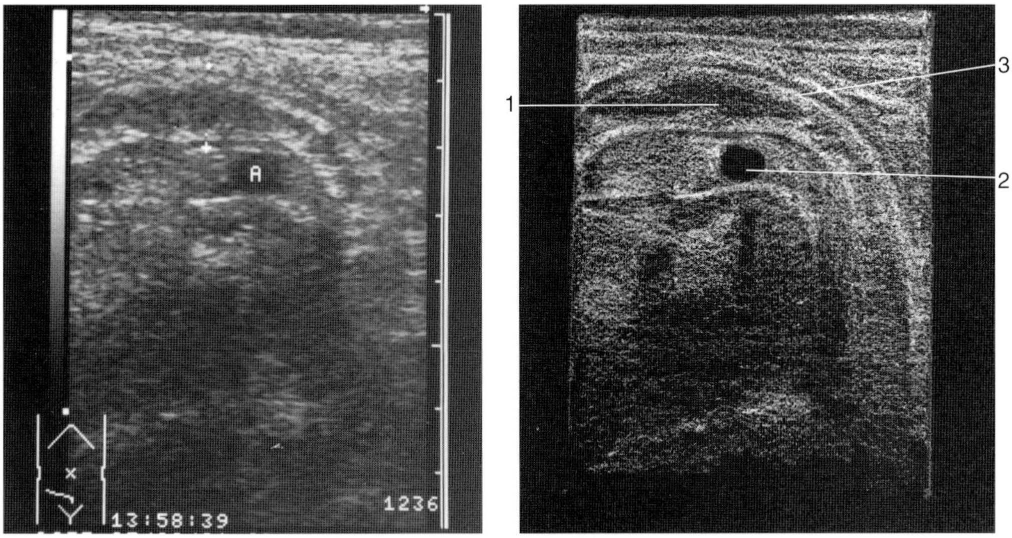

1. Inflamed, dilated appendix 2. Iliac artery
3. Submucosa

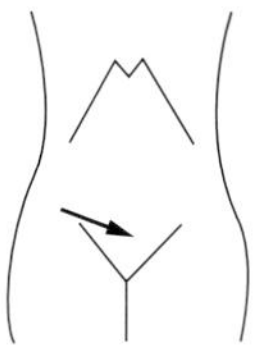

Figure 8-25. Acute appendicitis, catarrhal stage.
The intestinal appendix, an organ rich in lymphatics, is often involved in acute serous or catarrhal inflammation and acute appendicitis, which sometimes leads to the severe suppurative inflammation. In this stage, typical clinical symptoms of acute abdominal pain with nausea, and vomiting, and leukocytosis appear. This sonogram shows the first stage of inflammation in a slightly enlarged appendix.

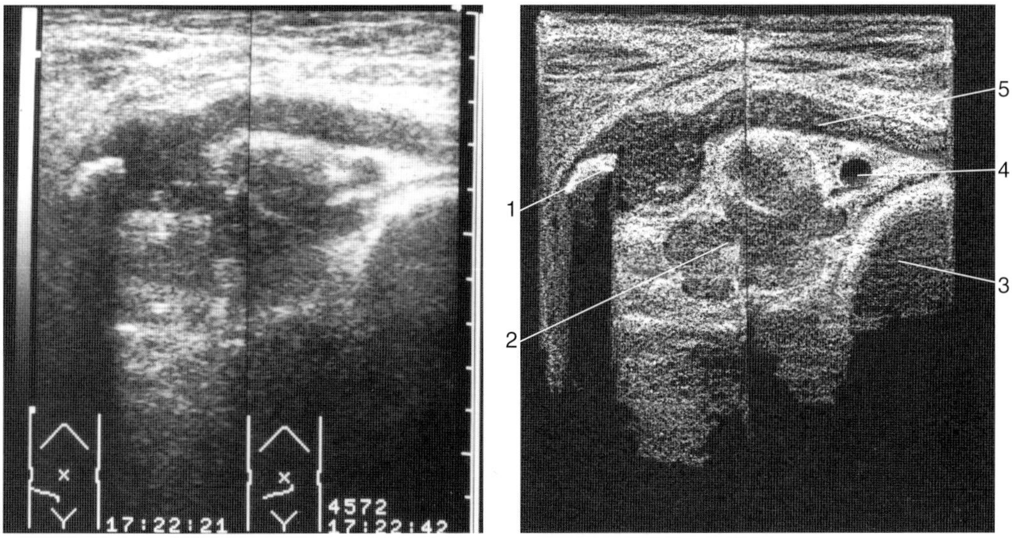

1. Fecolith 2. Psoas muscle 3. Vertebra
4. Iliac artery 5. Dilated appendix

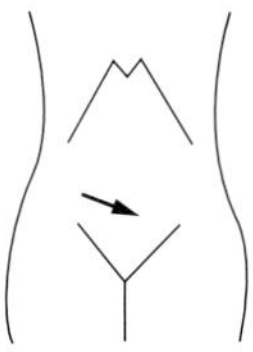

Figure 8-26. Acute appendicitis with a fecolith.
Acute appendicitis frequently occurs when the appendix is obstructed by a fecolith. This sonogram is from a patient with moderate leukocytosis; a careful search has demonstrated an engorged appendix with a fecolith, which casts a characteristic acoustic shadowing distally. The loss of the normal layered structure is due to inflammatory changes in the appendix wall. At laparotomy the patient was found to have localized peritonitis around a markedly inflamed appendix.

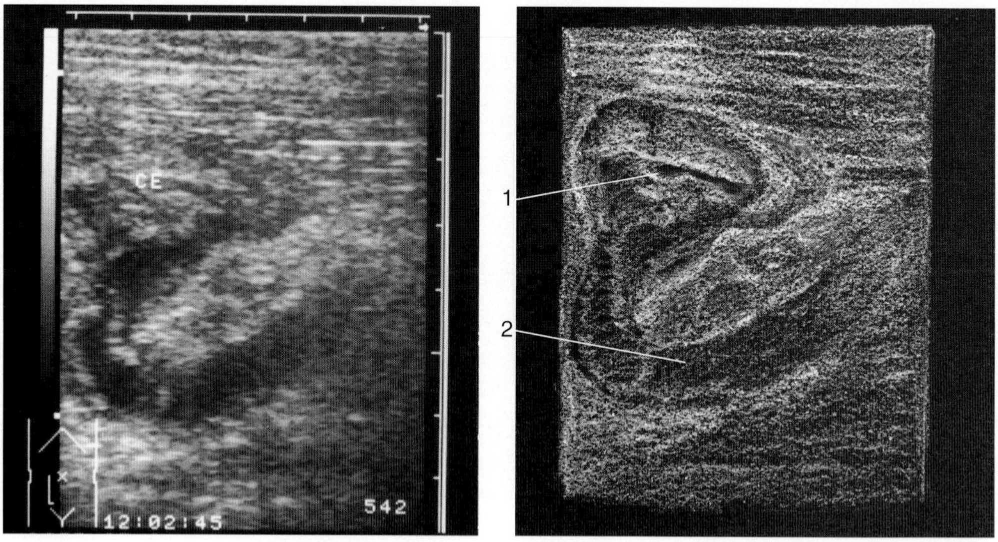

1. Cecum 2. Severely inflamed, necrotic appendix

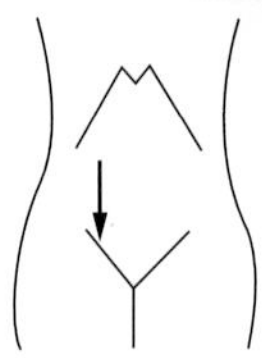

Figure 8-27. Acute necrotic and perforating appendicitis.
This sonogram of the appendix was recorded in a young man with the typical clinical picture of severe acute appendicitis. He had a leukocyte count of 17,000 with a marked left shift. The sonogram revealed loss of the echogenic third layer, indicating necrotic inflammatory changes of the mucosa. At laparotomy, severe inflammation of the appendix was confirmed. It was found to have extended into the colon, so that partial resection of the cecum had to be performed.

a

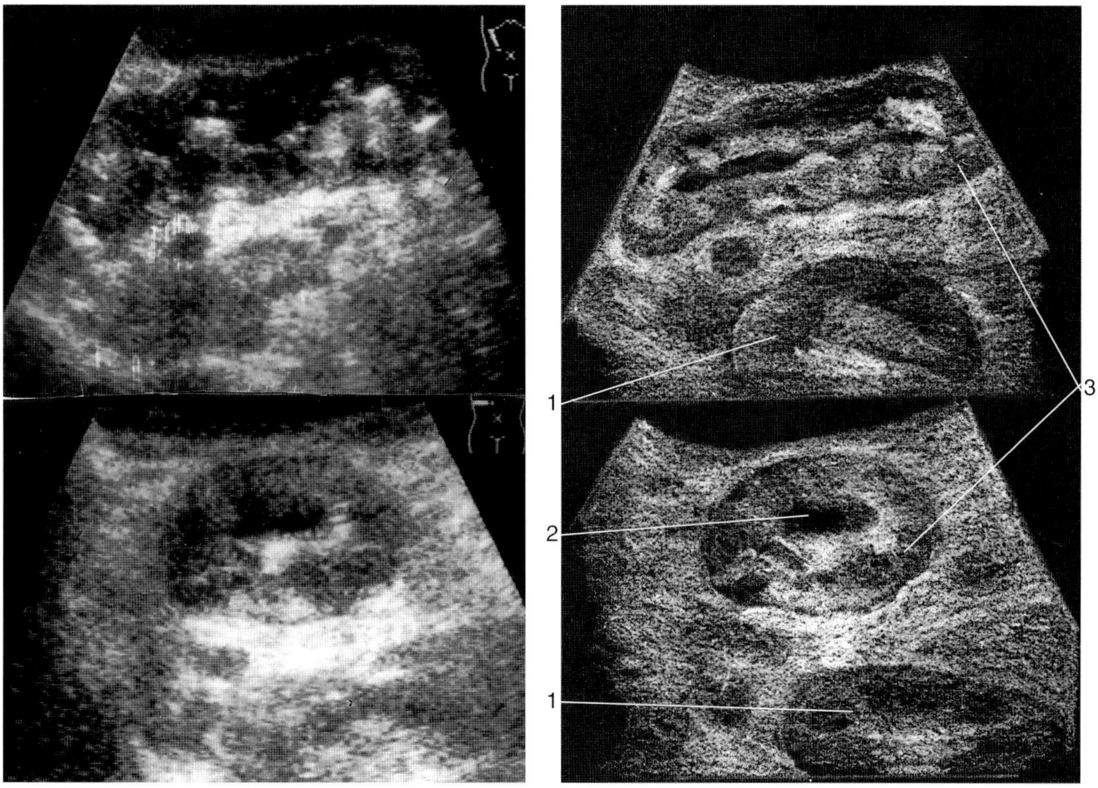

b

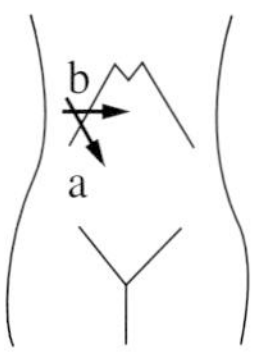

1. Right kidney 2. Intestinal lumen 3. Edematous thickening of colonic wall

Figure 8-28. Acute hemorrhagic enterocolitis.
Acute exudative inflammation of the colon occurs relatively frequently in a variety of clinical conditions especially following the use of antibiotics such as oral synthetic penicillins. The resultant growth of *Clostridium difficile* (the most common causative agent) leads to mucosal thickening with bleeding erosions. Following successful treatment, the change rapidly disappeared and the scan returned to normal.

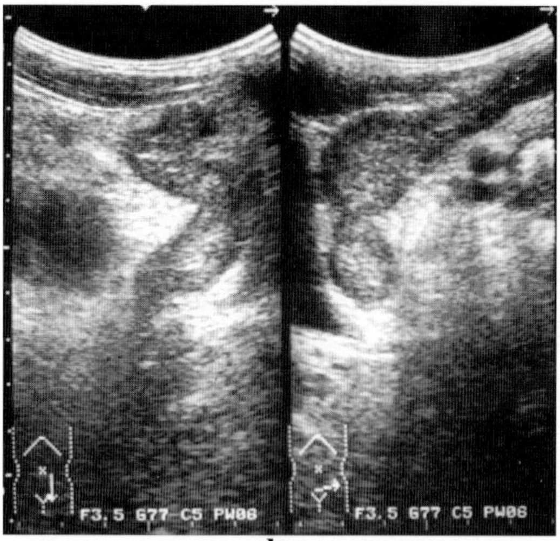

a b

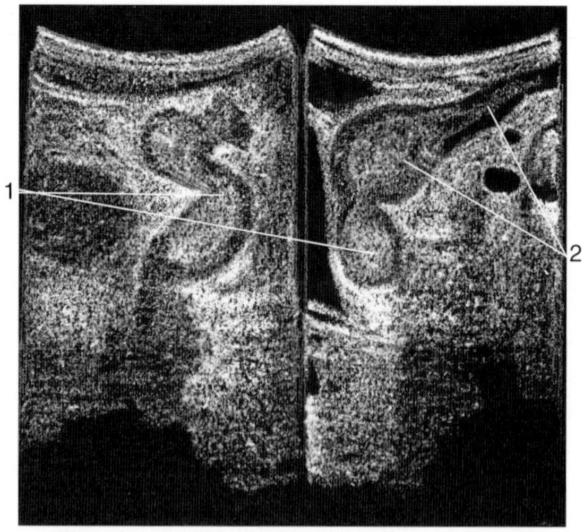

1. Sigmoid colon 2. Descending colon

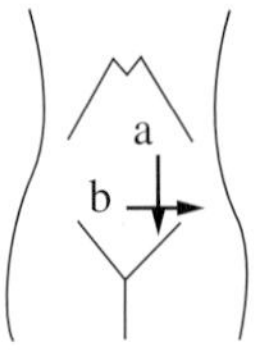

Figure 8-29. Crohn's disease.
Crohn's disease presents with variable symptoms depending on the site and extent of the intestinal changes. This profound changes affect the entire length of the colon, with sausage-shaped, inflammatory thickening characteristic of Crohn's disease. The disease tends to run a chronic course; however, in this patient, recovery followed complete parenteral nutrition and prolonged medical treatment.

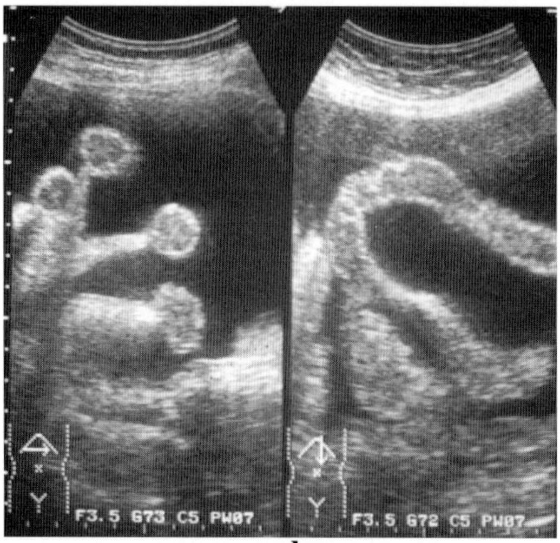

a b

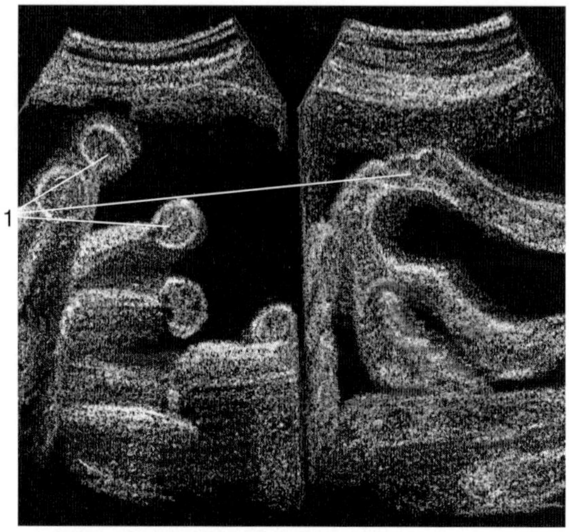

1. Floating intestinal loops

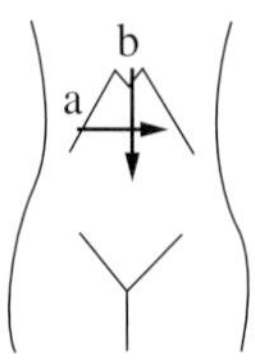

Figure 8-30. Intestinal loops of ascites.
Intestinal loops are seldom imaged unless they are fluid-filled, for example, in intestinal obstruction or ileus. In patients with ascites, loops of intestine, both large and small, are well demonstrated together with the mesocolon that connect the loops to the posterior abdominal wall.

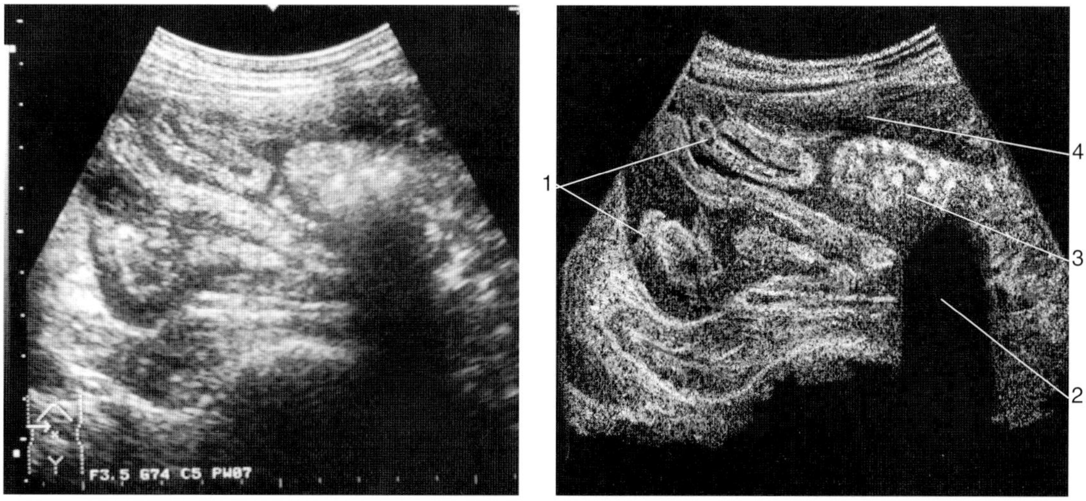

1. Floating intestinal loops 2. Acoustic shadow
3. Calcified mesentrial tissues 4. Ascites

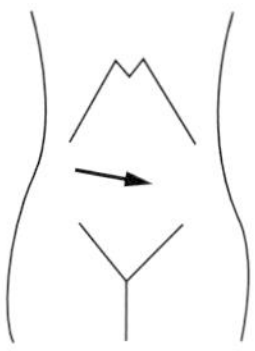

Figure 8-31. Intestinal loops in tuberculous peritonotis.
Intestinal loops visualized by virtue of ascitic fluid fill the abdominal cavity. The low-level echoes observed throughout the ascitic fluid are caused by minute echogenic particles of cholesterol crystal cause by the prolonged chronic peritonitis of tuberculous origin. There was also involvement of both kindneys and the spleen.

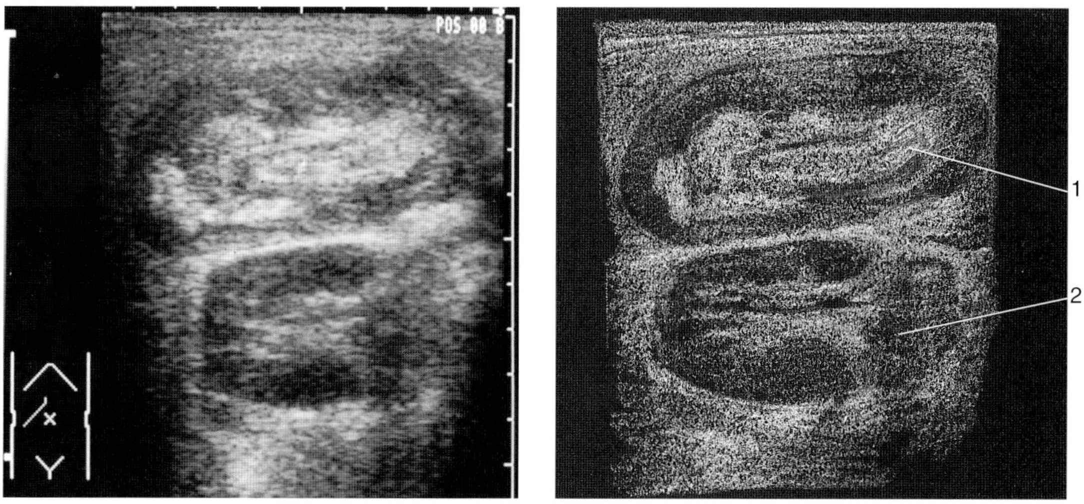

1. Cancer of ascending colon 2. Right kidney

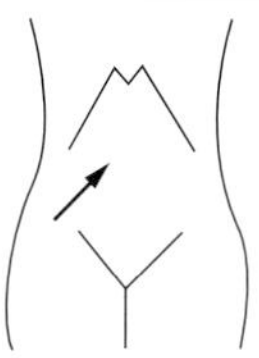

Figure 8-32. Colonic carcinoma demonstrating the pseudokidney sign.
In the pseudokidney sign, a well-documented finding in gastrointestinal tract walls characterized by a hypoechoic periphery representing the tumor tissue with a central echogenic portion mimicking the calices of the kidney. This large tumor mass of the ascending colon was visualized along with the sonogram of the real kidney posteriorly.

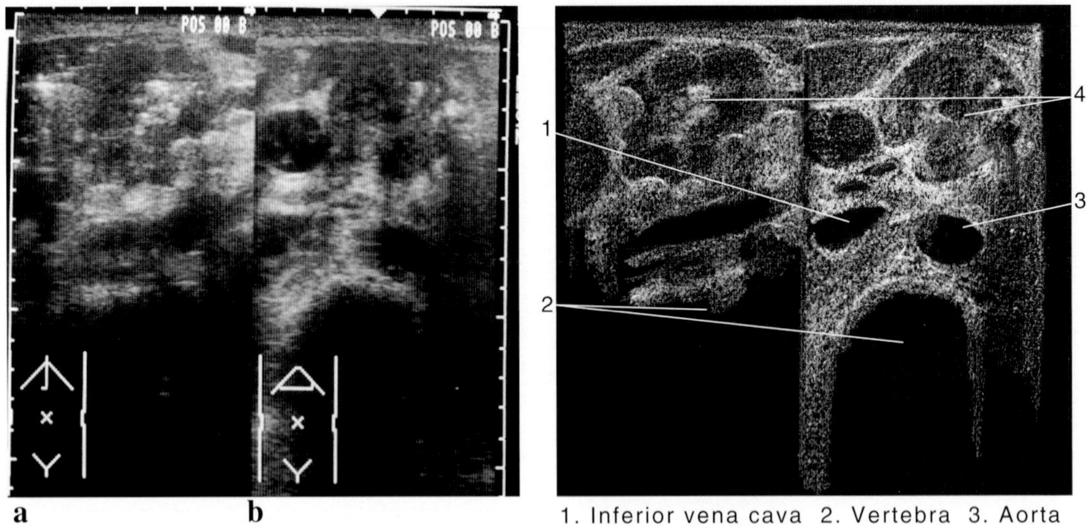

1. Inferior vena cava 2. Vertebra 3. Aorta
4. Cancer of transverse colon

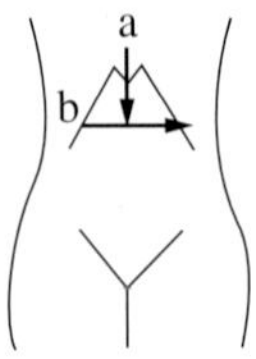

Figure 8-33. Carcinoma of the transverse colon.
Typical sonograms of carcinoma of the transverse colon are visualized in transverse and sagittal scans. The echogenicity of the mass is low. The margins are irregular and the mass central echo cluster, indicating the luminal echoes characteristic of an intestinal mass.

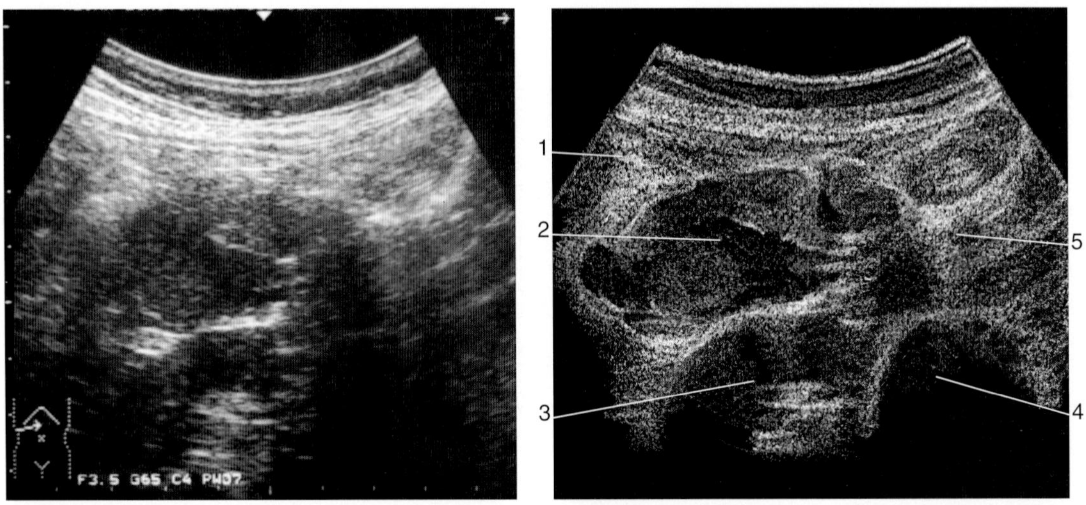

1. Gas 2. Cancer of colon 3. Right kidney
4. Vertebra 5. Colon

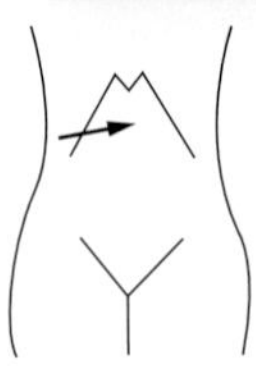

Figure 8-34. Carcinoma of the colon.
A large, echo-poor mass was visualized in the upper portion of the ascending colon. Both the contour and the internal texture are irregular and heterogeneous, suggesting the malignant nature of the mass. Directly below the tumor mass, part of the right kidney is visualized, with acoustic shadowing from its lower pole of the kidney. Ill-defined multiple echogenic, metastatic nodules were found throughout the liver.

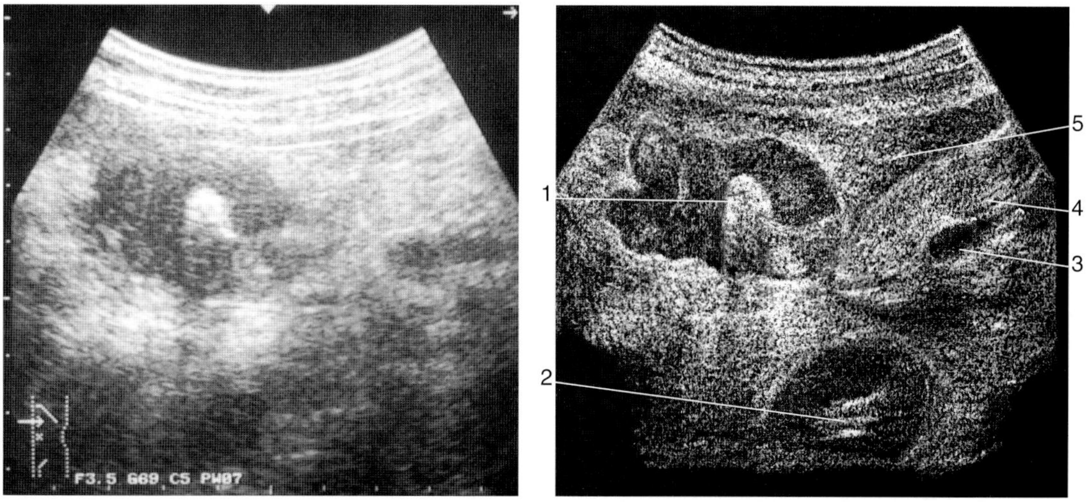

1. Tumor of transverse colon 2. Left kidney
3. Splenic vein 4. Pancreas 5. Liver

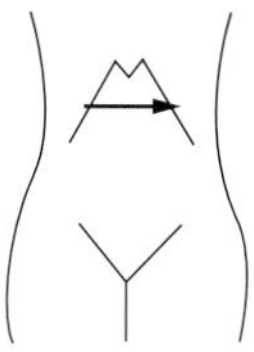

Figure 8-35. Cancer of the transverse colon.
An oval-shaped, hypoechoic mass with luminal echoes in its center was demonstrated at the mid-epigastrium when scanning in the right decubitus position. At the right, next to the tumor, the upper part of the head and body of the pancreas were also visualized. The mass showed irregularity in contour, suggesting its malignant nature. A slight degree of echo enhancement behind the mass was noted.

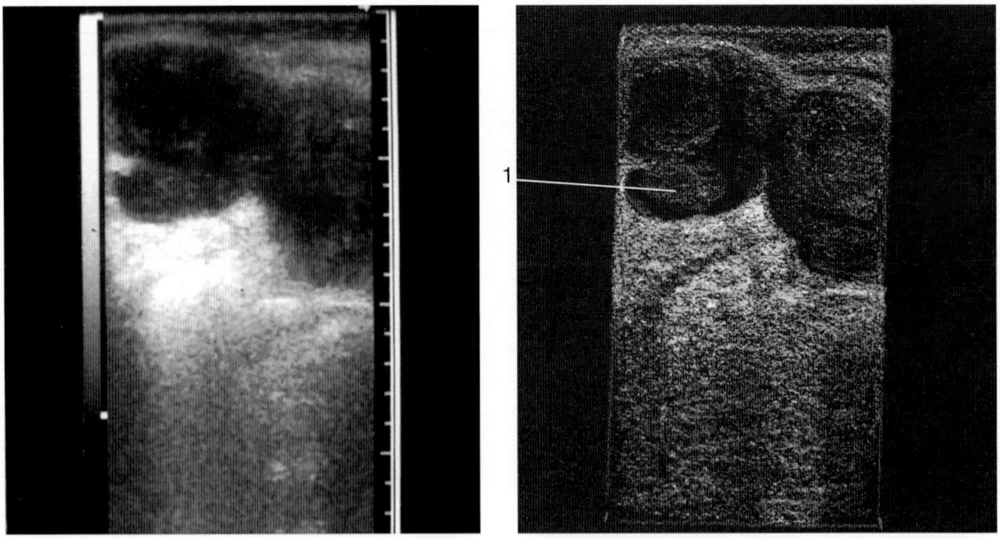

a

1. Malignant lymphoma (NHL)

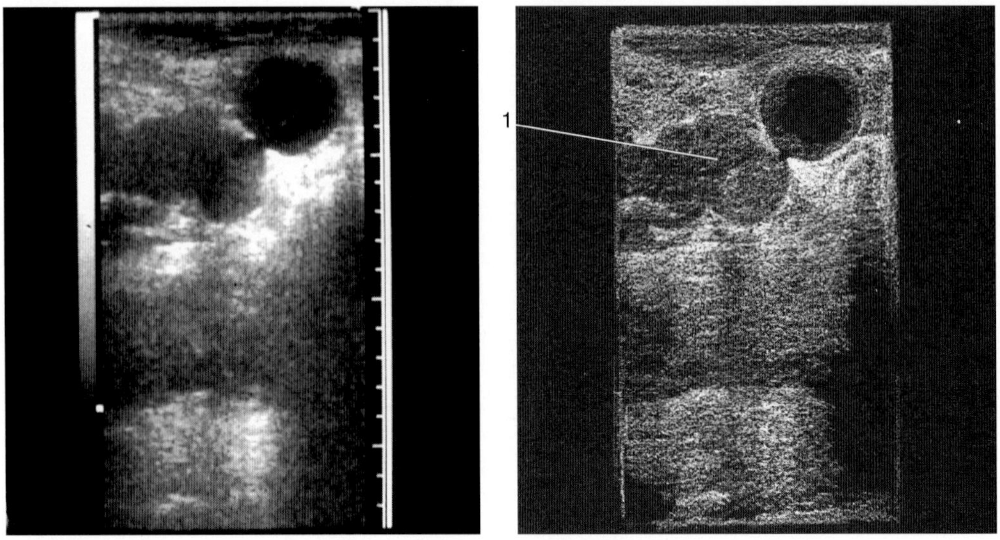

b

1. Malignant lymphoma (NHL)

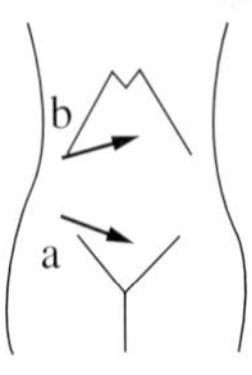

Figure 8-36. Lymphoma of the colon.
Lymphoma can also occur in the colon, where it produces anechoic tumor masses. This 82-year-old woman developed a hard mass in the ileocecal region. The first sonographic examination revealed two cystic lesions with signs of partial intestinal obstruction. At necropsy, the masses proved to be large lymphomas with enlarged regional lymph nodes extending to the midtransverse colon; the colonic tumor was accompained by ulcerative change. Posterior echo enhancement, as seen in these figures, is not caused by cystic change in the mass but is a typical finding of malignant lymphomas.

a

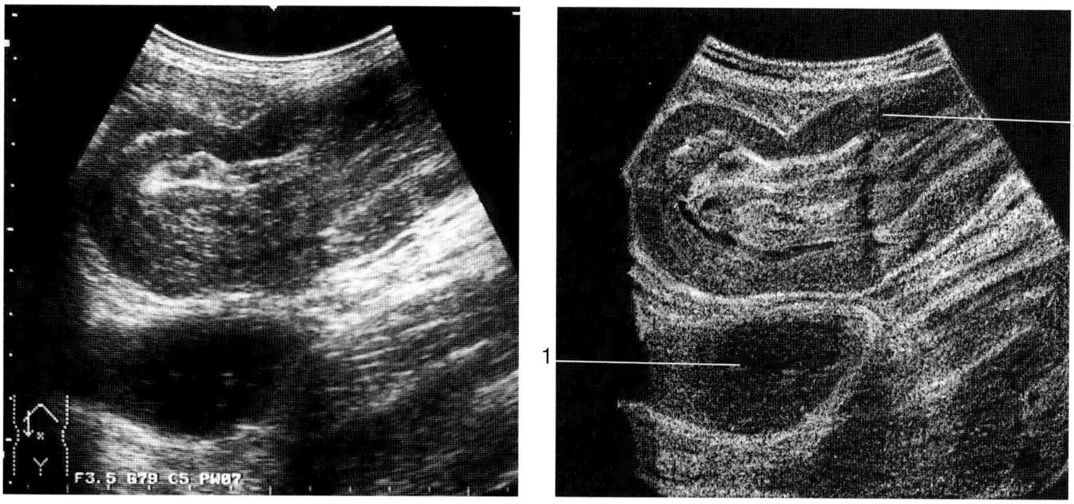

1. Dilated loop 2. Colonic loop with metastasis

b

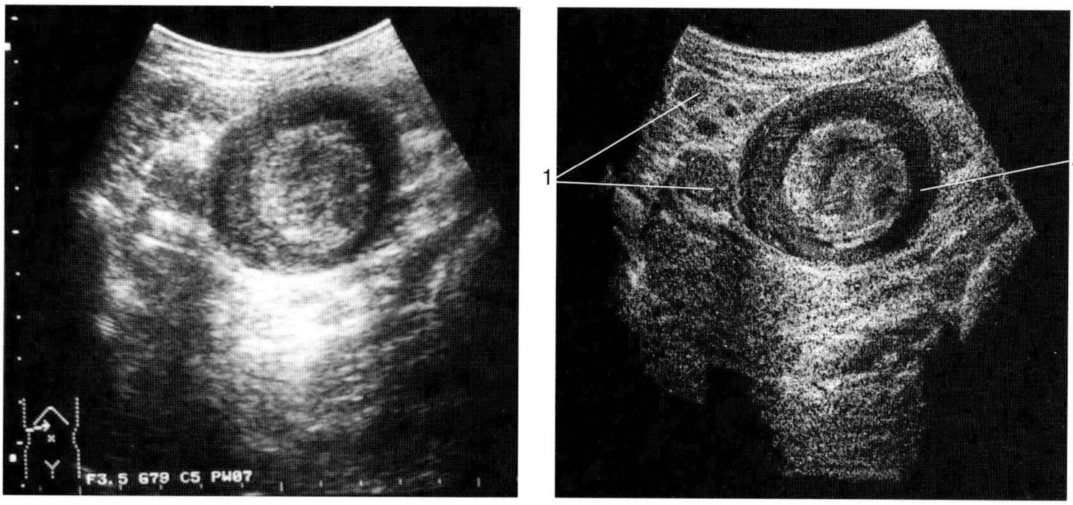

1. Lymph nodes 2. Colonic loop with metastasis

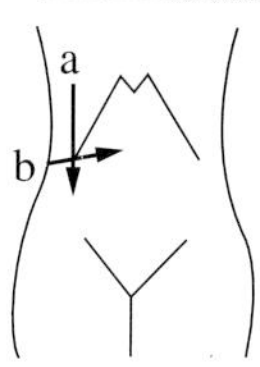

Figure 8-37. Metastasis of renal carcinoma to the ascending colon.
In addition to primary carcinoma of the colon, metastases from malignant tumor of adjacent organs can occur. These figures show a large tumor involving the upper one third of the ascending colon, producing partial ileus of the proximal intestinal loops. The primary was a carcinoma of the left kidney, and the colon was diffusely infiltrated from its serosal surface.

REFERENCES

1. Allmendinger G, Blaich E, Hofgartner F, et al: Correlation between endoscopic biopsy findings and sonograms of the abdomen in stomach cancer. Gastroenterology 22 : 62-65, 1984.
2. Ball TI, Atkinson GO Jr, Gay BB Jr: Ultrasound diagnosis of hypertrophic pyloric stenosis: Real-time application and the demonstration of a new sonographic sign. Radiology 147 : 499-502, 1983.
3. Bluth EI, Merritt CRB, Sullivan MA: Ultrasonic evaluation of the stomach, small bowel and colon. Radiology 133 : 677-680, 1979.
4. Burke LF, Clark EG: Ileocolic intussusception: A case report. JCU 5 : 346-347, 1977.
5. Carroll BA, Ta HN: The ultrasonic appearance of extranodal abdominal lymphoma. Radiology 136 : 419-425, 1980.
6. Carroll BA: US of the gastrointestinal tract. Radiology 172 : 605-608, 1989
7. Derchi LE, Biggi E, Rollandi GA: Sonographic staging of gastric cancer. AJR 140 : 273-276, 1983.
8. Derchi LE, Banderali A, Bossi MC, et al: The sonographic appearance of gastric lymphoma. J Ultrasound Med 3 : 251-256,1984.
9. Deutsch A, Leopold GR: Ultrasonic demonstration of the inflamed appendix. Case report. Radiology 140 : 163-164, 1981.
10. Dinkel E, Grosser G, Beck A: Sonographic diagnosis of the gastrointestinal tract. Radiologie 26 : 144-153, 1986.
11. Dragsted J, Gammelgaard J: Endoluminal ultrasonic scanning in the evaluation of rectal cancer: A preliminary report of 13 cases. Gastrointest Radiol 8 : 367-369, 1983.
12. Fleischer AC, Dowling AD, Weinstein ML, et al: Sonographic pattern of distended, fluid-filled bowel. Radiology 133 : 681-685, 1979.
13. Fleischer AC, Muhletaler CA, James AE Jr: Sonographic assessment of the bowel wall. AJR 136 : 887-891,1981.
14. Gooding GAW: Ultrasonography of the cecum. Gastrointest Radiol 6 : 243-246, 1981.
15. Gonzalez AC, Hanes JD: Retrorenal abscess secondary to a ruptured retrocecal appendix diagnosed by ultrasound B scan and 67 Ga radionuclide scan. JCU 5 : 114-116, 1977.
16. Graif M, Itzchak Y, Avigad I, et al: The pylorus in infancy: Overall sonographic assessment. Pediatr Radiol 14 : 14-17, 1984.
17. Hauser JB, Stanley RJ, Geisse G: The ultrasound findings in an obstructed afferent loop. JCU 2 : 287-289, 1974.
18. Hayden CK Jr, Boulden TF, Swischuk LE, et al: Sonographic demonstration of duodenal obstruction with midgut volvulus. AJR 143 : 9-10, 1984.
19. Hayden CK Jr: Gastrointestinal tract. Clin Diagn Ultrasound 24 : 77-101, 1989.
20. Hollmann JP, Goebel N: Computerized tomography and sonography in the diagnosis of recurrent colorectal tumors. ROFO 143 : 665-671, 1985.
21. Hopens T, Coggs GC, Goldstein HM, et al: Sonographic diagnosis of afferent loop obstruction. AJR 138 : 967-969, 1982.
22. Kimmey MB, Martin RW, Hagitt RC, et al: Histologic correlates of gastrointestinal ultrasound images. Gastroenterology 96 : 433-441, 1989.
23. Kremer H, Lohmoeller G, Zollner N: Primary ultrasonic detection of a double carcinoma of the colon. Radiology 124 : 481-482, 1977.
24. Kurihara M, Aoki K, Hisamichi S (eds): UICC Cancer Motality Statistics in the World, 1950-1985. University of Nagoya Press, 1989, pp 1-93.
25. Limberg B: Diagnosis of acute ulcerative colitis and colonic Crohn's disease by colonic sonography. JCU 17 : 25-31, 1989.
26. Lix G, Heycder N, Lutz H: Ultrasound tomography of the upper gastrointestinal tract. Orientation and diagnostic possibilities. Scand J Gastroenterol 19 (Suppl) 94 : 13-20, 1984.
27. Madrazo BL, Hricak H, Sandler MA, et al: Sonographic findings in complicated peptic ulcer disease. Radiology 140 : 457-461, 1981.
28. Miller JH, Kemberling CR: Ultrasound scanning of the gastrointestinal tract in children: Subjective review. Radiology 152 : 671-677, 1984.
29. Miller JH, Hindman BW, Lam AH: Ultrasound in evaluation of small bowel lymphoma in children. Radiology 135 : 409-414, 1980.
30. Montali G, Croce F, DePra L, et al: Intussusception of the bowel: A new sonographic pattern. Br J Radiol 56 : 621-623, 1983.
31. Morin ME, Panella J, Baker DA, et al: Ultrasound detection of a carcinoid tumor. Gastrointest Radiol 4 :

359-360, 1979.
32. Peterson LR, Cooperberg PL: Ultrasound demonstration of lesions of the gastrointestinal tract. Gastrointest Radiol 3 : 303-306, 1978.
33. Parulekar SG: Ultrasonographic findings in disease of the appendix. J Ultrasound Med 2 : 59-64, 1983.
34. Pozderac RV, Doust BD: Confusing appearance of a dilated jejunal loop. JCU 6 : 165-166, 1978.
35. Rao BK, Fleischer AC: Sonography of the gastrointestinal tract. Curr Opin Radiol 2 : 207-212, 1990.
36. Rubin C, Kurtz AB, Goldberg BB: A new ultrasound technique in defining pelvic anatomy. JCU 6 : 28-33, 1978.
37. Salem S, O'Malley BP, Hiltz CW: Ultrasonographic appearance of gastrointestinal masses. J Can Assoc Radiol 31 : 163-167, 1980.
38. Salem S, Hiltz CW: Ultrasonographic appearance of gastric lymphosarcoma. JCU 6 : 429-430, 1978.
39. Sandler MA, Ratanaprakarn S, Madrazo BL: Ultrasonic findings in intramural exogenic lesions. Radiology 128 : 189-192, 1978.
40. Sauerbrei EE, Paloschi GGB: The ultrasonic features of hypertrophic pyloric stenosis with emphasis on the post operative appearance. Radiology 147 : 503-506, 1983.
41. Schabel SI, Rittenberg GM, Johnson EG: Carcinoma of the colon demonstrated by ultrasound. JCU 6 : 436-437, 1978.
42. Scheible W, Goldberg BB: Diagnosis of small bowel obstruction: The contribution of diagnostic ultrasound. AJR 133 : 685-688, 1979.
43. Schoelmerich J, Diaz A, Volk BA, et al: Clinical significance of abnormalities of the gastrointestinal tract detected by abdominal ultrasound. Dig Dis Sci 33 : 257-262, 1988.
44. Schwerk W, Braun B, Dombrowski H: Real-time ultrasound examination in the diagnosis of gastrointestinal tumors. JCU 7 : 425-431, 1979.
45. Subramanyam BR, Balthazar EJ, Raghavendra BN, et al: Sonography of exophytic gastrointestinal leiomyosarcoma. Gastrointest Radiol 7 : 47-51, 1982.
46. Swobodnik W: Sonography in gastroenterology. Established and new procedures. Internist 33 : 822-833, 1992.
47. Teele RL, Smith EH: Ultrasound in the diagnosis of idiopathic hypertrophic pyloric stenosis. N Engl J Med 296 : 1149-1150, 1977.
48. Tan A, Lau PH: Sonography of primary adenocarcinoma of the appendix with pathological correlation. Am J Gastroenterol 78 : 488-492, 1983.
49. Walecki JK, Hales ED, Chung EB, et al: Ultrasound contribution to diagnosis of Peutz-Jeghers syndrome. Pediatr Radiol 14 : 62-64, 1984.
50. Weighall SL, Wolfman NT, Weatson N: The fluid-filled stomach: A new sonic window. JCU 7 : 353-356, 1979.
51. Weissberg DL, Scheible W, Leopold GR: Ultrasonographic appearance of adult ileocolic intussusception. Radiology 124 : 791-792, 1977.
52. Worlicek H, Dunz D, Engelhard K: Ultrasonic examination of the wall of the fluid-filled stomach. JCU 17 : 5-14, 1989.

CHAPTER 9

ENDOSCOPIC SONOGRAPHY OF GASTROINTESTINAL DISORDERS

ENDOSCOPIC SONOGRAPHY OF THE GASTROINTESTINAL TRACT

Until very recently, investigations of diseases of the gastrointestinal tract were restricted to roentgenologic and endoscopic examinations. In routine practice, these exams were performed in conjunction with appropriate biochemical studies. Endoscopy is extremely effective for evaluating mucosal lesions of the gastrointestinal tract such as ulcers, polyps, carcinomas, and inflammation.

However, these standard approaches have limitations in diseases involving the submucosal and extramural layers of the gastrointestinal tract. For example, precise staging of gastric carcinomas in terms of the depth of penetration is almost impossible. Furthermore, diseases of organs adjacent to the gastrointestinal tract, such as the pancreas, biliary tract, and retroperitoneal spaces, are extremely difficult to diagnose by these standard procedures. To overcome the limitations, noninvasive imaging methods such as x-ray CT and ultrasound were developed. The limited resolution of the former method and the difficulty of penetration of sonic waves into air-containing, hollow viscera of the latter have significantly limited their diagnostic application in gastroenterology.

The situation changed significantly following the introduction of high-resolution real-time scanners and, more recently, of endosonographic methods, using mechanical or electronic sonoendoscope[5-8, 11, 12, 15, 26] (Figures 9-1 and 9-2).

These diagnostic methods created a new arena in diagnostic methodology in gastroenterology. Although experience with them is still rather limited, they have already yielded impressive results in the diagnosis of a variety of diseases involving the gastrointestinal tract, including malignant tumors, both intramural as well as nonmalignant disorders such as gastric ulcers, acute gastric mucosal lesions, chronic gastritis, Crohn's disease, ulcerative colitis and colonic polyposis.[14, 25, 29] Above all, endosonography has solved the problem of TNM staging of gastrointestinal malignancies[27], since it visualizes and assesses the size, extent, and depth of penetration of the tumor to the wall of the gastrointestinal tract and in adjacent organs, including lymph nodes.

Scanning Techniques for the Stomach and Esophagus

To obtain clear ultrasonic images of the stomach, the patient fasts overnight; preferably, a laxative is also given the night before. An antispasmodic may be injected prior to the examination to suppress peristalsis. After mild pharyngeal anesthesia, a sonoendoscope is inserted with the patient in the left decubitus position. After insertion of the scope, and the tip is gently advanced until it reaches the cardia of the stomach. Guided by visual observation through the fiberoptics of the scope, the tip is gently advanced toward the greater curvature of the stomach, with continuous inflation of air as for routine endoscopy. With further insertion, the tip passes through the gastric antrum to reach the pylorus. Mucosal lesions or tumors, if present, should be recorded photographically. After completion of the endoscopic observations, sufficient degassed water to distend the gastric lumen is gently infused through the fine water channel in the scope (Figure 9-3). The patient is then asked to lie in the right decubitus position to allow the lower half of the stomach to fill with water, and ultrasonic scanning is started. Sonographic images of the stomach wall, gallbladder, pancreas and liver are recorded on videotape for archiving while careful observation of the images on the video screen is carried out.[3, 9, 10, 14]

The scope may be advanced into the descending duodenum for further investigation of the lower part of the common bile duct and the head of the pancreas. If the balloon method is not used, the patient is asked to lie supine to ensure that the instilled water stays in the descending duodenum to facilitate sonographic observation.

The balloon over the tip of the scope can be used to ensure good acoustic contact between the scan head and the duodenal wall by manipulating the scan head in the left decubitus position.[1, 4, 31] After the tip of the scope is withdrawn to the antrum through the pyloric canal, the patient is asked to lie in the right decubitus position to continue observation of the head and body of the pancreas, as well as part of the liver and the gallbladder. Then the patient is turned into the left decubitus position to continue observation of the upper parts of the stomach wall together with the spleen, left kidney, left adrenal and left lobe of the liver. The scope is gently withdrawn from the gastric cavity to the esophagus, and continuous observation and recording are carried out over the entire length of the esophagus.

If a sonoendoscope is not available, examination of the stomach may be made using a real-time scanner following water ingestion, as described in Chapter 8. Although the technique is simpler for routine diagnosis, resolution is poorer and interpretation is difficult even with high-resolution equipment. Furthermore, image quality is seriously degraded if the lesion is located anywhere other than the gastric angulus or the antral region of the stomach. It is much more satisfactory to use the sonoendoscopic approach when fine details and precise diagnosis are required.

The Normal Structure of the Gastric Wall

The sonographic appearance of the gastrointestinal tract wall is almost identical over its entire length, the tubular structure of the wall consisting of the following layers: mucosa, submucosa, muscularis propria with serosal layers, outermost layers.

It is now well established that the stomach wall can be resolved into five distinct layers on endosonography. A number of published reports have confirmed that the innermost layer, with increased echogenicity and a thin, echo-poor layer immediately deep to it, corresponds mainly to the mucosa and partly to the muscularis mucosae, and that the next echogenic layer corresponds to the submucosa. The fourth echo-poor layer is the muscularis propria layer, and the outermost echogenic layer is the serosal layer[1-3, 17] (Figure 9-4).

A high-resolution sonogram obtained by routine abdominal scanning displays the same sonographic pattern, with slightly lower resolution. The stomach wall at the antrum usually displays three echogenic layers interspersed by thin, echo-poor layers. It is often difficult, however, to recognize the complete layeres in the anterior wall of the stomach because of multiple reflection artifacts arising from the reflective abdominal wall structures. Similarly, thorough examination of the body and cardia are almost impossible even after positioning the patient, underlining the advantages of endoscopic sonography for more detailed examinations.

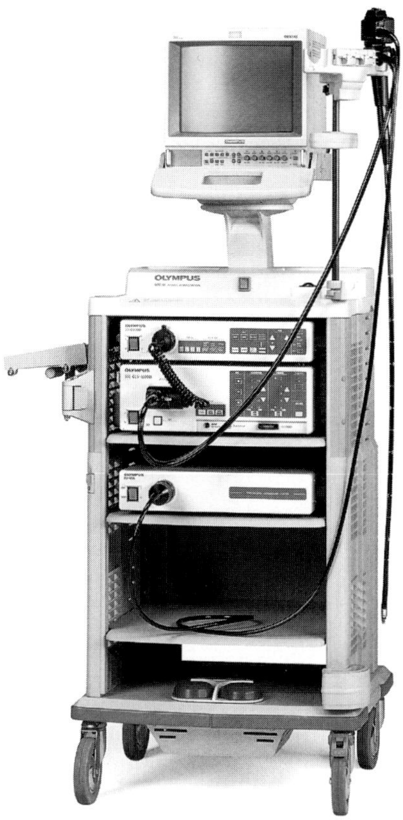

Figure 9-1. Endoscopic ultrasonograph (mechanical radial scanner).
A sonogastrofiberscope equipped with a mechanically rotating radial scanner is shown together with the imaging unit (Olympus GFUM3/EUM3).

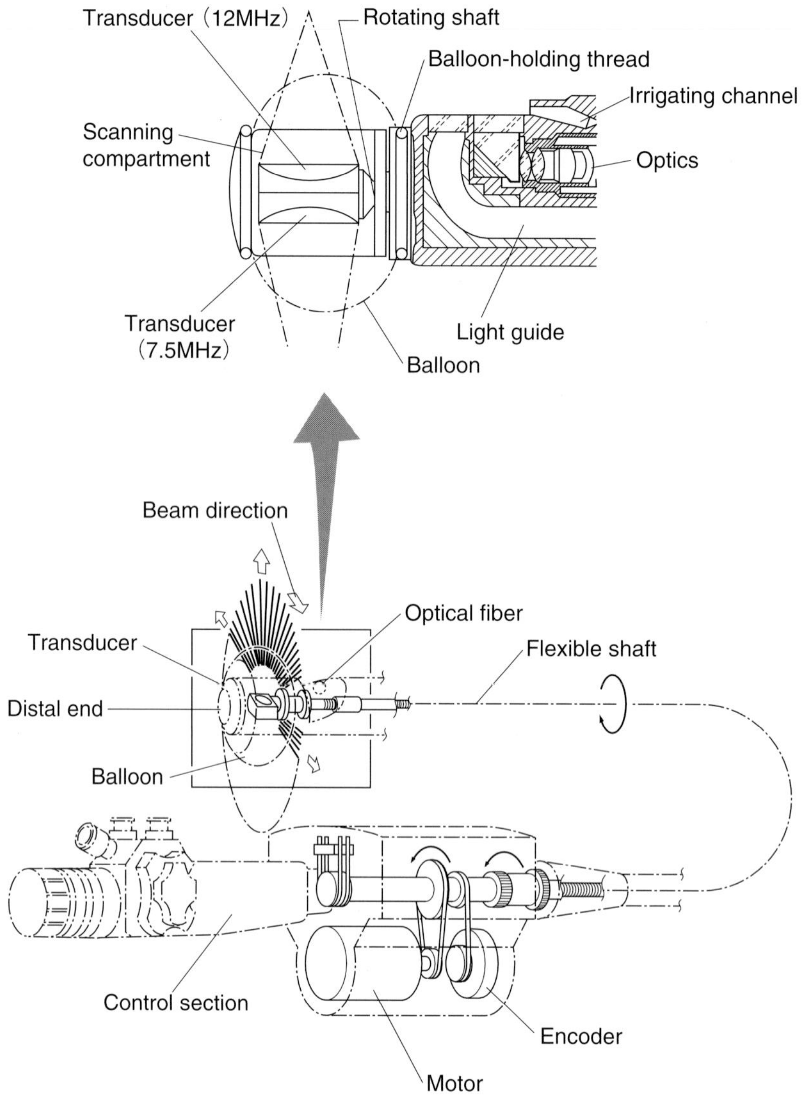

Figure 9-2. Schematic drawing of sonoendoscope, Olympus GFUM3.
A disc transducer (dual-disc) in the scanning chamber is rotated by the motor unit housed in the proximal end of the scope via a flexible steel shaft in the scope. The system gives real-time cross-sectional sonograms of the gastrointestinal tract, perpendicular to the axis of the scope.

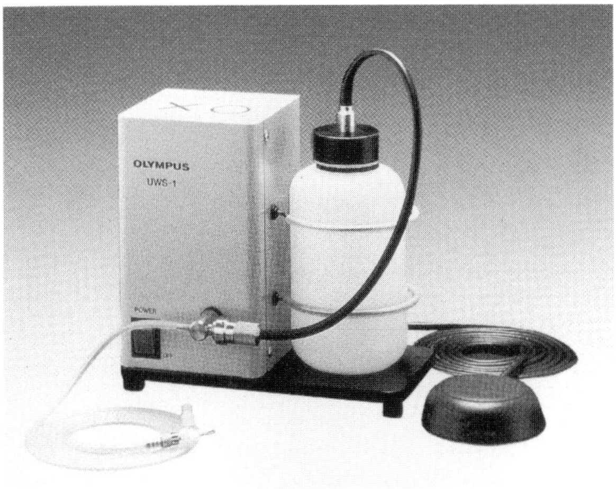

Figure 9-3. Automatic fluid infusion pump, positive-pressure type.
To obtain a complete 360° cross-sectional image by endoscopic ultrasound degassed water is infused to fill the lumen to be scanned. The speed of infusion is 1ml/sec and 500-700 ml of degassed water is required for a single examination. Alternatively, a rubber balloon covering the scan head may be inflated by water to secure acoustic contact with the wall of gastrointestinal tract.

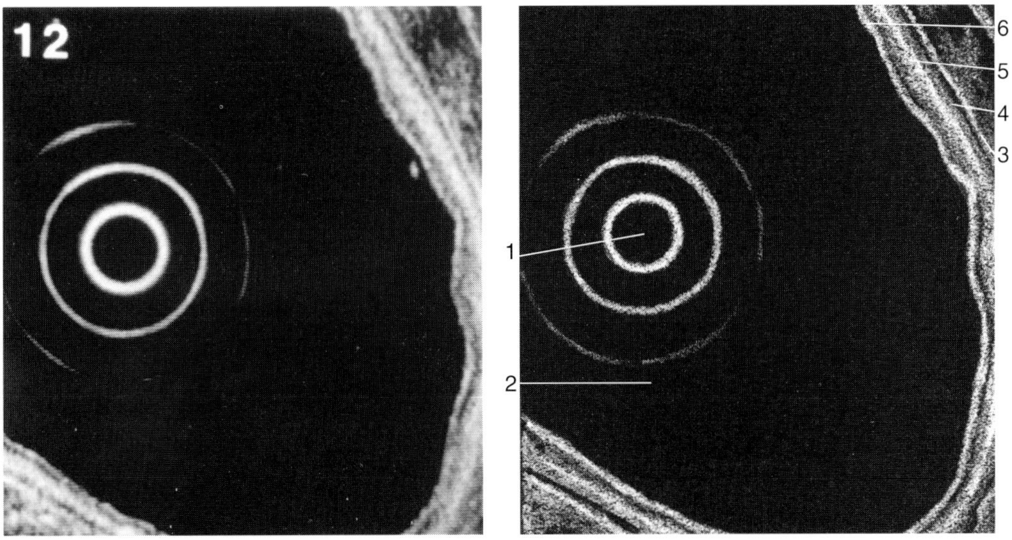

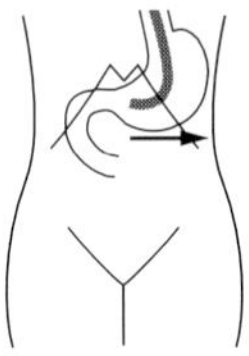

1. Transducer 2. Gastric lumen 3. Serosa (s)
4. Muscularis propria (pm; proper muscle)
5. Submucosa (sm) 6. Mucosa (m)

Figure 9-4. Normal gastric wall visualized by endosonography.
This image of normal gastric mucosa was obtained by scanning the water-filled stomach with a 12-MHz transducer. The high resolution demonstrating the basic five-layered structure of the wall, namely, the echogenic and echo-poor layers of the mucosa, followed by highly echogenic submucosa, the echo-poor muscularis propria and the echogenic serosal layer.

ABNORMAL FINDINGS IN THE ULTRASONOENDOSCOPIC EXAMINATION

The diagnostic indications for endoscopic ultrasound (EUS) are expanding rapidly; the established uses are summarized in Table 9-1. These will be presented briefly.

Table 9-1. Indications for endoscopic sonography.

1. **Transesophageal Scanning**
   - Diagnosis and staging of esophageal carcinoma
   - Diagnosis of esophageal submucosal tumors
   - Esophageal varices, including assessment of results of sclerotheraphy
   - Detection and differentiation of mediastinal tumors
   - Diagnosis of abnormalities of the heart and great vessels
2. **Gastric or Transgastric Scanning**
   - Diagnosis and staging of gastric carcinoma
   - Diagnosis of gastric lymphoma
   - Diagnosis of gastric submucosal tumors
   - Gastric varices
   - Differential diagnosis of extragastric compressions
   - Assesment of response to antitumor chemotherapy or laser treatment
   - Diagnosis and staging of pancreatic cancer
   - Differential diagnosis of chronic pancreatitis and pancreatolithiasis
   - Differential diagnosis of cystic lesions of the pancreas
3. **Transduodenal Scanning**
   - Differential diagnosis of duodenal submucosal tumors
   - Tumors of the duodenal papilla
   - Differential diagnosis of obstructive jaundice
   - Diagnosis and staging of carcinoma of the head and uncinate process of the pancreas
   - Differential diagnosis and staging of gallbladder carcinoma
4. **Examination of the Lower Colon**
   - Diagnosis and staging of colon cancer, including the rectum and sigmoid colon
   - Evaluation of colonic polyps
   - Diagnosis of submucosal tumors in the colorectal region
   - Guidance for biopsy of mucosal and submucosal tumors
   - Evaluation and differential diagnosis of Crohn's disease and ulcerative colitis
5. **Laparoscopic Sonography**
   - Detection and evaluation of hepatocellular carcinomas
   - Differential diagnosis of space-occupying lesions
   - Ultrasound-guided biopsy of liver tumors
   - Differential diagnosis of gallbladder tumors
   - Diagnosis of pancreatic carcinomas

Gastric Diseases

Extragastric compression

Elucidation of the exact cause of extragastric compression is often difficult with routine gastroscopy. Ultrasonic examination can readily demonstrate most of the underlying causes of compression, examples include enlargment of the left lobe of the liver (Figure 9-5), polycystic kidneys, an enlarged spleen or splenic masses, and pancreatic tumors. Endoscopic ultrasound can solve the problem more simply than routine abdominal sonography because of the direct imaging and increased resolution provided by high frequency transducers.

Gastric submucosal tumors

Leiomyoma is the most common submucosal tumor, and its position in relation to layers of the normal gastric mucosa can be identified with endosonography. These tumors are mostly benign, but they can grow so large as to be palpable. In general, the larger the tumor, the greater the possibility of malignancy (Figures 9-6 to 9-8). Sonographically, the diagnosis of gastric submucosal tumor is made by demonstrating the echogenic submucosal layer over the tumor together with a thin, echo-poor layer or a slit separating it from extragastric organs.[14, 21, 25, 28] By contrast, an extragastric mass is always covered by the full thickness of the gastric wall, with all five layers covering it. (see Figure 9-4) Respiratory movement of the tumor during real-time imaging often gives a better perception of the precise site of origin of the tumors.

Although sonoendoscopic examination generates superb images with high resolution, it cannot establish the histopathological diagnosis of gastric submucosal tumors; biopsy is still required. It may, however, be possible to suggest the true diagnosis by observing the ultrasonic characteristics of the mass in detail. Gastric leiomyomas are typically rather uniform in echo texture with a round or semiovoid outline. Occasionally they show multiple echo-poor, cystic changes due to liquefaction producing a complex echo pattern. Differentiation between benign and malignant tumors is, therefore, often difficult. As described above, the size of the mass is reliable indicator, but irregularity of the contour or margin of the mass is the most reliable sign of malignancy.[14]

Less frequent causes of gastric submucosal tumors, such as neurogenic tumors or aberrant pancreatic tissue often demonstrate cystic changes. Diagnosis of a simple cyst is straightforward, and the sonographic appearance gives a direct clue to the final diagnosis.

Malignant tumors of the stomach

Among malignant tumors of the stomach, the one most frequently encountered is gastric carcinoma. In advanced carcinoma, routine ultrasound is frequently able to reveal the so-called "pseudokidney sign" apparent in the empty stomach. Much smaller masses can also be identified by sonoendoscopy (Figures 9-9 and 9-10). Carcinomas in a less advanced stage is generally identified as localized thickening of the gastric wall, with distortion or complete destruction of its normal layered structure (Figure 9-11). Not infrequently, an echogenic ulcer crater is found at the center of the echo-poor carcinoma (Figure 9-12). Metastatic lymph nodes may be visualized in the vicinity of the mass, as shown in Figure 9-13.

Another type of gastric carcinoma, scirrhous variety, invading entire layers of the stomach producing diffuse thickening, can be precisely visualized by endoscopic sonography (Figure 9-14).

Because of the marked improvement in spatial as well as contrast resolution of endoscopic ultrasound, it is now possible to apply the technique to the staging of gastric carcinomas. Very early stages of m (mucosal type) and sm (extending to the submucosal layer) cancers, both of which correspond to T1 carcinoma by UICC-TNM classification are clearly differentiated from more advanced T2 and T3 stage carcinomas.[15,27,31] Good correlations are obtained between sonoendoscopic and histopathological diagnosis.

A less frequent type of malignant gastric tumor, the lymphoma is seen as a discrete, hypoechoic mass or as diffuse thickening of the gastric wall (Figure 9-15). A lymphomatous masses may be accompanied by slight mucosal erosion or may even produce deep ulceration, depending upon the grade of mucosal involvement.[12,14,19,27] The final diagnosis can only be made by histopathological examination of a biopsy specimen.

Assessment of gastric ulceration

The diagnosis of gastric ulcer is established rather precisely by standard diagnostic approaches employing either x-ray or endoscopic examinations. Sonoendoscopy provides a more direct assessment of disease status, such as the size of the ulcer crater, the depth of ulcer penetration, repair status in terms of reorganizing layers of the gastric wall, and inflammatory changes surrounding the ulceration (Figure 9-16).

Accumulating clinical experience suggests that the sonoendoscopic findings may be utilized as good prognostic indices, including monitoring of the therapeutic effects.

Identification of gastric varices

Gastric varices can occur with or without concomitant esophageal varices. Endoscopically, mucosal varices are easily detected, especially if they are large. However, it is very important to confirm the presence of varices using endoscopic sonography, since submucosal varices can be identified as anechoic chains of engorged vessels with a connecting to deeper vessels which are slso engorged as collaterals[14] (Figure 9-17). Enlargement of the submucosal vessels may be assessed using colorflow Doppler which provides the most reliable evidence of varices. This method can also be used to confirm the therapeutic effect of sclerosing therapy of varices.

Diseases of the Esophagus

Endoscopic ultrasound examination of the esophagus is much simpler than that of other parts of the gastrointestinal tract. Because of the limited size of the esophagus lumen, the balloon method is often necessary to obtain ultrasonic images with high resolution.

First, the scope is inserted deep into the esophagus, as far as the cardia and the balloon is inflated by instilling a little of water. The layers of the esophagus are almost identical to those of the other parts of the gastrointestinal tract, with five layers, but they are not as distinct as in the gastric wall, where the echogenic submucosal layer appears as a discrete echogenic zone.[2, 3, 7, 21, 25]

The indications for esophageal endosonography are similar to those for the stomach, the main application being assessment of the extent of malignant tumors. This method is highly accurate in detecting carcinomatous infiltration of the thoracic aorta and involvement of regional lymph nodes. The findings are frequently critical in assessing the feasibility of resection (Figure 9-18).

Benign lesions, such as leiomyomas (Figure 9-19) and cysts, are easily identified by their characteristic sonographic findings. Among other indications, the diagnosis of esophageal varices have recently been introduced.[4]

Disease of the Pancreas and Biliary System

The pancreas and biliary tree may be imaged by intragastric or intraduodenal scanning [10, 31] (Figures 9-20 and 9-21). The former method is similar to the maneuver described in the previous section on gastric scanning. The gallbladder and pancreas can be imaged by placing the scanning head in the pylorus and antrum of the stomach, respectively. The shape, location, and characteristic internal echo textures identify the organ. Detailed cross-sectional images of the lower part of the common duct and the head of the pancreas can be obtained by inserting the tip of the scope into the descending duodenum, with the inflated balloon covering the scanning compartment.

Figures 9-22 and 9-23 show the normal gallbladder with a cholesterol polyp, a pancreatic pseudocyst in its maximal dimension, and the shape of the pancreas. Internal echo textures are well visualized together with identifying landmarks.

The indication for the examination are summarized in Table 9-1. Among these, the identification of malignant tumors is of prime importance due to the resolving power of the method in defining the location and size of the tumor mass lesion and the presence or absence of invasion or dissemination (see Figure 9-20). The method is particularly well suited to early detection of pancreatic carcinomas including those arising in the tail, as well as carcinoma of the gallbladder or bile duct at sites that are difficult to image. Benign tumors can also be diagnosed with considerable accuracy. Cysts and stones are instantly diagnosed by their typical sonographic characteristics.

Striking personal findings have been the clear differential diagnosis of pancreatic carcinoma located in the tail of the organ, and also of small tumors obstructing the duct system located near the head of the pancreas (Figures 9-24 to 9-26).

Intraduodenal scanning is more effective in defining the lower portion of the common duct and the papilla of Vater, where it has proved superior to imaging by the transgastric route.

The differential diagnosis of chronic pancreatitis from pancreatic carcinoma that is such a problem to routine ultrasound examinaiton. However, chronic inflammatory masses of the pancreas can often be differentiated by the lack of a discrete tumor mass and by inhomogeneity of parenchymatous echo textures.

Diseases of the Colon

Routine sonographic examination of the rectum and sigmoid colon requires meticulous technique to yield satisfactory diagnostic results. The purpose of sonography here is similar to that in the upper gastrointestinal tract. Endosonography can be applied successfully for clinical staging of colonic malignancies, since it demonstrates the size of the tumor, the extent of infiltration, and even dissemination to adjacent organs or lymph nodes (Figures 9-27 and 9-28).[16-18, 20, 28] It can also be used to differentiate between benign and malignant tumors, intramural and extramural changes, involvement of the colon by nonmalignant diseases such as periproctal abscesses, bleeding, Crohn's disease, and tumor invasion from outside of the colon.

Scanning technique

Endosonography can be used effectively for scanning of the lower parts of the colon and rectum either alone or combined with endoscopy. The balloon method ensures complete contact of the scan head to the wall of the large intestine. Either mechanical or electronic scanning systems are available for examining the rectum, however, for scanning of the other parts of the colon, a specifically designed sonofiberscope is required to ensure safe manipulation during examination procedure.

The sonogram of the normal rectum wall and those of the colon also has the five layer structure common to the other parts of the gastrointestinal tract. The examination of the rectum is much more simple and often endosonography can suffice the purpose of examination, and a number of reports are available.

Recently the use of convex-array transducers are used for the similar purpose with excellent resolution to the perirectal tissue discriminations. 2D colorflow Doppler examinations are also introduced for the discriminations of the malignant tumor of the rectal wall with very promising results. In EUS examination of the colon and rectum, however, diagnostic capability and image quality produced are yet definitely superior in the mechanical scanner equipped with the disc transducer of higher frequency of 12 MHz to 20 MHz due to the better recognition of mucosal structure and also of perirectal tissues including lymph nodes.

The indication of the EUS had been largely limited to diseases of the rectum, the introduction of sonocolonofiberscope, UCF series, extended the EUS examination to the entire length of the colon.

Disease of the Liver: Laparoscopic Sonography

Sonographic examination of localized lesions of the liver has advanced rapidly following the wide-spread use of high resolution real-time ultrasound. The method has resulted in the detection of liver cancer at an early-stage and the discovery of small liver masses of indeterminate appearance. To resolve these differential diagnostic problems, a special method using laparoscopic sonography has been introduced [13,14] (Figure 9-29).

Two types of sonolaparoscope are available, one mechanical and the other with a linear-array electronic scanner. The former employs a rotating mirror instead of rotating the transducer itself in order to obtain good resolution in the very near field. Both types employ an optical system to observe the tip of the scope during insertion into the abdominal cavity via a trocar to avoid trauma to the intraperitoneal organs. The scanning compartment is gently placed on the liver and moved across its surface to locate the lesion. If a lesion is identified, sonolaparoscopic images are recorded on a videotape.

The high-resolution images yielded by high-frequency transducers are particularly helpful for detailed diagnosis of doubtful masses in the liver.

Hepatocellular carcinomas are clearly differentiated from cavernous hemangiomas or benign hyperplastic lesions (Figures 9-30 to 9-32). The information supplied by this technique is not limited to the cross-sectional images of the tumor itself but also includes the feeding vessels, frequently giving information that is useful in planning surgery.

The distinction of malignant from nonmalignant lesions is sometimes difficult, although the specific features of hepatocellular carcinoma are demonstrable in a significantly higher percentage of cases when compared to transabdominal scanning. In selected cases, biopsy guided by sonolaparoscopy has been successful in benign-malignant differentiation.

Endoscopic sonography is still a relatively new technique. However, the equipment and fundamental technology are now well established and promise to expand the applications of diagnostic ultrasound along with the other intraluminal scanning methods that have recently become available.

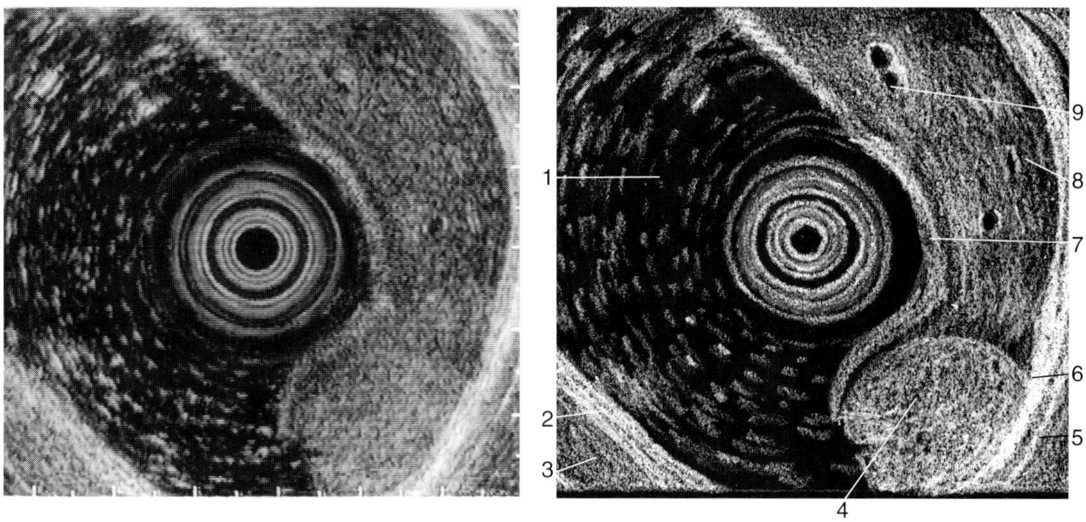

1. Gastric lumen 2. Gastric wall 3. Spleen
4. Hemangioma 5. Abdominal wall 6. Diaphragm
7. Gastric wall 8. Liver 9. Vessels

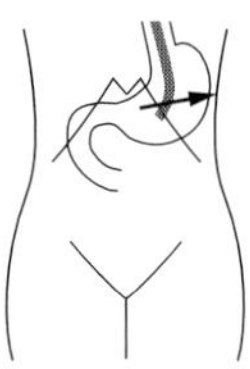

Figure 9-5. Extragastric compression by a hepatic hemangioma.
Extragastric compression of the cardia was found during routine endoscopic examination and was reexamined by endoscopic ultrasound. The normal mucosa was found to cover the weakly echogenic tumor, which showed a direct connection to the left lobe of the liver. The finding was confirmed by angiographic examination, revealing a small cavernous hemangioma at the lateral end of the left lobe of the liver.

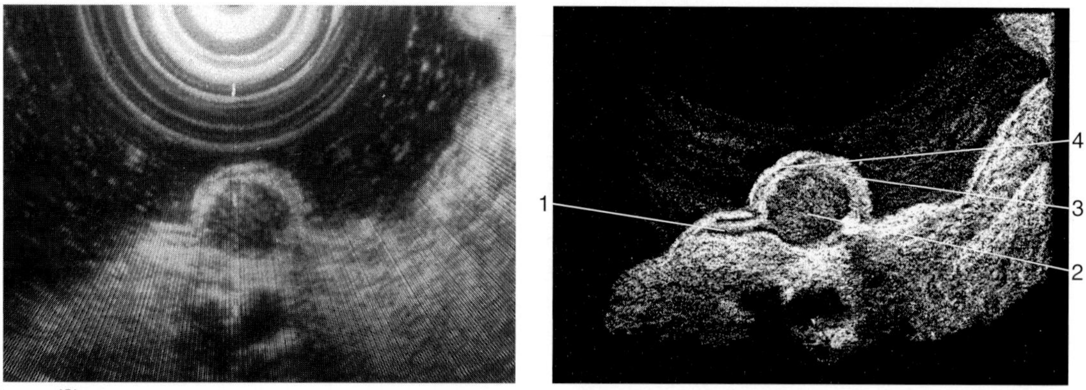

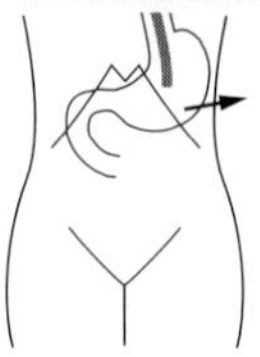

1. Muscularis propria (pm) 2. Leiomyoma
3. Submucosa (sm) 4. Mucosa (m)

Figure 9-6. A small submucosal tumor of the stomach.
A patient with a round, small elevation of the greater curvature of the stomach was examined by endoscopic ultrasound. An echo-poor, round tumor covered by intact mucosal and submucosal layers was demonstrated. A small leiomyoma of the stomach was suspected; the diagnosis was confirmed 2 years later, when the mass showed minimal enlargement, surgical resection was perfomed and the diagnosis was confirmed.

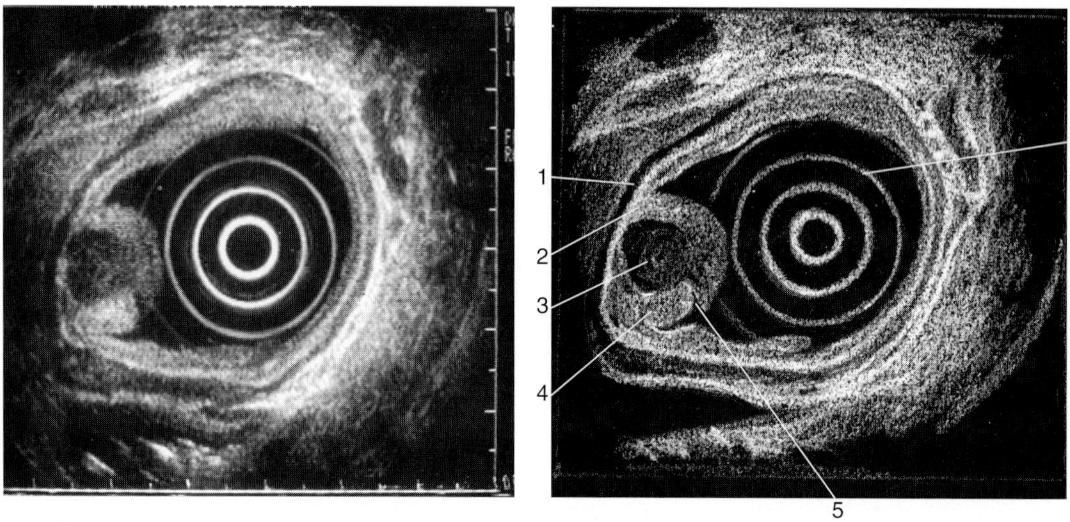

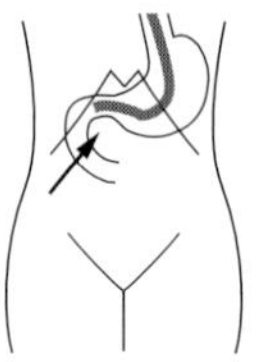

1. Muscularis propria (pm) 2. Muscularis mucosae (mm) 3. Submucosal tumor 4. Mucosa (m)
5. Small ulcer 6. Gastric lumen

Figure 9-7. A small submucosal tumor of the stomach.
On routine endoscopy, this tumor had appearances identical to findings to those of lesion in Figure 9-6. Endoscopic ultrasound showed a clearly defined, small, echo-poor mass originating from the muscularis mucosae (mm). The histological diagnosis was benign leiomyoma originating in the muscularis mucosae.

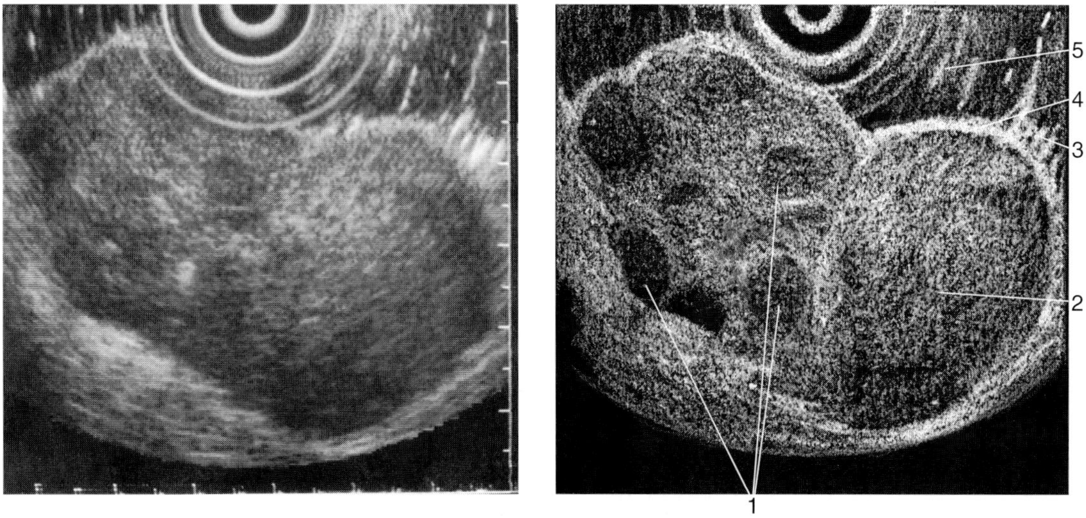

1. Tumor nodules 2. Leiomyoma 3. Mucus
4. Mucosa (m) 5. Gastric lumen

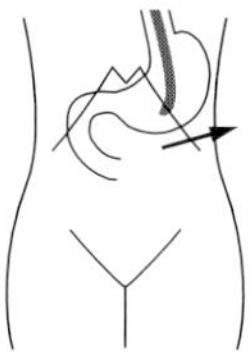

Figure 9-8. A large submucosal tumor of the stomach.
An oval-shaped, circumscribed tumor with a slightly irregular contour was found on the greater curvature of the stomach. The tumor was large, measuring 6.0 × 4.5 cm, and showed a heterogenous echo texture with a few nodules. Because of its size and irregularity, both in its contours and internal echo distribution, the possibility of malignant tumor was suspected. The tumor proved to be leiomyosarcoma of the stomach.

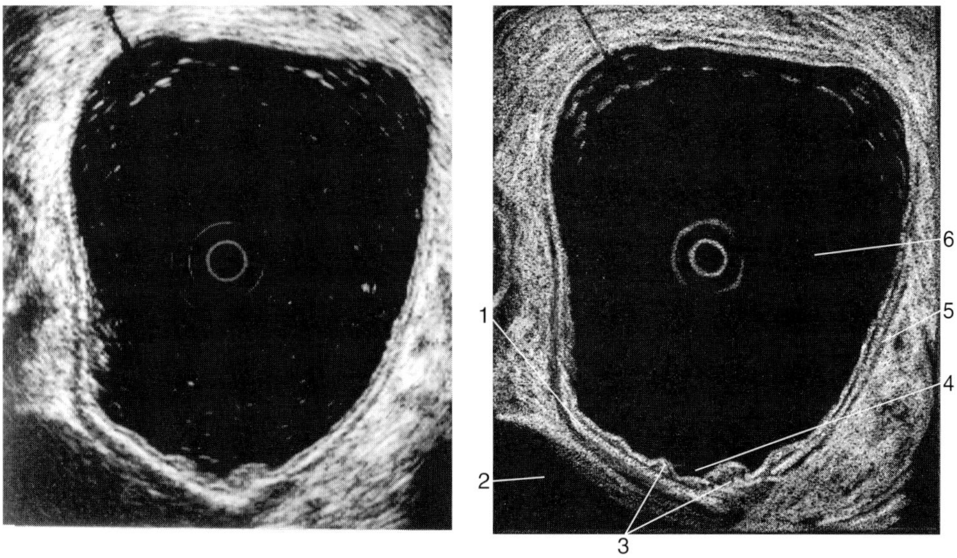

1. Gastric angulus 2. Antrum of stomach
3. Mucosal carcinoma with slight elevation
4. Ulceration 5. Normal mucosa 6. Gastric lumen

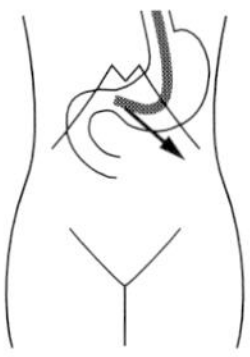

Figure 9-9. Mucosal carcinoma of the stomach.
In the early stage, the changes in the mucosa of gastric carcinoma involved are subtle, consisting of slight elevation of the mucosa or shallow ulceration surrounded by a thin, rim-like structure as seen in this example. Endoscopy with biopsy of the lesion generally establishes the diagnosis; however, the extent of tumor invasion can be accurately assessed only by endoscopic ultrasound.

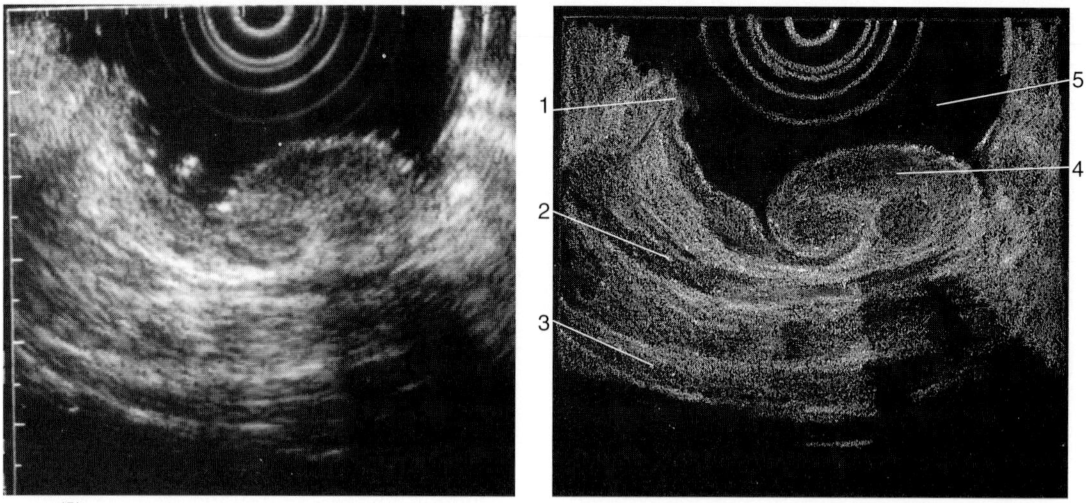

1. Gastric mucosa 2. Body of pancreas 3. Splenic vein 4. Polypoid tumor 5. Gastric lumen

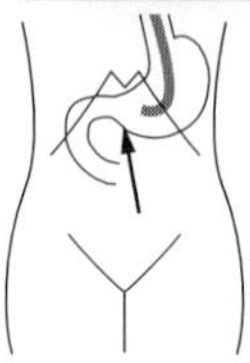

Figure 9-10. Carcinoma of the stomach.
This sonogram demonstrates an early gastric carcinoma of the polypoid type. It is diffusely echo-poor and extends to the echogenic submucosal layer of the stomach. No regional lymph node involvement was found. Histological study confirmed the ultrasonographic findings.

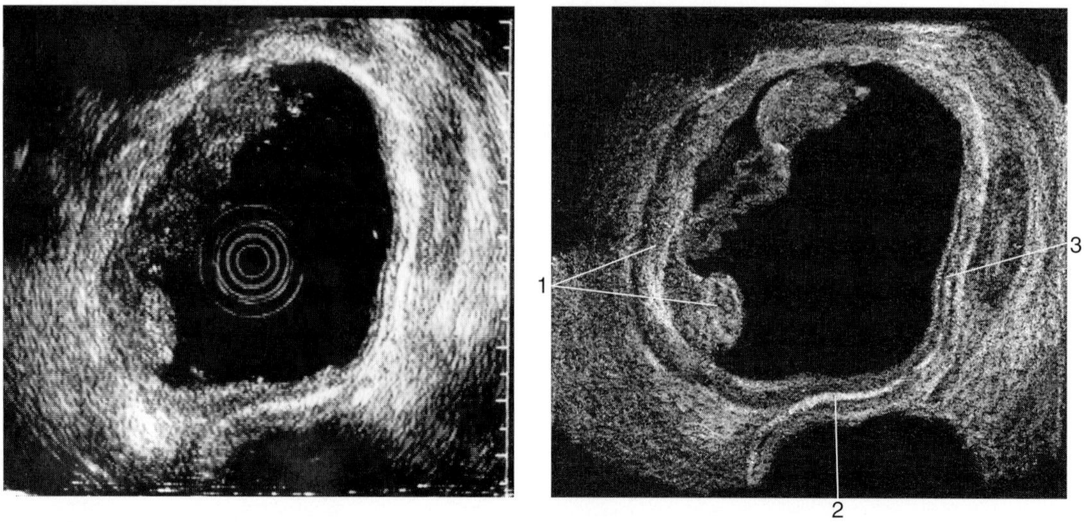

1. Gastric carcinoma 2. Gastric angulus 3. Normal mucosa

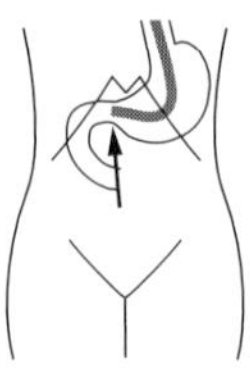

Figure 9-11. Carcinoma of the stomach.
This sonogram was obtained from a patient with an advanced gastric carcinoma on the posterior wall of the gastric antrum. Approximately two-fifths of the gastric mucosa in this cross-section appeared to be intact; in the remainder the normal architecture is completely lost. In addition, there is massive exophytic tumor protruding into the gastric lumen.

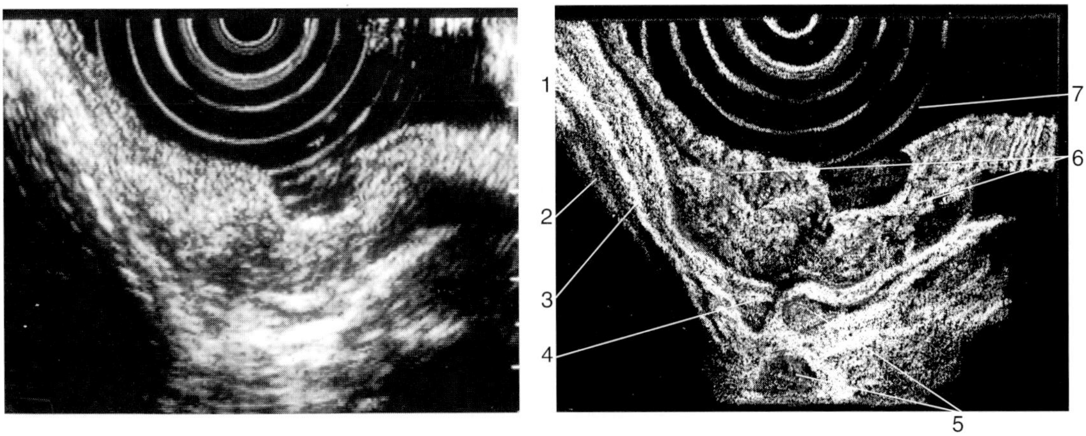

1. Submucosa 2. Serosa 3. Muscularis propria 4. Tumor protruding beyond serosa 5. Lymph nodes 6. Tumor 7. Gastric lumen

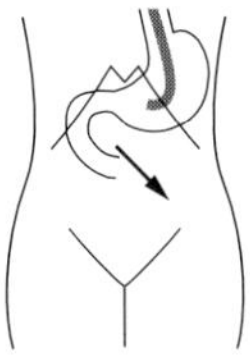

Figure 9-12. Advanced gastric carcinoma.
A massive tumor at the posterior portion of the angulus is imaged by intragastric scanning. A weakly echogenic tumor with a centrally located ulcer crater invaded the gastric wall, penetrating to the serosal layer of the stomach. A small protrusion of the mass to the adventitia is visualized, together with enlarged metastatic lymph nodes, close to the primary carcinoma.

a

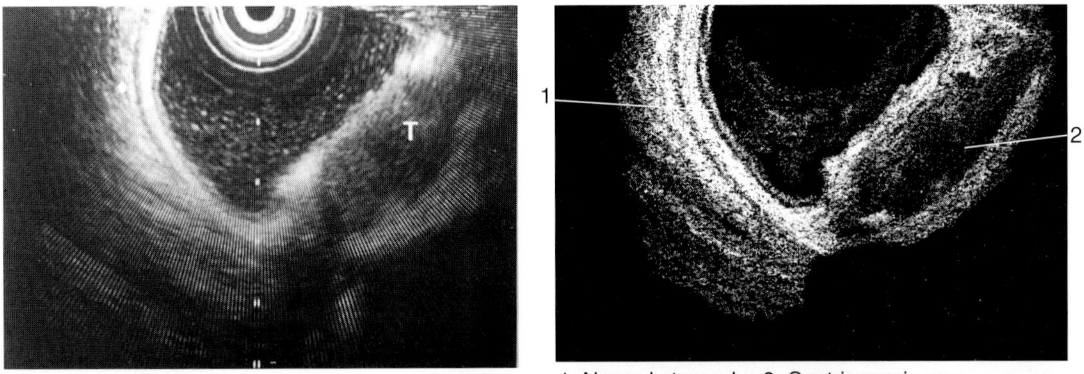

1. Normal stomach 2. Gastric carcinoma

b

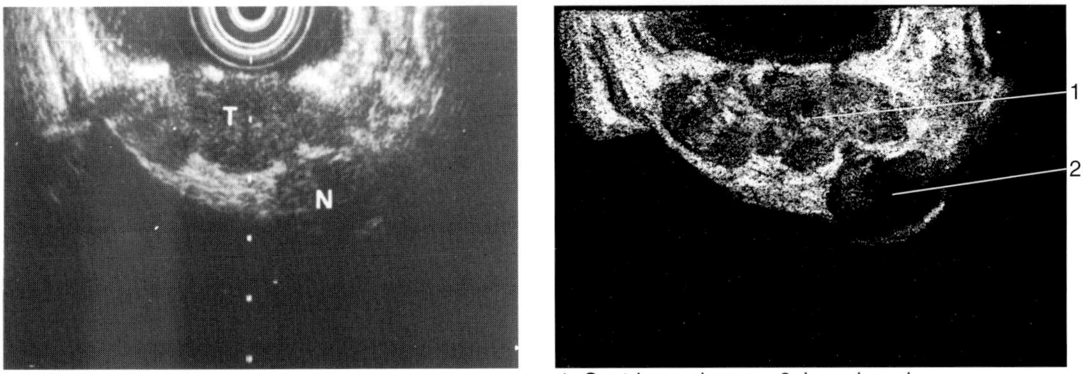

1. Gastric carcinoma 2. Lymph node

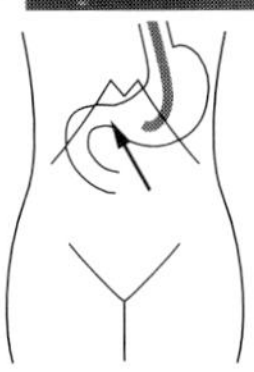

Figure 9-13. Advanced gastric carcinoma.
Endoscopic ultrasound clearly demonstrated the size of this primary tumor (T) at the lesser curvature and the extent of the lymph node involvement (N). Extensive dissemination of the tumor beyond the level of the cardia excluded the possibility of surgery. The tumor was treated with anticancer chemotherapy, though with little success.

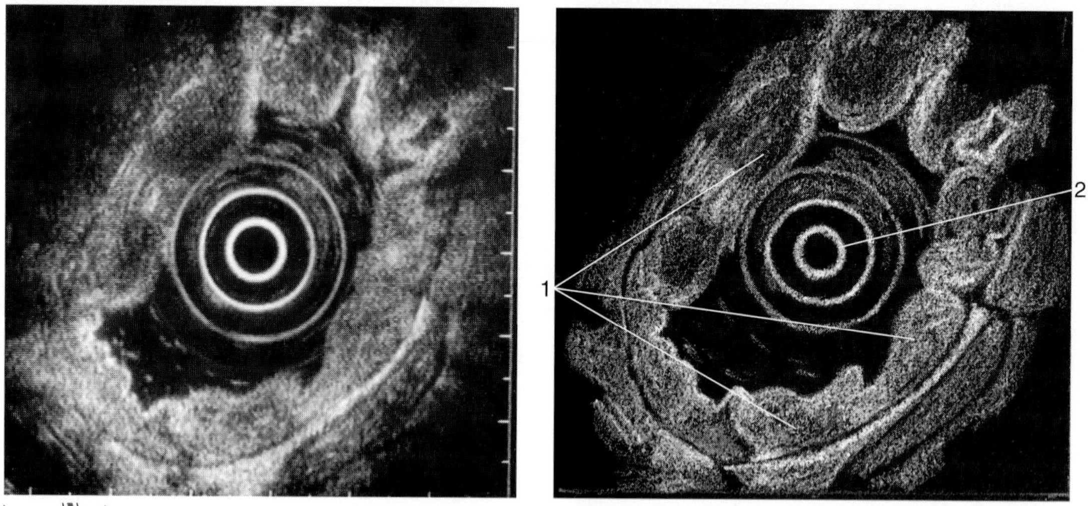

1. Carcinoma (scirrhous type) 2. Gastric lumen

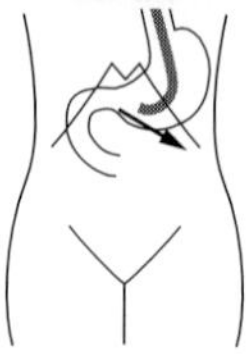

Figure 9-14. Advanced gastric carcinoma , scirrhous type.
This patient suffered from indigestion and general malaise. An endoscopic study disclosed the typical findings of scirrhous carcinoma of the stomach. Thickening of the wall and changes in the internal echo texture, including complete loss of normal layering structure are shown.

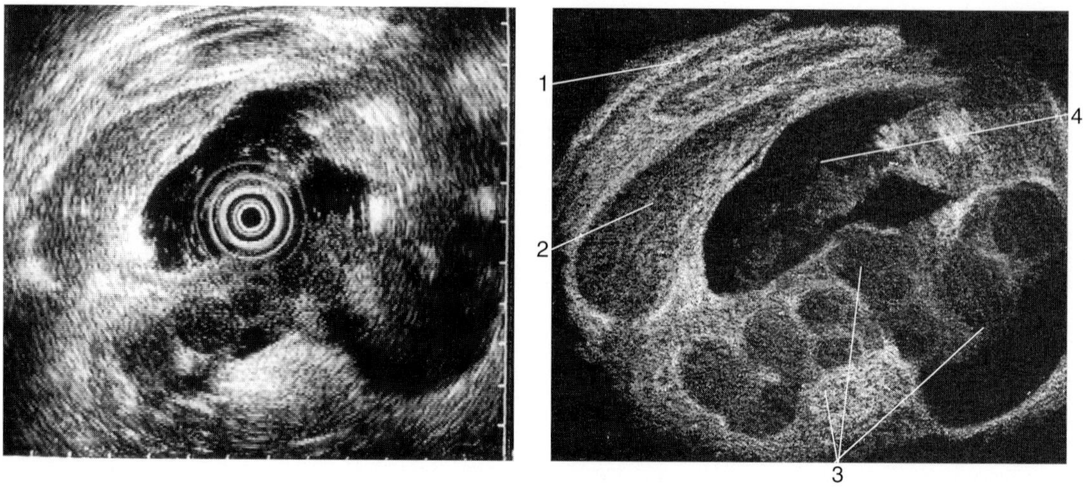

1. Abdominal wall 2. Liver 3. Gastric malignant lymphoma 4. Deformed gastric lumen

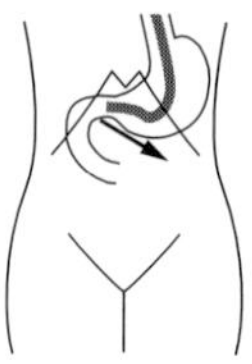

Figure 9-15. Lymphoma of the stomach.
Massive infiltration of the gastric mucosa by lymphomatous tissue is often difficult to differentiate from that of gastric carcinoma. In this patient, the tumor tissue was uniformly echo-poor, a characteristic of sarcomas. Sonoendoscopy clearly demonstrated its size and the extent of lymph node involvement.

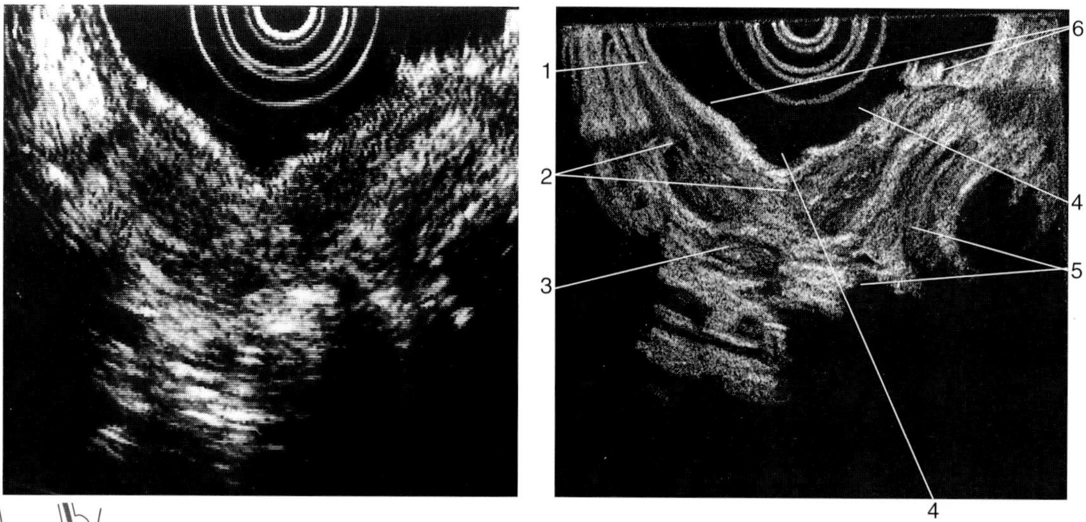

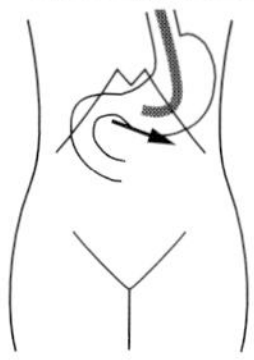

1. Normal gastric wall 2. Granulation tissue (symmetric tapering) 3. Lymph node 4. Ulcer crater 5. Adhesion of surrounding tissue 6. Mucus

Figure 9-16. Gastric ulcer.
This sonogram shows the typical pattern of a chronic gastric ulcer at the gastric angulus. A symmetrically tapering echo-poor lesion corresponds to the granulation tissue surrounding the ulcer crater. The diagnosis is usually straightforward on endoscopy with biopsy. The size of ulcer and the changes during healing are best depicted by endoscopic ultrasound.

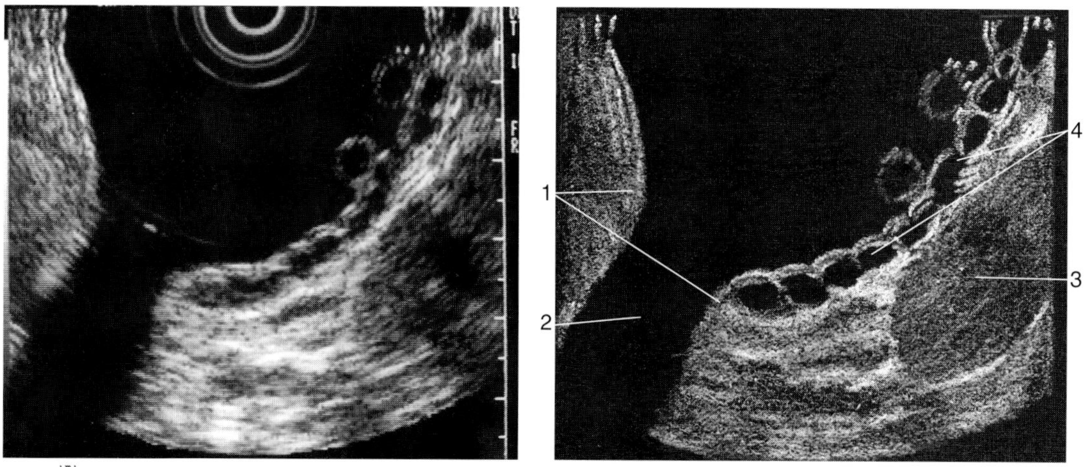

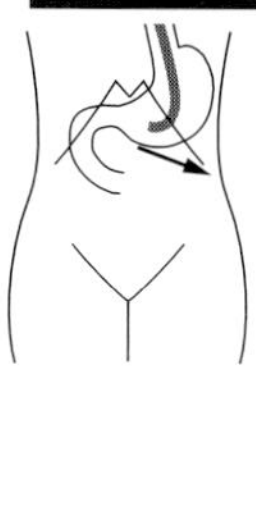

1. Gastric angulus 2. Antrum of stomach 3. Varices 4. Pancreas

Figure 9-17. Gastric varices.
A 39-year-old female was referred for endoscopic ultrasound because of irregularity of the gastric mucosa on routine endoscopy. Since the patient had no history of previous liver disease, and negative x-ray findings suggestive of esophageal varices, sonoendoscopic study was performed. In clear contrast to the normal gastric mucosa, numerous echo-free, dilated gastric varices were found. In the absence of esophageal varices, these gastric varices were unexpected. The patient underwent surgery, with a favorable outcome. The varices were confined mainly to the greater curvature of the stomach, and moderate splenomegaly was found.

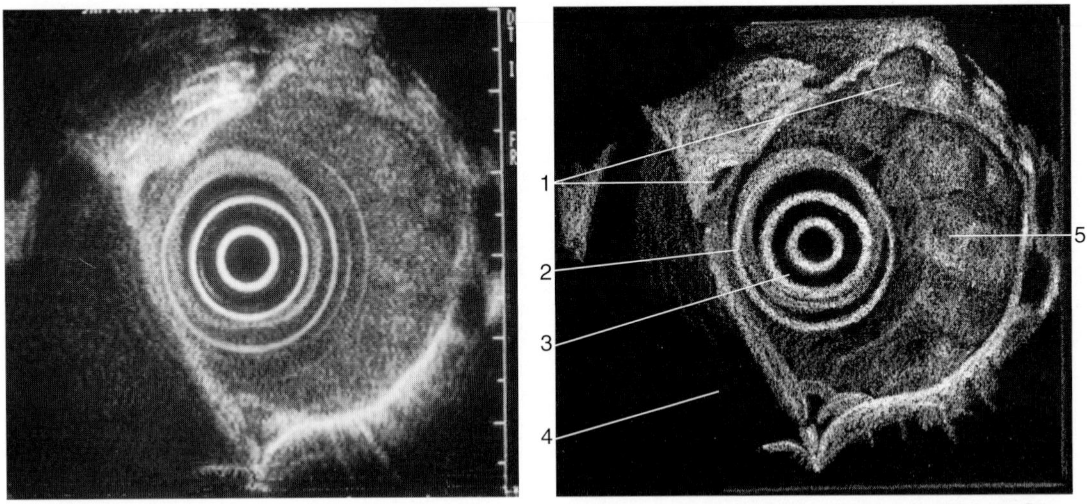

1. Lymph node metastasis 2. Inflated balloon 3. Scan head 4. Right auricle of heart 5. Esophageal cancer

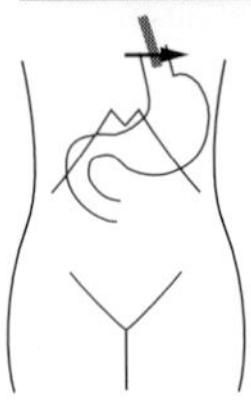

Figure 9-18. Esophageal cancer.
Examination of the esophagus is better with the balloon method because of its limited distensibility on fluid infusion. Though scanned without balloon, the resolution on this image was satisfactory. It showed diffuse thickening of the esophageal wall, forming localized nodular mass. Lymph node metastases are evident around the mass.

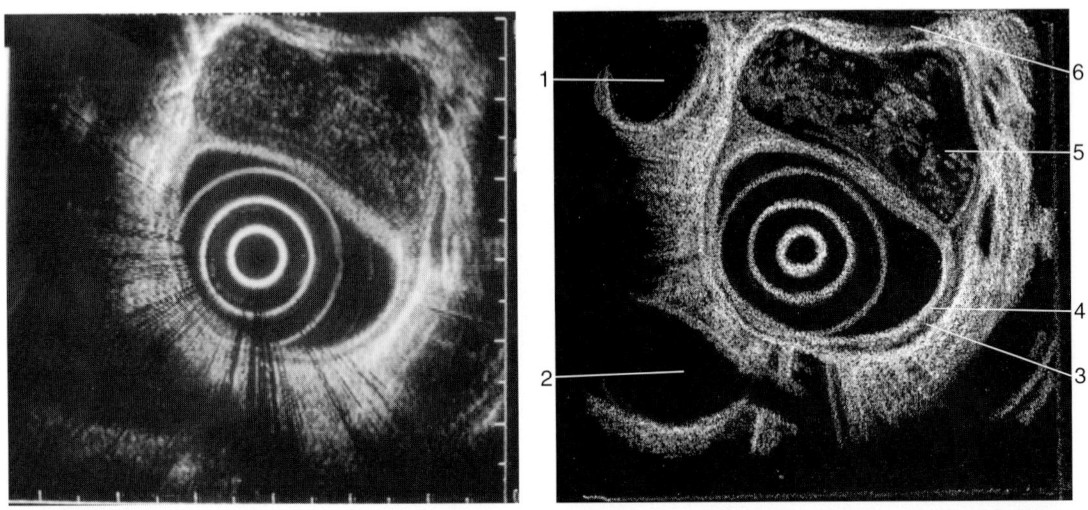

1. Aorta 2. Pulmonary artery 3. Esophageal mucosae 4. Balloon 5. Leiomyoma 6. Vertebra

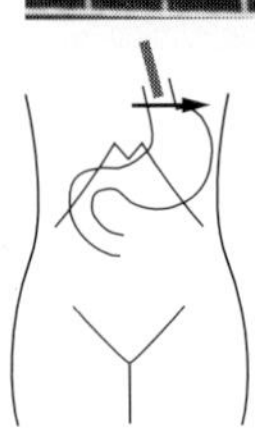

Figure 9-19. Submucosal tumor of the esophagus.
Benign leoimyoma in the esophagus has an echo texture to that of other organs. This scan was obtained from the lower esophagus of a patient suffering from dysphagia of relatively long duration. The clear boundaries and the absence of any signs of invasive support the diagnosis of leiomyoma of the esophagus.

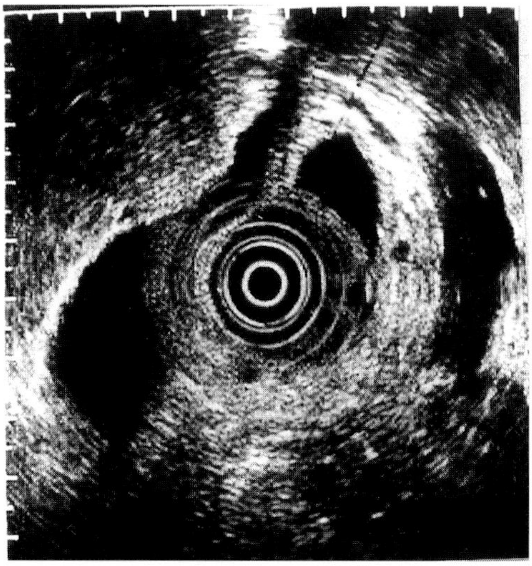

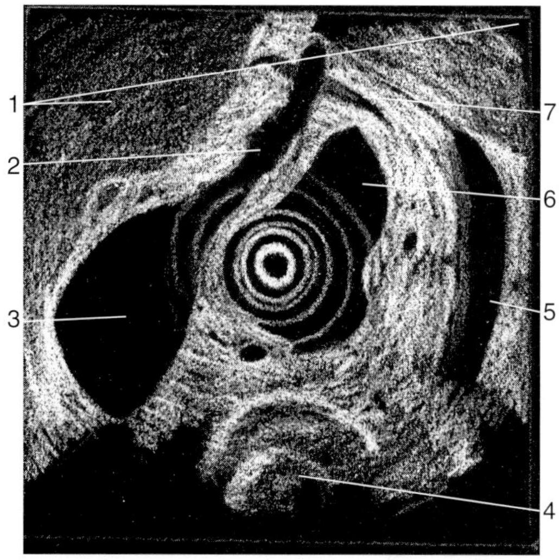

1. Liver 2. Neck of gallbladder 3. Fundus of gallbladder 4. Colon 5. Superior mesenteric vein 6. Duodenum 7. Common hepatic duct

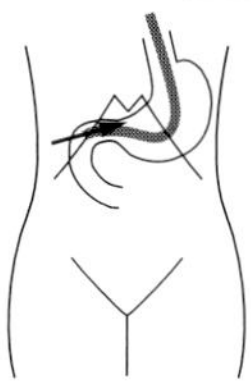

Figure 9-20. Normal gallbladder.
A normal gallbladder is imaged by placing the scan head in the duodenal bulb. A pear-shaped, configuration is typical and identifies the organ without difficulty. On the right-hand side, a thick, anechoic, tubular structure, the superior mesenteric vein, is imaged. The normally distended gallbladder wall usually appears as a single echogenic layer on scanning with a 7.5-MHz transducer. It is usually difficult to identify the junction of cystic duct with the common hepatic duct by routine extracorporeal sonography, it is also possible to identify the common hepatic duct by tracing the cystic duct during EUS examination by scanning to its point of fusion with common duct.

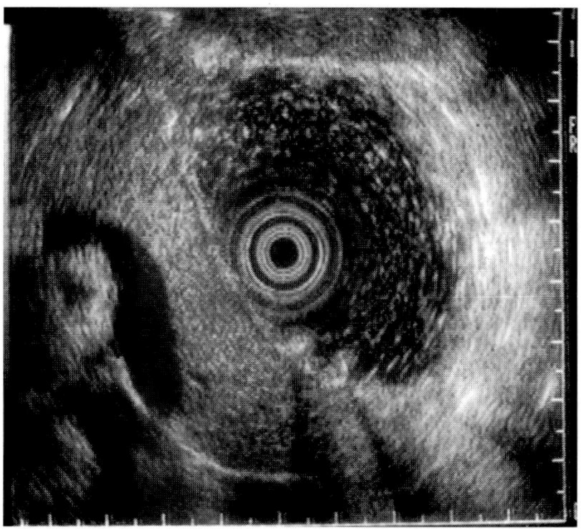

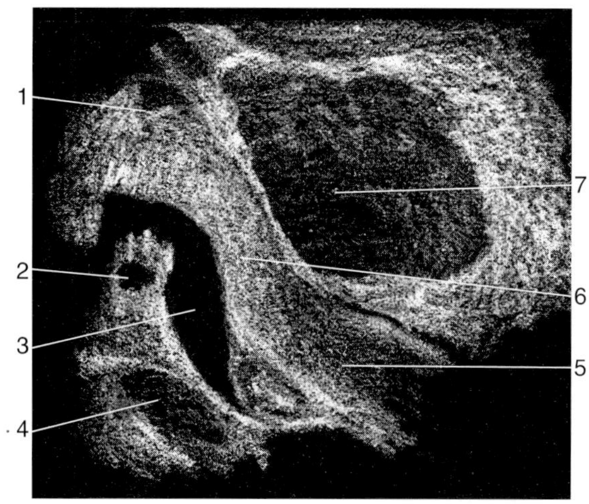

1. Gastroduodenal artery 2. Superior mesenteric artery 3. Splenic vein 4. Left kidney 5. Tail of pancreas 6. Body of pancreas 7. Gastric lumen

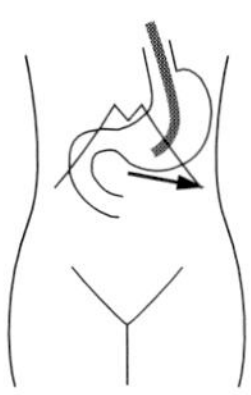

Figure 9-21. Normal pancreas.
Imaging of the normal pancreas can be performed either by transgastric or transduodenal scanning because of absence of intervening intestinal gas and the characteristic sonographic appearance of the organ. Directly below the gastric wall, pancreatic parenchyma is visualized and identified by its characteristic texture of evenly distributed fine echogenic foci. The vascular landmarks are well demonstrated without difficulty. During respiratory movement of the organ, the main pancreatic duct can be demonstrated running the central portion of the organ.

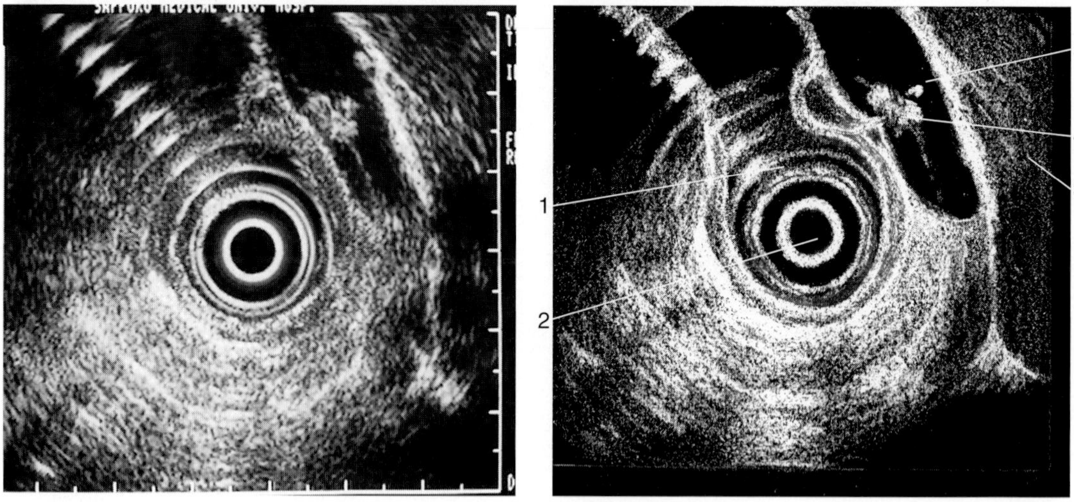

1. Duodenal lumen 2. Scan head 3. Liver 4. Polyp 5. Gallbladder

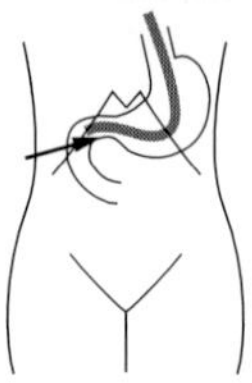

Figure 9-22. Cholesterol polyp of the gallbladder.
A small, papillomatous, echogenic polyp with a thin stalk is demonstrated on the posterior wall of the gallbladder. Absence of any echo-poor portion and the general granular texture clearly indicated its benign nature.

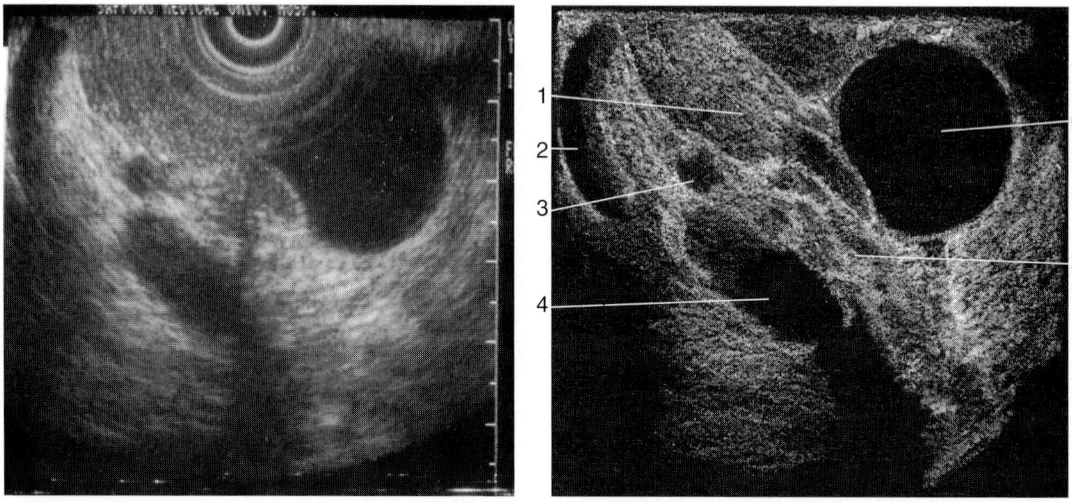

1. Pancreas 2. Portal vein 3. Superior mesenteric artery 4. Aorta 5. Tail of pancreas 6. Pseudocyst

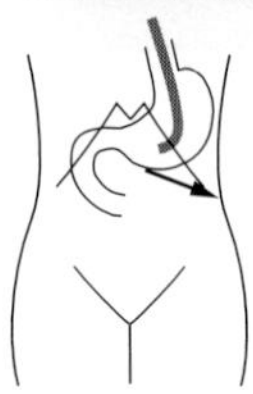

Figure 9-23. Pancreatic pseudocyst, tail.
A round, cystic mass is visualized in the tail of the pancreas. The cyst is approximately 4 cm in diameter, the wall is smooth, with no solid lesions. This pseudocyst was missed on routine ultrasound examination because of air in the intestine.

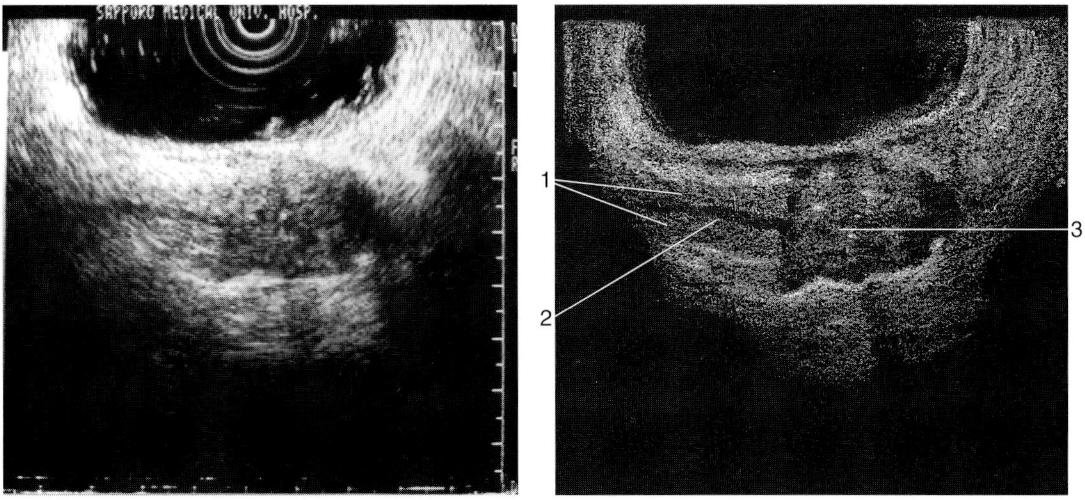

1. Body of pancreas 2. Pancreatic duct 3. Cancer of tail of pancreas

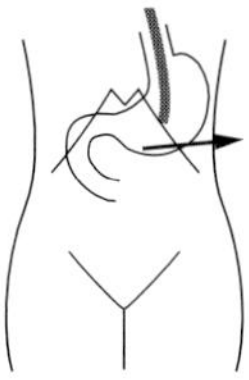

Figure 9-24. Carcinoma in the tail of the pancreas.
A mass found in the tail of the pancreas showed the typical sonographic pattern of pancreatic cancer: an echo-poor mass with irregular contours. The main pancreatic duct penetrates the tumor mass, suggesting the diagnosis of duct cell carcinoma, which was confirmed by surgery.

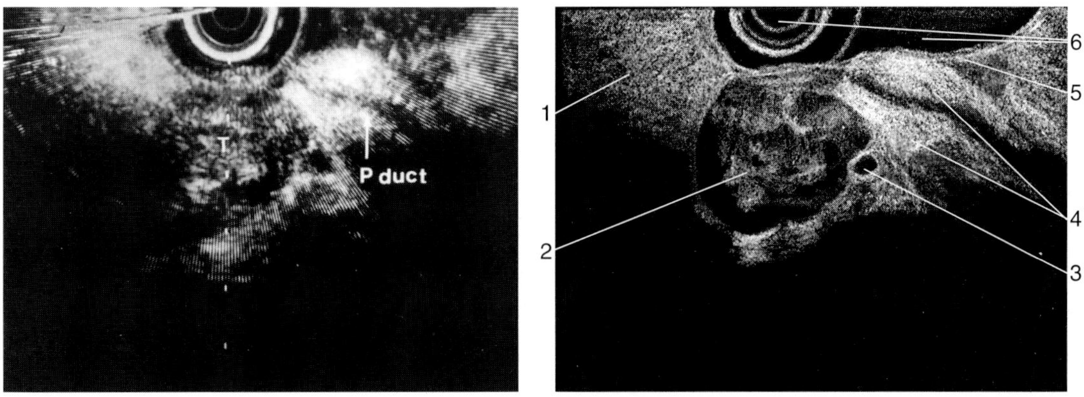

1. Gas echoes 2. Tumor 3. Superior mesenteric artery 4. Tail of pancreas 5. Gastric mucosa 6. Gastric lumen

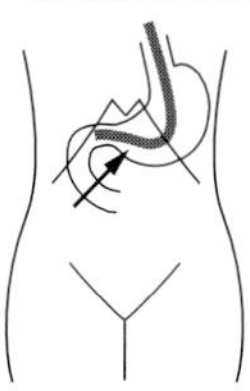

Figure 9-25. Carcinoma of the head of the pancreas.
A characteristic echo-poor mass with irregular boundaries adjacent to the descending duodenum is clearly imaged by endoscopic ultrasound of the pancreas via the gastric wall. The tumor compresses the adjacent normal pancreas and the portal vein.

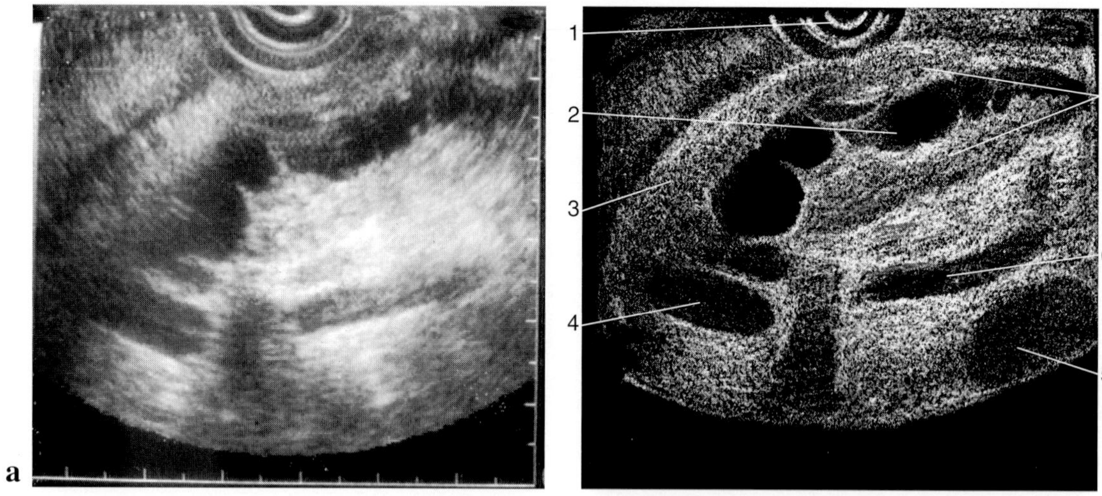

1. Stomach wall 2. Dilated main pancreatic duct 3. Head of pancreas 4. Inferior vena cava 5. Aorta 6. Left renal vein 7. Body of pancreas

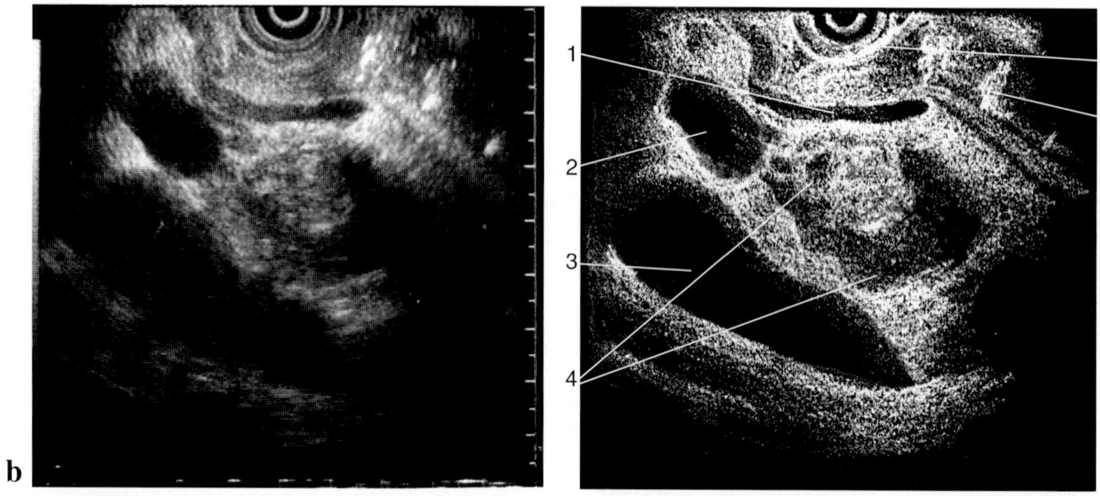

1. Pancreaticoduodenal artery 2. Dilated common bile duct 3. Inferior vena cava 4. Cancer of head of pancreas 5. Duodenojejunal junction 6. Gastric wall

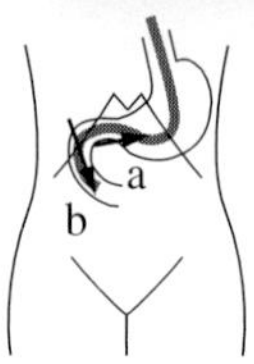

Figure 9-26. Pancreatic carcinoma.
A small carcinoma of the head of the pancreas is visualized by endoscopic ultrasound. Besides a hypoechoic, rounded tumor mass in the vicinity of the head of the pancreas, there is a marked dilatation of the common bile duct and the main pancreatic duct. This is the "double duct sign", a hallmark of the pancreatic head cancer.

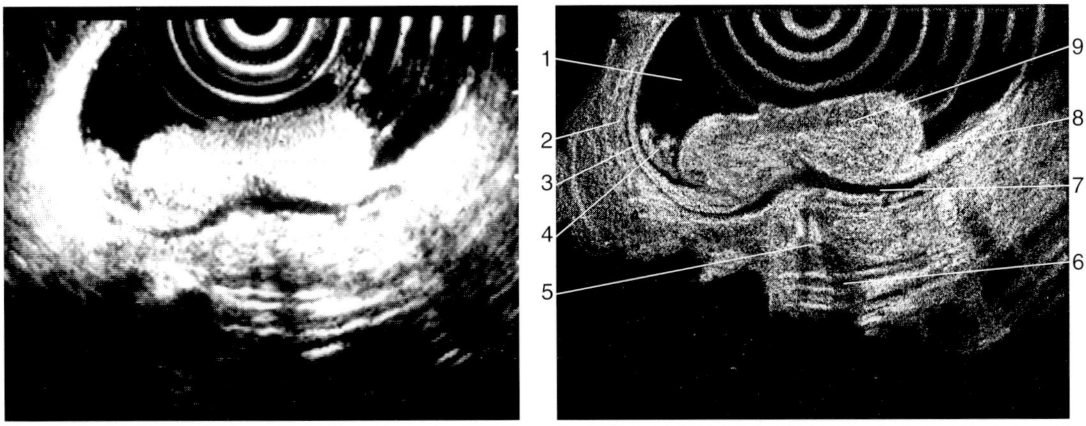

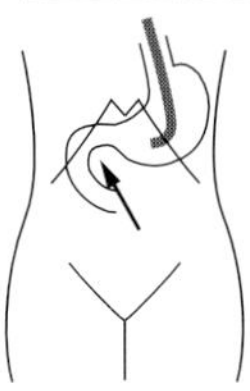

1. Rectal lumen 2. Submucosa 3. Rectal wall (mucosa) 4. Feces 5. Fatty tissue 6. Sacrum 7. pm layer 8. Submucosal layer 9.Tumor

Figure 9-27. Carcinoma of the rectum with invasion to the submucosa.
Endoscopic ultrasound of the rectum gives a clear cross-sectional image of the normal rectal mucosa, as well as of various neoplastic changes including polypoid lesions. This figure shows a sonogram of rectal carcinoma limited to the submucosal layer of the rectum, T1 stage. The tumor itself is relatively flat, and invasion confined to the submucosa. Surgery confirmed the endosonographic findings.

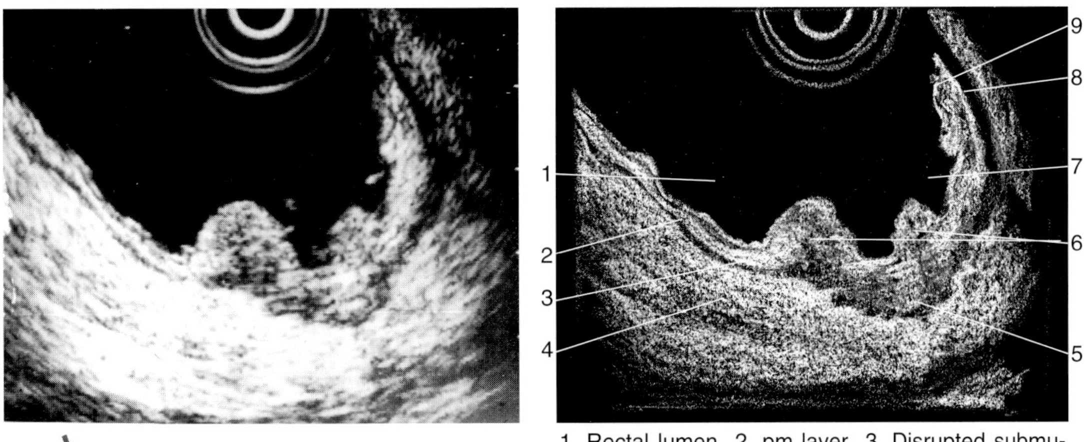

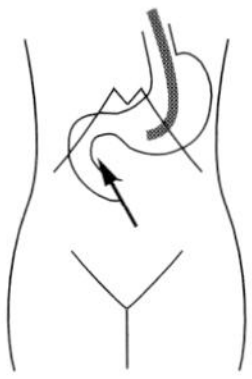

1. Rectal lumen 2. pm layer 3. Disrupted submucosal layer 4. Fat tissue 5. Tumor infiltration penetrating serosa 6. Tumor 7. Ulcers 8. Proper muscle (pm) layer 9. Tumor edge

Figure 9-28. Advanced carcinoma of the rectum.
This scan shows a typical ulcerating rectal carcinoma invading the serosal layer of the rectum. The echo-poor tumor tissue disrupted the pm layer and infiltrated part of the thin serosal layer surrounding the rectum. Lymph node involvement was absent. On histological examination a well-differentiated adenocarcinoma was found to invade the serosal layer of the rectum, supporting the ultrasonic findings.

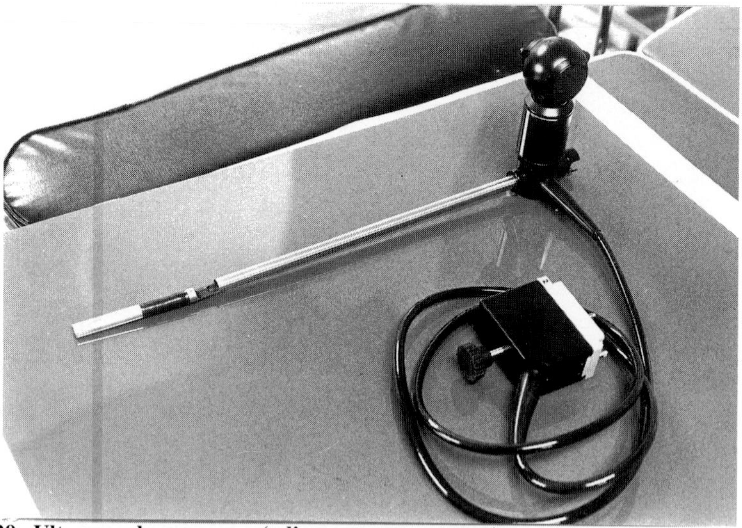

Figure 9-29. Ultrasono laparoscope (a linear-array scanner).
A linear array probe placed at the tip of a laparoscope can be bent 90° to either side. During peritoneoscopy, the sterilized scope is inserted into the inflated peritoneal cavity and an ultrasonic survey is made by gently contacting the probe to the surface of the organ to be explored.

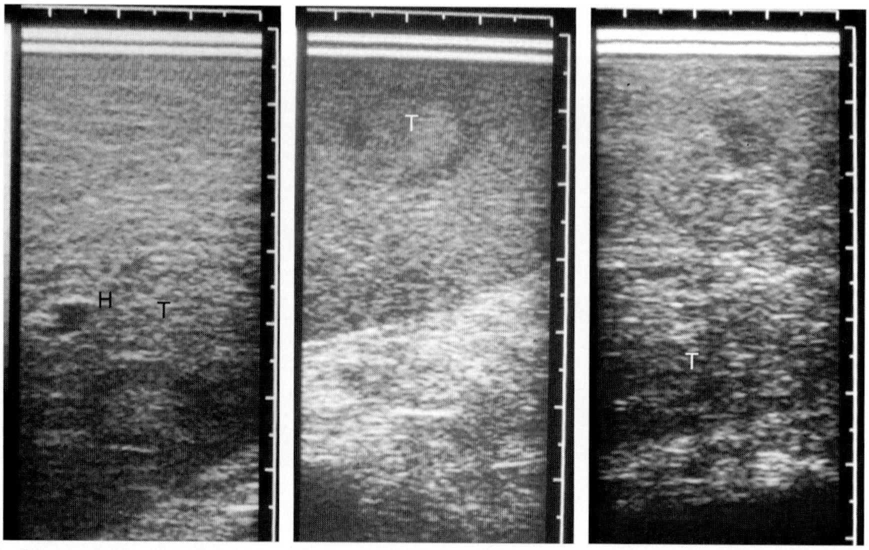

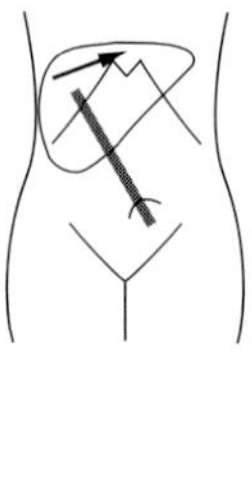

Figure 9-30. Small hepatocellular carcinoma (linear-array laparoscopic scanner).
Three cases of small hepatocellular carcinoma, each with a single tumor nodule in the liver, are shown. The echo-poor halo surrounding the tumor is rather indistinct but is a constant finding. Though these small tumors already show irregularity in contour, the echogenicities of these tumors appear to be seemingly different, reflecting rapid attenuation of 7.5-MHz ultrasound beam through the overlying liver tissues. H: halo, T: HCC.

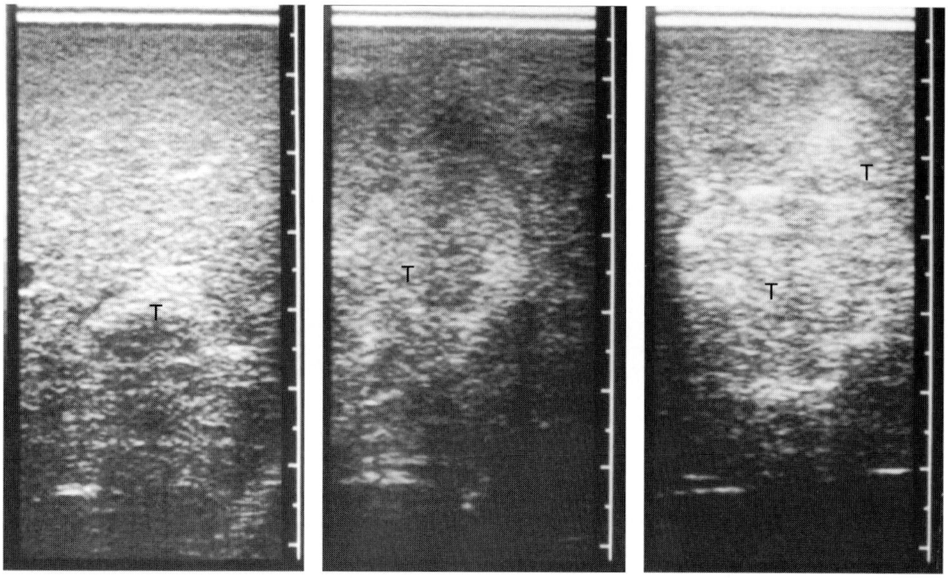

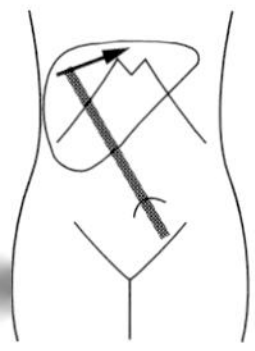

Figure 9-31. Large hepatoma nodules examined by sonolaparoscopy.
Three cases of hepatocellular carcinoma with larger tumor nodules are shown. Unlike a small nodule, which is uniformly echo-poor, these carcinomas show quite variable appearance, ranging from a mixed to a largely echo-poor pattern. Here the small size of the linear array preclude visualization of the entire mass. However, penetration is generally adequate compared to that of smaller tumors, demonstrating the reduced attenuation in larger tumors.

a

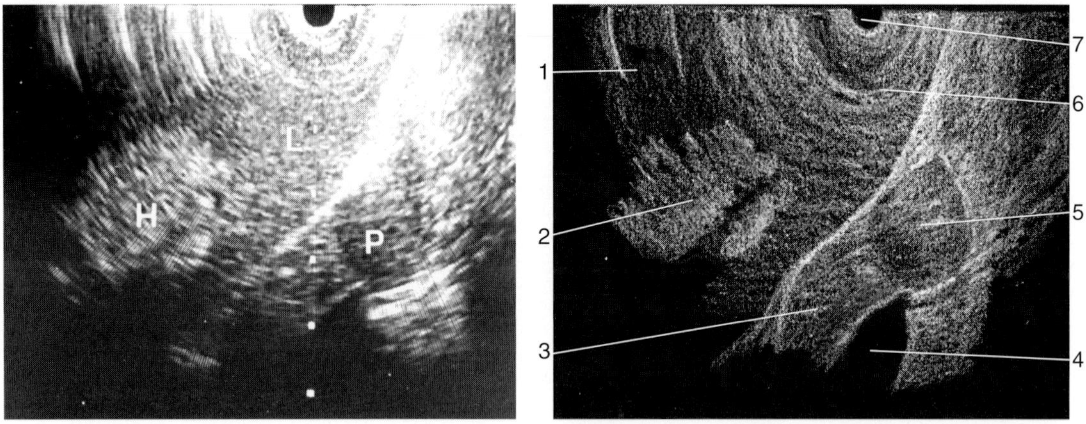

1. Reverberation artifact 2. Echogenic cavernous hemangioma 3. Head of pancreas 4. Splenic vein 5. Body of pancreas 6. Left lobe of liver 7. Scan head

b

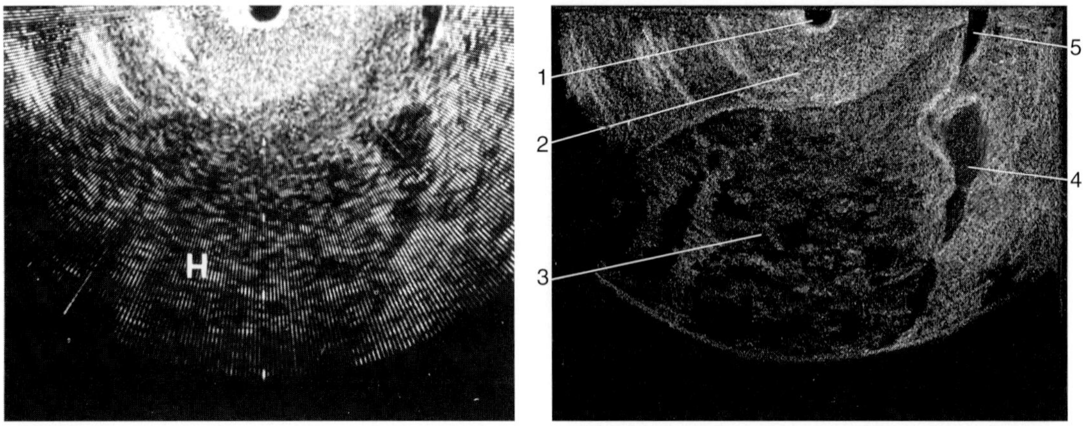

1. Scan head 2. Intact hepatic parenchyma 3. Hypoechoic cavernous hemangioma 4. Umbilical portion of left portal vein 5. Small branch of portal vein

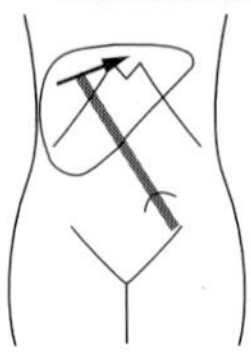

Figure 9-32. Hemangioma of the liver.
Hepatic hemangiomas often exhibit a characteristic appearance on laparoscopic ultrasound. The boundaries are somewhat indistinct and often irregular, there is no halo and the internal echo intensity varies according to the thickness of the wall and the width of the blood vessels in the cavernous hemangioma. The thicker the wall, the more echogenic the tumor, and thinner the wall and wider the sinusoidal space the more hypoechoic in its appearance. Two images of echogenic (a) and echo-poor hemangiomas (b) show the critical features. These images were obtained with a mechanically driven laparoscopic ultrasound transducer operating at 10 MHz.

REFERENCES

1. Aibe T, Fujii T, Okita K, et al: A fundamental study of normal layer structure of the gastrointestinal wall visualized by endoscopic ultrasonography. Scand J Gastroenterol 21(Suppl 123) : 6-15, 1986.
2. Bolondi L, Caletti G, Casanova P, et al: Problems and variations in the interpretation of the ultrasound feature of the normal upper and lower GI tract wall. Scand J Gastroenterol 21(Suppl 123) :16-26, 1986.
3. Caletti G, Bolondi L, Labo G: Ultrasonic endoscopoy. The gastrointestinal wall. Scand J Gastroenterol 19(Suppl 102) : 5-8, 1984.
4. Caletti G, Bolondi L, Zani L, et al: Detection of portal hypertension and esophageal varices by means of endoscopic ultrasonography. Scand J Gastroenterol 21(Suppl 123) : 74-77, 1986.
5. Classen M, Strohm WD, Kurtz WG: Pancreatic pseudocysts and tumors in endosonography. Scand J Gastroenterol 19(Suppl 94) : 77-84, 1984.
6. Dancygier H, Classen M: Endosonographic diagnosis of benign pancreatic and biliary lesions. Scand J Gastroenterol 21(Suppl 123) : 119-122, 1986.
7. DiMagno EP, Buxtoin JL, Regan PT, et al: Ultrasonic endoscopy. Lancet 1 : 629-631, 1980.
8. DiMagno EP, Regan PT, Clain JE, et al: Human endoscopic ultrasonography. Gastroenterology 83 : 824-829, 1982.
9. Fukuda M, Hirata K, Saito K, et al: On the diagnostic use of echoendoscope in abdominal disease. I. Diagnostic experience with a new type of echoendoscope on gastric diseases. Proc Jpn J Med Ultrason 37 : 409-410, 1980.
10. Fukuda M, Ohmi N, Terada S, et al: On the diagnostic use of echoendoscope in abdominal disease. II. Diagnostic experience with a new model of echoendoscope. Proc Jpn J Ultrason 39 : 405-406, 1981.
11. Fukuda M, Nakano Y, Saito K, et al.: Endoscopic ultrasonography in the diagnosis of pancreatic carcinoma. The use of a liquid-filled stomach method. Scand J Gastroenterol 19(Suppl 94) : 65-76, 1984.
12. Fukuda M: Use of the echoendoscope and echolaparoscope in the diagnosis of intraabdominal cancer. Intraluminal scanning, in Kossoff G, Fukuda M (eds), Ultrasonic Differential Diagnosis of Tumors. New York, Igaku-Shoin, 1984, pp186-199.
13. Fukuda M, Mima S, Tanabe T, et al: Endoscopic sonography of the liver. Diagnostic application of the echolaparoscope to localize intrahepatic lesions. Scand J Gastroenterol 21(Suppl 102) : 24-38, 1986.
14. Fukuda M: Endoscopic ultrasonography, in Gill RW, Dadd MJ (eds), Proceedings of the 4th Meeting of WFUMB, Sydney, Pergamon Press, 1985, pp13-16.
15. Fukuda M: Endoscopic sonography: Use of the echoendoscope and echolaparoscope in the diagnosis of intra-abdominal disorders, in Sanders RC, Hill M (eds), Ultrasound Annual 1986, New York, Raven Press, 1986, pp141-170.
16. Hayashi Y, Nakazawa S, Kimoto E, et al: Clinicopathologic analysis of endoscopic ultrasonograms in pancreatic mass lesions. Endoscopy 21 : 121-125, 1989.
17. Hisanaga K, Hisanaga A, Hibi N, et al: High speed rotation scanner for trans-esophageal cross-sectional echocardiography. Am J Cardiol 46 : 837-842, 1980.
18. Holm HH, Northved A: Transurethral ultrasonic scanner. J Urol 111 : 238-241, 1971.
19. Kimmey MB, Silverstein FE, Martin RW: Ultrasound interaction with the intestinal wall: Esophagus, stomach and colon, in Kawai K (ed), Endoscopic Ultrasonography in Gastroenterology. Tokyo, Igaku-Shoin, 1988, pp35-43.
20. Kimmey MB, Silverstein FE, Haggitt RC, et al: Cross-sectional imaging method: A system to compare ultrasound, computed tomography, and magnetic resonance with histologic findings. Invest Radiol 22 : 227-231, 1987.
21. Kimmey MB, Haggitt RC: Histologic correlates of gastrointestinal wall. Gastroenterology 96 : 433-441, 1989.
22. Lees WR: Endoscopic ultrasonography of chronic pancreatitis and pancreatic pseudocysts. Scand J Gastroenterol 21(Suppl 123) : 123-129, 1986.
23. Machi J, Takeda J, Sigel B, et al: Normal stomach wall and gastric cancer: Evaluation with high-resolution operative US. Radiology 159 : 85-87, 1986.
24. Rifkin MD, McGlynn ET, Marks G: Endorectal sonographic prospective staging of rectal cancer. Scand J Gastroenterol 21(Suppl 123) : 99-103, 1986.
25. Rifkin MD, Gordon SJ: Sonoendoscopic evaluation of extraesophageal and extragastric abnormalities: A review. Scand J Gastroenterol 21(Suppl 123) : 68-73, 1986.
26. Silverstein F, Kimmey M, Martin R, et al: Ultrasound and the intestinal wall: Experimental methods. Scand J Gastroenterol 21(Suppl 123) : 34-40, 1986.

27. Spiessl B, Beahrs OH, Hermanek P, et al (eds): UICC-TNM Atlas, 3rd Edition, 1989, pp 71-81.
28. Strohm WD, Phillip J, Hagenmueller F, et al: Ultrasonic tomography by means of an ultrasonic fiberendoscope. Endoscopy 12 : 241-244, 1980.
29. Strohm WD, Classen M: Endoscopisch-sonographische Diagnostik der Magenwand. Dtsch Med Wschr 108 : 1425-1427, 1983.
30. Tanaka Y, Yasuda K, Aibe T, et al: Anatomical and pathological aspects in ultrasonic endoscopy of GI tract. Scand J Gastroenterol 94(Suppl) : 43-50, 1984.
31. Tio TL, Tytgat GHJ: Endoscopic sonography in the assessment of intra- and transmural infiltration of tumours in the esophagus, stomach, and papilla of Vater and in the detection of extraesophageal lesions. Endoscopy 16 : 203-210, 1983.
32. Tio TL, Tytgat GNJ: Endoscopic sonography of normal and pathologic upper gastrointestinal wall structure. Comparison of studies in vivo and in vitro with histology. Scand J Gastroenterol 123(Suppl) : 27-33, 1986.
33. Tio TL, Tytgat GNJ: Endoscopic ultrasonography of the bile duct malignancy and the preoperative assessment of local resectability. Scand J Gastroenterol 123(Suppl) : 151-157, 1986.
34. Watanabe H, Igari D, Tanahashi Y, et al: Development and applicaiton of new equipment for transrectal ultrasonography. JCU 2 : 91-98, 1974.
35. Wild JJ, Reid JM: Progress in the techniques of soft tissue examination by 15 megacycle pulsed ultrasound, in Kelly E (ed), Ultrasound in Biology and Medicine. Washington, DC, American Institute of Biological Sciences, 1957, pp30-45.
36. Yasuda K, Nakajima M, Mukai H, et al: The detection of small pancreatic cancers by endoscopic ultrasonography, in Dancygier H, Classen M (eds), 5th International Symposium on Endoscopic Ultrasonography, Graefelfing, Demeter Verlag, 1987, pp 86-91.

INDEX

Page numbers in *italics* refer to figures or tables.

Q, R

S